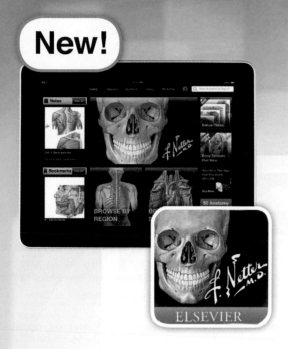
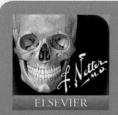

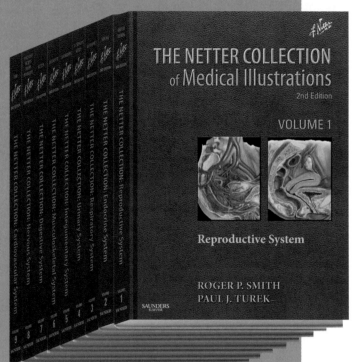

Netter's Illustrated Pharmacology

UPDATED EDITION

Robert B. Raffa, PhD
Scott M. Rawls, PhD
Temple University School of Pharmacy
Philadelphia, Pennsylvania

Elena Portyansky Beyzarov, PharmD
Director of Scientific Affairs
Pharmacy Times
Plainsboro, NJ

Illustrations by Frank H. Netter, MD

Contributing Illustrators
James A. Perkins, MS, MFA
John A. Craig, MD
Carlos A. G. Machado, MD
Dragonfly Media Group

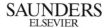

Elsevier Inc.
1600 John F. Kennedy Boulevard
Suite 1800
Philadelphia, PA 19103-2899

Notices

ISBN: 978-0-323-22091-0

Content Strategist: Elyse O'Grady
Content Development Manager: Marybeth Thiel
Publishing Services Manager: Patricia Tannian
Project Manager: Carrie Stetz

Printed in China

Last digit is the print number: 9 8 7 6 5 4 3 2

 Working together
to grow libraries in
developing countries

www.elsevier.com • www.bookaid.org

DEDICATION

To my family; to Temple University School of Pharmacy;
and to Dr. Ronald J. Tallarida, mentor and friend.

Robert B. Raffa

To my mother, whose support, love, dedication, and
sacrifices over the years have made this book possible,
and to my readers, whose thanks and suggestions for
improvement are appreciated.

Scott M. Rawls

To my parents, who gave me their spirit,
encouragement, and guidance when I needed it most
and who convinced me that pharmacy is a far better
career choice than aerospace engineering. To my
husband and daughter, for their infinite patience and
support while I barricaded myself with books and a
computer.

Elena Portyansky Beyzarov

PREFACE

Nothing enhances the efficient learning of scientific material more than good artwork. Personal teaching experience has shown us the power of visual learning in the classroom and the positive effect it has on students. A well-done, accurate, and eye-catching illustration captures one's attention and stimulates one's imagination. Visualization of a concept enhances and solidifies one's understanding and internalization of it, and a good illustration becomes the template upon which future learning can be superimposed. We were thus excited when we were approached with the idea of publishing a visual pharmacology book. That is the intent of this book—to provide high-quality illustrative aids that will enhance the learning of the basic principles of pharmacology and present them in a manner that is both scientifically rigorous and enjoyable. It is designed for the visual learner in all of us.

But can there be illustrations of pharmacology? Isn't the study of pharmacology the memorization of innumerable drugs, their trade names, their doses, and other nonvisual material? Hardly. Just as all other basic sciences have their practical side, pharmacology has its application in the use of drugs for treatment of diseases and disorders. But in the past couple of years, there has been a virtual explosion in understanding of the biologic features and events that underlie the therapeutic action of a drug. It is now possible, with the creative input and insight of an artist's eye, to visualize the anatomical, physiologic, biochemical, and molecular underpinnings of pharmacology. This exciting new aspect of pharmacology is the focus of this book.

We believe that this is the first book to place such emphasis on artwork for the explanation of pharmacologic principles. There is, of course, no better starting point for this task than the renowned work of physician-artist Frank H. Netter, MD, whose illustrations have educated generations of students. Having access to the Netter collection of illustrations was a rare opportunity to approach the subject of pharmacology visually. To provide illustrations of more recently discovered concepts, we called upon James A. Perkins, MS, MFA, and other talented artists to create dynamic new illustrations of the detailed molecular events that underlie drug action. The translation by these artists of recent complex research findings into clear, precise, and engaging artwork was a pleasure to observe and is a highlight of this book.

Three authors with different but complementary backgrounds and expertise jointly wrote this book. Our collaboration was intended to provide the most authoritative and broadest possible coverage of both the basic science and the clinical applications of pharmacology.

We have written this book with medical, pharmacy, dental, nursing, and other professional students in mind, hoping that it will serve as a valuable adjunct to their more comprehensive textbooks. Each of us has found the illustrations to be useful in our own learning or teaching of the material. However, this book was also designed to be a stand-alone, discussing pharmacologic principles in a manner that allows a great deal of material to be covered in a concise fashion. It is thus also appropriate for use in an introductory course for undergraduate students or even for the interested general reader. We sincerely hope that all find the book useful and the presentation enjoyable.

Robert B. Raffa, PhD
Scott M. Rawls, PhD
Elena Portyansky Beyzarov, PharmD

ABOUT THE AUTHORS

Frank H. Netter, MD, was born in 1906, in New York City. He studied art at the Art Student's League and the National Academy of Design before entering medical school at New York University, where he received his MD degree in 1931. During his student years, Dr. Netter's notebook sketches attracted the attention of the medical faculty and other physicians, allowing him to augment his income by illustrating articles and textbooks. He continued illustrating as a sideline after establishing a surgical practice in 1933, but he ultimately opted to give up his practice in favor of a full-time commitment to art. After service in the United States Army during World War II, Dr. Netter began his long collaboration with the CIBA Pharmaceutical Company (now Novartis Pharmaceuticals). This 45-year partnership resulted in the production of the extraordinary collection of medical art so familiar to physicians and other medical professionals worldwide.

In 2005, Elsevier, Inc. purchased the Netter Collection and all publications from Icon Learning Systems. There are now over 50 publications featuring the art of Dr. Netter available through Elsevier, Inc. (in the US: www.us.elsevierhealth.com/Netter and outside the US: www.elsevierhealth.com)

Dr. Netter's works are among the finest examples of the use of illustration in the teaching of medical concepts. The 13-book *Netter Collection of Medical Illustrations,* which includes the greater part of the more than 20,000 paintings created by Dr. Netter, became and remains one of the most famous medical works ever published. *The Netter Atlas of Human Anatomy,* first published in 1989, presents the anatomical paintings from the Netter Collection. Now translated into 16 languages, it is the anatomy atlas of choice among medical and health professions students the world over.

The Netter illustrations are appreciated not only for their aesthetic qualities, but, more importantly, for their intellectual content. As Dr. Netter wrote in 1949, ". . . clarification of a subject is the aim and goal of illustration. No matter how beautifully painted, how delicately and subtly rendered a subject may be, it is of little value as a *medical illustration* if it does not serve to make clear some medical point." Dr. Netter's planning, conception, point of view, and approach are what inform his paintings and what makes them so intellectually valuable.

Frank H. Netter, MD, physician and artist, died in 1991.

Learn more about the physician-artist whose work has inspired the Netter Reference collection: http://www.netterimages.com/artist/netter.htm

Carlos Machado, MD, was chosen by Novartis to be Dr. Netter's successor. He continues to be the main artist who contributes to the Netter collection of medical illustrations.

Self-taught in medical illustration, cardiologist Carlos Machado has contributed meticulous updates to some of Dr. Netter's original plates and has created many paintings of his own in the style of Netter as an extension of the Netter collection. Dr. Machado's photorealistic expertise and his keen insight into the physician/patient relationship informs his vivid and unforgettable visual style. His dedication to researching each topic and subject he paints places him among the premier medical illustrators at work today.

Learn more about his background and see more of his art at: http://www.netterimages.com/artist/machado.htm

ABOUT THE AUTHORS

Robert B. Raffa, PhD, is Professor of Pharmacology at Temple University School of Pharmacy and Research Professor at Temple University School of Medicine in Philadelphia. He has earned bachelor's degrees in Chemical Engineering and Physiological Psychology, master's degrees in Biomedical Engineering and Toxicology, and a PhD in Pharmacology. Dr. Raffa has published more than 150 research articles in refereed journals and more than 70 abstracts and symposia presentations. He is an associate editor of the *Journal of Pharmacology and Experimental Therapeutics* and is founder and editor of the journal *Reviews in Analgesia.* Dr. Raffa is a past president of the Mid-Atlantic Pharmacology Society, the recipient of the Hofmann Research Award, the Lindback teaching award, and other honors. He maintains an active research effort and teaching load. He is author of *Quick-Look Review of Pharmacology;* coauthor of *Principles in General Pharmacology;* editor of *Antisense Strategies for the Study of Receptor Mechanisms* and *Drug-Receptor Thermodynamics: Introduction and Applications;* and is a contributor to *Pain: Current Understanding, Emerging Therapies, and Novel Approaches to Drug Discovery, Molecular Recognition in Protein-Ligand Interactions,* and *Remington: the Science and Practice of Pharmacy.*

Scott M. Rawls, PhD, is Assistant Professor of Pharmacodynamics in the Department of Pharmaceutical Sciences at Temple University School of Pharmacy. Dr. Rawls received his PhD (1999) from East Carolina University School of Medicine in neuroscience. He completed 2 years of postdoctoral training in the Department of Pharmacology at Temple University. In 2003, Dr. Rawls was Assistant Professor of Biology at Washington College in Maryland, where he was the recipient of an undergraduate distinguished teaching award. Dr. Rawls joined the faculty at Temple University School of Pharmacy in the fall of 2004, where he currently teaches in the Pharmacology, Biochemistry, and Anatomy and Physiology courses. Dr. Rawls investigates the effects of cannabinoid, vanilloid, and opioid systems on brain neurotransmitter levels in rats and the role these interactions play in thermoregulation and drug abuse.

Elena Portyansky Beyzarov, PharmD, is a clinical pharmacist at Newark Beth Israel Medical Center. Dr. Beyzarov received her BS degree in pharmacy in 1996 from Arnold and Marie Schwartz College of Pharmacy and Health Sciences at Long Island University and received her PharmD in 1999 from the College of Pharmacy at the University of Arkansas for Medical Sciences. Dr. Beyzarov's career began in medical publishing, where she authored hundreds of clinical articles for *Drug Topics* magazine on a broad range of pharmacotherapeutic subjects. In 2002, she held an academic appointment as adjunct associate professor of pharmacology in the Department of Professional Nursing at Felician College. After deciding to become more involved in clinical practice, Dr. Beyzarov joined Newark Beth Israel Medical Center in 2003 as a clinical pharmacist. Her major activities include performing daily clinical interventions based on review of patient charts and physician orders and providing drug information to staff pharmacists, physicians, and nurses. She also attends daily medical rounds, conducts drug utilization studies, and presents lectures to other health care professionals on pharmacologic management of various disease states.

ACKNOWLEDGMENTS

This book was a team effort from beginning to end. The idea for the book originated at Icon Learning Systems and was developed in a meeting with Paul Kelly, Executive Editor. The access to Netter art made the proposal irresistible.

It is fair to say that the project might not have been completed without the help of Judith B. Gandy, who, with skilled questioning and patience, transformed our rough early drafts into what we were truly trying to say.

We knew that this book was going to attain its goal when we began to work with James A. Perkins, MS, MFA. We had seen his artwork in previous publications, so his artistic talents were known, but the pleasant interactions and his contributions to the subject matter were an unexpected bonus. The arrival of each new illustration was something looked forward to.

He and the other talented artists created illustrations that capture not only the visual aspect of the topic, but also its educational essence. It is anticipated that class after class of students will remember this artwork when they think of pharmacologic principles.

Jennifer Surich, Managing Editor, did a yeoman's job in keeping things going and made sure that this project was actually accomplished. Thanks also go to Greg Otis, Nicole Zimmerman, and all of the others at Icon who converted an idea into reality.

Thanks also to the staff at Elsevier for providing us an opportunity to update the text and add Student Consult access.

Robert B. Raffa, PhD
Scott M. Rawls, PhD
Elena Portyansky Beyzarov, PharmD

CONTENTS

CONTENTS

CONTENTS

CONTENTS

CONTENTS

CONTENTS

ABBREVIATIONS

5-FU	5-fluorouracil
5-HT	5-hydroxytrypyamine
5-ISMN	isosorbide-5-mononitrate
6-MP	mercaptopurine
6-TG	thioguanine
ACE	angiotensin-converting enzyme
ACh	acetylcholine
ACTH	corticotropin
ADH	antidiuretic hormone
ADME	absorption, distribution, metabolism, and elimination
AIDS	acquired immunodeficiency syndrome
AMI	acute myocardial infarction
AMP	adenosine monophosphate
ANS	autonomic nervous system
Asp	aspartate
ATP	adenosine triphosphate
ATPase	adenosine triphosphatase
AV	atrioventricular
cAMP	cyclic adenosine monophosphate
CCB	calcium channel blocker
CCK	cholecystokinin
CDC	Centers for Disease Control
cGMP	cyclic guanosine monophosphate
CHF	congestive heart failure
CML	chronic myeloid leukemia
CMV	cytomegalovirus
CNS	central nervous system
CoA	coenzyme A
COC	combination oral contraceptive
COPD	chronic obstructive pulmonary disease
COX	cyclooxygenase
CRH	corticotropin-releasing hormone
CSF	cerebrospinal fluid
CTZ	chemoreceptor trigger zone
DM	diabetes mellitus
DNA	deoxyribonucleic acid
DRC	dose-response curve
DRSP	drug-resistant *Streptococcus pneumoniae*
DUMBELS	diarrhea, urination, miosis, bronchoconstriction, excitation (skeletal muscles and central nervous system), lacrimation, and salivation and sweating
ED_{50}	median effective dose
EDTA	ethylenediaminetetraacetic acid
EGFR	epidermal growth factor receptor
EPI	epinephrine
EPSP	excitatory postsynaptic potential

ER	estrogen receptor
ESWL	extracorporeal shock wave lithotripsy
FDA	Food and Drug Administration
FPG	fasting plasma glucose
FSH	follicle-stimulating hormone
GABA	γ-aminobutyric acid
$GABA_A$	γ-aminobutyric acid receptor type A
$GABA_B$	γ-aminobutyric acid receptor type B
GDP	guanosine diphosphate
GERD	gastroesophageal reflux disease
GFR	glomerular filtration rate
GH	growth hormone
GHRH	growth hormone–releasing hormone
GI	gastrointestinal
Glu	glutamate
Gly	glycine
GnRH	gonadotropin-releasing hormone
GPCR	G protein–coupled receptor
GTN	glyceryl nitrate
GTP	guanosine triphosphate
GTPase	guanosine triphosphatase
H_2CO_3	carbonic acid
Hb	hemoglobin
HCO_3^-	bicarbonate
HDL	high-density lipoprotein
HER	human epidermal growth factor receptor
HIV	human immunodeficiency virus
HMG-CoA	hydroxymethylglutaryl-coenzyme A
HPA	hypothalamic-pituitary-adrenal
HRT	hormone replacement therapy
HSV	herpes simplex virus
IBS	irritable bowel syndrome
Ig	immunoglobulin
IGF	insulinlike growth factor
IPSP	inhibitory postsynaptic potential
IV	intravenous
LD_{50}	median lethal dose
LDL	low-density lipoprotein
L-DOPA	levodopa
LFT	liver function test
LH	luteinizing hormone
LT	leukotriene
mAChR	muscarinic cholinergic receptor
MAOI	monoamine oxidase inhibitor
MoAb	monoclonal antibody
MPA	medroxyprogesterone acetate
mRNA	messenger ribonucleic acid

MRSA	methicillin-resistant *Staphylococcus aureus*
MTX	methotrexate
nAChR	nicotinic cholinergic receptor
NANC	nonadrenergic-noncholinergic
NE	norepinephrine
NERD	nonerosive esophageal reflux disease
NHL	non-Hodgkin lymphoma
NK	natural killer
NMDA	N-methyl-D-aspartate
NNRTI	nonnucleoside reverse transcriptase inhibitor
NO	nitric oxide
NRTI	nucleoside reverse transcriptase inhibitor
NSAID	nonsteroidal antiinflammatory drug
OC	oral contraceptive
OCD	obsessive-compulsive disorder
PD	pharmacodynamic
PDE	phosphodiesterase
Ph	Philadelphia chromosome
PI	protease inhibitor
PK	pharmacokinetic
PNS	peripheral nervous system
PPAR	peroxisome proliferator-activated receptor
PPI	proton pump inhibitor
PRL	prolactin
PTU	propylthiouracil
PUVA	psoralen plus ultraviolet A light
RAI	radioactive iodine
RNA	ribonucleic acid
SA	sinoatrial
SAR	structure-activity relation
SERM	selective estrogen receptor modulator
SNS	somatic nervous system
SSRI	selective serotonin reuptake inhibitor
T_3	triiodothyronine
T_4	thyroxine
TCA	tricyclic antidepressant
TRF	thyrotropin-releasing factor
TRH	thyrotropin-releasing hormone
TSH	thyroid-stimulating hormone
TZD	thiazolidinedione
UTI	urinary tract infection
UV	ultraviolet
VC	vomiting center
VZV	varicella-zoster virus

CHAPTER 1

BASIC PRINCIPLES OF PHARMACOLOGY

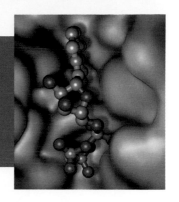

OVERVIEW

Pharmacology is the study of drug action at both the molecular and the whole-organism levels. At the molecular level, *drug action* refers to the mechanism by which a drug or other molecule produces a biologic effect. At the whole-organism level, *drug action* refers to the therapeutic effects of a drug and its unwanted (ie, adverse, or side) effects. Drugs can produce biologic effects in several ways, eg, killing harmful invading organisms such as bacteria and viruses; killing the body's own cells that have gone awry (eg, cancer cells); neutralizing acid (mechanism of action of antacids); modifying ongoing underactive or overactive physiologic processes. In the last case, direct replacement of chemicals (eg, insulin) or indirect or more subtle modulation of biochemical processes (eg, inhibition of enzyme action) may be required.

Drugs can be said to modify the communication system within an organism. The modification should not interfere with the fidelity of the signal and should not activate unwanted compensatory responses. Drugs should selectively target specific cellular components that function in the normal signaling process. The study of molecular, biochemical, and physiologic effects of drugs on cellular systems and drug mechanisms of action is termed *pharmacodynamics*.

Equally important to drug action are the absorption, distribution, metabolism, and elimination (ADME) of drugs. The study of these processes (which involves the movement of the drug molecules through various physiologic compartments) and how they affect drug use and usefulness is termed *pharmacokinetics*. Complete understanding of the action of a drug involves knowledge of both pharmacodynamic (PD) and pharmacokinetic (PK) properties. In addition, the physical characteristics of an individual patient (eg, age, sex, weight, liver function, kidney function) dictate how the PD and PK characteristics of the drug are manifested.

Pharmacognosy is the study of drugs from natural sources. *Pharmacy* is the clinical practice devoted to the formulation and proper and safe distribution and use of therapeutic agents.

Therapeutic drug action involves interaction between an exogenous chemical and the endogenous biochemical target. The study of chemical structures of drugs and the study of normal and abnormal physiology are thus interrelated. Only by a clear understanding of the anatomy, physiology, and pathology of the organism can the proper drugs be designed and administered. The study of pharmacology therefore involves broad-based knowledge of the drug molecule, the organism, and the interaction between them.

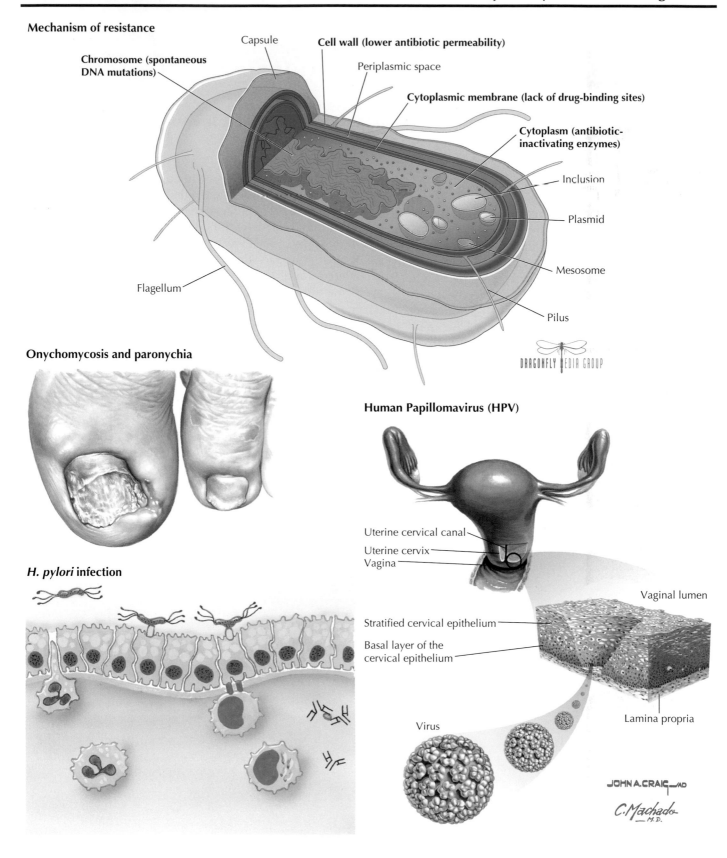

Mechanism of resistance

Chromosome (spontaneous DNA mutations)

Capsule

Cell wall (lower antibiotic permeability)

Periplasmic space

Cytoplasmic membrane (lack of drug-binding sites)

Cytoplasm (antibiotic-inactivating enzymes)

Inclusion

Plasmid

Mesosome

Flagellum

Pilus

Onychomycosis and paronychia

Human Papillomavirus (HPV)

Uterine cervical canal

Uterine cervix

Vagina

Vaginal lumen

Stratified cervical epithelium

Basal layer of the cervical epithelium

Lamina propria

H. pylori infection

Virus

JOHN A. CRAIG_MD

C. Machado_M.D.

DRAGONFLY MEDIA GROUP

FIGURE 1-1 EXTERNAL AND INTERNAL THREATS

Invading organisms such as bacteria, viruses, fungi, and helminths can threaten the health of the host. Cancer cells are abnormal and differ from normal cells in terms of chromosome alterations, uncontrolled proliferation, dedifferentiation and loss of function, and invasiveness. Drug therapy (chemotherapy) aims to kill invading organisms or aberrant cells directly or to reduce their numbers to a level that can be managed by a host-mounted defense. Typical drug targets for invading organisms include

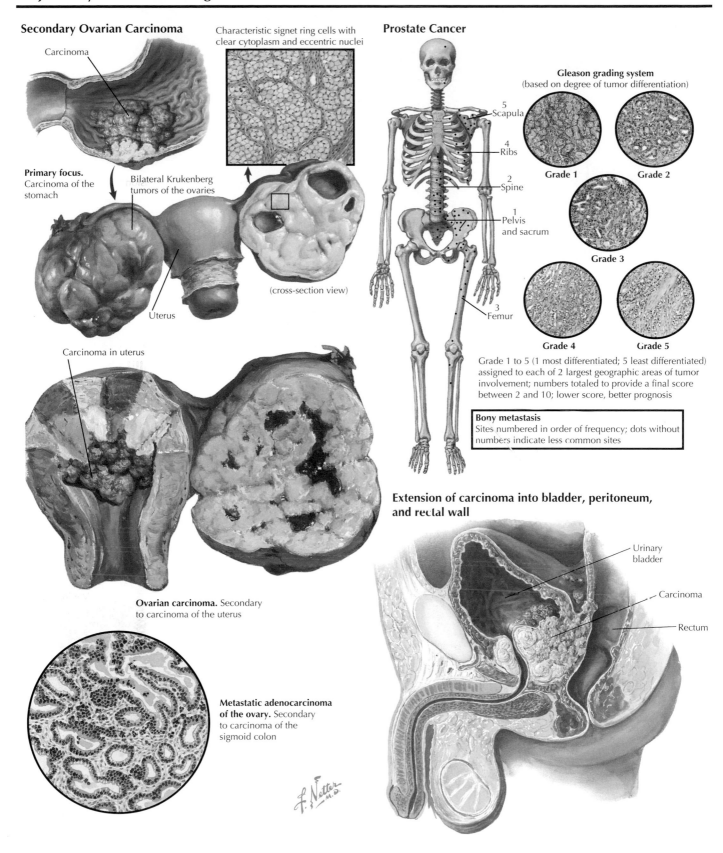

Secondary Ovarian Carcinoma

Carcinoma

Primary focus. Carcinoma of the stomach

Bilateral Krukenberg tumors of the ovaries

Uterus

(cross-section view)

Characteristic signet ring cells with clear cytoplasm and eccentric nuclei

Carcinoma in uterus

Ovarian carcinoma. Secondary to carcinoma of the uterus

Metastatic adenocarcinoma of the ovary. Secondary to carcinoma of the sigmoid colon

Prostate Cancer

5 Scapula
4 Ribs
2 Spine
1 Pelvis and sacrum
3 Femur

Gleason grading system
(based on degree of tumor differentiation)

Grade 1　　Grade 2

Grade 3

Grade 4　　Grade 5

Grade 1 to 5 (1 most differentiated; 5 least differentiated) assigned to each of 2 largest geographic areas of tumor involvement; numbers totaled to provide a final score between 2 and 10; lower score, better prognosis

Bony metastasis
Sites numbered in order of frequency; dots without numbers indicate less common sites

Extension of carcinoma into bladder, peritoneum, and rectal wall

Urinary bladder

Carcinoma

Rectum

FIGURE 1-1 EXTERNAL AND INTERNAL THREATS (continued)

biochemical processes needed for cell wall synthesis or integrity. Drug targets for abnormal cells include cell-cycle regulation and enzymes involved in protein synthesis, so as to inhibit cancer cell replication. In both cases, optimal treatment occurs when a drug or combination of drugs displays selectivity against invaders or cancer cells. Such therapy—with separation between a desired therapeutic effect and unwanted (adverse or side) effects—minimizes harmful drug effects.

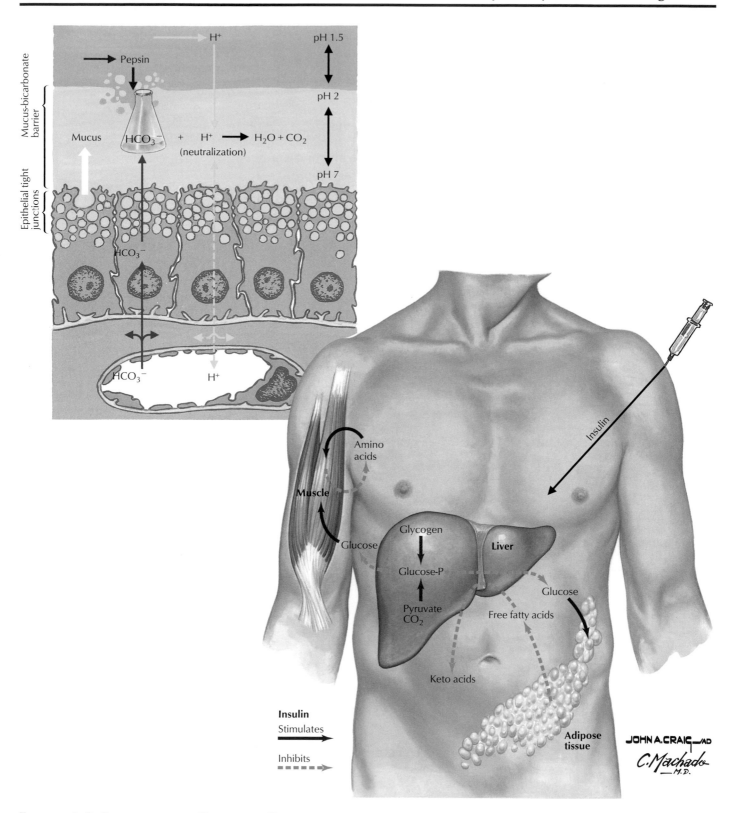

FIGURE 1-2 ENDOGENOUS CHEMICAL BALANCE

When the amount of an endogenous substance is insufficient for normal functions, it may be possible to supply it from sources outside of the body (exogenous supply). Examples include insulin used for diabetes and dopamine used for parkinsonism. The exogenous material may originate from humans, animals, microorganisms, or minerals or it may be synthesized—a product of technology. It can be the substance itself or a precursor metabolized to the substance (eg, levodopa is metabolized to dopa-

mine). Excess amounts can also be harmful, eg, excess stomach acid can cause or exacerbate ulcer formation. Gastric acid levels can be reduced directly by using an antacid (a base such as calcium carbonate or magnesium hydroxide). An alternative approach—inhibiting acid secretion—can be achieved by antagonizing the action of histamine on H_2 receptors of parietal cells (eg, with cimetidine) or by interfering with the proton pump that transports acid across parietal cells (eg, with omeprazole).

Interdependent and Interacting Factors in Blood Pressure Regulation

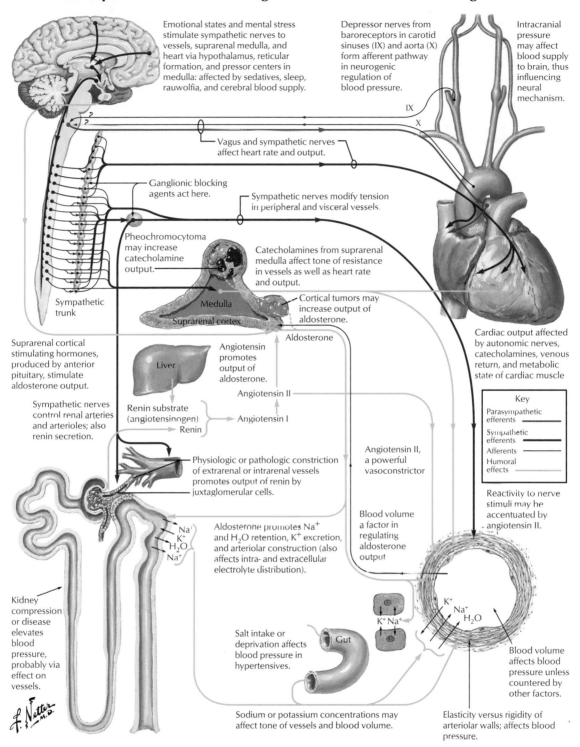

Emotional states and mental stress stimulate sympathetic nerves to vessels, suprarenal medulla, and heart via hypothalamus, reticular formation, and pressor centers in medulla: affected by sedatives, sleep, rauwolfia, and cerebral blood supply.

Depressor nerves from baroreceptors in carotid sinuses (IX) and aorta (X) form afferent pathway in neurogenic regulation of blood pressure.

Intracranial pressure may affect blood supply to brain, thus influencing neural mechanism.

IX

X

Vagus and sympathetic nerves affect heart rate and output.

Ganglionic blocking agents act here.

Sympathetic nerves modify tension in peripheral and visceral vessels.

Pheochromocytoma may increase catecholamine output.

Catecholamines from suprarenal medulla affect tone of resistance in vessels as well as heart rate and output.

Sympathetic trunk

Medulla

Suprarenal cortex

Cortical tumors may increase output of aldosterone.

Aldosterone

Cardiac output affected by autonomic nerves, catecholamines, venous return, and metabolic state of cardiac muscle

Suprarenal cortical stimulating hormones, produced by anterior pituitary, stimulate aldosterone output.

Liver

Angiotensin promotes output of aldosterone.

Angiotensin II

Sympathetic nerves control renal arteries and arterioles; also renin secretion.

Renin substrate (angiotensinogen)

Renin

Angiotensin I

Physiologic or pathologic constriction of extrarenal or intrarenal vessels promotes output of renin by juxtaglomerular cells.

Angiotensin II, a powerful vasoconstrictor

Key
Parasympathetic efferents
Sympathetic efferents
Afferents
Humoral effects

Reactivity to nerve stimuli may be accentuated by angiotensin II.

Blood volume a factor in regulating aldosterone output

Na^+
K^+
H_2O
Na^+

Aldosterone promotes Na^+ and H_2O retention, K^+ excretion, and arteriolar construction (also affects intra- and extracellular electrolyte distribution).

Kidney compression or disease elevates blood pressure, probably via effect on vessels.

Salt intake or deprivation affects blood pressure in hypertensives.

Gut

$K^+ Na^+$

K^+
Na^+
H_2O

Blood volume affects blood pressure unless countered by other factors.

f. Netter M.D.

Sodium or potassium concentrations may affect tone of vessels and blood volume.

Elasticity versus rigidity of arteriolar walls; affects blood pressure.

FIGURE 1-3 MODULATE PHYSIOLOGIC PROCESSES

Drugs use different mechanisms to modify normal homeostatic and biochemical communication in cellular and physiologic processes. They mimic (eg, carbachol) or block neurotransmitters that transmit information across synapses. Chemical substances such as hormones also act over long distances in the body. Drugs that mimic hormones include oxandrolone; mifepristone blocks hormone action. Drugs selectively modify physiologic processes by targeting enzymes, DNA, neurotransmitters, or other chemical mediators or components of signaling processes

such as receptors. The total effect depends on whether a drug promotes or reduces endogenous activity. Drugs with other mechanisms of action are chelating agents (contain metal atoms that form chemical bonds with toxins or drugs), antimetabolites (masquerade as endogenous substances but are inactive or less active than these substrates), irritants (stimulate physiologic processes), and nutritional or replacement agents (eg, vitamins, minerals).

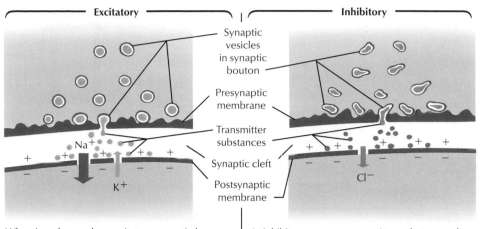

Excitatory	Inhibitory

Synaptic vesicles in synaptic bouton

Presynaptic membrane

Transmitter substances

Synaptic cleft

Postsynaptic membrane

Na^+ K^+ Cl^-

When impulse reaches excitatory synaptic bouton, it causes release of a transmitter substance into synaptic cleft. This increases permeability of postsynaptic membrane to Na^+ and K^+. More Na^+ moves into postsynaptic cell than K^+ moves out, due to greater electrochemical gradient.

At inhibitory synapse, transmitter substance released by an impulse increases permeability of the postsynaptic membrane to Cl^-. K^+ moves out of postsynaptic cell, but no net flow of Cl^- occurs at resting membrane potential.

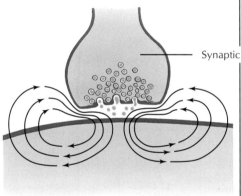

Synaptic bouton

Resultant net ionic current flow is in a direction that tends to depolarize postsynaptic cell. If depolarization reaches firing threshold, an impulse is generated in postsynaptic cell.

Resultant ionic current flow is in direction that tends to hyperpolarize postsynaptic cell. This makes depolarization by excitatory synapses more difficult—more depolarization is required to reach threshold.

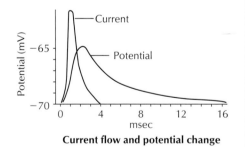

Current flow and potential change

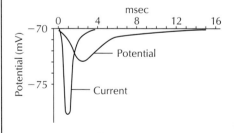

Current flow and potential change

FIGURE 1-4 CHEMICAL TRANSMISSION AT THE SYNAPSE

Communication (transmission of information) across synapses occurs via chemical messengers—neurotransmitters—stored in vesicles in presynaptic neurons. Action potentials at presynaptic axon terminals initiate steps that release neurotransmitter molecules into a synapse, which cross the synaptic cleft and bind reversibly to postsynaptic receptors. Receptor activation leads to cellular response. Receptor activators (eg, drugs) are *agonists*; *antagonists* are drugs that combine with but do not activate receptors. Transmitters are removed from synapses by enzymatic destruction, diffusion, and active reuptake into presynaptic neurons. Major peripheral neurotransmitters are acetylcholine and catecholamines (eg, epinephrine, dopamine). In the brain and spinal cord, major excitatory neurotransmitters are glutamate and aspartate; major inhibitory neurotransmitters are GABA and glycine. 5-HT, or serotonin, and neuropeptides are other neurotransmitters.

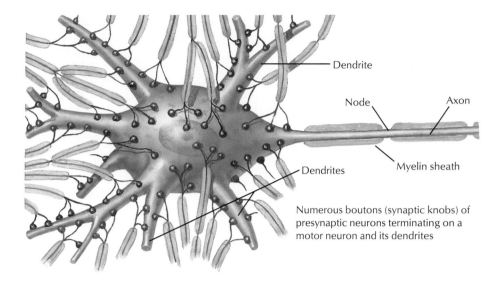

Dendrite

Node

Axon

Dendrites

Myelin sheath

Numerous boutons (synaptic knobs) of
presynaptic neurons terminating on a
motor neuron and its dendrites

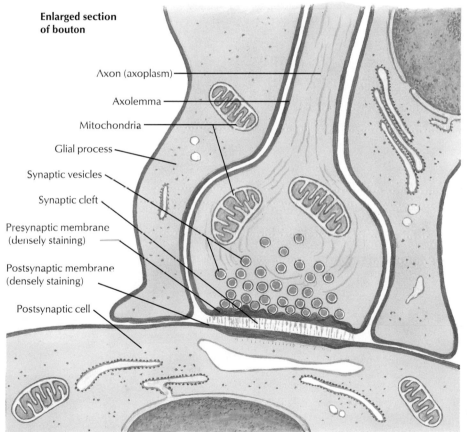

**Enlarged section
of bouton**

Axon (axoplasm)

Axolemma

Mitochondria

Glial process

Synaptic vesicles

Synaptic cleft

Presynaptic membrane
(densely staining)

Postsynaptic membrane
(densely staining)

Postsynaptic cell

FIGURE 1-5 SYNAPSE MORPHOLOGY

A *synapse* is a region including the axon terminal of a presynaptic neuron, the plasma membrane of the postsynaptic (receiving) cell, and the physical space between the cells (synaptic cleft). Postsynaptic cells can be neurons or other cells (eg, effector cells in muscle). At synapses, electrical transmissions—action potentials along presynaptic neurons—are translated into chemical signals, which lead to postsynaptic cell responses: increase (excitation), decrease (inhibition), or modulation of neuron activity or biochemistry. Synaptic transmission involves many steps, all possible drug targets. Steps occur in presynaptic neurons (eg, neurotransmitter synthesis and storage in vesicles), at presynaptic membranes (eg, vesicle docking with membranes, neurotransmitter exocytosis), in synaptic clefts (eg, enzymatic reuptake), on postsynaptic membranes (eg, binding to receptors, change in ion channel function), and in postsynaptic neurons (eg, effects on second-messenger transduction).

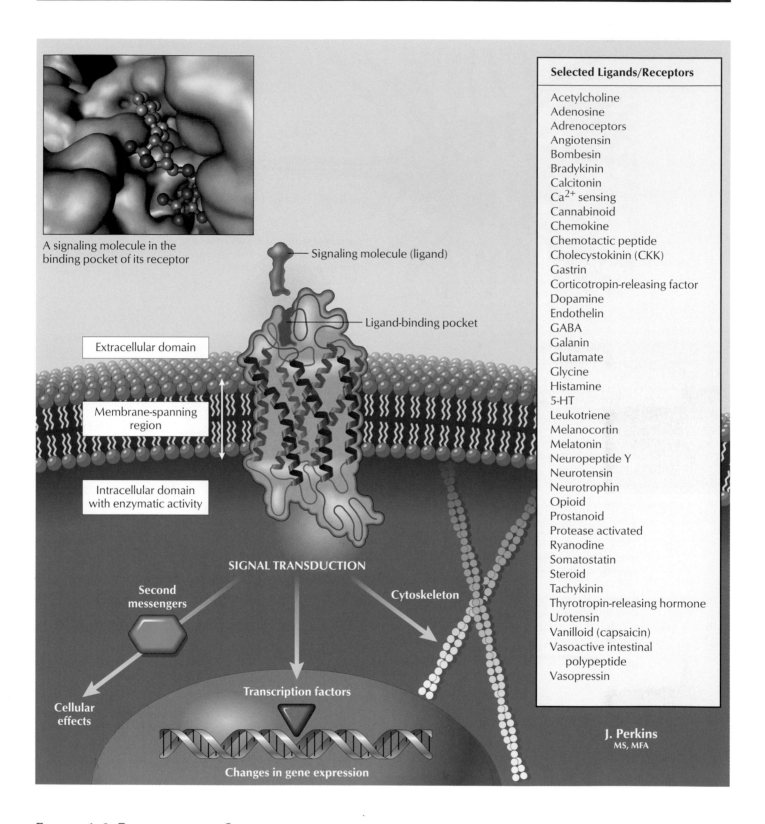

A signaling molecule in the binding pocket of its receptor

Signaling molecule (ligand)

Ligand-binding pocket

Extracellular domain

Membrane-spanning region

Intracellular domain with enzymatic activity

SIGNAL TRANSDUCTION

Second messengers

Cytoskeleton

Cellular effects

Transcription factors

Changes in gene expression

J. Perkins
MS, MFA

Selected Ligands/Receptors

Acetylcholine
Adenosine
Adrenoceptors
Angiotensin
Bombesin
Bradykinin
Calcitonin
Ca^{2+} sensing
Cannabinoid
Chemokine
Chemotactic peptide
Cholecystokinin (CKK)
Gastrin
Corticotropin-releasing factor
Dopamine
Endothelin
GABA
Galanin
Glutamate
Glycine
Histamine
5-HT
Leukotriene
Melanocortin
Melatonin
Neuropeptide Y
Neurotensin
Neurotrophin
Opioid
Prostanoid
Protease activated
Ryanodine
Somatostatin
Steroid
Tachykinin
Thyrotropin-releasing hormone
Urotensin
Vanilloid (capsaicin)
Vasoactive intestinal
    polypeptide
Vasopressin

FIGURE 1-6 RECEPTORS AND SIGNALING

Receptors are the first molecules in or on a cell that respond to a neurotransmitter, a hormone, or another endogenous or exogenous signaling molecule (ligand) and transmit messages (via transduction) from the molecule to the cell machinery. Receptors ensure fidelity of the intended communication by responding only to the intended signaling molecule or to molecules with closely related chemical structures (such as drugs with the required shape). Receptors are composed primarily of long sequences (typically hundreds) of amino acids. The body has dozens of receptor types to maintain communication pathways that must be differentiated from each other and serve different purposes. An individual cell may express one or many types of receptors, with the number depending on age, health, or other factors.

D₁ Amino Acid Sequence

```
1    MRTLNTSAMD GTGLVVERDF SVRILTACFL SLLILSTLLG NTLVCAAVIR
51   FRHLRSKVTN FFVISLAVSD LLVAVLVMPW KAVAEIAGFW PFGSFCNIWV
101  AFDIMCSTAS ILNLCVISVD RYWAISSPFR YERKMTPKAA FILISVAWTL
151  SVLISFIPVQ LSWHKAKPTS PSDGNATSLA ETIDNCDSSL SRTYAISSSV
201  ISFYIPVAIM IVTYTRIYRI AQKQIRRIAA LERAAVHAKN CQTTTGNGKP
251  VECSQPESSF KMSFKRETKV LKTLSVIMGV FVCCWLPFFI LNCILPFCGS
301  GETQPFCIDS NTFDVFVWFG WANSSLNPII YAFNADFRKA FSTLLGCYRL
351  CPATNNAIET VSINNNGAAM FSSHHEPRGS ISKECNLVYL IPHAVGSSED
401  LKKEEAAGIA RPLEKLSPAL SVILDYDTDV SLEKIQPITQ NGQHPT
```

D₂ Amino Acid Sequence

```
1    MDPLNLSWYD DDLERQNWSR PFNGSDGKAD RPHYNYYATL LTLLIAVIVF
51   GNVLVCMAVS REKALQTTTN YLIVSLAVAD LLVATLVMPW VVYLEVVGEW
101  KFSRIHCDIF VTLDVMMCTA SILNLCAISI DRYTAVAMPM LYNTRYSSKR
151  RVTVMISIVW VLSFTISCPL LFGLNNADQN ECIIANPAFV VYSSIVSFYV
201  PFIVTLLVYI KIYIVLRRRR KRVNTKRSSR AFRAHLRAPL KGNCTHPEDM
251  KLCTVIMKSN GSFPVNRRRV EAARRAQELE MEMLSSTSPP ERTRYSPIPP
301  SHHQLTLPDP SHHGLHSTPD SPAKPEKNGH AKDHPKIAKI FEIQTMPNGK
351  TRTSLKTMSR RKLSQQKEKK ATQMLAIVLG VFIICWLPFF ITHILNIHCD
401  CNIPPVLYSA FTWLGYVNSA VNPIIYTTFN IEFRKAFLKI LHC
```

Alternative splice sequence ------------------------

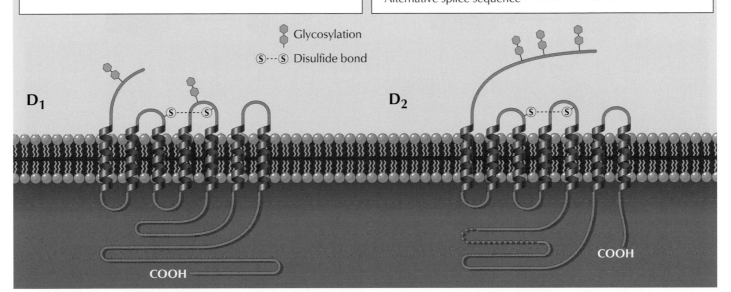

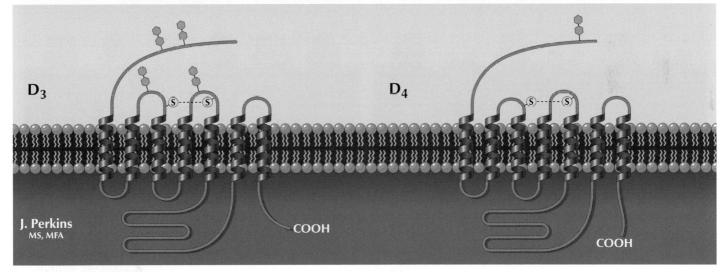

J. Perkins
MS, MFA

FIGURE 1-7 RECEPTOR SUBTYPES

Receptors can be classified into subtypes, as first noted for receptors for the structurally related catecholamines epinephrine, isoproterenol, and norepinephrine. The order of potency (structure-activity relation, or SAR) of these drugs in some tissues is norepinephrine > epinephrine > isoproterenol; in other tissues, it is the reverse. Catecholamine receptors (adrenoceptors) exist in pharmacologically distinct types (α and β) and subtypes (eg, α₁, α₂, and so on). Subtypes are differentiated by amino acid sequence and posttranslational processing, as shown for dopamine receptor subtypes. A clinical example of receptor subtype targeting involves asthma treatment. Activation of adrenoceptors in the lung relaxes smooth muscles and dilates bronchioles to ease breathing. To avoid stimulation of heart adrenoceptors, β₂-selective drugs (eg, albuterol, metaproterenol, ritodrine, terbutaline) were developed to activate only lung adrenoceptors; β₁-selective drugs would affect the heart.

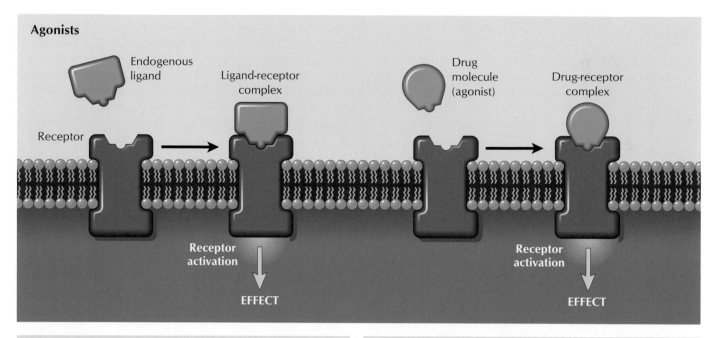

Agonists

Endogenous ligand

Receptor

Ligand-receptor complex

Receptor activation

EFFECT

Drug molecule (agonist)

Drug-receptor complex

Receptor activation

EFFECT

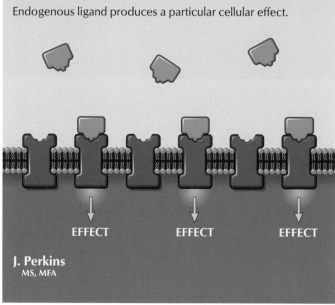

Endogenous ligand produces a particular cellular effect.

EFFECT **EFFECT** **EFFECT**

J. Perkins
MS, MFA

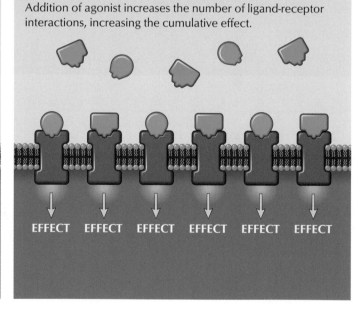

Addition of agonist increases the number of ligand-receptor interactions, increasing the cumulative effect.

EFFECT **EFFECT** **EFFECT** **EFFECT** **EFFECT** **EFFECT**

FIGURE 1-8 AGONISTS

Certain molecules have physiochemical and stereochemical (3-dimensional) characteristics that impart *affinity* for a receptor, affinity being the quantifiable tendency of a drug molecule to form a complex with (bind to) a receptor. Binding involves interaction between a ligand molecule (L) and a receptor molecule (R) to form a ligand-receptor complex (LR): $L + R \leftrightarrow LR$. Affinity is quantified by the reciprocal of the equilibrium constant of this interaction and is commonly reported (often designated K_d or K_i);

the greater the affinity is, the smaller the K value is. Drugs can activate receptors and thus elicit a biologic effect (ie, have intrinsic activity, or efficacy). Such molecules have shapes complementary to receptor shapes and somehow alter the activity of a receptor. Full agonists possess high efficacy and can elicit a maximal tissue response, whereas partial agonists have intermediate levels of efficacy (the tissue response is submaximal even when all receptors are occupied).

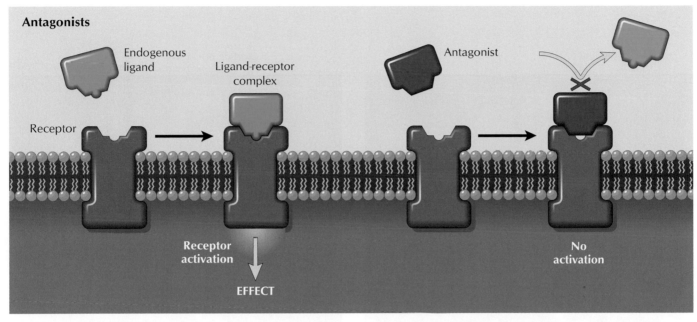

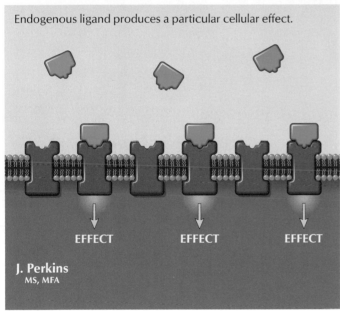

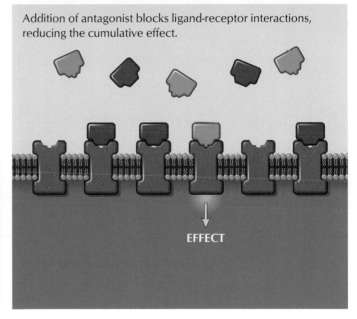

FIGURE 1-9 ANTAGONISTS

Some molecules have physiochemical and stereochemical traits that impart affinity for a receptor but cannot activate it. Such molecules bind to (occupy) receptors and block access of agonists, thereby reducing the effects of agonists. Such pharmacologic antagonists do not elicit biologic effects directly; they modify the physiologic process that is maintained by agonist action (eg, by neurotransmitters). Examples of drugs that are receptor antagonists are atropine (muscarinic cholinergic),

d-tubocurarine (nicotinic cholinergic), atenolol (adrenoceptor), spironolactone (mineralocorticoid), diphenhydramine (histamine H_1), ondansetron (5-HT), flumazenil (benzodiazepine), haloperidol (dopamine), and naloxone (opioid). Chemical antagonism (eg, neutralization of gastric acid by chemical bases) or physiologic antagonism, in which an effect of one drug opposes an effect of another agent (eg, epinephrine used to counteract the histamine response to a bee sting), of drug effects can also occur.

Binding pocket

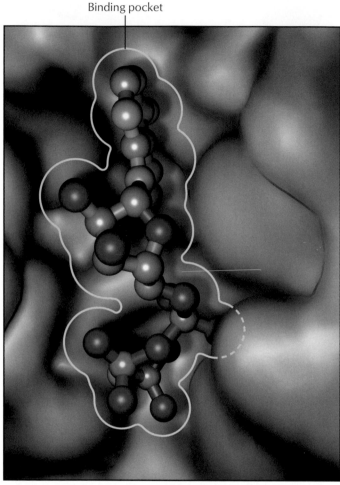

One enantiomer fully occupies the receptor binding pocket...

Binding pocket

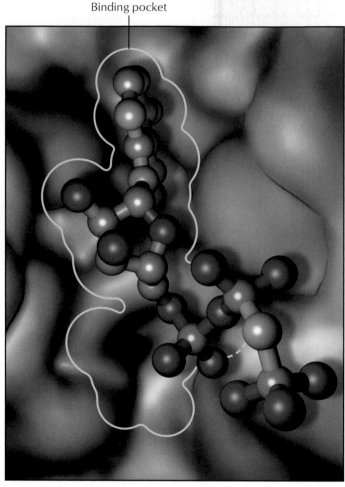

... while the other enantiomer is only a partial match.

J. Perkins
MS, MFA

FIGURE 1-10 STEREOCHEMISTRY AND 3-DIMENSIONAL FIT

One enantiomer of a racemic pair is often observed to bind more avidly to (has greater affinity for) a receptor than does the other enantiomer of the pair. Because the only difference between them is the stereochemistry, the 3-dimensional shape of a molecule must be a crucial characteristic for binding affinity. The relation between chemical structure and biologic response is known as the *SAR* and is a common focus of drug discovery efforts. Computer modeling of the ligand-receptor fit provides a visual representation of the fit of a ligand into the receptor pocket. It can also be used for virtual screening for goodness of fit of potential drug candidates before they are synthesized.

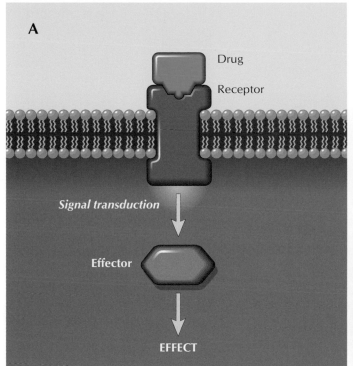

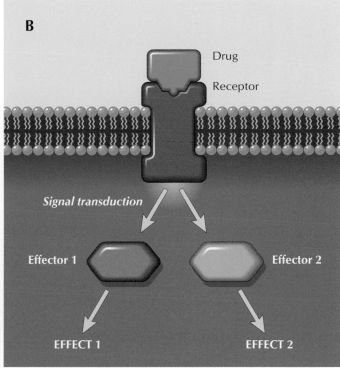

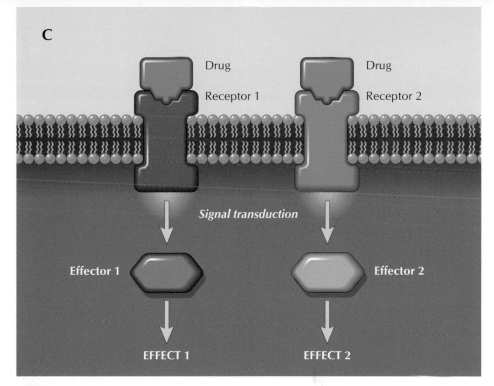

J. Perkins
MS, MFA

FIGURE 1-11 RECEPTOR-EFFECTOR COUPLING

In most cases, a drug activates or inhibits only 1 molecule in a long series of biochemical reactions. When a drug binds to a receptor on a cell membrane, the extracellular drug signal must be passed to the intracellular physiologic processes, ie, it must be converted (transduced) to an intracellular message, the process termed *signal transduction*, which occurs via many mechanisms. The effect of a drug depends on its receptors, the transduction pathways to which it is coupled, its level of receptor expression in cells, and its cellular response capacity. In the simplest case (**A**), a drug binds to 1 receptor coupled to 1 effector (transduction pathway) and produces 1 effect. A drug can bind to 1 receptor coupled to more than 1 effector (**B**) so it produces more than 1 effect in the same or different cells. A drug can also have affinity for more than 1 receptor (**C**), with each receptor coupled to a different effector. Effect 2 can be a therapeutic end point or an adverse effect.

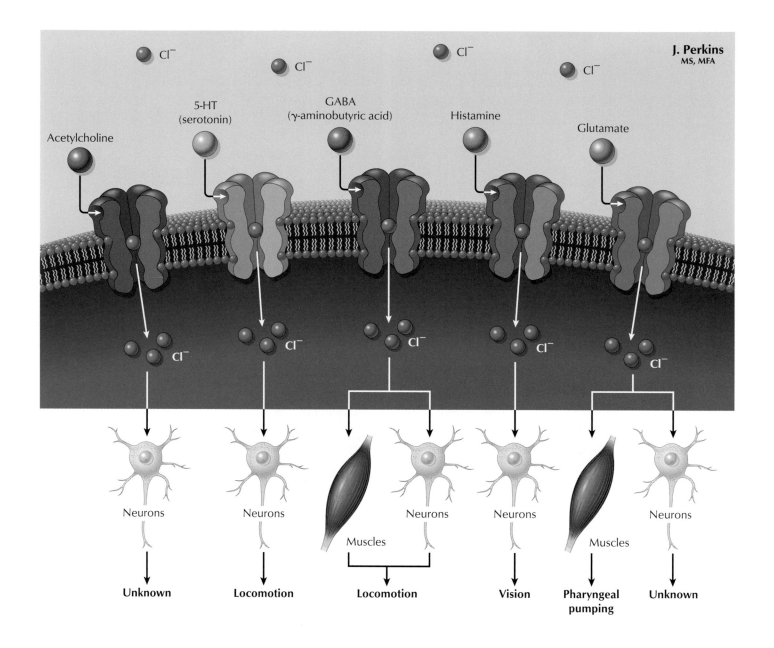

FIGURE 1-12 SIGNAL TRANSDUCTION AND CROSS TALK

Receptors provide specificity for cell responses to only certain extracellular chemical signals. Different receptor types can have 1 or more intracellular second-messenger transduction mechanisms without loss of ligand specificity. Different ligands acting through different receptors can thus have the same or different effects via 1 messenger system. In some invertebrate organisms all ionotropic (ion channel) receptors shown here regulate Cl⁻ influx and have the effects shown. In mamals only the GABA receptor regulates Cl⁻ influx. The others have other transduction mechanisms and produce different effects. The effect depends on ligand concentration, cell type, and expression of receptor and second messenger system components. Integrated communication between and within cells thus occurs. A cell with multiple receptor types can be regulated by various ligands and by interaction among receptor types. Interaction among receptor types constitutes receptor cross talk, which allows cells diverse and sophisticated response possibilities.

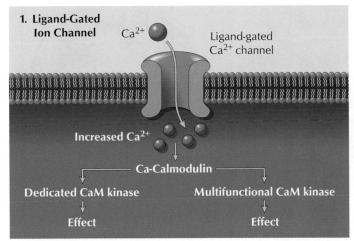

1. Ligand-Gated Ion Channel

Ca^{2+}

Ligand-gated Ca^{2+} channel

Increased Ca^{2+}

Ca-Calmodulin

Dedicated CaM kinase — Effect

Multifunctional CaM kinase — Effect

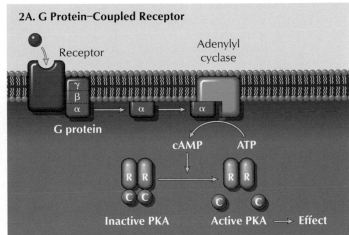

2A. G Protein–Coupled Receptor

Receptor

Adenylyl cyclase

γ β α

G protein

α

α

cAMP   ATP

R R
C C
Inactive PKA

R R
C   C
Active PKA ⟶ Effect

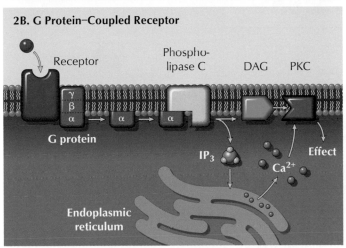

2B. G Protein–Coupled Receptor

Receptor

Phospho-lipase C   DAG   PKC

γ β α

G protein

α

α

IP$_3$

Ca^{2+}

Effect

Endoplasmic reticulum

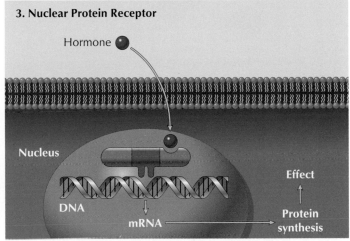

3. Nuclear Protein Receptor

Hormone

Nucleus

DNA

mRNA ⟶ Protein synthesis

Effect

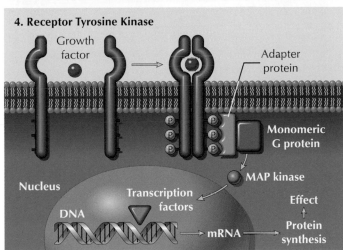

4. Receptor Tyrosine Kinase

Growth factor

Adapter protein

Monomeric G protein

MAP kinase

Nucleus

Transcription factors

DNA

mRNA ⟶ Protein synthesis

Effect

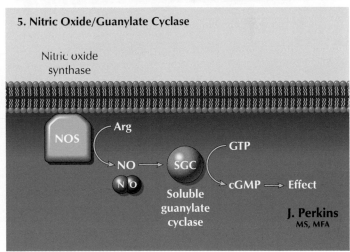

5. Nitric Oxide/Guanylate Cyclase

Nitric oxide synthase

NOS   Arg

NO ⟶ SGC

GTP

NO

Soluble guanylate cyclase

cGMP ⟶ Effect

J. Perkins
MS, MFA

FIGURE 1-13 SECOND-MESSENGER PATHWAYS

Signal transduction commonly occurs by means of several general mechanisms: (1) ligand-gated ion channels modulate the influx or outflow of ions that alter transmembrane potential or modulate intracellular biochemical reactions (eg, the calcium-calmodulin system); (2) ligand binding to GPCRs modulates enzyme activity (eg, adenylyl cyclase or phospholipase C); (3) ligand binding activates a catalytic portion of the receptor (eg, tyrosine kinase activity); (4) a ligand enters the cell nucleus and alters protein (receptor) synthesis; and (5) a ligand amplifies or attenuates nitric oxide synthesis and the subsequent production of cGMP.

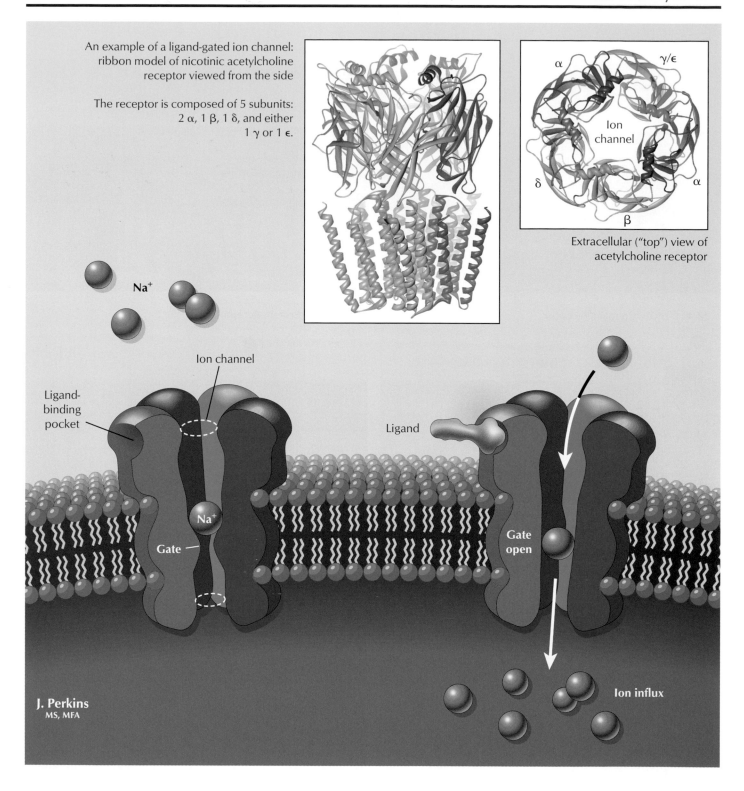

An example of a ligand-gated ion channel: ribbon model of nicotinic acetylcholine receptor viewed from the side

The receptor is composed of 5 subunits: 2 α, 1 β, 1 δ, and either 1 γ or 1 ε.

α   γ/ε

Ion channel

δ   α

β

Extracellular ("top") view of acetylcholine receptor

Na⁺

Ion channel

Ligand-binding pocket

Ligand

Na⁺

Gate

Gate open

J. Perkins
MS, MFA

Ion influx

FIGURE 1-14 LIGAND-GATED ION CHANNELS

Some drugs bind to molecules (ion channels) that form transmembrane pores for ions (usually Na^+, K^+, Ca^{2+}, Cl^-), the channels being composed of many subunits. A drug's binding to 1 or more subunits modifies the receptor function (ion passage), ie, the channels are ligand gated. A single ion channel can accommodate multiple drugs, with each drug binding to a different subunit or site on or within (extracellular, transmembrane, or intracellular) the channel. Membrane-bound channels include nicotinic cholinergic, ionotropic glutamate, $GABA_A$, 5-HT_3 (serotonin), and glycine receptors. Intracellular channels include those for Ca^{2+} on the sarcoplasmic reticulum, endoplasmic reticulum, and mitochondria. Barbiturates, for example, bind to sites on the $GABA_A$ receptor complex, which increases Cl^- influx and produces increased resting transmembrane potential difference and decreased cell excitability. One drug that modifies activity of an intracellular ligand-gated ion (Ca^{2+}) channel is caffeine.

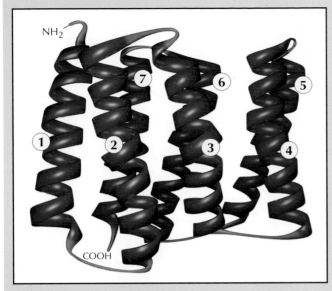

Selected G Protein–Coupled Receptors/Ligands

5-HT	Histamine
Acetylcholine	Interleukins
(muscarinic)	Leukotrienes
Adenosine	Luteinizing hormone
Adrenocorticotropic	Melatonin
hormone	Neuropeptide Y
Angiotensin	Neurotensin
Bradykinin	Norepinephrine
CCK	Opioids
Dopamine	Purines
Epinephrine	Somatostatin
Follicle-stimulating	Tachykinins
hormone	Thrombin
GABA	Thyroid hormone
Glucagon	Parathyroid hormone
Glutamate	Vasopressin

α-Adrenergic receptor, a G protein–coupled receptor with 7 transmembrane α helices

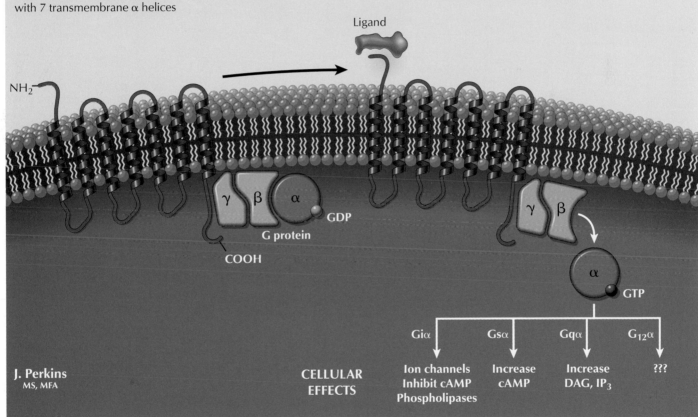

J. Perkins
MS, MFA

FIGURE 1-15 G PROTEIN–COUPLED RECEPTORS

Some drugs bind to receptors whose transduction involves a physical association of a receptor with G proteins—the GPCRs. GPCRs, a large family of receptors, mediate effects of neurotransmitters, hormones, and drugs. GPCRs are large proteins that span a cell membrane many times; many drug-related GPCRs, the 7-TM GPCRs, do this 7 times (amino terminus is outside the cell; carboxy terminus is inside). Examples are receptors for epinephrine, norepinephrine, dopamine, 5-HT, ACh (muscarinic),

histamine, adenosine, purines, GABA, glutamate, opioids, and vasopressin. Binding of an agonist (drug or endogenous ligand) to a GPCR activates associated G proteins by GTP-GDP exchange, which stimulates dissociation of α from βγ subunits. Inherent GTPase activity within the α subunit restores the initial conditions. One receptor can be coupled to more than 1 type of G protein. Some G proteins activate and others inhibit biochemical steps in signal transduction.

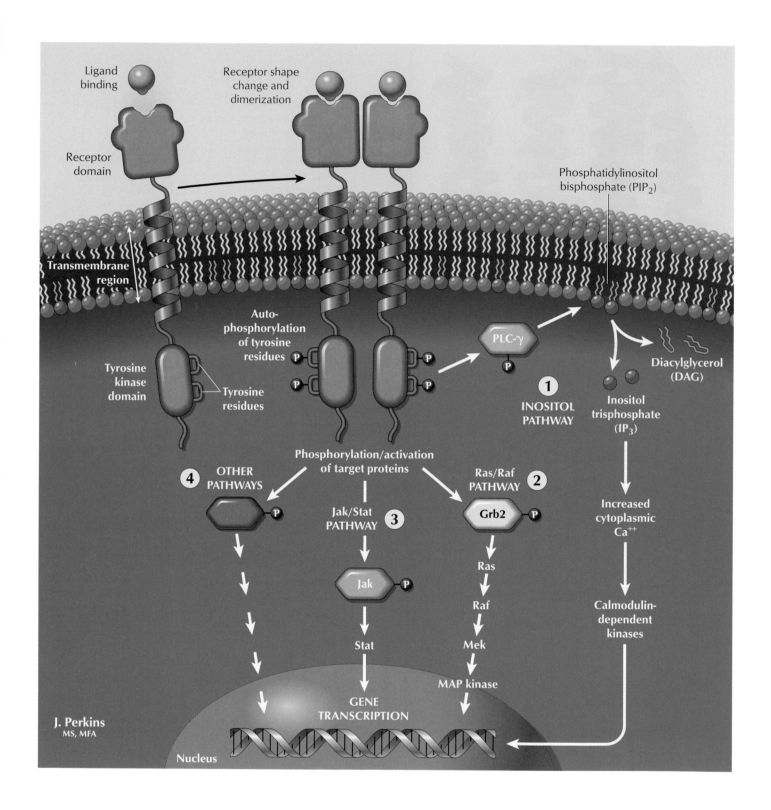

FIGURE 1-16 *TRK* RECEPTORS

Some drugs bind to receptors that are composed of an extracellular ligand-binding domain, a transmembrane region, and an intracellular domain that has tyrosine kinase (trk) activity. When activated, these receptors catalyze the intracellular phosphorylation of tyrosine residues in target proteins that are important for cellular growth and differentiation and responses to metabolic stimuli. Examples of ligands (and drug mimetics) that bind to *trk* receptors include insulin, nerve growth factor, platelet-derived growth factor, cytokines, and other growth factors. It is hypothesized that agonists cause a change in the conformation of the receptor, thereby promoting its action as a tyrosine kinase.

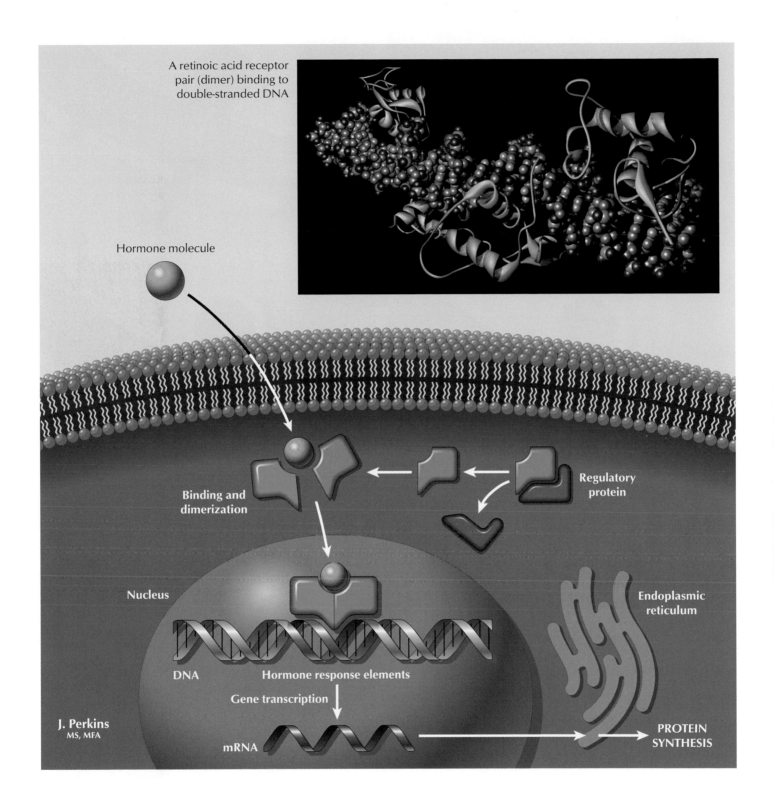

A retinoic acid receptor pair (dimer) binding to double-stranded DNA

Hormone molecule

Binding and dimerization

Regulatory protein

Nucleus

Endoplasmic reticulum

DNA   Hormone response elements

Gene transcription

J. Perkins
MS, MFA

mRNA

PROTEIN SYNTHESIS

FIGURE 1-17 NUCLEAR RECEPTORS

Some drugs produce their effects by binding to receptors located in the cytoplasm or the nucleus of the cell. For example, steroid hormones, thyroid hormone, corticosteroids, vitamin D, and retinoids diffuse through the plasma membrane of the cell and bind to their respective receptors in the cytoplasm. The complex or activated receptors then act as transcription factors by entering the nucleus and binding to DNA hormone-response elements within the nucleus. The DNA-binding domain recognizes certain base sequences, which leads to promotion or repression of particular genes. Regulation of gene transcription by this mechanism can lead to long-term effects. One class of nuclear receptors functions in increased expression of drug-metabolizing enzymes induced by many drugs.

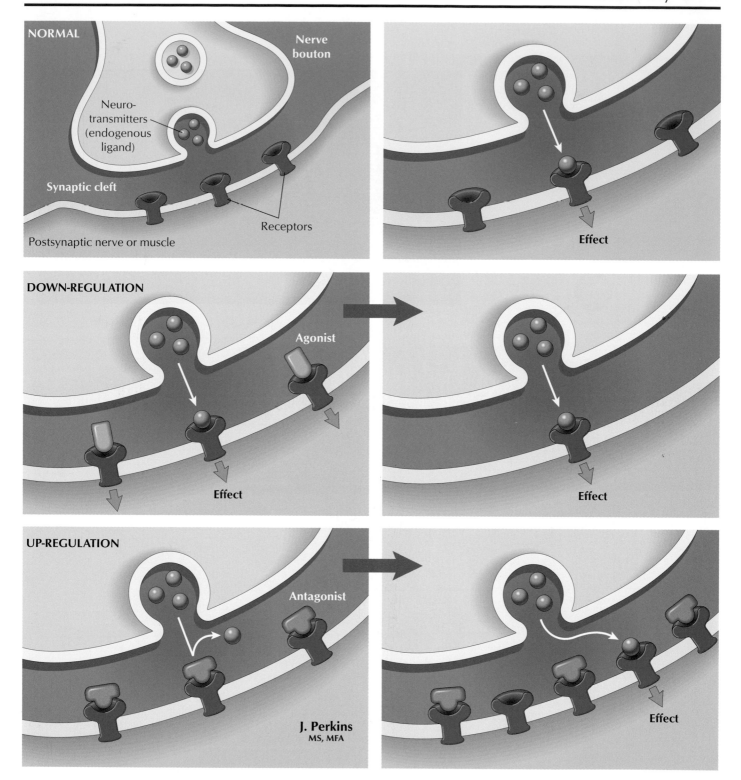

FIGURE 1-18 UP-REGULATION AND DOWN-REGULATION OF RECEPTORS

The type and number of receptors that a cell expresses are the net effect of simultaneous receptor synthesis and destruction. In addition to other factors, the number of receptors is modified by long-term exposure to drugs. Chronic stimulation by agonists tends to decrease receptor number (down-regulation), whereas chronic inhibition by antagonists tends to increase the number of receptors (up-regulation). The cellular response opposes the drug-induced effect and may be a defense mechanism. Also, the effect of subsequent administration of drug is greater (or less) than that of initial exposure, and abrupt withdrawal of drug leaves the cell overresponsive or underresponsive to the endogenous ligand. Down-regulation is one mechanism by which pharmacologic tolerance can occur, in which increasing doses of a drug must be used to achieve the same effect.

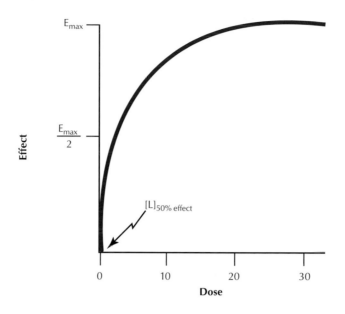

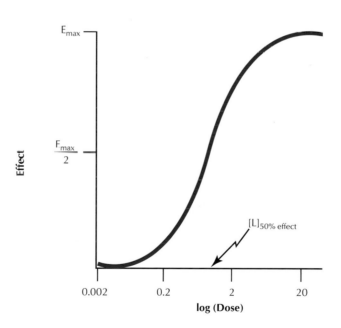

FIGURE 1-19 DOSE-RESPONSE CURVES

A direct relation exists between the concentration or dose of a drug and the magnitude of its biologic effect. As a graph, this relation is commonly referred to as a *DRC*. A DRC can be plotted by using a continuous (graded) or binary (quantal) measure of effect and a linear or logarithmic representation of dose (the latter producing the familiar S-shaped DRC). Each of a drug's usually multiple effects can be represented by a DRC. When the effect is mediated by receptors, the shape of the DRC is consistent with a reversible interaction between ligand (L) and receptor (R): $nL + mR \leftrightarrow L^nR^m$, where m and n usually equal 1. The general relation between ligand $[L]$ (drug concentration) and effect E is given by

$$E = \frac{E_{max} \cdot [L]}{[L] + [L]_{50\% \ effect}}.$$

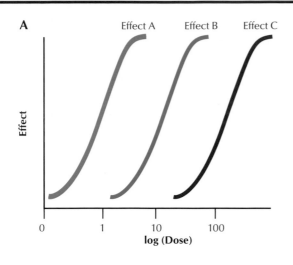

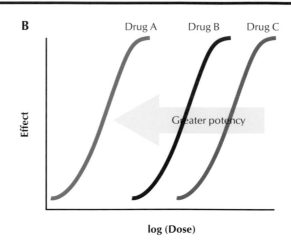

FIGURE 1-20 POTENCY

Potency is the drug quantity required for a specified level of a specified effect. For the drug with a DRC given by line A (**A**), potency is 1 mg/kg for the 50% level of effect A. The 50% level is usually used, with potency shown as an ED_{50} value. Potency represents ADME and PD properties. Potency for desirable and adverse effects can be established: the potency of one drug for effects A, B, and C (**A**) is 1, 10, and 100 mg/kg. Potency is thus related to the relative position of a DRC along the horizontal axis. Potency is also used to compare drugs with similar effects (**B**): 1 mg/kg of drug A is needed for 50% of the effect. Ten times the amount of drug B (10 mg/kg) is required for this level, so drug A is more potent than drug B; both are more potent than drug C. Potency is clinically important only if a drug is expensive or the amount needed is too large. The ED_{50}/LD_{50} ratio (therapeutic index) is used to compare potency (ED_{50}) with lethality (LD_{50}).

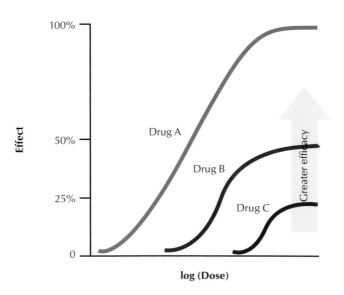

FIGURE 1-21 EFFICACY

At a molecular level, *efficacy* is the ability of a drug to produce an effect (agonists have positive efficacy, and antagonists have zero efficacy) and the degree of effect per drug molecule bound. At an organism level, it refers to the maximum effect of a drug. Maximum effects of drugs whose DRCs are given by lines A, B, and C is 100%, 50%, and 25%, with the order of efficacy being A > B > C. Efficacy is thus associated with the position of a DRC along the vertical axis. Drugs with a maximal possible effect are *full agonists*; *partial agonists* are drugs whose effect is less than maximal. Some agonists elicit this effect by occupying less than 100% of available receptors, and the other receptors are called *spare receptors*. Efficacy is associated with the molecular actions of a drug, not its PK properties. Efficacy can be determined for each of a drug's effects. Unlike potency, efficacy is relatively important clinically because it indicates the maximum attainable effect of a drug.

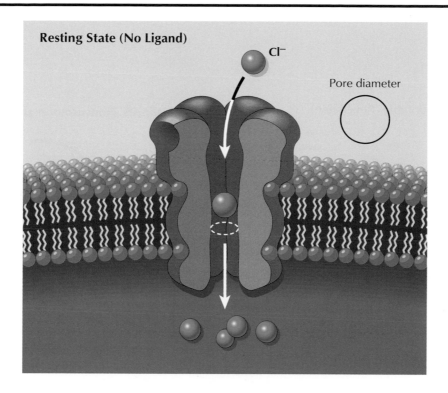

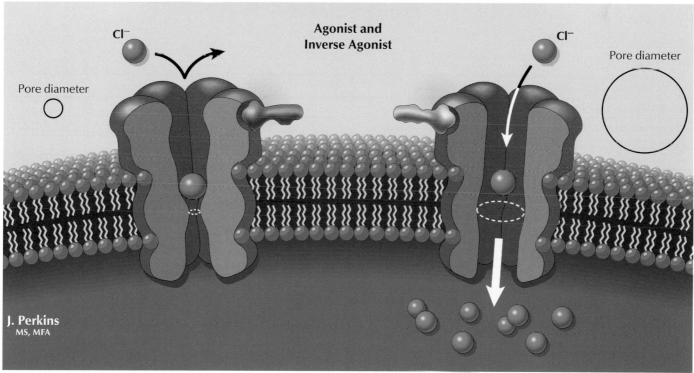

J. Perkins
MS, MFA

FIGURE 1-22 INVERSE AGONISTS

Drug receptors were first thought to be binary switches—either on (activated) or off (resting). Agonists turned the switch on; antagonists blocked agonists' access to receptors. Today, a receptor is viewed as a continuous switch, with the resting state between on or off. Two types of agonists can exist at these receptors: those that move the receptor from resting toward on and those that move it toward off. Both types are agonists, because both have affinity and intrinsic activity. For example, the channel pore of a ligand-gated ion-channel receptor may have a certain resting diameter; some agonists bind to the receptor and increase pore size (increase ion flux), whereas others decrease pore size (decrease ion flux). Which agonist is said to be the inverse of another is arbitrary and depends on which was discovered first. Classic examples of inverse agonists reduce Cl^- flow through a $GABA_A$ receptor and cause rather than inhibit anxiety. The same antagonist should block both types of agonist.

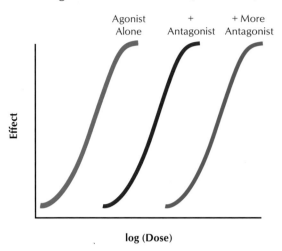

Antagonists: Surmountable (Reversible)

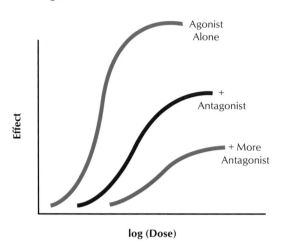

Antagonists: Nonsurmountable (Irreversible)

	Function	**Example**
Surmountable antagonist		
Muscarinic cholinergic antagonists	Reduce secretions	Atropine
	Treat asthma	Ipratropium
	Manage parkinsonism	Trihexyphenidyl
Adrenoceptor antagonists	Treat hypertension	Atenolol, propranolol
	Treat asthma	Albuterol, terbutaline
Dopamine antagonists	Manage schizophrenia	Haloperidol
Histamine H_2-receptor antagonists	Treat duodenal and gastric ulcers	Cimetidine, famotidine, nizatidine, ranitidine
Nonsurmountable antagonist (α adrenoceptor)	Control hypertension caused by excess catecholamine release from an adrenal tumor (pheochromocytoma)	Phenoxybenzamine

FIGURE 1-23 ANTAGONISTS: SURMOUNTABLE (REVERSIBLE) AND NONSURMOUNTABLE (IRREVERSIBLE)

The ability of an antagonist to alter an agonist effect depends on the affinity of the antagonist for the shared receptor. With weak, reversible antagonist binding (eg, hydrogen bonds), thermal agitation causes some antagonist molecules to uncouple from receptor and agonists successfully compete for receptor sites. If the agonist DRC with surmountable antagonists shifts to the right along the horizontal (dose) axis, the same maximal effect can occur. If antagonist molecules bind to a receptor irreversibly (eg, covalent chemical bonds) or irreversibly alter receptor sites, those sites are unavailable for agonist molecules. Antagonist molecules do not uncouple from a receptor; agonist molecules cannot compete for unoccupied sites. Fewer drug-receptor complexes mean diminished drug effect. The agonist DRC with irreversible antagonists shifts to the right along the dose axis and downward. The same maximal effect cannot be achieved by the agonist at any dose (nonsurmountable antagonism).

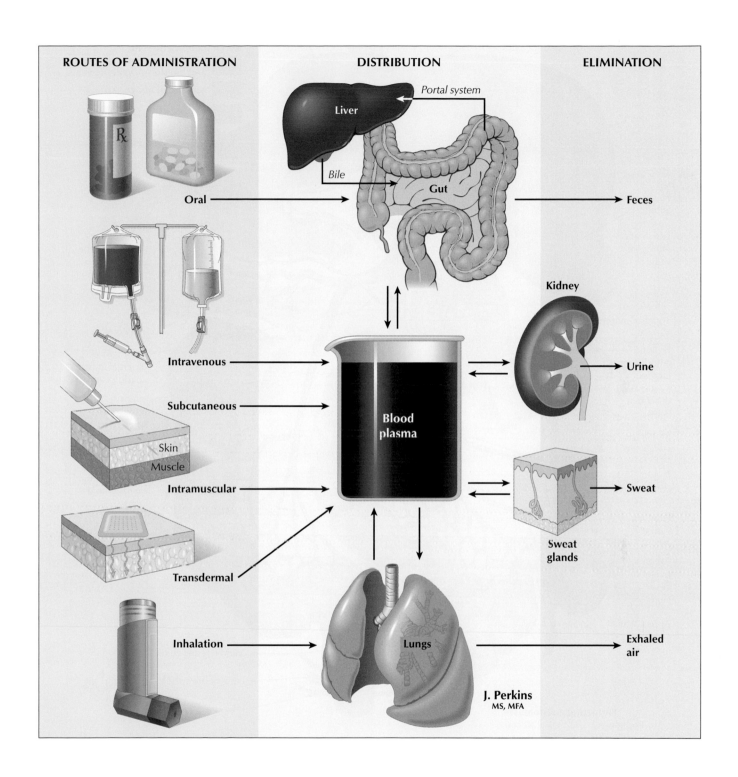

FIGURE 1-24 ROUTES OF ADMINISTRATION

The oral route is generally the most convenient, economic, and safe. Most drugs are rapidly and well absorbed along the GI tract, although some (eg, insulin) are not because of inactivation by enzymes. Drugs given intravenously enter the systemic circulation rapidly; drugs given intra-arterially reach a target site in high concentration. Subcutaneous and intramuscular routes rely on diffusion of the drug into the bloodstream, which can be influenced by warming or cooling the area or by other drugs.

Inhalation produces a rapid response to a drug because of the large surface area of the lungs and their extensive blood supply. Transdermal application is becoming an increasing popular mode of administration. Other routes or sites of drug administration include dermal (for local action), mucous membranes (for systemic action), insufflation (lungs), intraneural (nerves), optic (eyes), otic (ears), intraperitoneal (abdomen), and epidural (spinal cord).

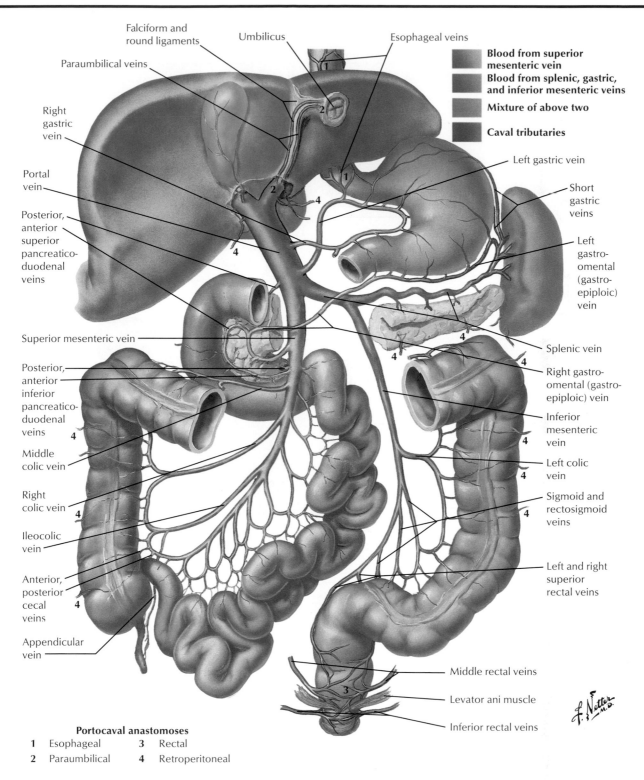

Falciform and round ligaments
Umbilicus
Esophageal veins
Paraumbilical veins

Blood from superior mesenteric vein

Blood from splenic, gastric, and inferior mesenteric veins

Mixture of above two

Caval tributaries

Right gastric vein

Left gastric vein

Portal vein

Short gastric veins

Posterior, anterior superior pancreatico-duodenal veins

Left gastro-omental (gastro-epiploic) vein

Superior mesenteric vein

Splenic vein

Posterior, anterior inferior pancreatico-duodenal veins

Right gastro-omental (gastro-epiploic) vein

Inferior mesenteric vein

Middle colic vein

Left colic vein

Right colic vein

Sigmoid and rectosigmoid veins

Ileocolic vein

Left and right superior rectal veins

Anterior, posterior cecal veins

Appendicular vein

Middle rectal veins

Levator ani muscle

Inferior rectal veins

Portocaval anastomoses

| 1 | Esophageal | 3 | Rectal |
| 2 | Paraumbilical | 4 | Retroperitoneal |

FIGURE 1-25 FIRST-PASS EFFECT

Drugs that are administered into the GI tract (orally or rectally) are subject to a first-pass effect. Venous drainage of blood from most portions of the GI tract enters the portal circulation, which delivers blood to the liver. In the liver (sometimes the gut wall), drug molecules can be biotransformed (term preferred to *metabolized*) to less active substances (usually). The amount of active drug that enters the systemic circulation after GI administration is thus less—by the amount of the first-pass effect—than that after another route of administration. The magnitude of this effect on a drug's systemic bioavailability (*F*) is expressed as the extraction ratio (*ER*):

$$F = f \times (1 - ER) = f \times (1 - Cl_{liver}/Q),$$

where *f* is the extent of absorption, Cl_{liver} is the hepatic clearance, and *Q* is the hepatic blood flow (normally approximately 90 L/h in a 70-kg person). Two related drugs that have comparable bioavailability and similar t_{max} (time to peak concentration) are said to be *bioequivalent*.

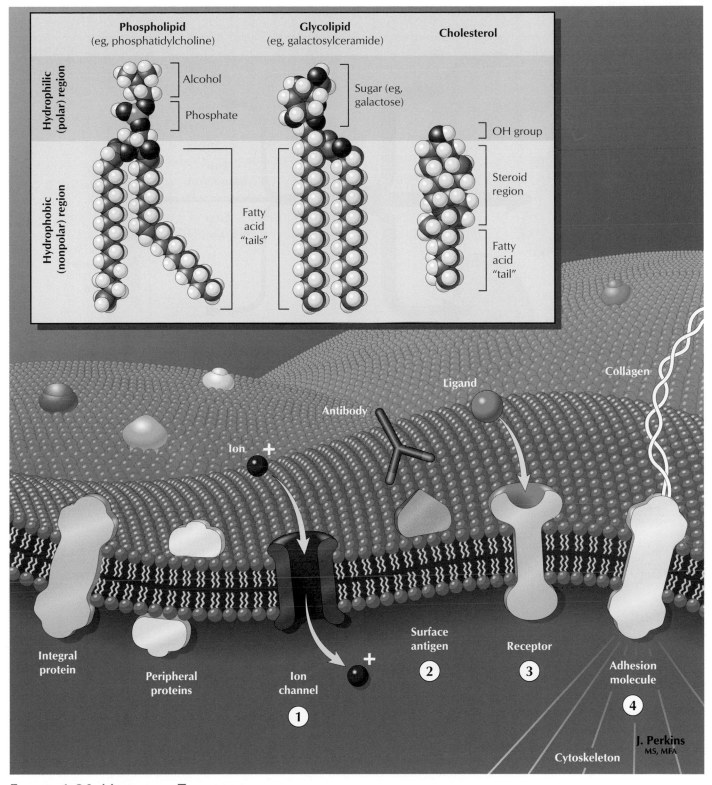

FIGURE 1-26 MEMBRANE TRANSPORT

The biologic membrane is a phospholipid bilayer, a hydrophobic core (lipid layer) between 2 hydrophilic portions (phospho groups). Small molecules can pass through membrane pores. Drugs can pass across membranes by passive diffusion (through lipid or aqueous channels), by active transport (combining with carriers), or by pinocytosis. To cross membranes, most drugs must be both water soluble (hydrophilic or lipophobic) and fat soluble (lipophilic or hydrophobic), which is achieved by weak acids (HA ↔ H⁺ + A⁻) and weak bases (BH⁺ ↔ B + H⁺), whose charged (hydrophilic) and uncharged (lipophilic) forms are in equilibrium. The extent of drug absorption is a function of pK_a of the drug and pH of the local environment. Equations for determining distribution of protonated and nonprotonated forms of a drug across a membrane are

$$\text{Acids:}\quad pK_a = pH + \log(HA/A^-)$$
$$\text{Bases:}\quad pK_a = pH + \log(BH^+/B).$$

For reference, pH values in the stomach are 1.0 to 1.5; that in blood plasma is approximately 7.4.

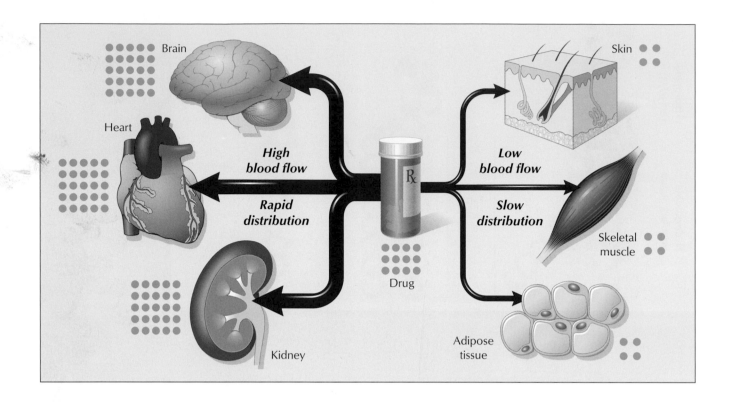

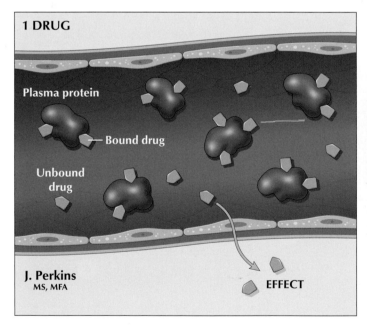

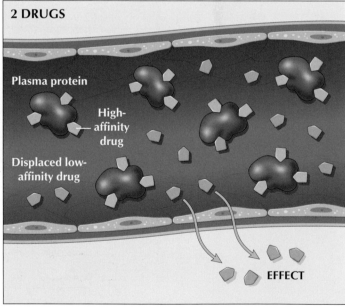

FIGURE 1-27 DISTRIBUTION

After absorption, drugs enter the systemic circulation and are distributed widely in the body; they leave the bloodstream and enter cells, with the amount entering depending on local blood flow, capillary permeability, and relative drug lipophilicity. Drugs in the blood are either unbound or bound reversibly to plasma proteins (eg, albumin) in equilibrium. The unbound portion is bioactive. Binding of drugs to these proteins is determined by affinity between drug and protein and protein binding capacity. Only a few binding sites are available, so a high dose can saturate binding sites, and additional drug circulates unbound in the bloodstream. If 2 or more drugs have affinity for the same binding sites, the one with highest affinity will bind, which increases plasma concentration of displaced drug. These effects, which may have clinical consequences, must be considered for the dosing regimen. Drugs with high plasma protein binding (≥95%) include lithium, midazolam, and warfarin (99%).

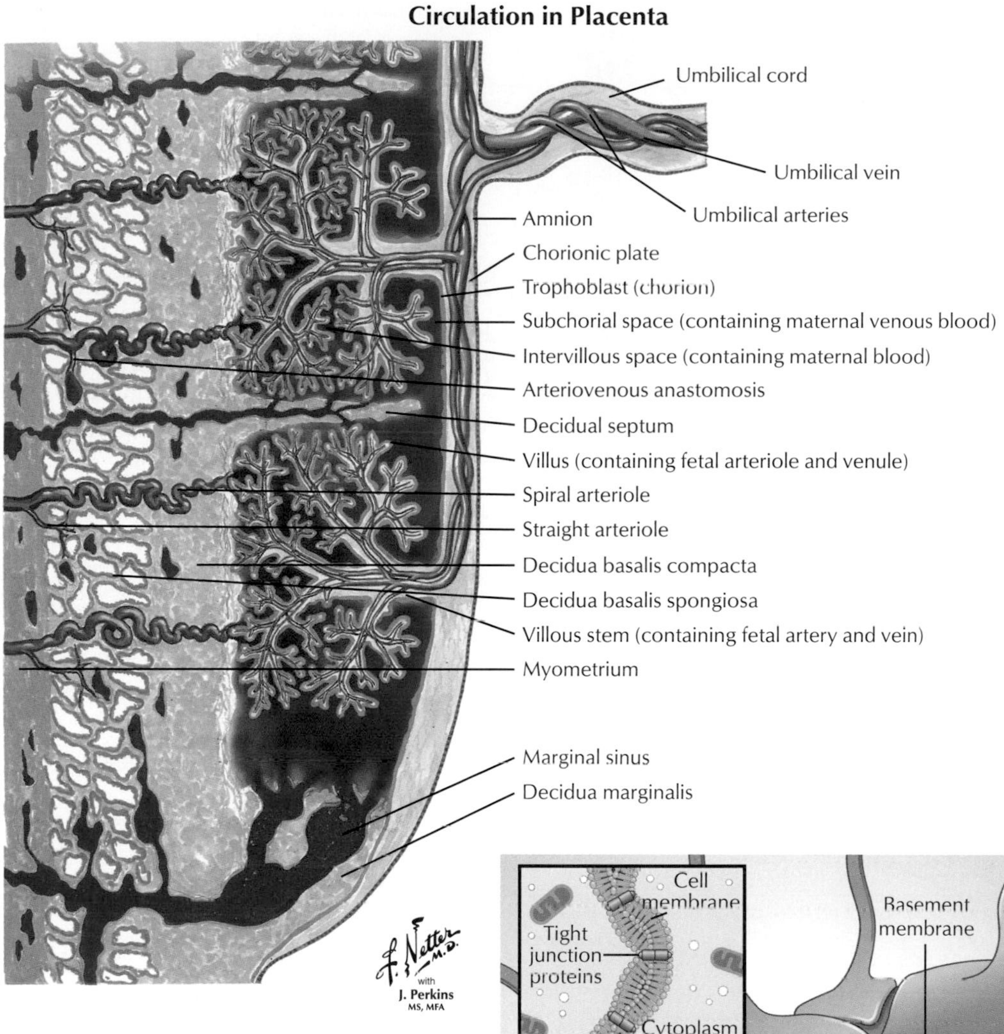

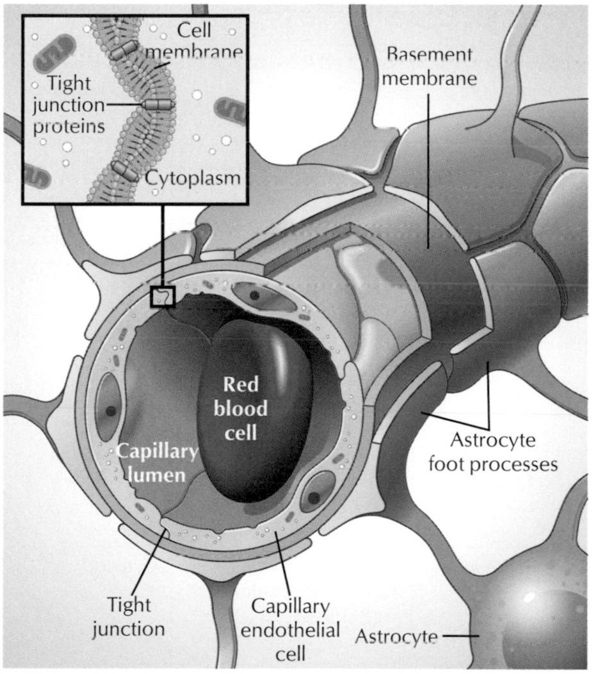

Circulation in Placenta

- Umbilical cord
- Umbilical vein
- Umbilical arteries
- Amnion
- Chorionic plate
- Trophoblast (chorion)
- Subchorial space (containing maternal venous blood)
- Intervillous space (containing maternal blood)
- Arteriovenous anastomosis
- Decidual septum
- Villus (containing fetal arteriole and venule)
- Spiral arteriole
- Straight arteriole
- Decidua basalis compacta
- Decidua basalis spongiosa
- Villous stem (containing fetal artery and vein)
- Myometrium

- Marginal sinus
- Decidua marginalis

- Cell membrane
- Tight junction proteins
- Cytoplasm
- Basement membrane
- Red blood cell
- Capillary lumen
- Astrocyte foot processes
- Tight junction
- Capillary endothelial cell
- Astrocyte

FIGURE 1-28 BARRIERS

Because of various anatomical and physiologic features, endothelial cells of the capillaries can limit passage of drugs from the bloodstream to tissues. For example, endothelial cells of brain capillaries, whose tight junctions merge into a continuous wall, are highly impermeable to many substances. Thus, a blood-brain barrier is established that generally limits accessibility of a good number of drugs, many of which are ionized in the blood at pH 7.4, to the brain. Water-soluble drugs, polar drugs, and ionized forms of drugs cannot cross this blood-brain barrier because they cannot pass through slit junctions and have difficulty traversing the lipid cell membrane. Lipid-soluble drugs pass more readily through cell membranes. In the liver, large fenestrations allow most drugs free access to the hepatic interstitium (with subsequent metabolism of the drugs). The placenta limits but does not prevent entry of drugs into the fetal circulation.

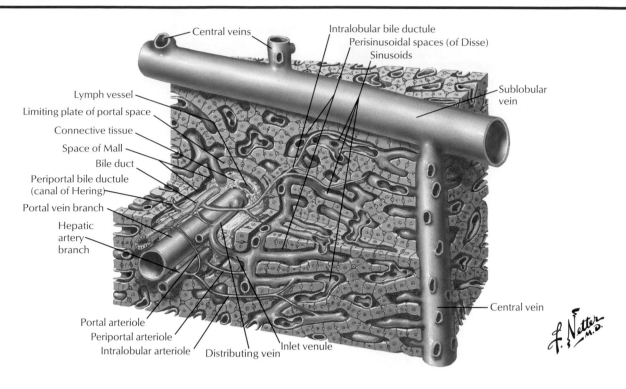

Conjugation Reaction	Endogenous Conjugant	Intracellular Sites	Common Substrates	Drug Examples
Acetylation	Acetyl-CoA	Cytosol	−OH, −COOH, −NH₂, −NR₂, −SH	Clonazepam, dapsone, isoniazid, sulfonamides, valproate
Glutathione conjugation	Reduced form of γ-Glu-Cys-Gly (the most common intracellular thiol)	Cytosol and microsomes	Electrophilic benzyl halides, aliphatic nitrate esters, epoxides, and quinines	Acetaminophen, ethacrynic acid
Gly (amino acid) conjugation	Gly, Glu, others	Mitochondria	−COOH	Benzoic and salicylic acid
Glucuronidation	UDPGA (uridine-5'-diphospho-α-D-glucuronic acid)	Microsomes	Hydroxyl, amino, or sulfhydryl groups	Acetaminophen, codeine, diazepam, disulfiram, ethinyl estradiol, fentanyl, galantamine, lorazepam, modafinil, morphine, propanolol, paroxetine, sulfonamides
Methylation (N-, O-, and S-)	CH₃ from S-adenosylmethionine (SAM)	Cytosol (eg, COMT)	−OH, −NH₂, −SH	Oxprenolol (N-), clomethiazole and isoproterenol (O-), captopril (S-)
Sulfate conjugation	3'-Phosphoadenosine-5'-phosphosulfate (PAPS)	Cytosol	−OH, −NH₂	Acetaminophen, ethinyl estradiol, methyldopa, paoxetine, steroids, triamterene

FIGURE 1-29 METABOLISM (BIOTRANSFORMATION) OF DRUGS

Drugs undergo biotransformation by many of the same reactions as endogenous compounds. Drugs are usually metabolized to less active and more ionized (water-soluble) forms, but equally or more active metabolites can also be created. An inactive parent drug that forms active metabolites is called a *prodrug*. Although drug metabolism occurs in almost all tissues, including the GI tract, the liver is the major site because of its strategic place in the portal circulation and its many metabolic enzymes.

Two general types of drug metabolic reactions occur: phase 1, involving chemical modification, typically by oxidation, reduction, or hydrolysis; and phase 2, in which an endogenous chemical is covalently attached (conjugated) (glucose conjugation, or glucuronidation, the most common). Drugs often undergo multiple phase 1 and 2 reactions, which produces many metabolites, each with its own pharmacologic profile. Liver disease alters drug metabolism, so appropriate dosage adjustment is required.

Cytochrome P-450

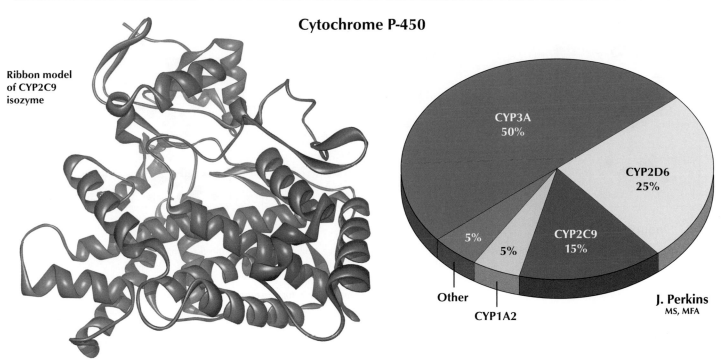

Ribbon model of CYP2C9 isozyme

J. Perkins
MS, MFA

CYP	Substrate
1A2	Acetaminophen, antipyrine, caffeine, clomipramine, olanzapine, ondansetron, phenacetin, rilozole, ropinirole, tamoxifen, theophylline, warfarin
2A6	Coumarin
2B6	Artemisinin, buproprion, cyclophosphamide, S-mephobarbital, S-mephenytoin, (N-demethylation to nirvanol), propofol, selegiline, sertraline
2C8	Pioglitazone
2C9	Carvedilol, celecoxib, fluvastatin, glimepiride, hexobarbital, ibuprofen, losartan, mefenamic, meloxicam, montelukast, nateglinide, phenytoin, tolbutamide, trimethadone, sulfaphenazole, warfarin, ticrynafen, zafirlukast
2C19	Citalopram, diazepam, escitalopram, esomeprazole (S isomer of omeprazole), irbesartan, S-mephenytoin, naproxen, nirvanol, omeprazole, pantoprazole, proguanil, propranolol
2D6	Almotriptan, bufuralol, bupranolol, carvedilol, clomipramine, clozapine, codeine, debrisoquin, dextromethorphan, dolasetron, fluoxetine (S-norfluoxetine), formoterol, galantamine, guanoxan, haloperidol, hydrocodone, 4-methoxy-amphetamine, metoprolol, mexlletine, olanzapine, oxycodone, paroxetine, phenformin, phenothiazines, propoxyphene, risperidone, selegiline, (deprenyl), sparteine, thioridazine, timolol, tolterodine, tramadol, tricyclic antidepressants, type 1C antiarrhythmics (eg, encainide, flecainide, propafenone), venlafaxine
2E1	Acetaminophen, chlorzoxazone, enflurane, halothane, ethanol (minor pathway)
3A4	Acetaminophen, alfentanil, almotriptan, amiodarone, astemizole, beclomethasone, bexarotene, budesonide, S-bupivacaine, carbamazepine, citalopram, cocaine, cortisol, cyclosporine, dapsone, delavirdine, diazepam, dihydroergotamine, dihydropyridines, diltiazem, escitalopram, ethinyl estradiol, fentanyl, finasteride, fluticasone, galantamine, gestodene, imatinab, indinavir, itraconazole, letrozole, lidocaine, loratadine, losartan, lovastatin, macrolides, methadone, miconazole, midazolam, mifepristone (RU-486), montelukast, oxybutynin, paclitaxel, pimecrolimus, pimozide, pioglitazone, progesterone, quinidine, rabeprazole, rapamycin, repaglinide, ritonavir, saquinavir, spironolactone, sulfamethoxazole, sufentanil, tacrolimus, tamoxifen, terfenadine, testosterone, tetrahydrocannabinol, tiagabine, triazolam, troleandomycin, verapamil, vinca alkaloids, ziprasidone, zonisamide
27	Doxercalciferol (activated)
No/ minimal involvement	Abacavir, acyclovir, alendronate, amiloride, benazepril, cabergoline, digoxin, disoproxil, hydrochlorothiazide, linezolid, lisinopril, olmesartan, oxaliplatin, metformin, moxifloxacin, raloxifene, ribavirin, risedronate, telmisartan, tenofovir, tiludronic acid, valacyclovir, valsartan, zoledronic acid

FIGURE 1-30 CYTOCHROME P-450 (CYP450) ENZYMES

A major enzyme system that catalyzes phase 1–type drug metabolism reactions is the microsomal CYP450 mixed-function oxidase (monooxygenase) system located in the endoplasmic reticulum in liver, GI tract, lungs, kidney, and other tissues. These enzymes catalyze an oxidation-reduction process that requires CYP450, CYP450 reductase, NADPH (reducing agent), and O_2. The only common feature of the many drugs metabolized by this pathway is lipid solubility. The pie chart shown above indicates the approximate percent of current drugs that are metabolized by the indicated CYP isozymes. Known polymorphisms in these enzymes require a drug dosage adjustment. If 2 drugs are metabolized by the same CYP isozyme, they can interfere with each other's normal route or rate of metabolism, and a drug interaction may decrease or increase plasma drug concentrations. An example is interaction between fluoxetine (a selective serotonin reuptake inhibitor) and St John's wort.

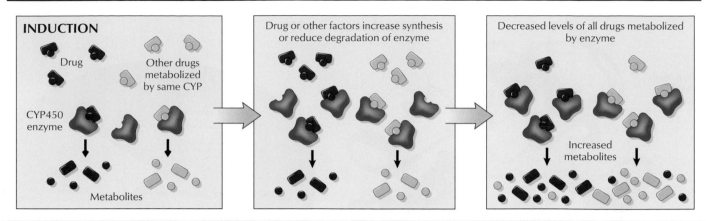

CYP	Inducers	Inhibitors
1A2	Smoking, charbroiled foods, cruciferous vegetables, insulin, modafinil, nafcillin, omeprazole, phenobarbital, primidone, rifampin	Amiodarone, anastrozole, cimetidine, ciprofloxacin, diltiazem, enoxacin, erythromycin, fluoroquinolones, fluvoxamine, grapefruit (juice), mexiletine, norfloxacin, ritonavir, tacrine, ticlopidine
2A6	Dexamethasone, phenobarbital	Methoxsalen, ritonavir, tranylcypromine
2B6	Cyclophosphamide, dexamethasone, phenobarbitol, phenytoin, primidone, rifampin	Efavirenz, nelfinavir, orphenadrine, ritonavir, thiotepa, ticlopidine
2C8/9	Dexamethasone, primidone, rifampin, secobarbital	Anastrozole, amiodarone, cimetidine, diclofenac, disulfiram, fluconazole, fluvoxamine, flurbiprofen, fluvastatin, isoniazid, ketoprofen, lovastatin, metronidazole, omeprazole, paroxetine, phenylbutazone, ritonavir, sertraline, sulfinpyrazone, sulfonamides, sulfamethoxazole, trimethoprim, troglitazone, zafirlukast
2C19	Barbituates, rifampin	Cimetidine, ketoconazole, modafinil, omeprazole, oxcarbazepine, ticlopidine
2D6	Dexamethasone, quinidine, rifampin	Amiodarone, buproprion, celecoxib, chlorpromazine, chlorpheniramine, cimetidine, clomipramine, cocaine, doxorubicin, fluoxetine, fluphenazine, fluvoxamine, haloperidol, lomustine, metoclopramide, methadone, norfluoxetine, paroxetine, perphenazine, propafenone, quinidine, ranitidine, ritonavir, sertindole, sertraine, terbinafine, thioridazine, venlafaxine, vinblastine, vinorelbine
2E1	Acetone, ethanol, isoniazid	Disulfiram, ritonavir
3A4	Barbituates, carbamazepine, dexamethasone, efavirenz, macrolides, glucocorticoids, modafinil, nevirapine, oxcarbazepine, phenobarbital, phenylbutazone, pioglitazone, phenytoin, primidone, rifabutin, rifampin, St John's wort, sulfinpyrazone, troglitazone	Amiodarone, anastrozole, chloramphenicol, cimetidine, ciprofloxacin, clarithromycin, clotrimazole, danazol, delavirdine, diltiazem, erythromycin, fluconazole, fluoxetine, fluvoxamine, grapefruit juice, indinavir, itraconazole, ketoconazole, metronidazole, mibefradil, miconazole, nefazodone, nelfinavir, nevirapine, norfloxacin, norfluoxetine, omeprazole, paroxetine, propoxyphene, quinidine, ranitidine, ritonavir, saquinavir, sertindole, troglitazone, troleandomycin, verapamil, zafirlukast, zileuton

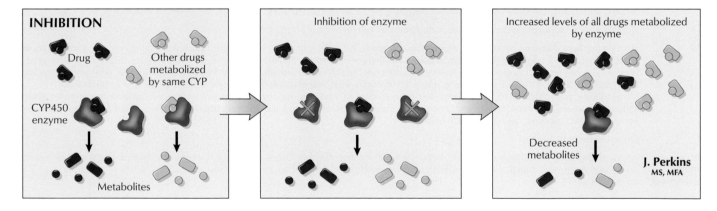

FIGURE 1-31 METABOLIC ENZYME INDUCTION AND INHIBITION

Multiple factors, including drugs, can either increase or decrease metabolic enzyme activity. Long-term administration of drugs often induces CYP450 activity dramatically by enhancing the rate of synthesis or reducing the rate of degradation of these hepatic microsomal enzymes. Enzyme induction results in more rapid metabolism of the drug and all other drugs metabolized by the same enzymes. As a result, plasma levels and biologic effects of the drugs decrease (except for prodrugs, whose biologic effects increase). Barbiturates are well-known strong inducers of CYP450 enzymes. Other substances can inhibit CYP450 enzymatic activity. In this case, the metabolism of other drugs through this pathway is reduced, which results in increased blood levels of these other drugs. The clinical consequences of the altered blood levels can be greater biologic effects (except for prodrugs) or increased toxicity.

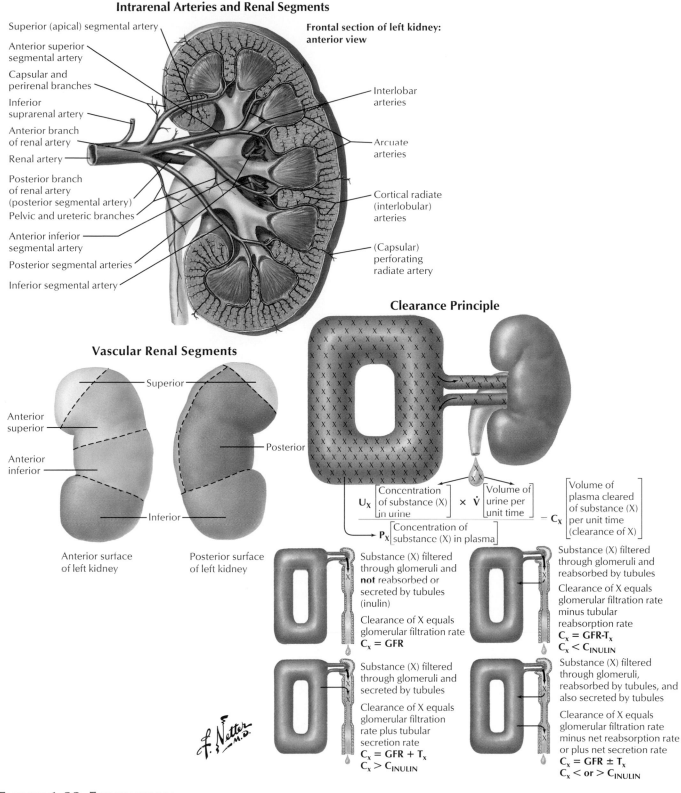

Intrarenal Arteries and Renal Segments

Frontal section of left kidney: anterior view

Superior (apical) segmental artery

Anterior superior segmental artery

Capsular and perirenal branches

Inferior suprarenal artery

Anterior branch of renal artery

Renal artery

Posterior branch of renal artery (posterior segmental artery)

Pelvic and ureteric branches

Anterior inferior segmental artery

Posterior segmental arteries

Inferior segmental artery

Interlobar arteries

Arcuate arteries

Cortical radiate (interlobular) arteries

(Capsular) perforating radiate artery

Vascular Renal Segments

Superior

Anterior superior

Anterior inferior

Posterior

Inferior

Anterior surface of left kidney

Posterior surface of left kidney

Clearance Principle

$$U_X \left[\begin{matrix} \text{Concentration} \\ \text{of substance (X)} \\ \text{in urine} \end{matrix} \right] \times \dot{V} \left[\begin{matrix} \text{Volume of} \\ \text{urine per} \\ \text{unit time} \end{matrix} \right] - C_X \left[\begin{matrix} \text{Volume of} \\ \text{plasma cleared} \\ \text{of substance (X)} \\ \text{per unit time} \\ \text{(clearance of X)} \end{matrix} \right]$$

$$P_X \left[\begin{matrix} \text{Concentration of} \\ \text{substance (X) in plasma} \end{matrix} \right]$$

Substance (X) filtered through glomeruli and **not** reabsorbed or secreted by tubules (inulin)

Clearance of X equals glomerular filtration rate

$C_X = GFR$

Substance (X) filtered through glomeruli and reabsorbed by tubules

Clearance of X equals glomerular filtration rate minus tubular reabsorption rate

$C_X = GFR\text{-}T_X$

$C_X < C_{INULIN}$

Substance (X) filtered through glomeruli and secreted by tubules

Clearance of X equals glomerular filtration rate plus tubular secretion rate

$C_X = GFR + T_X$

$C_X > C_{INULIN}$

Substance (X) filtered through glomeruli, reabsorbed by tubules, and also secreted by tubules

Clearance of X equals glomerular filtration rate minus net reabsorption rate or plus net secretion rate

$C_X = GFR \pm T_X$

$C_X < \text{or} > C_{INULIN}$

FIGURE 1-32 ELIMINATION

The major route of drug elimination is through the kidneys, which receive one fifth to one fourth of the cardiac output. Other routes are feces and lungs (especially for anesthetic gases). The rate of elimination of most drugs follows first-order kinetics (exponential decline). The time for the plasma levels of a drug to reach half the initial value is the *half-life* ($t_{1/2}$). A notable exception is ethanol, which follows zero-order (linear) kinetics at sub-intoxicating concentrations. The *clearance* of a drug from the body is the sum of clearances from all elimination routes, eg, clearance from the kidney is given by the volume of plasma that is completely cleared of the drug per unit time (usually 1 minute). In this case, the amount of drug in urine is measured. Kidney clearance of drug X (C_X) is calculated from drug concentrations in urine (U_X) and plasma (P_X), and urine volume (V): $CL_X = (U_X \times V)/P_X$. A kidney disorder alters the rate of drug elimination, so the dosage must be adjusted.

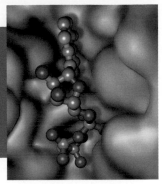

CHAPTER 2

DRUGS USED TO AFFECT THE AUTONOMIC AND SOMATIC NERVOUS SYSTEMS

OVERVIEW

The nervous system functions as a major communication system within the body. Information is transmitted by electrical conduction along axons of neurons to (via afferent nerves) and from (via efferent nerves) the central nervous system (CNS). Between neurons or between neurons and target cells are gaps termed *synapses* across which the signal is transmitted chemically rather than electrically (with some exceptions). The endogenous chemical substances that transmit these signals are termed *neurotransmitters*. Accuracy of signal transmission requires that the postsynaptic cell reliably receive the intended message from the presynaptic cell. The fidelity is ensured by neurotransmitter-specific receptors located on the postsynaptic cell membrane.

Because an action potential, or the change in membrane potential occurring in excitable tissue during excitation, relies on a chemical process (ion flux across the membrane) and the transmission across synapses is primarily chemical, exogenously administered chemicals or drugs can modify physiologic processes mediated by the nervous system. The major neurotransmitters in the periphery are acetylcholine (ACh) and norepinephrine, and drugs can be designed either to mimic or to inhibit their actions. The integrated arrangement of the nervous system and the special distribution of neurotransmitter receptors allow for a targeted drug effect. In most cases, the actual action of the drug—and even much of its unwanted action—is predictable on the basis of the anatomy and physiology of the nervous system. It is convenient for the understanding of drug action to subclassify the peripheral nervous system (PNS) into 2 components: the somatic nervous system (SNS) and the autonomic nervous system (ANS).

The nerves of the SNS innervate skeletal muscles, and drugs that act on this system thus affect skeletal muscle function such as tone (eg, muscle relaxants given before surgery). Because all skeletal neuromuscular junctions contain ACh as the neurotransmitter, ACh and its receptors are targets for drugs intended to modify skeletal muscle function. The cholinergic receptors at these skeletal neuromuscular junctions are sufficiently different structurally (3-dimensional shape) from those at other sites to allow drugs to be designed to bind to only this type (nicotinic) of cholinergic receptor.

The nerves of the ANS innervate the organs of the body and can be further classified into sympathetic and parasympathetic subdivisions. Sympathetic activity is increased by drugs that mimic or enhance the action of norepinephrine. Parasympathetic activity is increased by drugs that mimic or enhance the action of ACh. Both systems are tonically active. Hence, antagonism of one system results in enhanced activity of the other. The SNS and ANS together provide a mechanistic framework for understanding the effects (good and bad) of drugs.

Elucidation of additional roles for neurotransmitters and identification of other receptor subtypes will likely lead to development of more selective drugs. Such drugs will be found by using, for example, high-throughput screening assays or molecular modeling techniques—or even by serendipity. However they are discovered, they should permit more selective targeting of the therapeutic end point with fewer unwanted effects.

Some Cell Types of the Nervous System

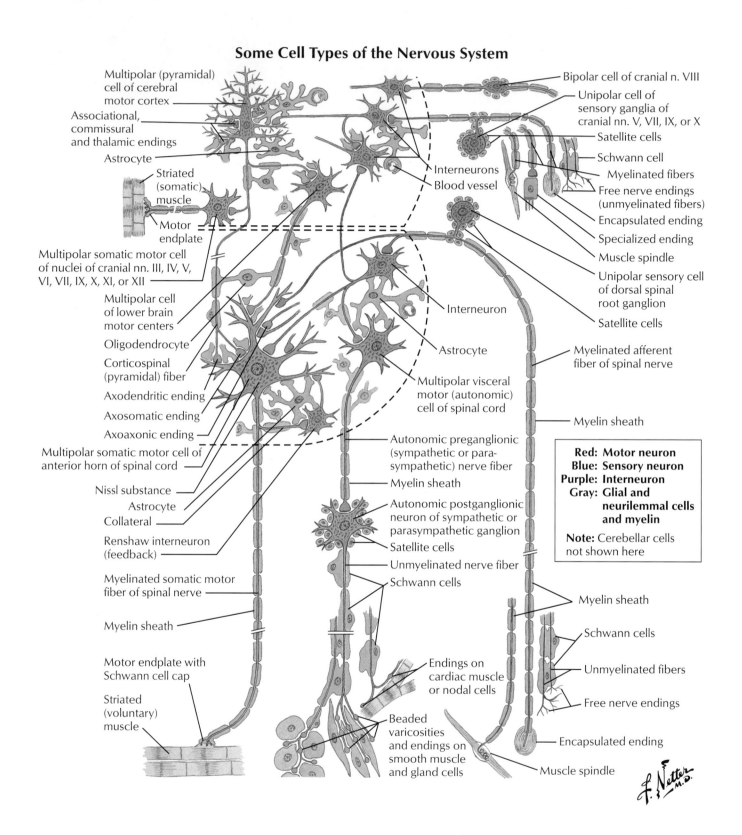

FIGURE 2-1 ORGANIZATION OF THE NERVOUS SYSTEM

The actions of many drugs can be understood as the modulation of the nervous system's control of physiologic processes. The CNS and PNS communicate via afferent and efferent neurons. As a result of this anatomical organization, drugs can affect sensory input (eg, local anesthetics for pain), skeletal muscle activity (eg, muscle relaxants for surgery), or autonomic output (eg, drugs that act on blood vessels or the heart to reduce high blood pressure).

Drug	Action on Membrane	Changes in Membrane Potential and Action Potential	Clinical Effects
Tetrodotoxin (puffer fish toxin) Saxitoxin (shellfish toxin)	Blocks voltage-sensitive Na$^+$ channels	Blocks action potential	Nerve block, paralysis, death
Tetraethylammonium (TEA)	Blocks K$^+$ permeability channels	Decreases resting potential (partial depolarization); prolongs action potential	?
Increased external potassium concentration	Makes K$^+$ equilibrium potential (E$_{K^+}$) less negative	Decreases resting potential (partial depolarization), thereby causing accommodation that decreases action potential size and increases threshold for action potential	Nerve block, plus action on many systems causing varied clinical picture
Metabolic inhibitors (cyanide) Cardiac glycosides (ouabain)	Block active transport, allowing Na$^+$ to accumulate in axoplasm, K$^+$ to leak out		
Low external calcium concentration	Destabilizes membrane: A. Ionic permeability increased B. Increases change in Na$^+$ permeability produced by depolarization	A. Resting potential shifts in depolarized direction (partial depolarization) B. Threshold level shifts in hyperpolarized direction A. and B. may induce repetitive firing	Hyperexcitability, tetany
Local anesthetics (procaine)	Stabilizes membrane: A. Ionic permeability produced by depolarization B. Decreases change in Na$^+$ permeability produced by depolarization	A. Resting potential constant B. Threshold level shifts in depolarized direction until approaching impulse can no longer trigger action potential	Nerve block

FIGURE 2-2 ACTION OF DRUGS ON NERVE EXCITABILITY

Efficient and effective transmission of neuronal action potentials relies on the unequal distribution of positive (primarily Na$^+$ and K$^+$) and negative (primarily Cl$^-$) ions across the axonal membrane. Selective, voltage-sensitive permeability of the membrane to these ions establishes the unequal distribution of the ions according to the Nernst equation and gives rise to a resting transmembrane potential difference. Drugs that alter the ion flux affect the resting transmembrane potential difference. The larger this difference, the further the neuron is from its firing threshold and the less likely that it will fire (ie, initiate an action potential). The smaller the transmembrane potential difference, the more likely it is that the neuron will reach this threshold and fire.

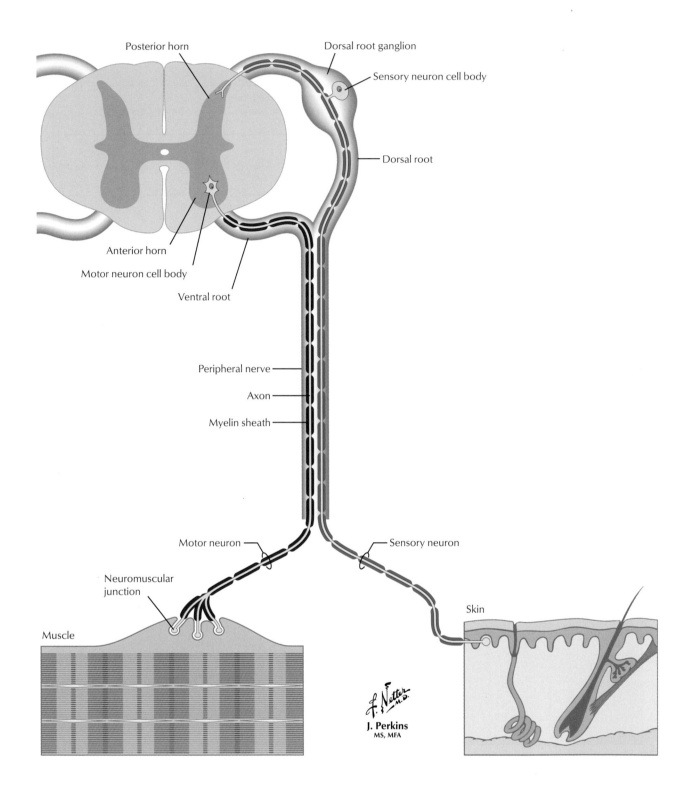

FIGURE 2-3 INTERFACE OF THE CENTRAL AND PERIPHERAL NERVOUS SYSTEMS AND ORGANIZATION OF THE SOMATIC DIVISION

Spinal nerve pairs enter and exit along segmented caudal, thoracic, lumbar, and sacral portions of the spinal cord and distribute throughout the body. Somatic afferent neurons transmit sensory information about normal status (eg, proprioception) or pathologic states (eg, heat and mechanical damage) to the spinal cord and brain. Efferent neurons carry motor signals from the spinal cord and brain to the somatic (striated or skeletal muscles: effectors) and autonomic (smooth muscle, cardiac muscle, glands) divisions of the PNS. Drugs can selectively modulate the activity of afferent or efferent pathways: those that excite afferent nociceptive neurons produce pain; those that inhibit afferent nociceptive neurons are analgesic. Those that excite efferent, or neuromuscular, junctions produce tetanus; those that inhibit these junctions cause paralysis.

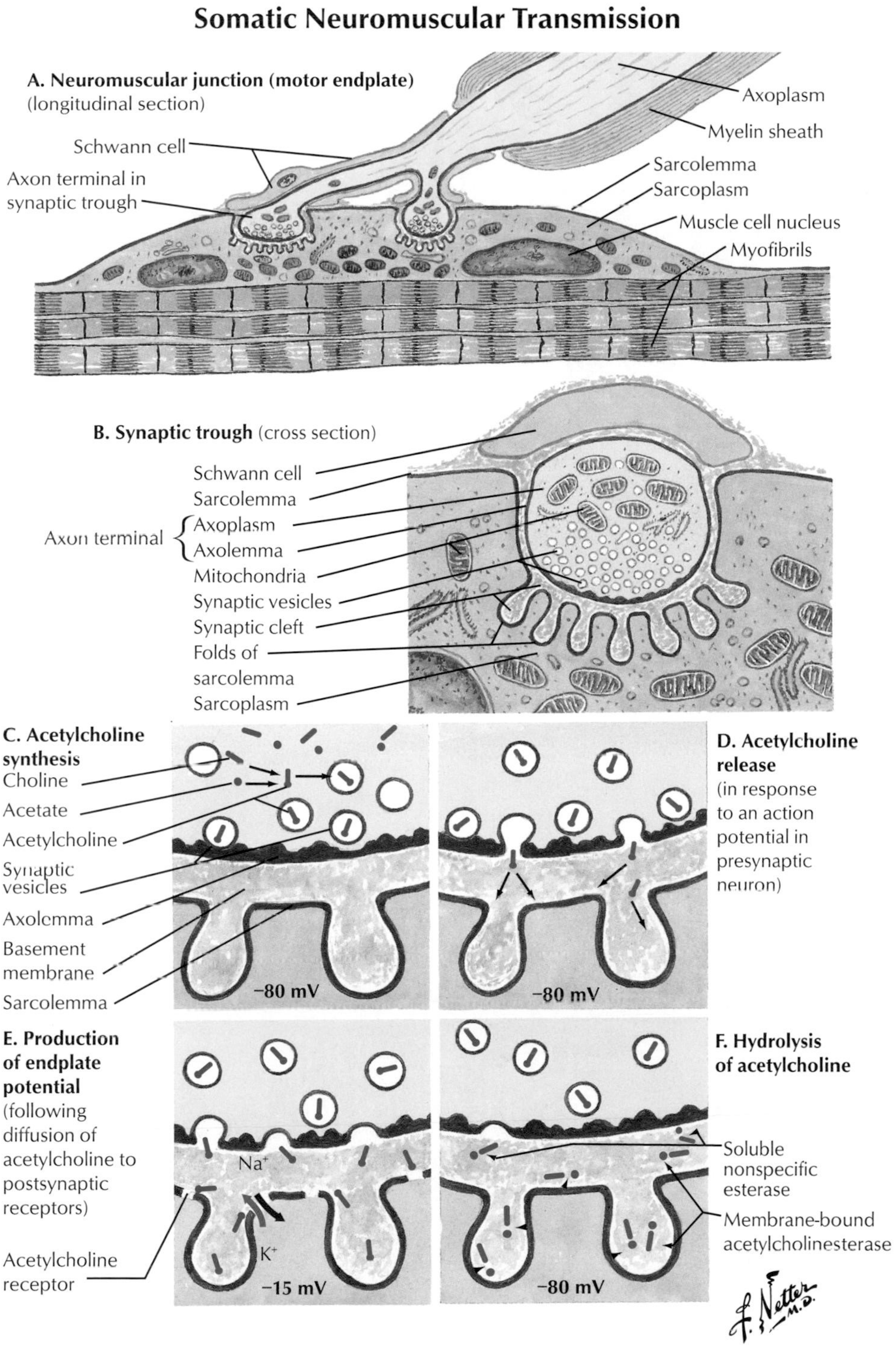

Somatic Neuromuscular Transmission

A. Neuromuscular junction (motor endplate) (longitudinal section)

- Schwann cell
- Axon terminal in synaptic trough
- Axoplasm
- Myelin sheath
- Sarcolemma
- Sarcoplasm
- Muscle cell nucleus
- Myofibrils

B. Synaptic trough (cross section)

Axon terminal {
- Schwann cell
- Sarcolemma
- Axoplasm
- Axolemma
- Mitochondria
- Synaptic vesicles
- Synaptic cleft
- Folds of sarcolemma
- Sarcoplasm

C. Acetylcholine synthesis
- Choline
- Acetate
- Acetylcholine
- Synaptic vesicles
- Axolemma
- Basement membrane
- Sarcolemma

−80 mV

D. Acetylcholine release (in response to an action potential in presynaptic neuron)

−80 mV

E. Production of endplate potential (following diffusion of acetylcholine to postsynaptic receptors)
- Acetylcholine receptor

Na⁺
K⁺
−15 mV

F. Hydrolysis of acetylcholine
- Soluble nonspecific esterase
- Membrane-bound acetylcholinesterase

−80 mV

F. Netter

FIGURE 2-4 NEUROMUSCULAR TRANSMISSION

Neurons innervate skeletal muscles at the neuromuscular junction (**A**). The axon-muscle interface forms at a synaptic trough, which has extensive foldings that increase the surface area of exposure to a neurotransmitter (**B**). ACh, the neurotransmitter at neuromuscular junctions, is synthesized in the presynaptic neuron from mitochondrial acetyl-CoA and extracellular choline via an enzyme-catalyzed reaction. ACh is stored in presynaptic vesicles (**C**) until release in response to an action potential in the presynaptic neuron (**D**), a Ca^{2+}-dependent process. ACh diffuses across the synaptic cleft and binds reversibly to specific receptor sites on the postsynaptic membrane. Ion flux then increases and the postsynaptic membrane depolarizes (**E**), which triggers an action potential that leads to muscle contraction. Released ACh is eliminated from the synapse by cholinesterase action (**F**).

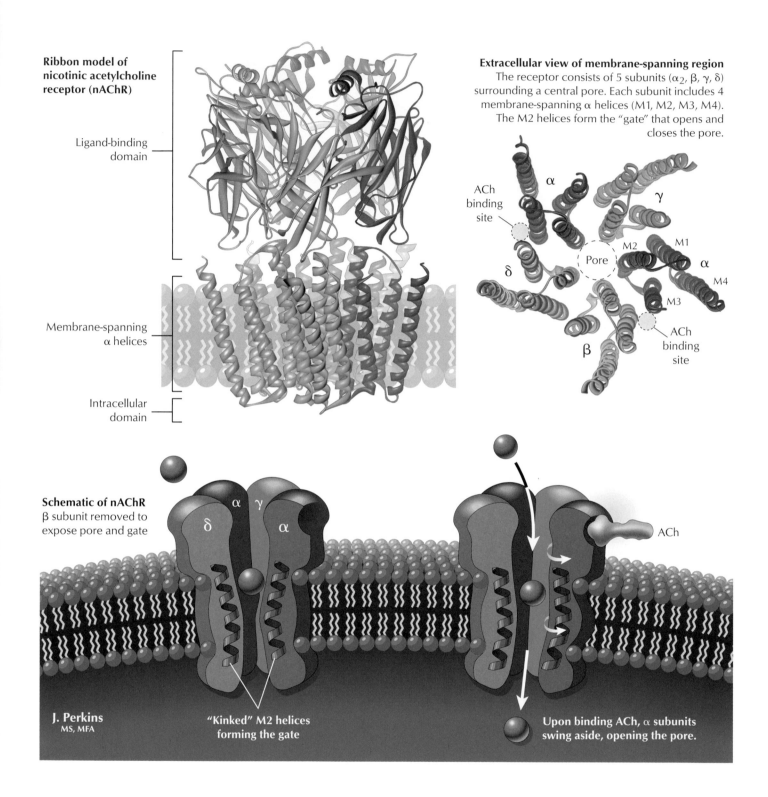

Ribbon model of nicotinic acetylcholine receptor (nAChR)

Ligand-binding domain

Membrane-spanning α helices

Intracellular domain

Extracellular view of membrane-spanning region
The receptor consists of 5 subunits (α_2, β, γ, δ) surrounding a central pore. Each subunit includes 4 membrane-spanning α helices (M1, M2, M3, M4). The M2 helices form the "gate" that opens and closes the pore.

α

γ

ACh binding site

δ

Pore

M2 M1

α

M4

M3

ACh binding site

β

Schematic of nAChR
β subunit removed to expose pore and gate

δ   α   γ   α

ACh

J. Perkins
MS, MFA

"Kinked" M2 helices forming the gate

Upon binding ACh, α subunits swing aside, opening the pore.

FIGURE 2-5 NICOTINIC ACETYLCHOLINE RECEPTOR

Drugs that block cholinesterases prolong the ACh residency time in the synapse and enhance the effect of ACh. Receptors at neuromuscular junctions are termed *nicotinic cholinergic receptors* (nAChRs) because nicotine is a relatively selective agonist at these sites. In an nAChR, 5 subunits (α_2, β, γ, σ) form a cluster around a central cation-selective pore. Two ACh-binding sites are in the extracellular part of the receptor between α and the other subunits. When ACh binds to the sites, the receptor conformation changes: α subunits swing out, and the channel opens. Charged amino acids lining the pore select ions that can pass into the cell.

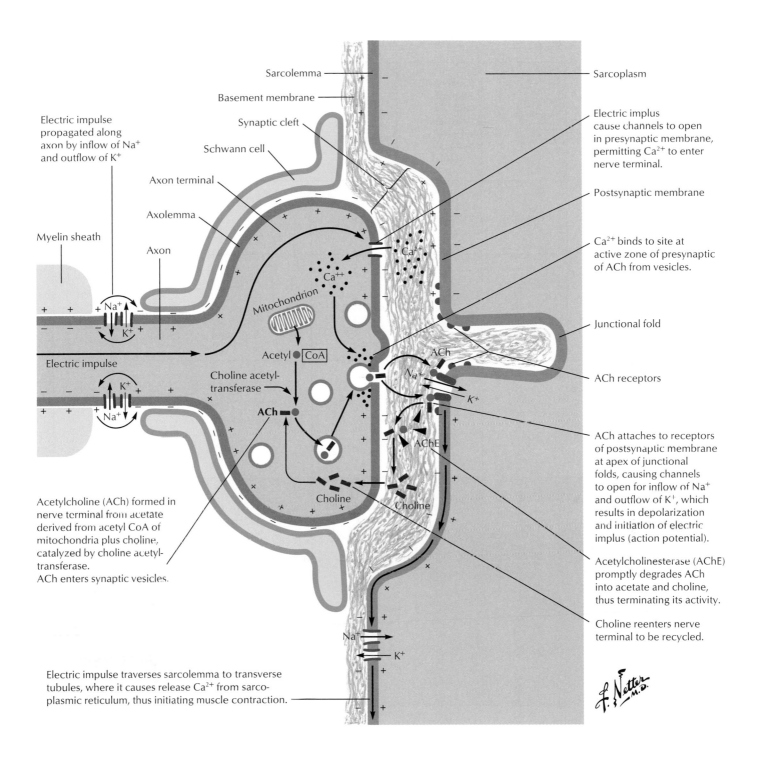

Sarcolemma

Basement membrane

Synaptic cleft

Schwann cell

Axon terminal

Axolemma

Axon

Myelin sheath

Electric impulse propagated along axon by inflow of Na⁺ and outflow of K⁺

Electric impulse

Mitochondrion

Acetyl CoA

Choline acetyl-transferase

ACh

Choline

Ca⁺⁺

Na⁺

K⁺

Na⁺

K⁺

ACh

AChE

Choline

Na⁺

K⁺

Sarcoplasm

Electric implus cause channels to open in presynaptic membrane, permitting Ca²⁺ to enter nerve terminal.

Postsynaptic membrane

Ca²⁺ binds to site at active zone of presynaptic of ACh from vesicles.

Junctional fold

ACh receptors

ACh attaches to receptors of postsynaptic membrane at apex of junctional folds, causing channels to open for inflow of Na⁺ and outflow of K⁺, which results in depolarization and initiation of electric implus (action potential).

Acetylcholinesterase (AChE) promptly degrades ACh into acetate and choline, thus terminating its activity.

Choline reenters nerve terminal to be recycled.

Acetylcholine (ACh) formed in nerve terminal from acetate derived from acetyl CoA of mitochondria plus choline, catalyzed by choline acetyl-transferase.
ACh enters synaptic vesicles.

Electric impulse traverses sarcolemma to transverse tubules, where it causes release Ca²⁺ from sarco-plasmic reticulum, thus initiating muscle contraction.

FIGURE 2-6 PHYSIOLOGY OF THE NEUROMUSCULAR JUNCTION

As Loewi demonstrated in the 1920s, a gap (synapse) exists between an ANS neuron's axon terminal and the adjacent neuron or effector cell. Information is transmitted across this gap via chemical transmitters (neurotransmission). Neurotransmitters are commonly stored in presynaptic vesicles; arrival of an action potential stimulates a Ca²⁺-dependent neurotransmitter release into the synapse. The neurotransmitter crosses the gap and binds to highly selective receptor molecules on the postsynaptic cell, thereby modifying the activity of the postsynaptic cell. Neurotransmission provides fidelity of signal transmission. ANS neurotransmitters are simple organic molecules, and exogenous chemicals (drugs) can modify (mimic or antagonize) the action of the endogenous ANS neurotransmitters.

Drug	Effect on Supply of ACh in Terminal	Effect on Amount of ACh Released in Terminal by Action Potential	Effect of Amplitude on Endplate Potential	Effect of Muscle Response to Application of ACh	Direct Effect on Muscle Membrane Resting Potential	Clinical Effect
Choline uptake inhibitors Hemicholinium Triethylcholine	Decreased	Decreased (smaller quanta)	Decreased	—	—	Paresis
ACh release blockers Botulinum toxin Low Ca^{2+} or high Mg^{2+} concentration	—	Decreased (fewer quanta)	Decreased	—	—	Paralysis (low Ca^{2+} concentration may also produce tetany by direct action on nerves)
ACh (nicotinic) antagonists D-Tubocurarine Gallamine triethiodide Dihydro-β-erythroidine	—	—	Decreased	Decreased	Depolarized (in high dosage)	Paralysis
Cholinomimetics Nicotine Carbamylcholine Succinylcholine	—	—	Decreased (by desensitization)	Decreased (by desensitization)	Strongly depolarized	Paralysis
Cholinesterase inhibitors Physostigmine Neostigmine Edrophonium Organophosphorous compounds (nerve gases)	— —	— —	Increased; prolonged	Increased; prolonged	Depolarized slightly in high doses No change	Muscle power and duration of contraction increased Convulsions

FIGURE 2-7 PHARMACOLOGY OF THE NEUROMUSCULAR JUNCTION

Pharmacologic agents can induce effects at the neuromuscular junction by altering steps involved in ACh synthesis, storage, release, receptor binding, and elimination from the synapse. They can also have direct actions on skeletal muscle. For example, inhibitors of choline uptake limit ACh synthesis and depress neuromuscular functioning (eg, paresis). Inhibitors of ACh release, such as botulinum toxin (food poisoning) and nAChR antagonists, have the same effect. With sufficient suppression of ACh, complete paralysis results. Neuromuscular stimulation is produced by substances that enhance ACh action or mimic its action at cholinergic receptor sites (cholinomimetics).

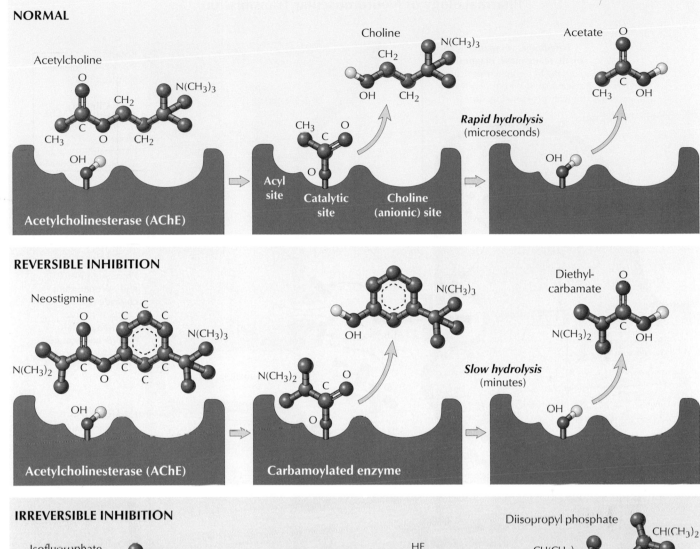

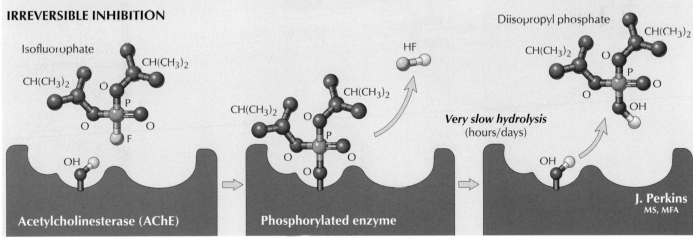

FIGURE 2-8 MECHANISM OF ACTION OF ACETYLCHOLINESTERASE INHIBITORS

Enhancement of endogenous ACh action results from increasing ACh release or inhibiting degradation of ACh by AChE. ACh binds to active subsites (choline, catalytic, and acyl) on AChE, choline is released by hydrolysis, acetylated enzyme is formed and rapidly hydrolyzed, and active enzyme is reformed by hydrolysis. Only nAChR agonists or antagonists selectively modify ACh action at the skeletal neuromuscular junction.

Neostigmine and other reversible inhibitors bind to the active site and form a carbamoylated enzyme that is hydrolyzed slowly by AChE; irreversible inhibitors such as organophosphates (eg, isofluorphate) form a stable, phosphorylated enzyme that is very slowly hydrolyzed. Effects of AChE inhibition persist until new enzyme is synthesized.

Pharmacology of Neuromuscular Transmission

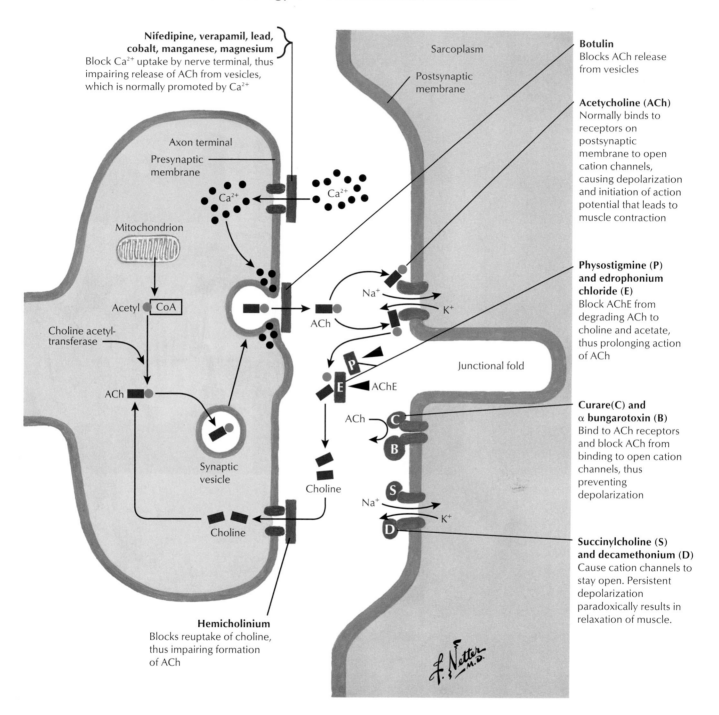

Nifedipine, verapamil, lead, cobalt, manganese, magnesium
Block Ca²⁺ uptake by nerve terminal, thus impairing release of ACh from vesicles, which is normally promoted by Ca²⁺

Botulin
Blocks ACh release from vesicles

Acetycholine (ACh)
Normally binds to receptors on postsynaptic membrane to open cation channels, causing depolarization and initiation of action potential that leads to muscle contraction

Physostigmine (P) and edrophonium chloride (E)
Block AChE from degrading ACh to choline and acetate, thus prolonging action of ACh

Curare(C) and α bungarotoxin (B)
Bind to ACh receptors and block ACh from binding to open cation channels, thus preventing depolarization

Succinylcholine (S) and decamethonium (D)
Cause cation channels to stay open. Persistent depolarization paradoxically results in relaxation of muscle.

Hemicholinium
Blocks reuptake of choline, thus impairing formation of ACh

FIGURE 2-9 NEUROMUSCULAR BLOCKING AGENTS: NONDEPOLARIZING AND DEPOLARIZING

Muscle relaxants inhibit ACh transmission at the skeletal neuromuscular junction; categorization as nondepolarizing or depolarizing agents depends on mechanism of action. The former (eg, pancuronium, atracurium, vecuronium, and now rarely used tubocurarine [curare] and gallamine) are reversible nAChR antagonists that bind to postsynaptic membrane nAChRs, block ACh access to nAChRs, and cause muscles to relax. Increasing nAChR occupation directly (via cholinomimetics) or indirectly (via AChE inhibitors) overcomes drug action. Adverse effects are

hypotension, tachycardia, and bronchospasm. Depolarizing agents are nAChR agonists and, like ACh, depolarize membranes (cause muscle twitching). These agents are not degraded by AChE; they stimulate nAChRs, muscle depolarization persists, and muscles relax. Cholinomimetics or AChE inhibitors do not affect these agents. Only succinylcholine is used currently. Unwanted effects are bradycardia, prolonged paralysis, and malignant hyperthermia.

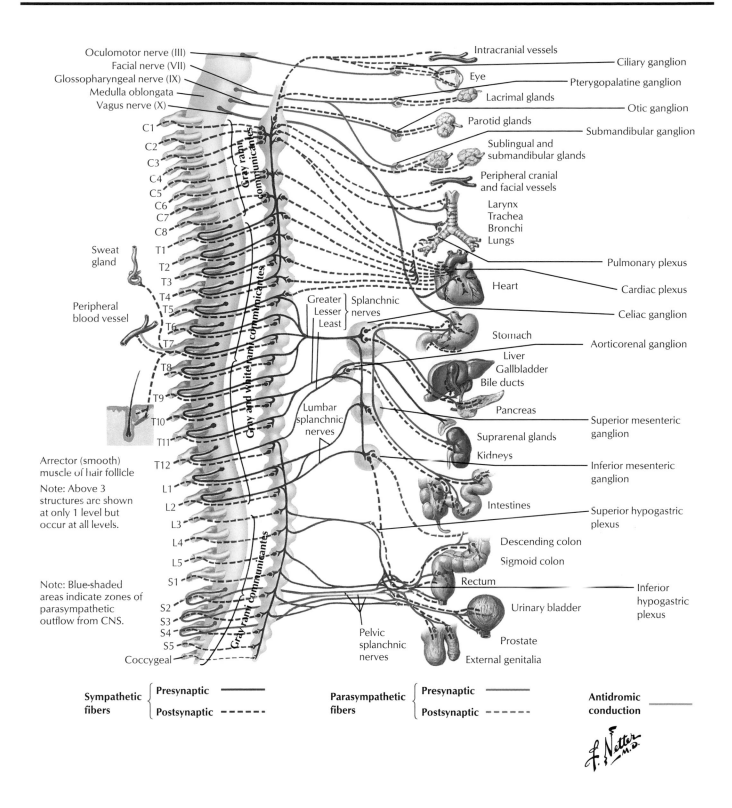

FIGURE 2-10 AUTONOMIC NERVOUS SYSTEM: SCHEMA

In contrast to SNS nerves, which innervate skeletal muscles, ANS nerves distribute to smooth muscle, cardiac muscle, and glands. The somatic division mainly controls the stability and voluntary movement of the body; the ANS primarily controls more autonomous internal body functions. The ANS consists of efferent (from CNS to periphery) and afferent (from periphery to CNS) components and is subclassified on the basis of anatomy and physiology into sympathetic and parasympathetic divisions. Sympathetic or parasympathetic fibers innervate almost all organs. The knowledge that most organs are innervated by both sympathetic and parasympathetic ANS neurons aids in understanding selective actions and adverse effects of drugs. Sympathetic neurons mediate fight or flight responses (pupil dilation, bronchodilation, increased heart rate). Parasympathetic neurons usually mediate the opposite response and control daily functions such as peristalsis, saliva flow, and near vision accommodation.

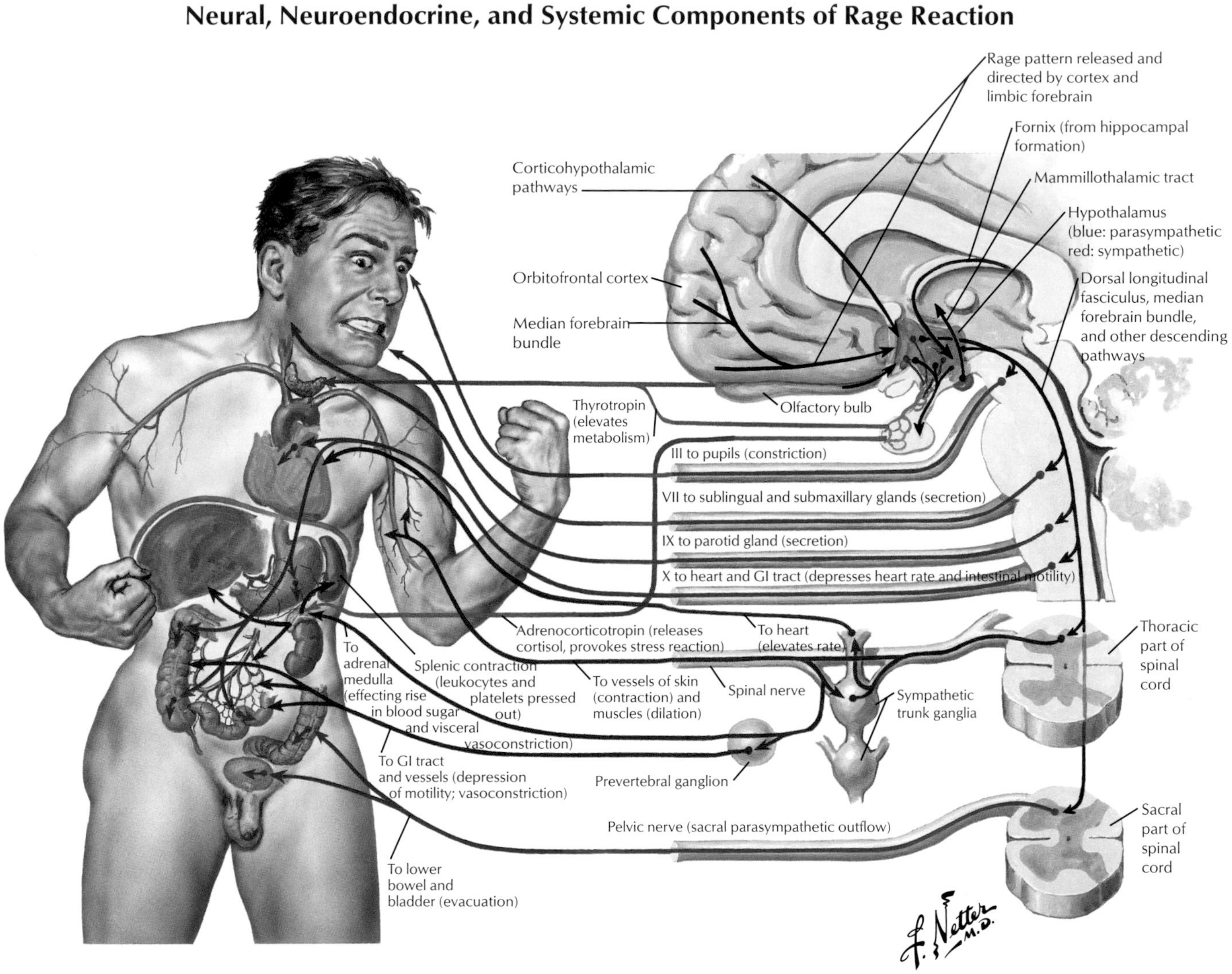

Neural, Neuroendocrine, and Systemic Components of Rage Reaction

Rage pattern released and directed by cortex and limbic forebrain

Fornix (from hippocampal formation)

Mammillothalamic tract

Hypothalamus (blue: parasympathetic red: sympathetic)

Dorsal longitudinal fasciculus, median forebrain bundle, and other descending pathways

Corticohypothalamic pathways

Orbitofrontal cortex

Median forebrain bundle

Olfactory bulb

Thyrotropin (elevates metabolism)

III to pupils (constriction)

VII to sublingual and submaxillary glands (secretion)

IX to parotid gland (secretion)

X to heart and GI tract (depresses heart rate and intestinal motility)

Adrenocorticotropin (releases cortisol, provokes stress reaction)

To heart (elevates rate)

Thoracic part of spinal cord

To adrenal medulla (effecting rise in blood sugar and visceral vasoconstriction)

Splenic contraction (leukocytes and platelets pressed out)

To vessels of skin (contraction) and muscles (dilation)

Spinal nerve

Sympathetic trunk ganglia

To GI tract and vessels (depression of motility; vasoconstriction)

Prevertebral ganglion

Pelvic nerve (sacral parasympathetic outflow)

Sacral part of spinal cord

To lower bowel and bladder (evacuation)

FIGURE 2-11 SYMPATHETIC FIGHT OR FLIGHT RESPONSE

A result of activating the sympathetic ANS has been viewed as an evolutionary adaptation for a fight or flight response to a real or perceived threat to the organism. The response is rapid and widespread and includes pupil dilation (mydriasis) for better vision, and increased heart rate, bronchodilation, and vasodilation of blood vessels supplying skeletal muscles for increased energy supply. Energy from fat stores is mobilized, and blood glucose levels increase. Simultaneously, parasympathetic activity is depressed, and functions not needed immediately for survival are dampened. The opposite reactions occur during times of rest. The release of the hormone epinephrine (also called *adrenaline*) from the adrenal (suprarenal) gland is part of the fight or flight response. Epinephrine in the bloodstream activates receptors located throughout the body. The closely related neurotransmitter norepinephrine (noradrenaline) elicits nearly the same effects but does so locally. Activation of these responses by a real threat elicits a beneficial, magnified, short-term response; prolonged activation (stress) has harmful effects. Most available sympathomimetics—ie, drugs or other chemicals that mimic fight or flight responses—target a subset of fight or flight responses. For example, phenylephrine, a common component of decongestants, produces vasodilation of nasal blood vessels but has relatively little effect on the heart. Some substances are sympathomimetic because they amplify epinephrine or norepinephrine release. Examples include ephedrine (the active ingredient of ephedra, or Ma-huang, which is banned in the United States because of adverse effects), amphetamines (synthesized in the 1930s as an alternative to ephedra), and tyramine (present in fermented foods). Interconnections among organs through ANS neurons explain some adverse effects of drugs on organs other than the intended targets.

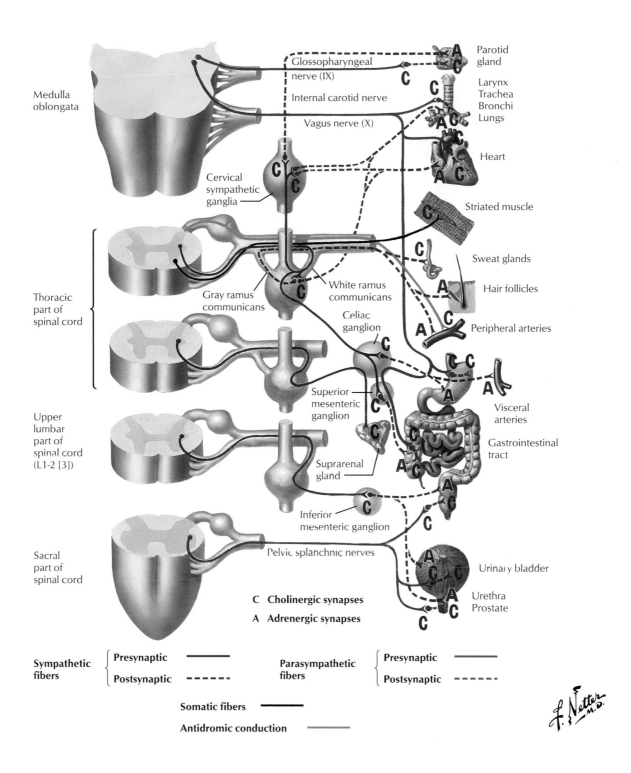

Medulla
oblongata

Glossopharyngeal
nerve (IX)

Internal carotid nerve

Vagus nerve (X)

Cervical
sympathetic
ganglia

Parotid
gland

Larynx
Trachea
Bronchi
Lungs

Heart

Striated muscle

Sweat glands

Hair follicles

Peripheral arteries

Visceral
arteries

Gastrointestinal
tract

Urinary bladder

Urethra
Prostate

Thoracic
part of
spinal cord

Gray ramus
communicans

White ramus
communicans

Celiac
ganglion

Superior
mesenteric
ganglion

Suprarenal
gland

Upper
lumbar
part of
spinal cord
(L1-2 [3])

Inferior
mesenteric ganglion

Sacral
part of
spinal cord

Pelvic splanchnic nerves

C Cholinergic synapses

A Adrenergic synapses

Sympathetic fibers { Presynaptic ——— Postsynaptic - - - - }

Parasympathetic fibers { Presynaptic ——— Postsynaptic - - - - }

Somatic fibers ———

Antidromic conduction ———

F. Netter M.D.

FIGURE 2-12 CHOLINERGIC AND ADRENERGIC SYNAPSES

Drugs affect organs innervated by the ANS and SNS by mimicking or antagonizing neurotransmitter action. Knowing the identity and synaptic distribution of neurotransmitters can offer insight into the therapeutic action or adverse effects of a drug, which can often be predicted. ACh is the neurotransmitter at neuromuscular junctions, preganglionic synapses (sympathetic and parasympathetic), and postganglionic parasympathetic synapses. Norepinephrine, or noradrenaline, is the neurotransmitter at most postganglionic sympathetic synapses. Drugs that mimic or potentiate norepinephrine produce sympathetic effects that resemble fight or flight responses such as increased heart rate. Drugs that mimic or potentiate ACh produce parasympathetic effects such as decreased heart rate. Nonadrenergic-noncholinergic (NANC) neurotransmitters in the ANS also exist, including peptides, nitric oxide, and serotonin.

PRIMARY CLOSED-ANGLE GLAUCOMA

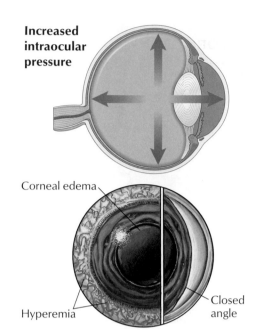

Normal

Outflow

Inflow

Equilibrium between aqueous production and drainage

Pupillary block

Outflow

Inflow

Pupil block

Secondary block at angle

Primary angle closure may result from pupillary block with bulging iris or from occlusion at periphery of iris. Both result in an imbalance between aqueous production and drainage.

Iris plateau

Outflow

Inflow

Primary block at angle

Increased intraocular pressure

Corneal edema

Hyperemia

Closed angle

Acute angle closure results in marked increase in intraocular pressure with conjunctival hyperemia, corneal edema, and fixed middilated pupil.

NERVE PATHWAYS AND DRUG TREATMENT

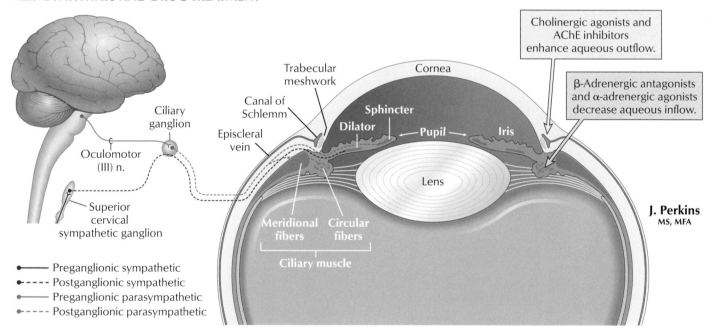

Ciliary ganglion

Oculomotor (III) n.

Superior cervical sympathetic ganglion

Trabecular meshwork

Canal of Schlemm

Episcleral vein

Cornea

Sphincter

Dilator

Pupil

Iris

Lens

Meridional fibers

Circular fibers

Ciliary muscle

Cholinergic agonists and AChE inhibitors enhance aqueous outflow.

β-Adrenergic antagonists and α-adrenergic agonists decrease aqueous inflow.

J. Perkins
MS, MFA

━━ Preganglionic sympathetic
┄┄ Postganglionic sympathetic
━━ Preganglionic parasympathetic
┄┄ Postganglionic parasympathetic

FIGURE 2-13 EXAMPLE OF CHOLINERGIC AND ADRENERGIC DRUG TREATMENT: GLAUCOMA

Certain types of glaucoma (excess intraocular pressure) can be treated with drugs that modify the activity of sympathetic or parasympathetic nerves in the eye. Parasympathetic activity opens pores in the trabecular meshwork and enhances outflow of aqueous humor into the canal of Schlemm. Sympathetic activity on the ciliary epithelium increases the secretion of aqueous humor. Cholinergic agonists such as pilocarpine, which enhance aqueous humor outflow, and adrenergic antagonists such as timolol, which decrease aqueous humor inflow, ameliorate symptoms of glaucoma. Adrenergic agonists such as apraclonidine that reduce aqueous humor production and irreversible AChE inhibitors such as echothiophate, an organophosphate, are also used.

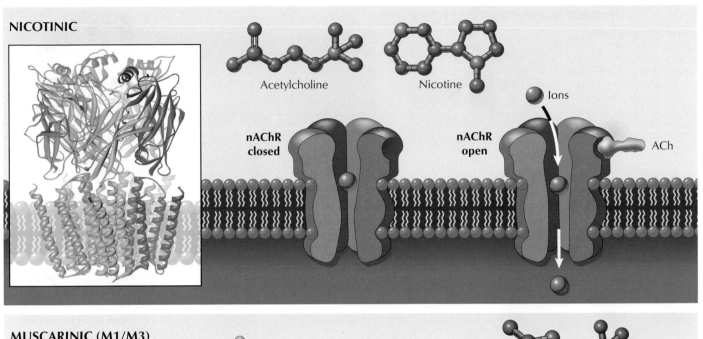

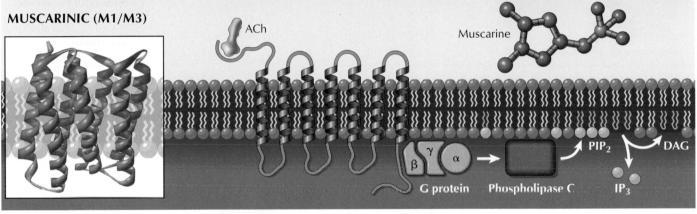

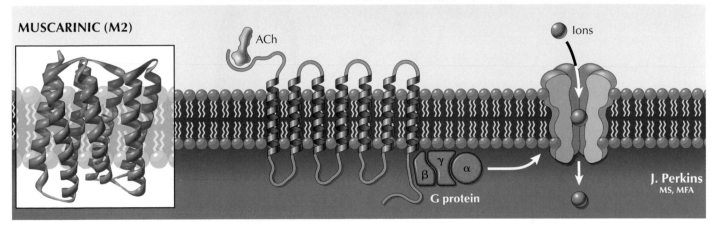

FIGURE 2-14 CHOLINERGIC RECEPTORS

Cholinergic receptors are classified into 2 major types: nicotinic (nAChR) and muscarinic (mAChR), each having several subtypes. nAChRs are ligand-gated ion channels, and mAChRs are GPCRs. The receptors were named on the basis of selective actions of nicotine and muscarine (from the mushroom *Amanita muscaria*).

Muscarinic agonists mimic the actions of ACh at the postganglionic mAChRs in synapses of the parasympathetic subdivision of the ANS; antagonists inhibit these actions. Nicotinic agonists mimic the actions of ACh at nAChRs at skeletal neuromuscular junctions (SNS; detailed earlier); antagonists inhibit these actions.

The pupils in poisoning

Miosis (pinhole pupils)
Seen in poisoning by morphine and morphine derivatives, some types of mushrooms, cholinesterase inhibitors, parasympathomimetics, nicotine, chloral hydrate, sympatholytics, and some other compounds

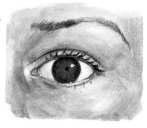

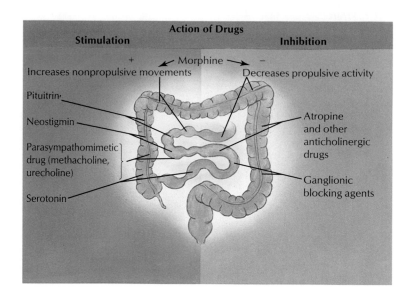

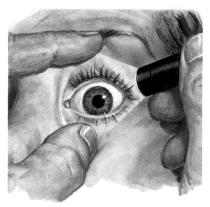

Mydriasis (pupils dilated and not reactive)
Seen in poisoning by barbiturates, carbon monoxide, methyl and other alcohols, oxalic acid, cocaine, belladonna derivatives, camphor, cyanide, sympathomimetics, parasympatholytics, and a number of other compounds

Motor unit (3 units illustrated)

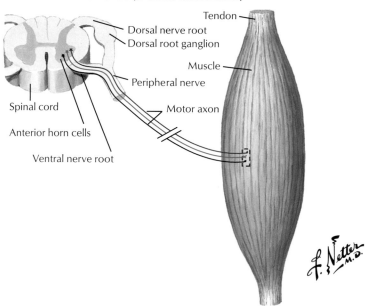

FIGURE 2-15 CHOLINERGIC DRUGS

Acetylcholine is rapidly broken down by cholinesterases in the blood and AChE in the synaptic cleft. AChE inhibitors (drugs such as physostigmine or poisons) enhance actions of ACh by decreasing its enzymatic breakdown and prolonging its synaptic residency time. Muscarinic agonists such as pilocarpine amplify parasympathetic actions and, for example, decrease pupil diameter (miosis), decrease heart rate, increase gastrointestinal motility and secretion, contract bronchiolar and urogenital smooth

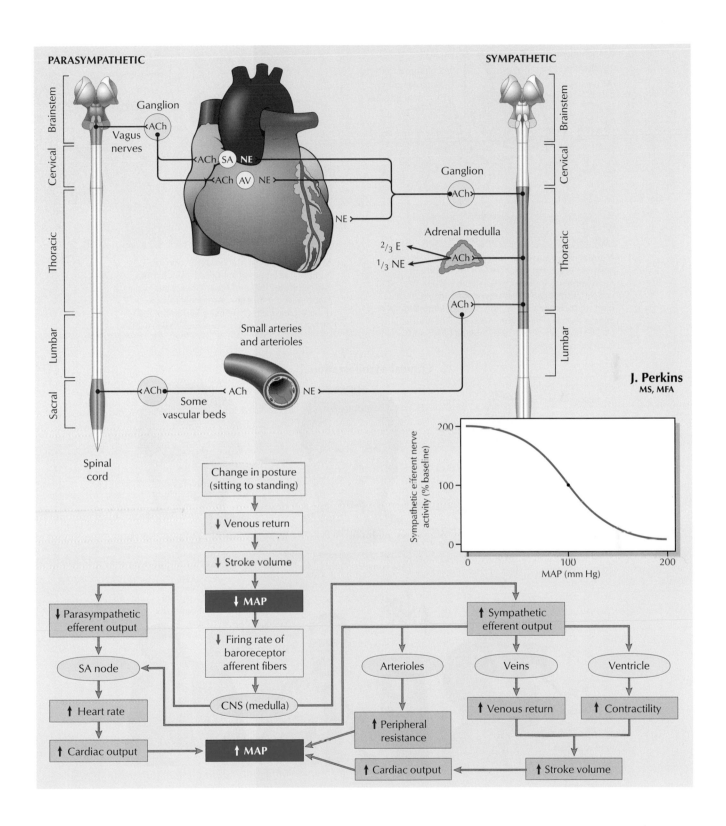

FIGURE 2-15 CHOLINERGIC DRUGS (continued)

muscles, and stimulate glandular secretions. Muscarinic antagonists such as atropine (derived from *Atropa belladonna*) and scopolamine have the opposite effects. Nicotinic agonists such as

succinylcholine stimulate, and nicotinic antagonists such as pancuronium inhibit, skeletal muscle contraction.

Myasthenia Gravis

Pathophysiologic Concepts

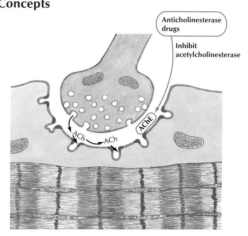

Nerve axon
Mitochondria
Synaptic vesicles
ACh receptors
Synaptic cleft
Sarcolemmal folds
Sarcolemma
Sarcoplasm
Myofibrils

Anticholinesterase drugs

Inhibit acetylcholinesterase

Normal neuromuscular junction: Synaptic vesicles containing acetylcholine (ACh) form in nerve terminal. In response to nerve impulse, vesicles discharge ACh into synaptic cleft. ACh binds to receptor sites on muscle sarcolemma to initiate muscle contraction. Acetylcholinesterase (AChE) hydrolyzes ACh, thus limiting effect and duration of its action.

Myasthenia gravis: Marked reduction in number and length of subneural sarcolemmal folds indicates that underlying defect lies in neuromuscular junction. Anticholinesterase drugs increase effectiveness and duration of ACh action by slowing its destruction by AChE.

Clinical Manifestations

Regional distribution of muscle weakness

95%
60%
30%
10%

Ptosis and weakness of smile are common early signs.

Improvement after edrophonium chloride

Patient with chin on chest cannot resist when physician pushes head back.

7:15

In early stages, patient may feel fine in the morning but develops diplopia and speech slurs later in the day.

FIGURE 2-16 EXAMPLE OF CHOLINERGIC DRUG TREATMENT: MYASTHENIA GRAVIS

Myasthenia gravis is characterized by progressive weakening of skeletal muscles. It preferentially affects women and is lethal if untreated. Symptoms are caused by an autoimmune-induced decrease (70-90%) in the number of nAChRs at the neuromuscular junction. In early stages of the disease, AChE inhibitors such as edrophonium produce a rapid recovery of function, which is diagnostic, and can be continued for therapy. Adverse effects of AChE inhibitors are those of excess ACh, known as DUMBELS: diarrhea, urination, miosis, bronchoconstriction, excitation (skeletal muscles and CNS), lacrimation, and salivation and sweating.

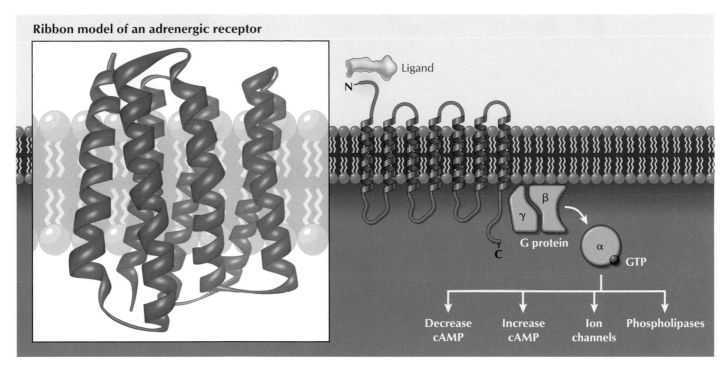

Ribbon model of an adrenergic receptor

Ligand

N

β

γ

G protein

α

GTP

C

Decrease cAMP | Increase cAMP | Ion channels | Phospholipases

Primary Tissue Locations of Adrenergic Receptor Subtypes

α_1: Postjunctional smooth muscle (contraction)

α_2: Presynaptic neurons, postsynaptic tissues (ocular, adipose, intestinal, hepatic, renal, endocrine), and blood platelets

β_1: Heart (stimulation)

β_2: Bronchial, uterine, and vascular smooth muscle (relaxation)

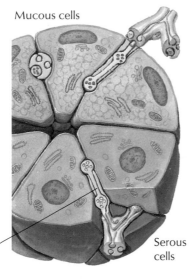

Smooth muscle cells

Mucous cells

Nerve axons

Serous cells

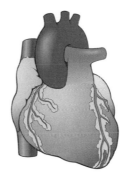

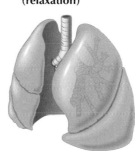

β_3: Causes lipolysis in adipose tissue

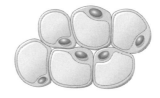

J. Netter
M.D.

J. Perkins
MS, MFA

FIGURE 2-17 ADRENERGIC RECEPTORS

Adrenergic receptors (adrenoceptors) are classified into 2 major types, α and β, each with multiple subtypes that differ in terms of their mechanism of signal transduction (eg, increased or decreased cAMP). All adrenoceptors are 7-transmembrane GPCRs: they cross the cell membrane 7 times (with the amino terminus of the receptor on the extracellular side) and are coupled to a guanine nucleotide-binding protein (G protein). When an agonist binds to a GPCR, it enhances the association of a

receptor with a G protein, which then stimulates (eg, G_s) or inhibits (e.g., G_i) a step in the second-messenger pathway, such as adenylyl cyclase, phospholipase C, or an ion channel. The same adrenergic agonist (eg, epinephrine, norepinephrine, or drug) can produce various effects depending on the G protein coupling in a cell. Effects of receptor activation include muscle contraction (α_1, α_2) and relaxation (α_1, α_2, β_2), increased heart rate and force (β_1), and lipolysis and thermogenesis (β_3).

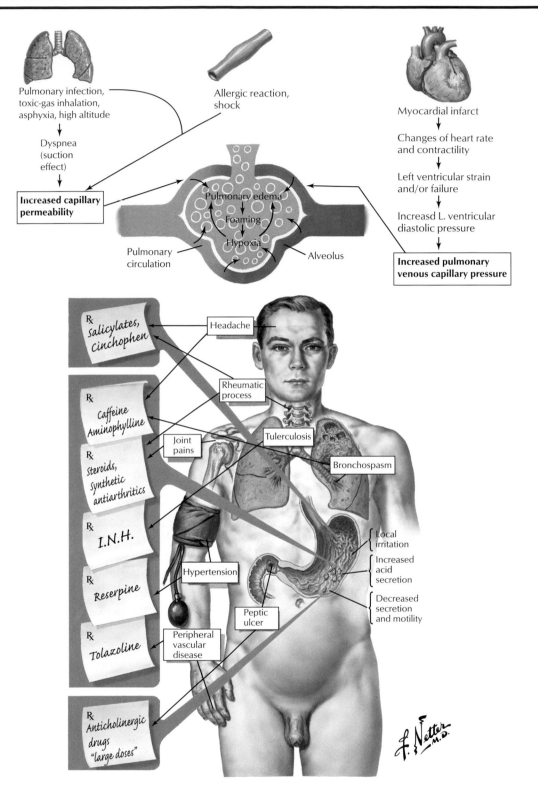

FIGURE 2-18 ADRENERGIC DRUGS

α_1-Adrenoceptor agonists (eg, phenylephrine) elicit vasoconstriction and mydriasis and are used as nasal decongestants and in eye examinations. α_2-Adrenoceptor agonists (eg, clonidine) bind to presynaptic receptors and activate a negative feedback loop that inhibits further release of norepinephrine; they serve as antihypertensive agents. α_1-Adrenoceptor antagonists (eg, doxazosin) are also used to treat hypertension. β_1-Adrenoceptor agonists (eg, dobutamine) augment sympathetic innervation of the heart and

are used as cardiac stimulants. β_1-Adrenoceptor antagonists (eg, atenolol) attenuate sympathetic innervation of the heart and function as antihypertensive agents. β_2-Adrenoceptor agonists (eg, albuterol) stimulate bronchodilation and are used to treat asthma. Certain drugs (eg, isoproterenol and labetalol) affect multiple receptor types. Adverse effects include vasoconstriction, vasodilation, and tachycardia.

	Sympathetic		Parasympathetic
	α-Adrenergic Receptors	β-Adrenergic Receptors	Muscarinic Cholinergic Receptors
Natural agonists			
Norepinephrine (released by sympathetic nerve endings)	+++	+	−
Epinephrine (released by adrenal medulla)	+	+++	−
Acetylcholine (released by parasympathetic nerve endings)	−	−	+++
Other (synthetic) agonists	Methoxamine Phenylephrine Oxymetazoline	Isoproterenol Methoxyphenamine Dobutamine Albuterol Terbutaline	Muscarine Pilocarpine Carbachol
Direct effects of agonists on:			
Heart	−	Increased rate and force of contraction	Decreased rate and force of contraction
Blood vessels	Vasoconstriction	Vasodilatation	Vasodilatation
Intestines	Decreased motility	Decreased motility	Increased motility
Antagonists (blocking agents)	Phentolamine Phenoxybenzamine Doxazosin Prazosin Terazosin Ergot alkaloids	Propranolol Pindolol Alprenolol Nadolol Timolol	Atropine Scopolamine 3-Quinuclidinyl benzylate
Agents that block enzymatic degradation of transmitter	Monoamine oxidase (MAO) inhibitors Catechol-O-methyltransferase (CCMT) inhibitors		Anticholinesterase

FIGURE 2-19 DRUGS THAT ACT ON THE AUTONOMIC NERVOUS SYSTEM

Actions of drugs affecting the PNS can be organized on the basis of ANS anatomy and the neurotransmitter receptors that mediate physiologic responses to endogenous ACh and norepinephrine. Sympathetic effects can be produced by drugs that either enhance sympathetic tone (sympathomimetics such as adreno-ceptor agonists) or depress parasympathetic tone (cholinergic receptor antagonists). Parasympathetic effects can be produced by drugs that either enhance parasympathetic tone or depress sympathetic tone. Drugs enhancing neurotransmitter action by activating receptors are known as *direct acting*; drugs enhancing neurotransmitter action by some other means, eg, by inhibiting enzymes that degrade the neurotransmitter, are known as *indirect acting*.

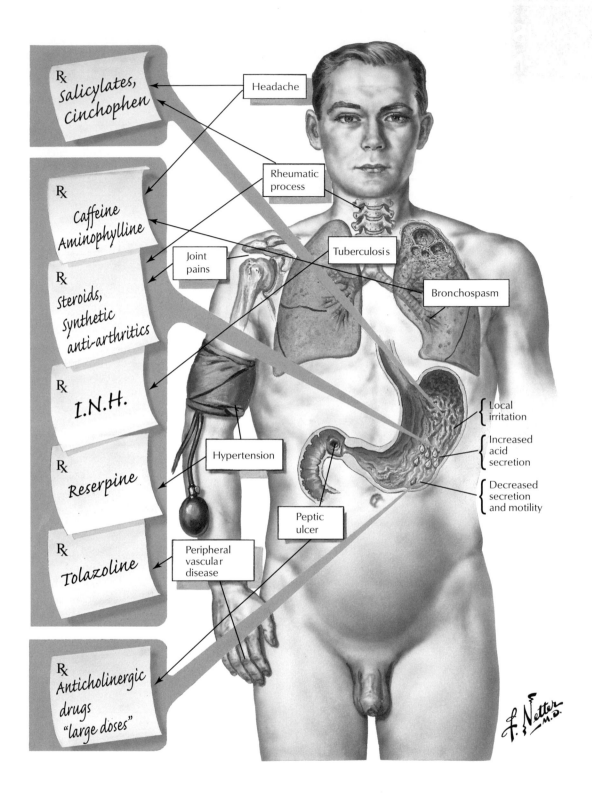

Rx Salicylates, Cinchophen

Rx Caffeine Aminophylline

Rx Steroids, Synthetic anti-arthritics

Rx I.N.H.

Rx Reserpine

Rx Tolazoline

Rx Anticholinergic drugs "large doses"

Headache

Rheumatic process

Joint pains

Tuberculosis

Bronchospasm

Local irritation

Increased acid secretion

Decreased secretion and motility

Hypertension

Peptic ulcer

Peripheral vascular disease

FIGURE 2-20 DRUG SIDE EFFECTS

The organization of the ANS permits an understanding of effects that drugs can have on organs other than those that are the intended targets of drug action. For example, drugs that are designed to reduce heart rate by activating mAChRs on the heart activate mAChRs throughout the ANS unless subtypes of mAChR were identified on the heart and the drug selectively activates that subtype. The therapeutic and adverse effects of a drug are sometimes a function of intended use. The same drug (eg, an mAChR antagonist) in one clinical setting may be given to treat diarrhea and cause sensitivity to light (mydriasis) as an adverse effect; in another clinical setting, the drug may be used therapeutically for an eye examination, but it could cause constipation as an adverse effect. The drug-induced effects are the same in both cases. Also, drugs that have different therapeutic targets can share a similar side effect.

CHAPTER 3

DRUGS USED IN DISORDERS OF THE CENTRAL NERVOUS SYSTEM AND TREATMENT OF PAIN

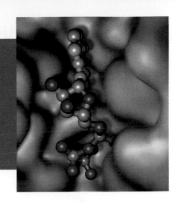

OVERVIEW

There is something special and inherently compelling about drugs that affect behavior or cognitive processes. However, in many ways the pharmacology of drugs that have effects (wanted or unwanted) on the CNS is similar to the pharmacology of drugs that have effects on peripheral organs. The properties of the CNS, like the properties of peripheral organs, are mediated by neurochemical transmitters acting at receptor sites. Hence, at the molecular level, the fundamental mechanisms of action of drugs affecting the CNS differ little from the mechanisms of action of drugs that act on the PNS.

Neurotransmitter pathways exist in the CNS (brain and spinal cord) just as they do in the PNS, although more CNS than PNS neurotransmitters have been identified, and amino acid transmitters and peptides play a more preeminent role in the CNS than they do in the PNS. As in the ANS, the CNS consists of opposing neurotransmitter systems. The major excitatory neurotransmitters are the amino acids glutamate (Glu) and aspartate (Asp); the major inhibitory neurotransmitters are GABA and glycine (Gly).

The etiology of CNS functional disorders is often difficult to determine. Psychosocial influences are important in many disorders, so they are best treated with a combination of pharmacotherapy and psychosocial intervention. Drug treatment of these disorders developed partly as the result of serendipity and, more recently, targeted drug discovery efforts. Many CNS disorders are imperfectly treated with current medications, and basic research findings continuously provide promising leads for new drugs.

More is also being learned about the disorders themselves. For example, it is now recognized that clinical depression and clinical anxiety are biochemically distinct from normally experienced feelings of sadness or apprehension. Schizophrenia is now known to consist of what are known as positive and negative symptoms. Pain is seen as multifaceted. Neuronal atrophy is implicated in conditions in which it was not previously suspected.

Drugs targeted to CNS disorders, like drugs used for conditions affecting the PNS but to a much larger extent, are subject to abuse—sometimes by patients but more often by nonpatients. Such abuse can adversely affect the availability of these drugs (such as opioids for relief of severe pain) to patients in need.

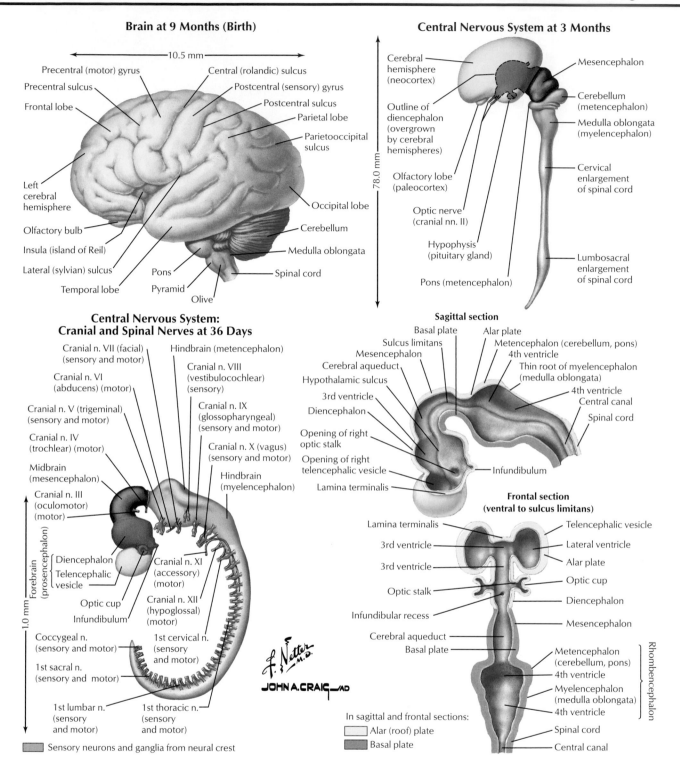

Brain at 9 Months (Birth)

— 10.5 mm —

Precentral (motor) gyrus
Precentral sulcus
Frontal lobe
Left cerebral hemisphere
Olfactory bulb
Insula (island of Reil)
Lateral (sylvian) sulcus
Temporal lobe
Pyramid
Olive
Central (rolandic) sulcus
Postcentral (sensory) gyrus
Postcentral sulcus
Parietal lobe
Parietooccipital sulcus
Occipital lobe
Cerebellum
Medulla oblongata
Spinal cord
Pons

Central Nervous System at 3 Months

Cerebral hemisphere (neocortex)
Outline of diencephalon (overgrown by cerebral hemispheres)
Olfactory lobe (paleocortex)
Optic nerve (cranial nn. II)
Hypophysis (pituitary gland)
Pons (metencephalon)
Mesencephalon
Cerebellum (metencephalon)
Medulla oblongata (myelencephalon)
Cervical enlargement of spinal cord
Lumbosacral enlargement of spinal cord
78.0 mm

**Central Nervous System:
Cranial and Spinal Nerves at 36 Days**

Cranial n. VII (facial) (sensory and motor)
Cranial n. VI (abducens) (motor)
Cranial n. V (trigeminal) (sensory and motor)
Cranial n. IV (trochlear) (motor)
Midbrain (mesencephalon)
Cranial n. III (oculomotor) (motor)
Diencephalon
Telencephalic vesicle
Optic cup
Infundibulum
Coccygeal n. (sensory and motor)
1st sacral n. (sensory and motor)
1st lumbar n. (sensory and motor)
1st thoracic n. (sensory and motor)
Hindbrain (metencephalon)
Cranial n. VIII (vestibulocochlear) (sensory)
Cranial n. IX (glossopharyngeal) (sensory and motor)
Cranial n. X (vagus) (sensory and motor)
Hindbrain (myelencephalon)
Cranial n. XI (accessory) (motor)
Cranial n. XII (hypoglossal) (motor)
1st cervical n. (sensory and motor)
Forebrain (prosencephalon)
1.0 mm

f. Netter
JOHN A. CRAIG

☐ Sensory neurons and ganglia from neural crest

Sagittal section

Basal plate
Sulcus limitans
Mesencephalon
Cerebral aqueduct
Hypothalamic sulcus
3rd ventricle
Diencephalon
Opening of right optic stalk
Opening of right telencephalic vesicle
Lamina terminalis
Alar plate
Metencephalon (cerebellum, pons)
4th ventricle
Thin root of myelencephalon (medulla oblongata)
4th ventricle
Central canal
Spinal cord
Infundibulum

**Frontal section
(ventral to sulcus limitans)**

Lamina terminalis
3rd ventricle
3rd ventricle
Optic stalk
Infundibular recess
Cerebral aqueduct
Basal plate
Telencephalic vesicle
Lateral ventricle
Alar plate
Optic cup
Diencephalon
Mesencephalon
Metencephalon (cerebellum, pons)
4th ventricle
Myelencephalon (medulla oblongata)
4th ventricle
Spinal cord
Central canal
Rhombencephalon

In sagittal and frontal sections:
☐ Alar (roof) plate
■ Basal plate

FIGURE 3-1 DEVELOPMENT OF THE NERVOUS SYSTEM

The nervous system, derived from ectoderm, begins with embryonic disk formation. The neural tube develops bulges, bends, and crevices that form mature brain structures and ventricles. Three major bulges appear by approximately day 28 of gestation: the forebrain (prosencephalon), midbrain (mesencephalon), and hindbrain (rhombencephalon). At approximately day 36, the posterior (caudal) portion of the forebrain develops into the diencephalon; the anterior part develops into the telencephalon (eventually cerebral hemispheres). The cerebral cortex has a

specific outline by 6 months but develops sulci and gyri only in the 3 months before birth. The developing brain is affected, especially in the first trimester, to injuries caused by various chemicals such as drugs. Various neurotransmitters and growth hormones play critical roles in development of normal CNS function and restoration of function after injury. Efforts aimed to identify these substances and design drugs that will facilitate or enhance their actions are ongoing.

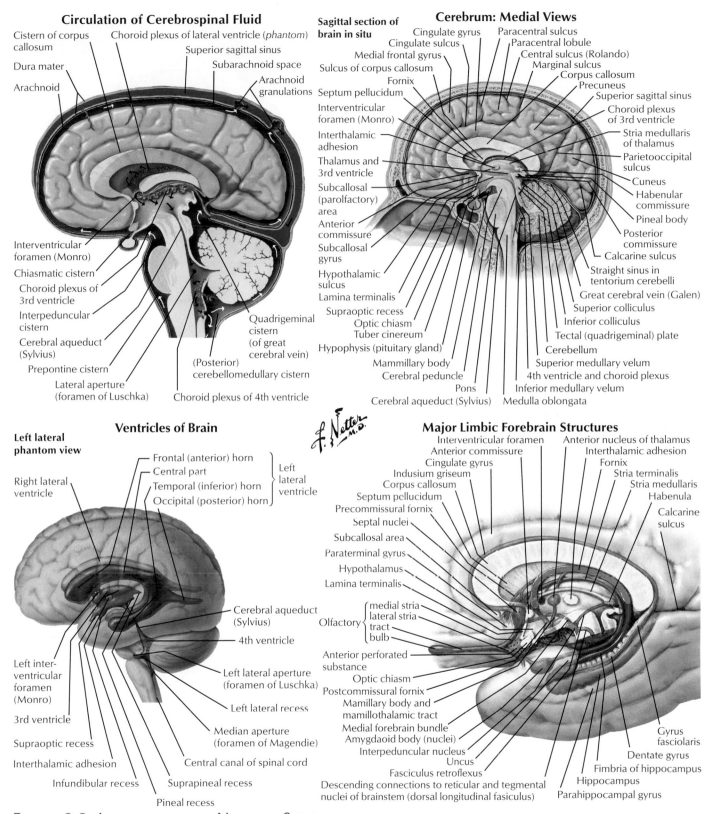

Circulation of Cerebrospinal Fluid

Cistern of corpus callosum
Dura mater
Arachnoid
Choroid plexus of lateral ventricle (*phantom*)
Superior sagittal sinus
Subarachnoid space
Arachnoid granulations
Interventricular foramen (Monro)
Chiasmatic cistern
Choroid plexus of 3rd ventricle
Interpeduncular cistern
Cerebral aqueduct (Sylvius)
Prepontine cistern
Lateral aperture (foramen of Luschka)
Quadrigeminal cistern (of great cerebral vein)
(Posterior) cerebellomedullary cistern
Choroid plexus of 4th ventricle

Cerebrum: Medial Views

Sagittal section of brain in situ

Cingulate gyrus
Cingulate sulcus
Medial frontal gyrus
Sulcus of corpus callosum
Fornix
Septum pellucidum
Interventricular foramen (Monro)
Interthalamic adhesion
Thalamus and 3rd ventricle
Subcallosal (parolfactory) area
Anterior commissure
Subcallosal gyrus
Hypothalamic sulcus
Lamina terminalis
Supraoptic recess
Optic chiasm
Tuber cinereum
Hypophysis (pituitary gland)
Mammillary body
Cerebral peduncle
Pons
Cerebral aqueduct (Sylvius)

Paracentral sulcus
Paracentral lobule
Central sulcus (Rolando)
Marginal sulcus
Corpus callosum
Precuneus
Superior sagittal sinus
Choroid plexus of 3rd ventricle
Stria medullaris of thalamus
Parietooccipital sulcus
Cuneus
Habenular commissure
Pineal body
Posterior commissure
Calcarine sulcus
Straight sinus in tentorium cerebelli
Great cerebral vein (Galen)
Superior colliculus
Inferior colliculus
Tectal (quadrigeminal) plate
Cerebellum
Superior medullary velum
4th ventricle and choroid plexus
Inferior medullary velum
Medulla oblongata

Ventricles of Brain

Left lateral phantom view

Right lateral ventricle
Frontal (anterior) horn
Central part
Temporal (inferior) horn
Occipital (posterior) horn
Left lateral ventricle
Cerebral aqueduct (Sylvius)
4th ventricle
Left interventricular foramen (Monro)
3rd ventricle
Supraoptic recess
Interthalamic adhesion
Infundibular recess
Left lateral aperture (foramen of Luschka)
Left lateral recess
Median aperture (foramen of Magendie)
Central canal of spinal cord
Suprapineal recess
Pineal recess

Major Limbic Forebrain Structures

Interventricular foramen
Anterior commissure
Cingulate gyrus
Indusium griseum
Corpus callosum
Septum pellucidum
Precommissural fornix
Septal nuclei
Subcallosal area
Paraterminal gyrus
Hypothalamus
Lamina terminalis
Olfactory {medial stria, lateral stria, tract, bulb}
Anterior perforated substance
Optic chiasm
Postcommissural fornix
Mamillary body and mamillothalamic tract
Medial forebrain bundle
Amygdaloid body (nuclei)
Interpeduncular nucleus
Uncus
Fasciculus retroflexus
Descending connections to reticular and tegmental nuclei of brainstem (dorsal longitudinal fasiculus)

Anterior nucleus of thalamus
Interthalamic adhesion
Fornix
Stria terminalis
Stria medullaris
Habenula
Calcarine sulcus
Gyrus fasciolaris
Dentate gyrus
Fimbria of hippocampus
Hippocampus
Parahippocampal gyrus

FIGURE 3-2 ANATOMY OF THE NERVOUS SYSTEM

Cerebral hemispheres are separated by a fissure and falx cerebri but are connected by commissures and other structures. The medial brain surface reveals complex, highly organized, structures of the hemispheres. The spinal cord and the brain (ie, the CNS) merge at the level of the brainstem. The major connection between the 2 hemispheres is the corpus callosum. Important sites of CNS drug effects are in the limbic system—communicating structures involved with smell, memory, and emotion. Four communicating cavities (ventricles) in the brain contain CSF produced by choroid plexuses. CSF circulation—from ventricles to central canal of spinal cord to drainage in venous sinuses—provides protection against trauma and a way to communicate chemically. Structures respond to circulating substances (eg, neurotransmitters, neuropeptides, hormones), as evidenced by introducing substances into CSF. The central action of a drug is studied by direct injection into ventricles.

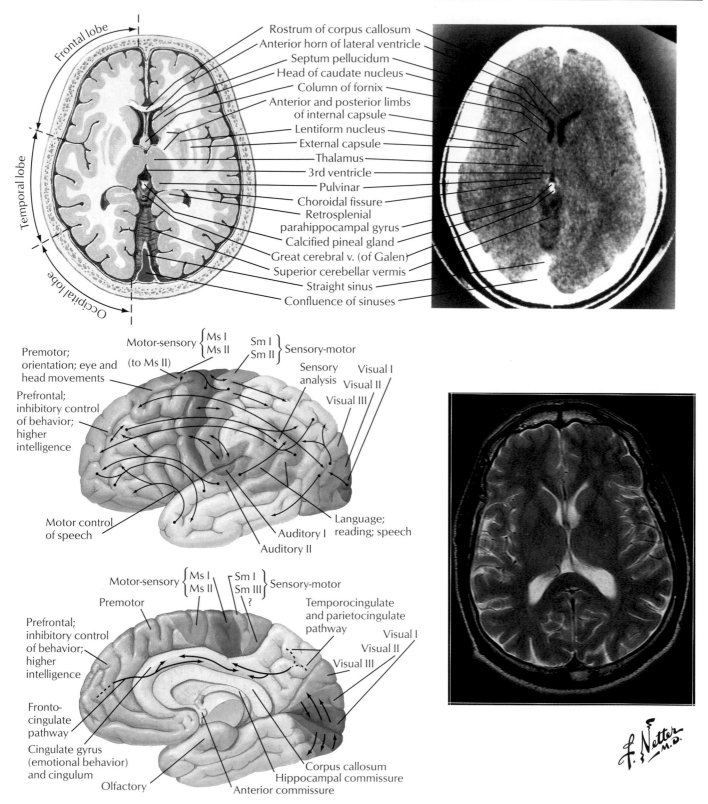

FIGURE 3-3 FUNCTIONAL CORRELATIONS AND VISUALIZATION OF BRAIN STRUCTURES

Although many, if not most, brain functions involve coordinated interaction among multiple brain structures and each portion of the brain is connected to almost every other portion, some functions are loosely associated with certain regions. For example, the somatosensory (motor-sensory and sensorimotor) regions of the frontal and parietal lobes and the premotor cortex of the frontal lobe are involved with initiation, activation, and performance of motor activity and reception of primary sensations.

Interconnections among parietal (integration and interpretation of sensory information), temporal (reception and interpretation of auditory information), and occipital (vision) lobes provide an organized, integrated system. The prefrontal cortex is involved with higher mental functions. Association pathways provide added organized communication via intrahemispheric and interhemispheric connections.

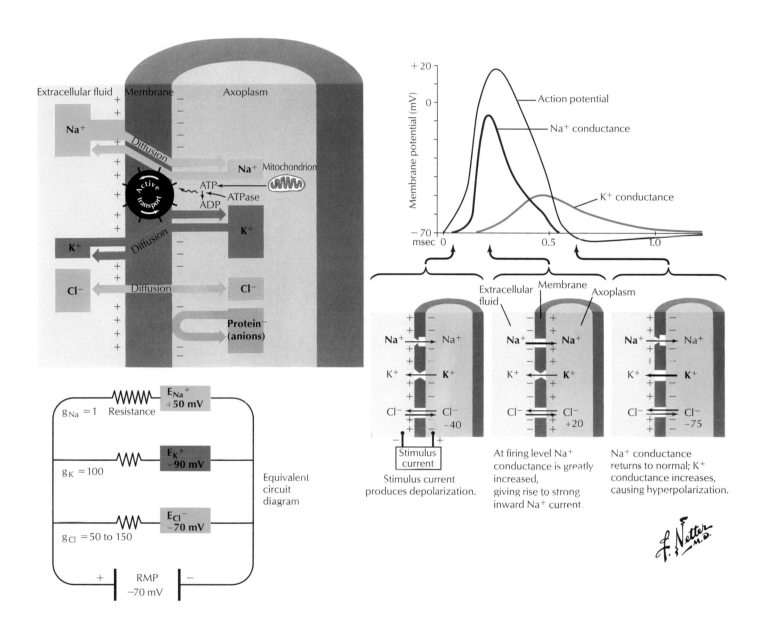

FIGURE 3-4 RESTING MEMBRANE AND ACTION POTENTIALS

The CNS comprises many types of neurons. In general, myelinated neurons conduct impulses more rapidly than do nonmyelinated neurons. The magnitude of the electrical potential difference across the neuronal membrane in the resting state, termed the *resting membrane potential*, depends on the relative intracellular and extracellular concentrations of Na^+ and Cl^- (higher on the outside) and K^+ (higher on the inside). The cytoplasmic electrical potential is more negative than the extracellular fluid by approximately -70 mV. The potential difference is partly maintained by

an Na^+/K^+ active transport exchange mechanism (ion pump). If the membrane is depolarized from its resting potential to approximately -40 mV (threshold potential), an action potential develops: the membrane potential continues to increase to approximately $+20$ to $+30$ mV and then returns to its resting level, in approximately one thousandth of a second. The frequency of a neuron's firing is one mechanism by which information is encoded within the CNS.

Temporal and Spatial Summation of Excitation and Inhibition

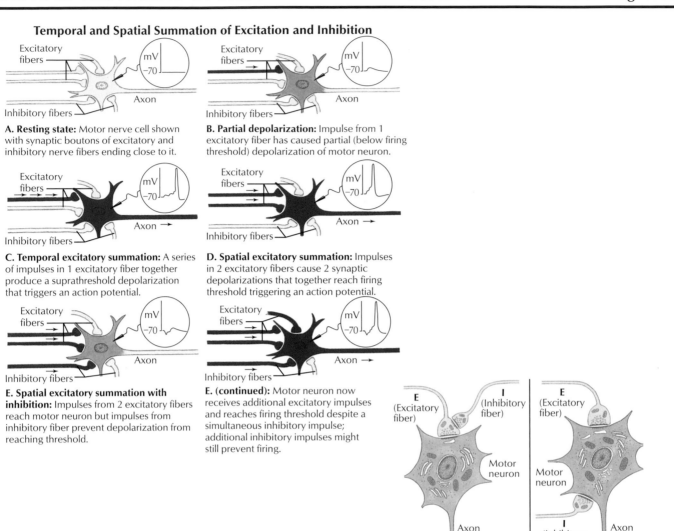

A. Resting state: Motor nerve cell shown with synaptic boutons of excitatory and inhibitory nerve fibers ending close to it.

B. Partial depolarization: Impulse from 1 excitatory fiber has caused partial (below firing threshold) depolarization of motor neuron.

C. Temporal excitatory summation: A series of impulses in 1 excitatory fiber together produce a suprathreshold depolarization that triggers an action potential.

D. Spatial excitatory summation: Impulses in 2 excitatory fibers cause 2 synaptic depolarizations that together reach firing threshold triggering an action potential.

E. Spatial excitatory summation with inhibition: Impulses from 2 excitatory fibers reach motor neuron but impulses from inhibitory fiber prevent depolarization from reaching threshold.

E. (continued): Motor neuron now receives additional excitatory impulses and reaches firing threshold despite a simultaneous inhibitory impulse; additional inhibitory impulses might still prevent firing.

A. Only E fires
90-mV spike in E terminal

EPSP in motor neuron

B. Only I fires
Long-lasting partial depolarization in E terminal

No response in motor neuron

C. I fires before E
Partial depolarization of E terminal reduces spike to 80 mV, thus releasing less transmitter substance

Smaller EPSP in motor neuron

A'. Only E fires
EPSP in motor neuron

B'. Only I fires
Motor neuron hyperpolarized

C'. I fires before E
Depolarization of motor neuron less than if only E fires

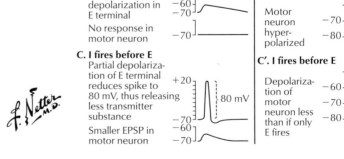

FIGURE 3-5 EXCITATORY AND INHIBITORY POSTSYNAPTIC POTENTIALS

Synaptic activation can either excite or inhibit a postsynaptic cell. During chemical synaptic transmission, neurotransmitters change postsynaptic membrane permeability to ions. For example, increased permeability to Na$^+$ produces excitation, and increased permeability to K$^+$ and Cl$^-$ produces inhibition. The former manifests as a depolarizing change in the transmembrane potential (EPSP), and the latter manifests as a hyperpolarizing change (IPSP). Each neuron receives input from many other neurons, so a membrane potential is a net influence of EPSPs and IPSPs. Excitatory neurotransmitters such as Glu and Asp produce EPSPs; inhibitory neurotransmitters such as GABA and Gly produce IPSPs. Drugs that enhance Glu or Asp action (or otherwise enhance EPSPs) (eg, low nicotine doses) have excitatory effects in the CNS; drugs that enhance GABA or Gly action (or otherwise enhance IPSPs) (eg, diazepam) have inhibitory CNS effects.

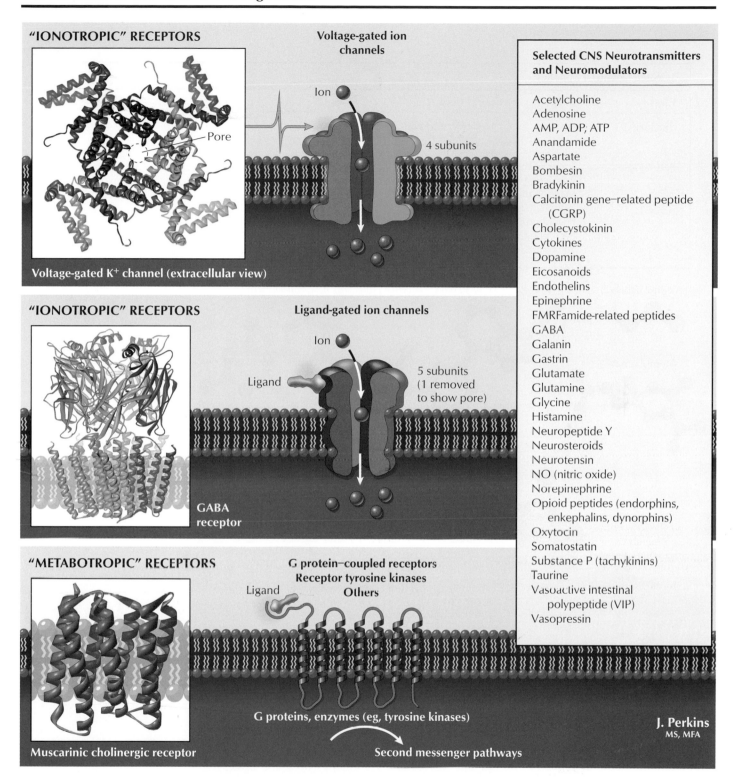

"IONOTROPIC" RECEPTORS

Voltage-gated ion channels

Ion

Pore

4 subunits

Voltage-gated K⁺ channel (extracellular view)

"IONOTROPIC" RECEPTORS

Ligand-gated ion channels

Ion

Ligand

5 subunits
(1 removed
to show pore)

GABA
receptor

"METABOTROPIC" RECEPTORS

G protein–coupled receptors
Receptor tyrosine kinases
Others

Ligand

G proteins, enzymes (eg, tyrosine kinases)

Second messenger pathways

Muscarinic cholinergic receptor

J. Perkins
MS, MFA

Selected CNS Neurotransmitters and Neuromodulators

Acetylcholine
Adenosine
AMP, ADP, ATP
Anandamide
Aspartate
Bombesin
Bradykinin
Calcitonin gene–related peptide
   (CGRP)
Cholecystokinin
Cytokines
Dopamine
Eicosanoids
Endothelins
Epinephrine
FMRFamide-related peptides
GABA
Galanin
Gastrin
Glutamate
Glutamine
Glycine
Histamine
Neuropeptide Y
Neurosteroids
Neurotensin
NO (nitric oxide)
Norepinephrine
Opioid peptides (endorphins,
   enkephalins, dynorphins)
Oxytocin
Somatostatin
Substance P (tachykinins)
Taurine
Vasoactive intestinal
   polypeptide (VIP)
Vasopressin

FIGURE 3-6 CENTRAL NERVOUS SYSTEM NEUROTRANSMITTERS, RECEPTORS, AND DRUG TARGETS

Many substances within the CNS modulate neurotransmitter actions. ACh and norepinephrine (NE), predominant in the PNS, also function in the CNS. Dopamine and 5-HT (serotonin)—more prominent in the CNS—and peptides such as endorphins are important in CNS function. Transduction mechanisms for neurotransmitter action are similar to those in the PNS: ionotropic types include voltage-gated ion channels (respond to membrane potential changes) and ligand-gated ion channels (alter membrane ion permeability in response to ligands such as neurotransmitters or drugs). Metabotropic types include GPCRs and involve second-messenger pathways (affect ion channels or biochemical reactions). Drugs affect various sites along neuronal pathways, including neurotransmitter synthesis, storage, and release; receptor activation and inhibition; modulation of intrasynaptic neurotransmitter metabolism or reuptake; and direct second-messenger pathway effects.

Selected Sedative-Hypnotics					
Class	**Drug**	**Class**	**Drug**	**Class**	**Drug**
Alcohols	Ethanol Chloral hydrate	Benzodiazepines	Alprazolam Chlordiazepoxide Clorazepate Diazepam Flurazepam Lorazepam Oxazepam Prazepam Temazepam Triazolam	Carbamates	Meprobamate
Barbiturates	Amobarbital Aprobarbital Mephobarbital Pentobarbital Phenobarbital Secobarbital Thiopental			Miscellaneous	Buspirone Zaleplon Zolpidem

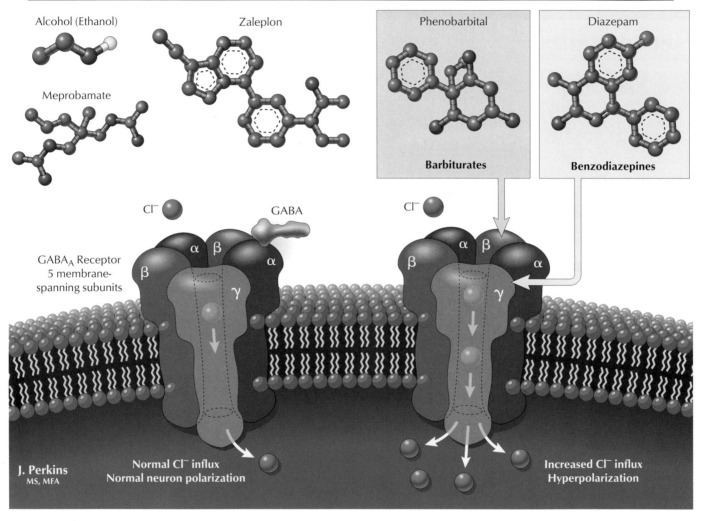

FIGURE 3-7 GABA_A RECEPTOR COMPLEX AND SEDATIVE-HYPNOTIC DRUGS

Many CNS depressants, including alcohols, barbiturates, benzodiazepines, and carbamates, produce sedation (reduction of anxiety) or hypnosis (induction of sleep). Sedative-hypnotics show considerable chemical diversity but share an ability to modulate Cl^- influx via interaction with the GABA_A receptor–Cl^- channel complex, a heteroligomeric glycoprotein comprising 5 or more membrane-spanning subunits. Various subunit combinations give rise to multiple receptor subtypes. GABA enhances Cl^- influx by binding to α or β subunits. Cl^- influx hyperpolarizes the neuron and makes it less likely to fire in response to stimulation (EPSPs). Barbiturates depress neuronal activity by facilitating and prolonging inhibitory effects of GABA and Gly by interacting with Cl^- channel sites and increasing the duration of GABA-mediated channel opening. Benzodiazepines (see Figure 3-9) bind to specific receptor sites on the complex and increase the frequency of GABA-mediated channel opening.

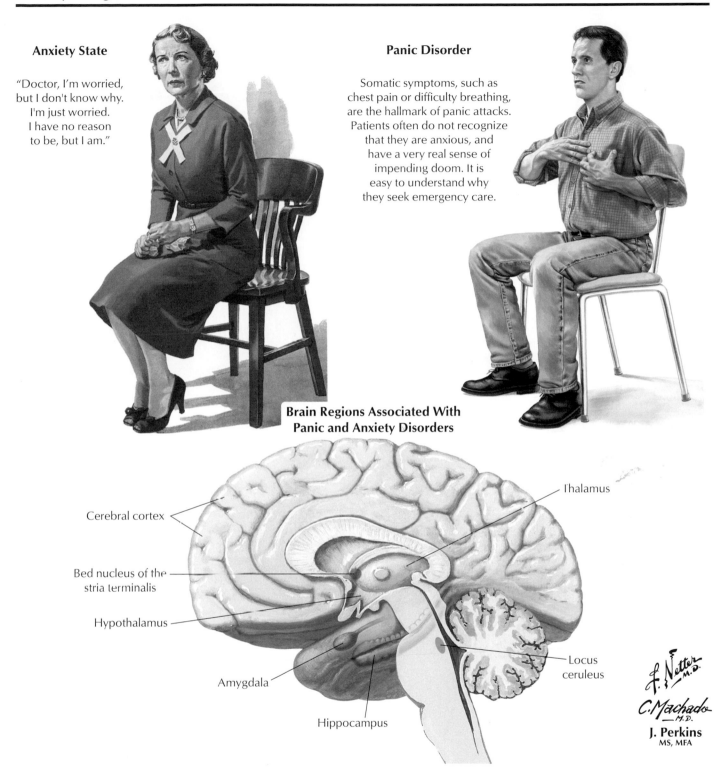

Anxiety State

"Doctor, I'm worried, but I don't know why. I'm just worried. I have no reason to be, but I am."

Panic Disorder

Somatic symptoms, such as chest pain or difficulty breathing, are the hallmark of panic attacks. Patients often do not recognize that they are anxious, and have a very real sense of impending doom. It is easy to understand why they seek emergency care.

Brain Regions Associated With Panic and Anxiety Disorders

Cerebral cortex

Bed nucleus of the stria terminalis

Hypothalamus

Amygdala

Hippocampus

Thalamus

Locus ceruleus

FIGURE 3-8 CLINICAL ANXIETY

To experience anxiety is normal. However, *clinical anxiety* is tension or apprehension that is grossly disproportionate to an actual or perceived stimulus. The source of anxiety may not be apparent and indeed may not be external; an underlying biochemical defect and genetic predisposition are hypothesized. Clinical anxiety, whether chronic or in the form of a panic attack, often produces somatic symptoms, impedes normal functioning, and adversely affects the quality of life. The disorders are approximately twice as common (possibly more often reported) in women than in men. The age at onset is usually between 20 and 30 years. Both endogenous and external factors likely contribute to susceptibility and expression of the clinical problem. Common adult anxiety disorders include generalized anxiety disorder, social phobia, OCD, panic disorder, and posttraumatic stress syndrome. Drugs for treating anxiety disorders, or anxiolytics, include benzodiazepines and buspirone.

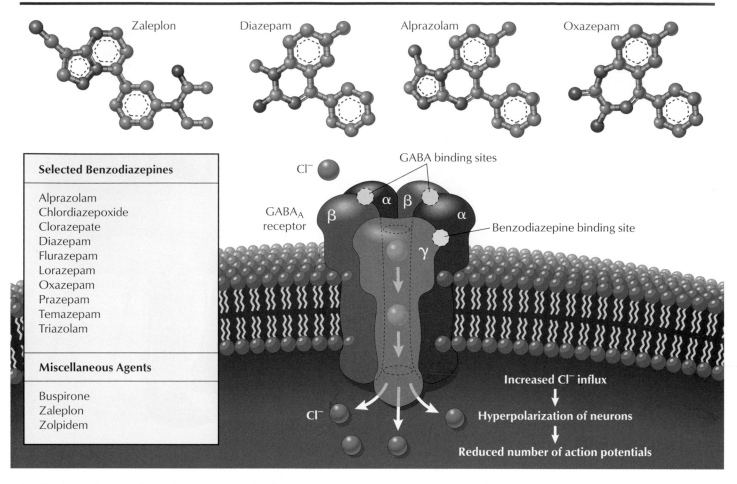

Zaleplon   Diazepam   Alprazolam   Oxazepam

Selected Benzodiazepines

Alprazolam
Chlordiazepoxide
Clorazepate
Diazepam
Flurazepam
Lorazepam
Oxazepam
Prazepam
Temazepam
Triazolam

Miscellaneous Agents

Buspirone
Zaleplon
Zolpidem

GABA binding sites

Cl⁻

GABA$_A$ receptor

Benzodiazepine binding site

β   α   β   α
γ

Increased Cl⁻ influx

Cl⁻

Hyperpolarization of neurons

Reduced number of action potentials

Distribution of Benzodiazepine Receptors in the Brain

Fornix and stria terminalis   Thalamus

Septal area

Hypo-thalamus

Olfactory bulb

Mamillary body

Pituitary

Amygdala

Hippocampus

Red nucleus

Periaqueductal gray matter

Midbrain tegmentum

Metabolism of Benzodiazepines

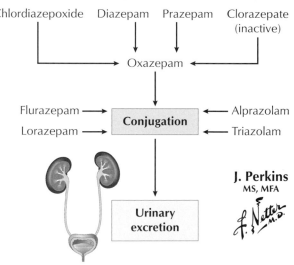

Chlordiazepoxide   Diazepam   Prazepam   Clorazepate (inactive)

Oxazepam

Flurazepam →   **Conjugation**   ← Alprazolam

Lorazepam →   ← Triazolam

Urinary excretion

J. Perkins
MS, MFA

f. Netter M.D.

FIGURE 3-9 ANXIOLYTIC AGENTS

Two main categories of anxiolytics are benzodiazepines and miscellaneous (eg, buspirone, zolpidem, zaleplon). Subclassification of benzodiazepines is based on speed of onset or duration of action, metabolism, and adverse effects. Benzodiazepines cross the blood-brain barrier and bind to specific receptors on the GABA$_A$ complex; these receptors occur in many brain regions. The drugs do not bind to the same sites as does GABA but potentiate GABA action. Benzodiazepines are safer than barbiturates (largely obsolete); adverse effects include dependence, ataxia, and drowsiness. Diazepam, chlordiazepoxide, prazepam, and the prodrug clorazepate undergo hepatic metabolism to the intermediate oxazepam. Alprazolam, flurazepam, lorazepam, and triazolam directly undergo conjugation before excretion. Zolpidem and zaleplon resemble benzodiazepines in pharmacology but differ chemically. Buspirone (an azapirone) acts on 5-HT$_{1A}$ receptors. These last drugs have fewer adverse effects and less abuse potential.

Causes of Seizures

Intracranial

Primary

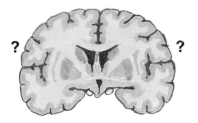

Unknown (genetic
or biochemical
predisposition)

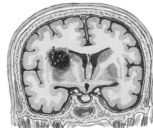

Tumor

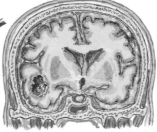

Vascular (infarct or hemorrhage)

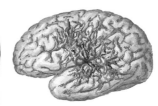

Arteriovenous
malformation

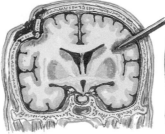

Trauma (depressed fracture,
penetrating wound)

Infection (abscess, encephalitis)

Congenital and hereditary
diseases (tuberous sclerosis)

Drugs for Treatment of:	Mechanism of Action
Tonic-clonic and partial seizures	
Carbamazepine, phenytoin	Block voltage-gated Na^+ channels in neuronal membranes and prolong neuronal refractory period
Primidone	Structural analog of phenobarbital, converted to phenobarbital (see below)
Valproic acid	Blocks voltage-gated Na^+ channels in neuronal membranes and prolong neuronal refractory period (high dose); inhibits T-type Ca^{2+} channels, particularly in the thalamus; may also enhance K^+ flux
Absence seizures	
Ethosuximide	Inhibits T-type Ca^{2+} channels, particularly in the thalamus
Valproic acid	Blocks voltage-gated Na^+ channels in neuronal membranes and prolongs neuronal refractory period (high dose); inhibits T-type Ca^{2+} channels, particularly in the thalamus; may also enhance K^+ flux
Clonazepam	Allosterically modulates GABA action at $GABA_A$ receptors, which increases frequency of Cl^- influx and hyperpolarizes neurons
Status epilepticus	
Diazepam, lorazepam	Allosterically modulate GABA action at $GABA_A$ receptors, which increases frequency of Cl^- influx and hyperpolarizes neurons
Additional drugs	
Felbamate, gabapentin	Uncertain
Lamotrigine	Blocks voltage-gated Na^+ channels in neuronal membranes and prolongs neuronal refractory period
Phenobarbital	Blocks voltage-gated Na^+ channels in neuronal membranes and prolongs neuronal refractory period (high dose); may be antagonist of Glu receptors
Tiagabine	Inhibits GABA transporters and may increase synaptic levels of GABA
Topiramate	May be antagonist of Glu receptors; may block Na^+ channels and potentiate GABA
Vigabatrin	Irreversibly blocks GABA transaminase (enzyme that terminates the action of GABA), enhancing its action

Extracranial

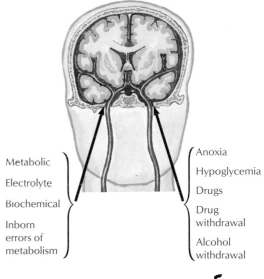

Metabolic
Electrolyte
Biochemical
Inborn
errors of
metabolism

Anoxia
Hypoglycemia
Drugs
Drug
withdrawal
Alcohol
withdrawal

FIGURE 3-10　CAUSES OF SEIZURES AND THEIR TREATMENT

Seizures have various causes, both internal (intracranial) and external (extracranial). However, many seizures, perhaps the majority, are idiopathic. Internal causes include congenital defects, inborn errors in metabolism, infection, trauma, fever, intracranial hemorrhage, and malignancy. External causes include metabolic, electrolyte, and other biochemical disorders; anoxia; and hypoglycemia as well as excess doses of drugs or abrupt cessation of drugs. Approximately 10% of the US population has a seizure by the age of 80 years. *Epilepsy*, a type of seizure disorder, is a heterogeneous symptom complex characterized by recurrent, unprovoked seizures and affects approximately 1% of the population. For optimal drug therapy, the specific type of epilepsy should be identified. The principal mechanism of action of most current antiepileptic drugs involves action on voltage-gated ion channels or on inhibitory or excitatory neurotransmitter function.

Generalized Tonic-Clonic Seizures

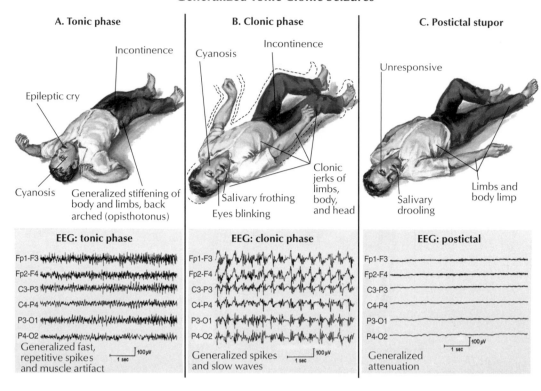

A. Tonic phase

Incontinence
Epileptic cry
Cyanosis
Cyanosis Generalized stiffening of body and limbs, back arched (opisthotonus)

EEG: tonic phase

Fp1-F3
Fp2-F4
C3-P3
C4-P4
P3-O1
P4-O2

Generalized fast, repetitive spikes and muscle artifact

100 μV
1 sec

B. Clonic phase

Incontinence
Cyanosis
Clonic jerks of limbs, body, and head
Salivary frothing
Eyes blinking

EEG: clonic phase

Fp1-F3
Fp2-F4
C3-P3
C4-P4
P3-O1
P4-O2

Generalized spikes and slow waves

100 μV
1 sec

C. Postictal stupor

Unresponsive
Limbs and body limp
Salivary drooling

EEG: postictal

Fp1-F3
Fp2-F4
C3-P3
C4-P4
P3-O1
P4-O2

Generalized attenuation

100 μV
1 sec

Status Epilepticus

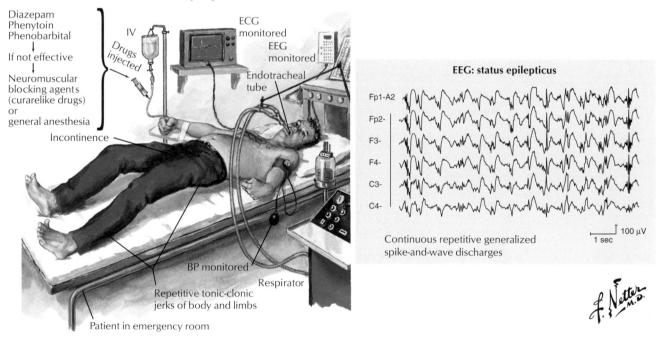

Diazepam
Phenytoin
Phenobarbital
↓
If not effective
↓
Neuromuscular blocking agents (curarelike drugs) or general anesthesia

IV
Drugs injected
Incontinence

ECG monitored
EEG monitored
Endotracheal tube

BP monitored
Respirator
Repetitive tonic-clonic jerks of body and limbs
Patient in emergency room

EEG: status epilepticus

Fp1-A2
Fp2-
F3-
F4-
C3-
C4-

Continuous repetitive generalized spike-and-wave discharges

100 μV
1 sec

f. Netter M.D.

FIGURE 3-11 EPILEPSY: GENERALIZED SEIZURES AND STATUS EPILEPTICUS

Primary generalized seizures, the most common type being generalized tonic-clonic (grand mal) seizures, involve both cerebral hemispheres. The seizure begins with tonic stiffening of the limbs in an extended position, with arching of the back, followed by synchronous clonic jerks of muscles of the limbs, body, and head. The tongue may be bitten, and incontinence may occur. A period of postictal lethargy, confusion, and disorientation follows the seizure. An unbroken cycle of seizures—termed *status epilepticus*—can develop. Generalized tonic-clonic status epilepticus is a life-threatening emergency and almost always requires intravenous medication for seizure control. Drugs for tonic-clonic (and partial) seizures include carbamazepine, phenytoin, valproic acid, and primidone; those for status epilepticus include diazepam and lorazepam. Adverse effects such as sedation, confusion, and hepatic toxicity and drug interactions occur.

Absence (Petit Mal) Seizures

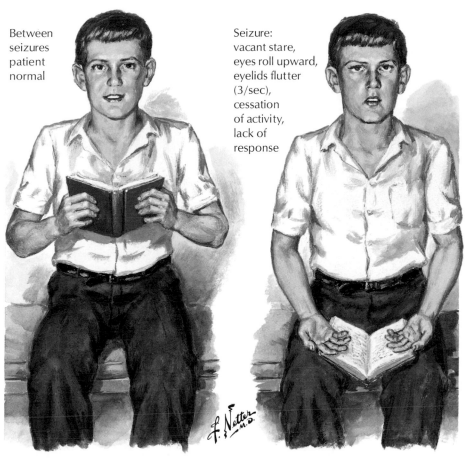

Between seizures patient normal

Seizure: vacant stare, eyes roll upward, eyelids flutter (3/sec), cessation of activity, lack of response

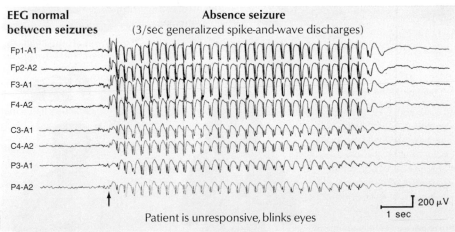

EEG normal between seizures

Absence seizure
(3/sec generalized spike-and-wave discharges)

Fp1-A1
Fp2-A2
F3-A1
F4-A2
C3-A1
C4-A2
P3-A1
P4-A2

Patient is unresponsive, blinks eyes

200 μV
1 sec

FIGURE 3-12 EPILEPSY: PARTIAL AND ABSENCE SEIZURES

Partial-onset seizures start in localized brain regions and may affect nearly any brain function, from motor or sensory involvement to complex repetitive, purposeless, undirected, and inappropriate motor activities. Patients can be unaware of these automatisms. Symptoms often represent the function of the underlying affected brain region. Postictal confusion and disorientation often occur. Drugs for these seizures include carbamazepine, phenytoin, valproic acid, and primidone. Absence

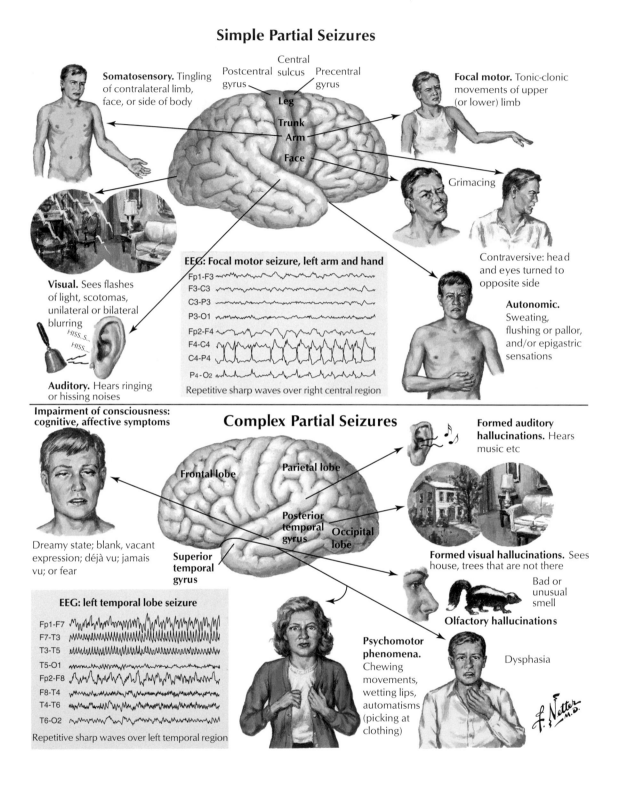

Simple Partial Seizures

Somatosensory. Tingling of contralateral limb, face, or side of body

Central sulcus
Postcentral gyrus   Precentral gyrus

Leg
Trunk
Arm
Face

Focal motor. Tonic-clonic movements of upper (or lower) limb

Grimacing

Contraversive: head and eyes turned to opposite side

Visual. Sees flashes of light, scotomas, unilateral or bilateral blurring

HISS...S...
HISS...

EEG: Focal motor seizure, left arm and hand
Fp1-F3
F3-C3
C3-P3
P3-O1
Fp2-F4
F4-C4
C4-P4
P4-O2
Repetitive sharp waves over right central region

Autonomic. Sweating, flushing or pallor, and/or epigastric sensations

Auditory. Hears ringing or hissing noises

Impairment of consciousness: cognitive, affective symptoms

Complex Partial Seizures

Formed auditory hallucinations. Hears music etc

Frontal lobe   Parietal lobe

Posterior temporal gyrus   Occipital lobe

Superior temporal gyrus

Dreamy state; blank, vacant expression; déjà vu; jamais vu; or fear

Formed visual hallucinations. Sees house, trees that are not there

Bad or unusual smell

Olfactory hallucinations

Dysphasia

EEG: left temporal lobe seizure
Fp1-F7
F7-T3
T3-T5
T5-O1
Fp2-F8
F8-T4
T4-T6
T6-O2
Repetitive sharp waves over left temporal region

Psychomotor phenomena. Chewing movements, wetting lips, automatisms (picking at clothing)

F. Netter M.D.

FIGURE 3-12 EPILEPSY: PARTIAL AND ABSENCE SEIZURES (continued)

(petite mal) seizures, characterized by periods of vacant staring or inattention (absence), occur without warning and last approximately 20 seconds. Hundreds may occur daily. Patients often have no memory of the events. These seizures usually occur in children, are often outgrown in adolescence, can disrupt academic performance, and are treated with ethosuximide and valproic acid and with clonazepam. Side effects of these drugs include sedation, leukopenia, and hepatic failure.

The Face of Depression

"Doctor, what's wrong with me?"

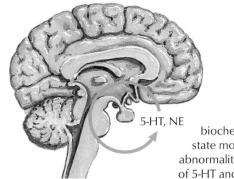

5-HT, NE

Depression is a biochemically mediated state most likely based on abnormalities in metabolism of 5-HT and norepinephrine.

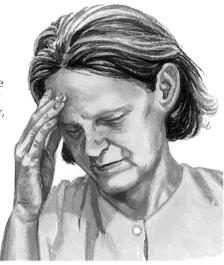

Clinical syndrome characterized by withdrawal, anger, frustration, and loss of pleasure

Associated Symptoms and Comorbidities

Depressed mood with feelings of worthlessness and guilt

Poor concentration

Fatigue

Withdrawal

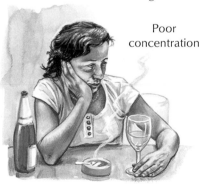

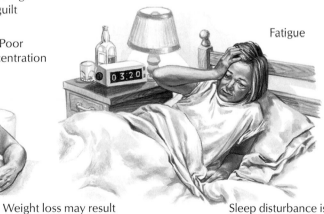

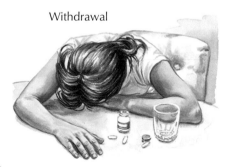

Substance abuse is a common comorbidity.

Weight loss may result from poor nutritional habits.

Sleep disturbance is a common complaint.

Increased suicide risk

FIGURE 3-13 CLINICAL DEPRESSION

Clinical (endogenous) depression, a heterogeneous biopsychologic disorder with genetic predisposition, can occur at any time in life, unrelated to obvious stressors. Treatment is required: approximately 15% of these patients commit suicide. Severe (major depression) and mild (dysthymic disorder) forms exist. Findings that clinical depression may be related to an imbalance in endogenous amines (5-HT or NE) in the CNS led to the amine hypothesis of etiology and spurred efforts to enhance synaptic action of these amines. Antidepressants are classified according to a presumed mechanism of action or chemical structure. TCAs and heterocyclics nonselectively inhibit both 5-HT and NE. SSRIs enhance drugs metabolized via the cytochrome P-450 pathway. MAOIs inhibit amine metabolism. Adverse effects (eg, mania, agitation, serotonin syndrome) and drug interactions (MAOIs used with TCAs or SSRIs) do occur.

Selected Antidepressants

Class	Drug	Mechanism of Action	Class	Drug	Mechanism of Action
Tricyclic agents	Amitriptyline Clomipramine Desipramine Doxepin Imipramine Nortriptyline Protriptyline	Nonselectively inhibit both 5-HT and NE reuptake	Heterocyclic agents	Amoxapine Bupropion Maprotiline Mirtazapine Nefazodone Trazodone Venlafaxine	Nonselectively inhibit both 5-HT and NE reuptake
SSRIs	Citalopram Fluoxetine Fluvoxamine Paroxetine Sertraline	Selectively inhibit 5-HT reuptake	MAOIs	Phenelzine Tranylcypromine	Inhibit amine metabolism

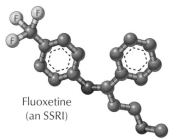

Fluoxetine
(an SSRI)

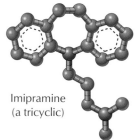

Imipramine
(a tricyclic)

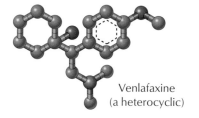

Venlafaxine
(a heterocyclic)

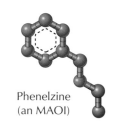

Phenelzine
(an MAOI)

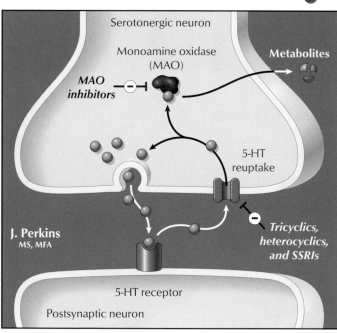

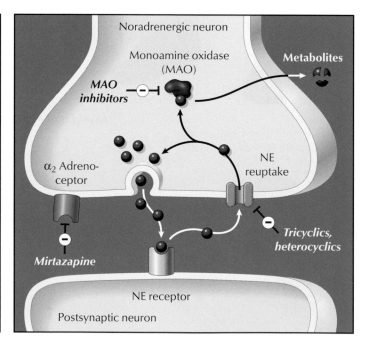

FIGURE 3-14 ANTIDEPRESSANTS: MECHANISMS OF ACTION

Most antidepressants primarily enhance the action of endogenous amine neurotransmitters; they act indirectly, not binding to 5-HT or NE receptors but enhancing neurotransmitter action by inhibiting metabolism or removing neurotransmitters from synapses. Increased synaptic 5-HT or NE levels then counteract the abnormally low levels that produce depression. 5-HT enhancement may be more important than enhancement of NE, so SSRIs have become popular. MAOIs inhibit metabolism of 5-HT and NE, thus increasing amine levels. Mechanisms of newer drugs include direct binding to 5-HT or NE receptor subtypes (eg, antagonist action at presynaptic α_2-adrenoceptors stimulates NE release). The action of bupropion does not seem to involve 5-HT or NE and therefore may represent a novel mechanism. The long-term mechanism of antidepressant action is unknown. All these drugs modify neurochemical pathways and can elicit adverse effects (eg, sedation and excitation).

Obsessive Compulsive Disorder

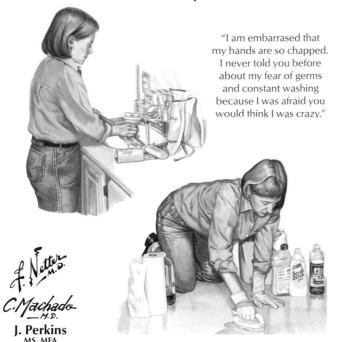

"I am embarrased that my hands are so chapped. I never told you before about my fear of germs and constant washing because I was afraid you would think I was crazy."

J. Netter M.D.
C. Machado M.D.
J. Perkins
MS, MFA

Bipolar Affective Disorder: Manic Episode

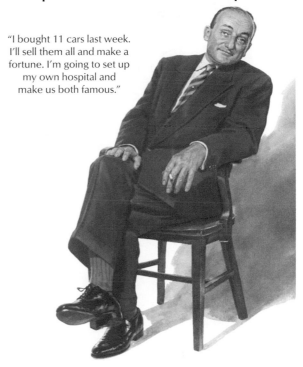

"I bought 11 cars last week. I'll sell them all and make a fortune. I'm going to set up my own hospital and make us both famous."

Lithium: Mechanism of Action

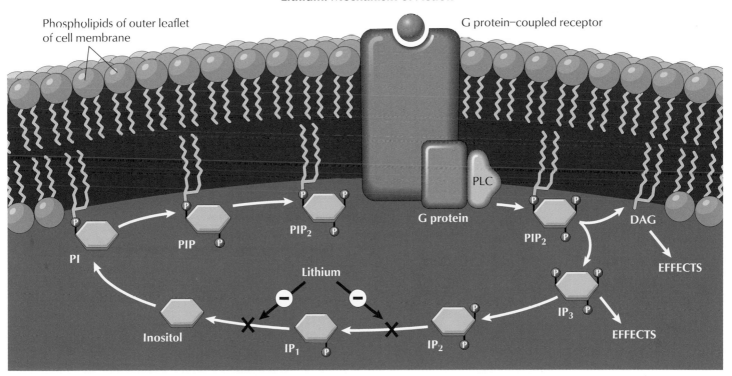

Phospholipids of outer leaflet of cell membrane

G protein–coupled receptor

PLC

G protein

PI

PIP

PIP_2

PIP_2

DAG

EFFECTS

Lithium

IP_3

EFFECTS

Inositol

IP_1

IP_2

FIGURE 3-15 BIPOLAR DISORDER AND COMPULSIVE BEHAVIOR

Bipolar disorder is characterized by alternating periods of mania and depression. The manic phase can be productive but can also be disruptive and physically exhausting. Bipolar disorder often responds to treatment with lithium, which is rapidly absorbed from the GI tract and is distributed throughout the body. Lithium may reduce neuronal activity by inhibiting cellular phosphoinositide pathways involving the second messengers inositol trisphosphate and diacylglycerol. Compulsive behaviors impair social interaction and disrupt daily activities. OCD affects at least 2% of the population (males and females approximately equally), with a genetic predisposition. The TCA clomipramine and SSRIs are usually chosen for OCD therapy. Other drugs, given individually or as combination therapy, include different TCAs, lithium, buspirone, clonazepam, dopamine antagonists (eg, haloperidol), and trazodone. Drugs used together with behavioral or psychosocial therapy are usually optimal.

Schizophrenia

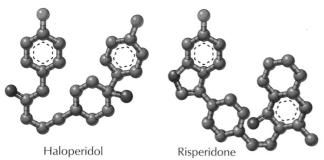

This patient exhibits the flat affect that is common to schizophrenia. She appears to be responding to internal stimuli—perhaps attending to auditory hallucinations. Alternatively, she may have significant negative symptoms including anhedonia, amotivation, and poverty of speech. Finally, she may have parkinsonism secondary to anti-psychotic medication.

Haloperidol   Risperidone

Neural Pathways Involved in Schizophrenia

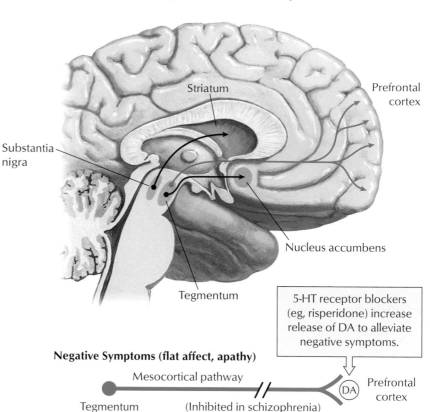

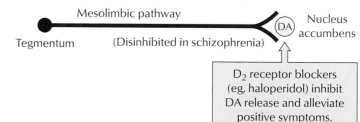

Negative Symptoms (flat affect, apathy)

Mesocortical pathway

Tegmentum   (Inhibited in schizophrenia)

5-HT receptor blockers (eg, risperidone) increase release of DA to alleviate negative symptoms.

DA   Prefrontal cortex

Positive Symptoms (delusions, hallucinations)

Mesolimbic pathway

Tegmentum   (Disinhibited in schizophrenia)

DA   Nucleus accumbens

D_2 receptor blockers (eg, haloperidol) inhibit DA release and alleviate positive symptoms.

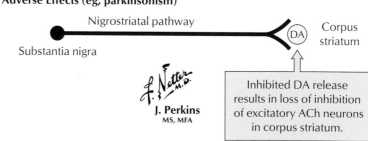

Adverse Effects (eg, parkinsonism)

Nigrostriatal pathway

Substantia nigra

DA   Corpus striatum

Inhibited DA release results in loss of inhibition of excitatory ACh neurons in corpus striatum.

J. Perkins
MS, MFA

FIGURE 3-16 PSYCHOSIS AND DOPAMINE PATHWAYS

Psychoses are psychogenic mental disorders involving a loss of contact with reality. The most common is schizophrenia, in which perception, thinking, communication, social functioning, and attention are altered. Caused by genetic and environmental factors, it affects approximately 10% of the population. Symptoms are called *positive* (eg, delusions, hallucinations) or *negative* (eg, flat affect, apathy); cognitive dysfunction may occur. Interest in dopamine, 5-HT, and Glu neurotransmitters led to

most early drugs' targeting the dopamine system, primarily as dopamine D_2 receptor antagonists. Typical antipsychotics (eg, chlorpromazine, haloperidol) are better for treating positive signs than negative signs. For treating negative signs, the newer (atypical) antipsychotic drugs (eg, clozapine, risperidone) target other receptors, particularly 5-HT. Neurologic (eg, dystonia, parkinsonism), anticholinergic (eg, blurred vision), and antiadrenergic (eg, hypotension) adverse effects can occur.

Horizontal Brain Section Showing Basal Ganglia

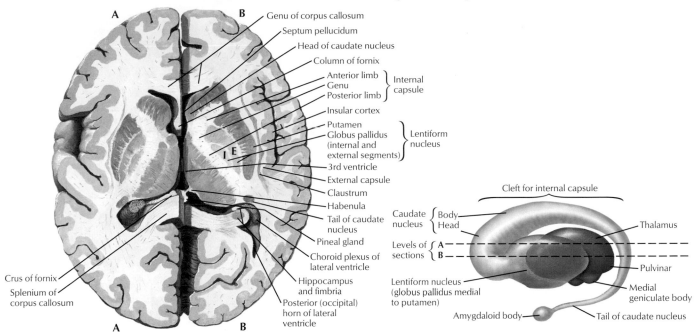

Connections of Basal Ganglia

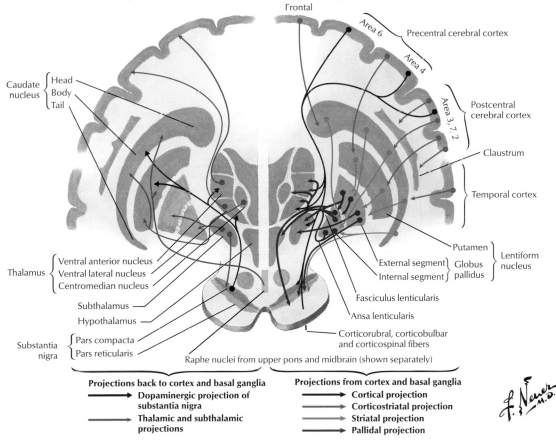

FIGURE 3-17 MOTOR TRACTS, BASAL GANGLIA, AND DOPAMINE PATHWAYS

Several major neuronal tracts coordinate somatic motor functions. One is the pyramidal tract, whose direct motor component goes from the precentral gyrus through the internal capsule and midbrain and terminates on motor neurons in the anterior horn of the spinal cord. Extrapyramidal tracts (eg, rubrospinal, reticulospinal, and corticoreticular) are also important for motor control. The basal ganglia (including caudate nucleus, putamen, and globus pallidus) are subcortical masses found between the

Pyramidal System

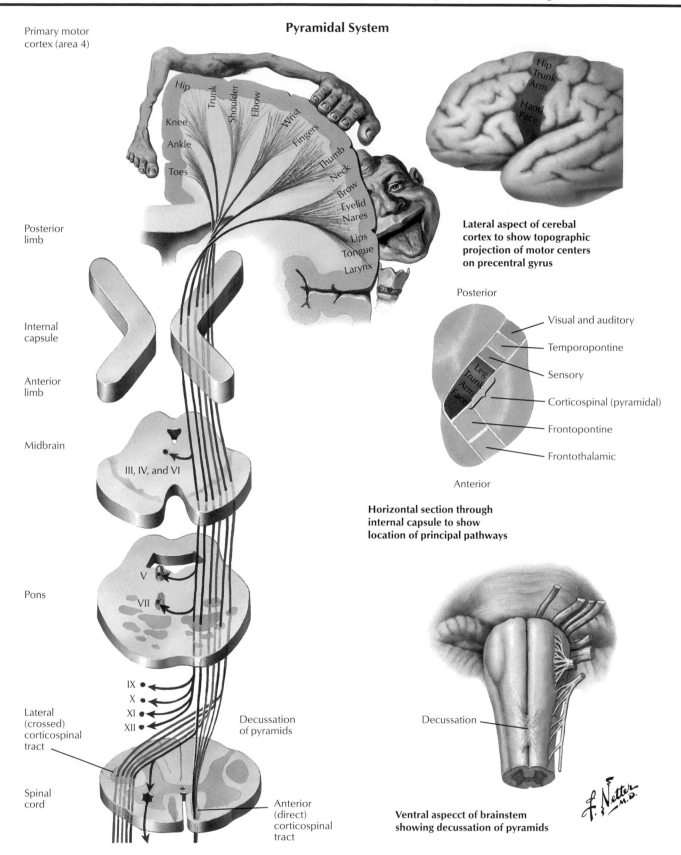

Primary motor cortex (area 4)

Posterior limb

Internal capsule

Anterior limb

Midbrain

III, IV, and VI

Pons

V

VII

IX
X
XI
XII

Lateral (crossed) corticospinal tract

Decussation of pyramids

Spinal cord

Anterior (direct) corticospinal tract

Lateral aspect of cerebral cortex to show topographic projection of motor centers on precentral gyrus

Posterior

Visual and auditory
Temporopontine
Sensory
Corticospinal (pyramidal)
Frontopontine
Frontothalamic

Anterior

Horizontal section through internal capsule to show location of principal pathways

Decussation

Ventral aspecct of brainstem showing decussation of pyramids

FIGURE 3-17 MOTOR TRACTS, BASAL GANGLIA, AND DOPAMINE PATHWAYS (continued)

cerebral cortex and thalamus that, together with the substantia nigra, help to coordinate movement. A major pathway, the nigrostriatal, originates in the substantia nigra and connects with basal ganglia and other structures. The substantia nigra receives reciprocal input from these structures plus others. Efferent pathways (nigrostriatal) are dopaminergic; afferent input is from neurons containing 5-HT, GABA, and substance P. Defects in these pathways lead to motor incoordination or incapacity.

Clinical Signs of Parkinson Disease

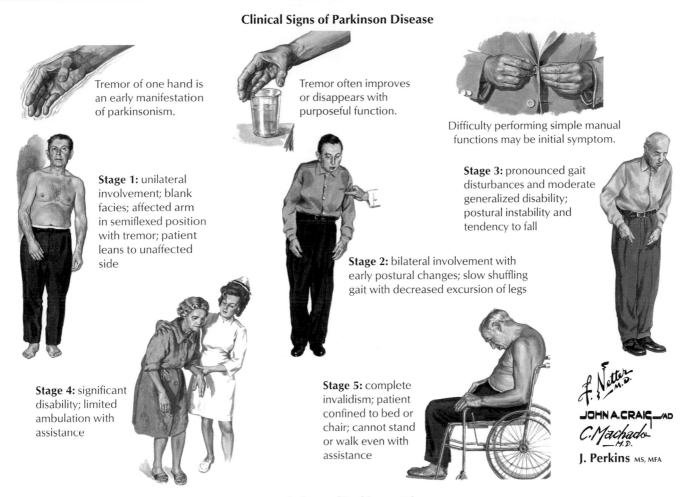

Tremor of one hand is an early manifestation of parkinsonism.

Tremor often improves or disappears with purposeful function.

Difficulty performing simple manual functions may be initial symptom.

Stage 1: unilateral involvement; blank facies; affected arm in semiflexed position with tremor; patient leans to unaffected side

Stage 3: pronounced gait disturbances and moderate generalized disability; postural instability and tendency to fall

Stage 2: bilateral involvement with early postural changes; slow shuffling gait with decreased excursion of legs

Stage 4: significant disability; limited ambulation with assistance

Stage 5: complete invalidism; patient confined to bed or chair; cannot stand or walk even with assistance

JOHN A. CRAIG —MD
C. Machado —M.D.
J. Perkins MS, MFA

Neuropathology of Parkinson Disease

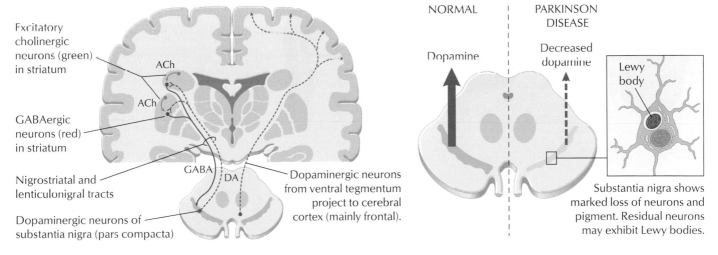

Excitatory cholinergic neurons (green) in striatum

ACh

ACh

GABAergic neurons (red) in striatum

Nigrostriatal and lenticulonigral tracts

GABA

DA

Dopaminergic neurons from ventral tegmentum project to cerebral cortex (mainly frontal).

Dopaminergic neurons of substantia nigra (pars compacta)

NORMAL | PARKINSON DISEASE

Dopamine

Decreased dopamine

Lewy body

Substantia nigra shows marked loss of neurons and pigment. Residual neurons may exhibit Lewy bodies.

FIGURE 3-18 PARKINSONISM: SYMPTOMS AND DEFECT

Parkinsonism is a progressive neurodegenerative disease that adversely affects motor neuron control. Major early symptoms are tremor at rest, bradykinesia, muscle rigidity, and flat facial affect. If untreated, the condition worsens, leading eventually to complete immobility and early mortality. The prevalence is approximately 2% in persons older than 65 years. A genetic predisposition seems likely, but environmental factors (including viral infections and neurotoxins) may play a role. The most distinctive neuropathologic finding is progressive loss of dopaminergic neurons of the pars compacta of the substantia nigra. Projections of dopaminergic neurons from the substantia nigra correlate with motor and cognitive deficits. Degeneration of dopaminergic neurons in the nigrostriatal tract causes loss of inhibitory dopamine action on striatal GABAergic neurons and leads to excessive cholinergic neuron excitation of these striatal neurons. Drugs such as levodopa (increases dopaminergic activity) can help.

Parkinsonism: Hypothesized Role of Dopa

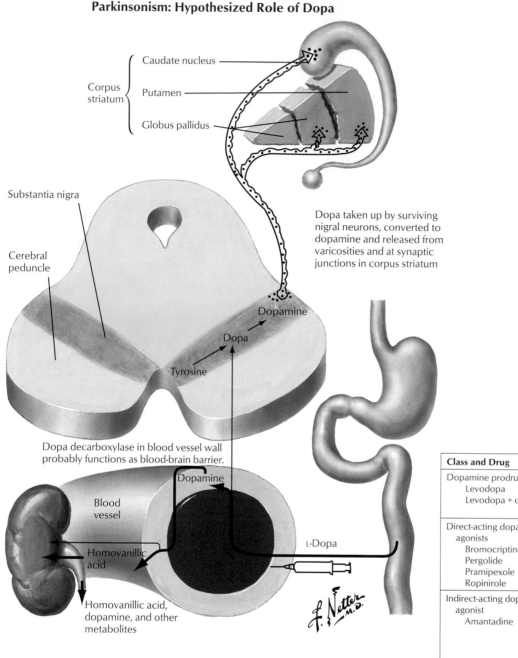

Corpus striatum
- Caudate nucleus
- Putamen
- Globus pallidus

Substantia nigra

Cerebral peduncle

Dopa taken up by surviving nigral neurons, converted to dopamine and released from varicosities and at synaptic junctions in corpus striatum

Dopamine

Dopa

Tyrosine

Dopa decarboxylase in blood vessel wall probably functions as blood-brain barrier.

Dopamine

Blood vessel

Homovanillic acid

Homovanillic acid, dopamine, and other metabolites

L-Dopa

Class and Drug	Mechanism of Action

Dopamine prodrugs
    Levodopa
    Levodopa + carbidopa
	Are rapidly converted to dopamine by dopa decarboxylase (which is inhibited by carbidopa)

Direct-acting dopamine agonists
    Bromocriptine
    Pergolide
    Pramipexole
    Ropinirole
	Bind to dopamine receptors and mimic the action of dopamine

Indirect-acting dopamine agonist Amantadine	Increases dopamine release and reduces dopamine reuptake into dopaminergic nerve terminals of substantia nigra neurons (by unknown mechanism)
MAOI Selegiline	Inhibits only type B isozyme

Muscarinic antagonists
    Benztropine
    Biperiden
    Orphenadrine
    Trihexyphenidyl
	Have central activity (brain) as anticholinergic agents

FIGURE 3-19 PARKINSONISM: LEVODOPA, CARBIDOPA, AND OTHER DRUGS

Treatment aims to replenish dopamine, or at least to reestablish the balance between dopamine and ACh influences on striatal neurons. Dopamine cannot cross the blood-brain barrier, so its metabolic precursor, levodopa, is used. Most of an oral dose is rapidly converted to dopamine by dopa decarboxylase located in blood vessel walls. Approximately 1% to 5% of the dose crosses the blood-brain barrier, enters metabolic pathways of dopaminergic neurons, and is converted to dopamine. To increase the amount of levodopa that enters the brain, it is usually given with an inhibitor of dopa decarboxylase (such as carbidopa) that does not easily cross the blood-brain barrier. Peripheral conversion of levodopa to dopamine is thus reduced, so more levodopa enters the brain. Adverse effects include the on-off effect, arrhythmias, and hypotension. Direct-acting dopamine receptor agonists, inhibitors of dopamine metabolism (eg, MAOIs), anticholinergic agents, and amantadine are other drug options.

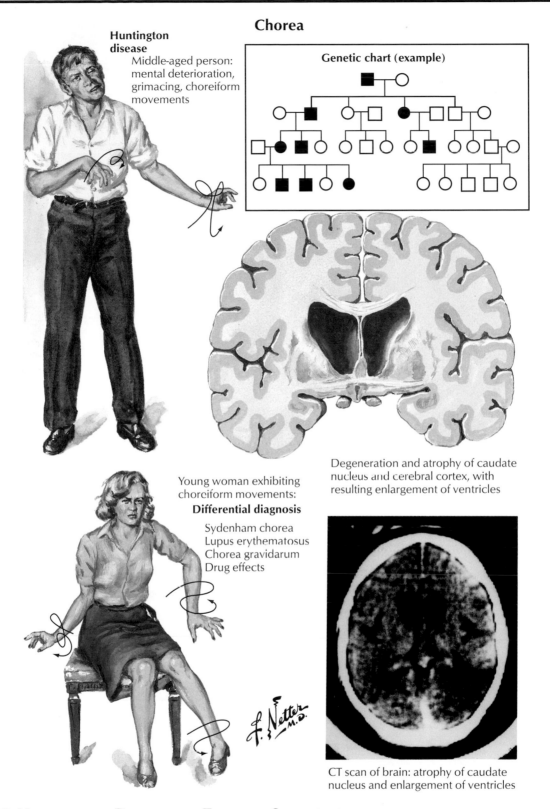

Huntington disease
Middle-aged person: mental deterioration, grimacing, choreiform movements

Chorea

Genetic chart (example)

Degeneration and atrophy of caudate nucleus and cerebral cortex, with resulting enlargement of ventricles

Young woman exhibiting choreiform movements:

Differential diagnosis

Sydenham chorea
Lupus erythematosus
Chorea gravidarum
Drug effects

CT scan of brain: atrophy of caudate nucleus and enlargement of ventricles

FIGURE 3-20 HUNTINGTON DISEASE AND TOURETTE SYNDROME

Various tremors (rhythmic oscillations around a joint), tics (repetitive, sudden, coordinated, abnormal movements), and chorea (irregular, unpredictable, involuntary muscle jerks) are components of disorders of coordinated movement. Gilles de la Tourette syndrome (which includes involuntary verbal outbursts) is a disorder of unknown cause. Current therapy consists primarily of haloperidol and other dopamine D_2 receptor antagonists. Huntington disease is a dominantly inherited disorder characterized by progressive chorea and dementia. It is typically associated with an adult onset and a shortened lifespan. GABA and enzymes for ACh and GABA synthesis are deficient in the basal ganglia of patients with Huntington disease. Current therapy consists usually of amine-depleting drugs, such as tetrabenazine, or haloperidol or other dopamine D_2 receptor antagonists. Hypotension, depression, sedation, restlessness, and parkinsonism are the most common adverse drug effects.

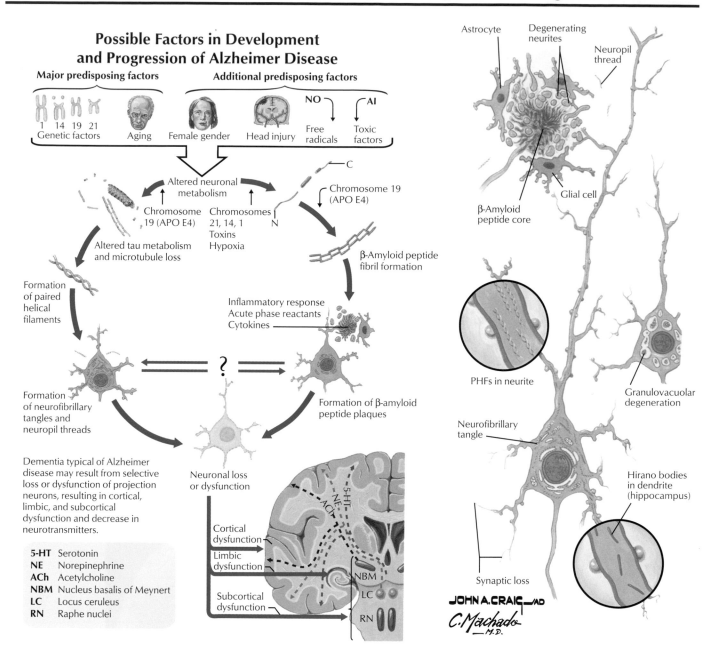

Possible Factors in Development and Progression of Alzheimer Disease

Phase and Dysfunction	Example
Early phase	
Memory loss	"Where is my checkbook?"
Spatial disorientation	"Could you direct me to my office? I have the address written down here somewhere, but I can't seem to find it."
Circumlocution	Asks husband, "John dear, please call that woman who fixes my hair."
More advanced phase	Sloppily dressed, slow, apathetic, confused, disoriented, stooped posture
Terminal phase	Bedridden, stiff, unresponsive, nearly mute, incontinent

FIGURE 3-21 ALZHEIMER DISEASE: SYMPTOMS, COURSE, AND PATHOLOGY

Alzheimer disease is a neurodegenerative disorder characterized by progressive impairment of short-term memory and other memory, language, and thought processes. Functions are typically lost in the reverse order in which they were attained. In advanced stages, patients cannot perform simple activities of daily life. Diagnosis is usually made 3 years or more after symptom onset, and life expectancy is approximately 7 to 10 years after diagnosis. Gross brain atrophy accompanies the progression of the disease, with characteristic high numbers of neuritic plaques (fragments of insoluble amyloid, type Aβ, protein) and neurofibrillary tangles (abnormal τ microtubule complexes), particularly in the hippocampus and posterior temporoparietal lobe areas. Predisposing factors include aging and genetics, with a possible contribution from environmental toxins. The neurodegeneration results in loss or dysfunction of neurotransmitter pathways.

Alzheimer disease: pathology

Regional atrophy of brain with narrowed gyri and widened sulci, but precentral and postcentral, inferior frontal, angular, supramarginal and some occipital gyri fairly well preserved; association cortex mostly involved

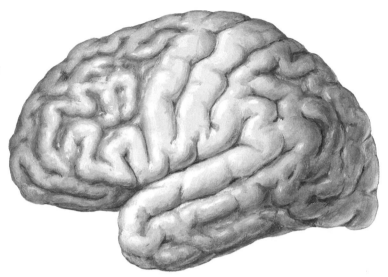

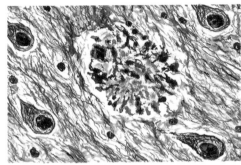

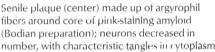

Senile plaque (center) made up of argyrophil fibers around core of pink-staining amyloid (Bodian preparation); neurons decreased in number, with characteristic tangles in cytoplasm

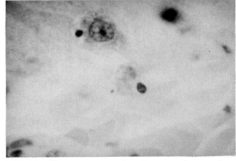

Section of hippocampus showing granulovacuolar inclusions and loss of pyramidal cells

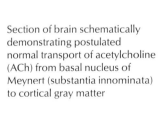

Section of brain schematically demonstrating postulated normal transport of acetylcholine (ACh) from basal nucleus of Meynert (substantia innominata) to cortical gray matter

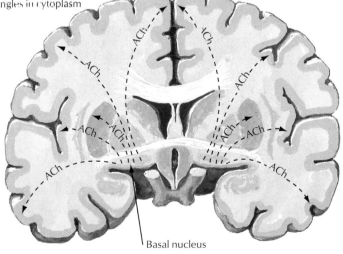

Basal nucleus

f. Netter M.D.

FIGURE 3-22 ALZHEIMER DISEASE: CHOLINERGIC INVOLVEMENT AND DRUGS

Although many neurotransmitter systems become disrupted in Alzheimer disease, cholinergic pathways become especially damaged. Functional cholinergic deficits, such as impairment in short-term memory, become apparent even in the early stages of the disease. Medication strategies to ameliorate the decline in cholinergic function include the administration of precursors (eg, lecithin); direct-acting cholinergic receptor agonists; and indirect-acting cholinomimetics. Indirect-acting agents, specifically

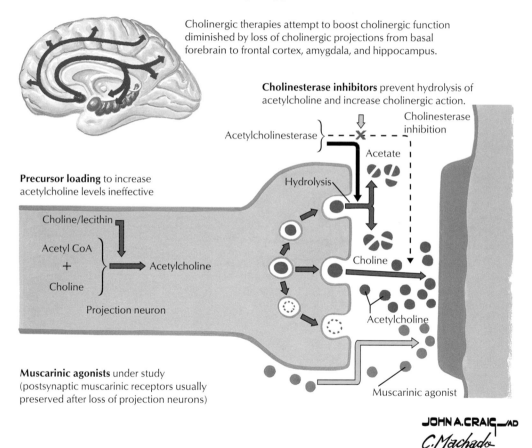

Pharmacologic Management Options in Alzheimer Disease
Cholinergic Approaches

Cholinergic therapies attempt to boost cholinergic function diminished by loss of cholinergic projections from basal forebrain to frontal cortex, amygdala, and hippocampus.

Cholinesterase inhibitors prevent hydrolysis of acetylcholine and increase cholinergic action.

Acetylcholinesterase

Cholinesterase inhibition

Acetate

Hydrolysis

Precursor loading to increase acetylcholine levels ineffective

Choline/lecithin

Acetyl CoA
+
Choline

→ Acetylcholine

Projection neuron

Choline

Acetylcholine

Muscarinic agonists under study (postsynaptic muscarinic receptors usually preserved after loss of projection neurons)

Muscarinic agonist

JOHN A. CRAIG—MD
C. Machado—M.D.

FIGURE 3-22 ALZHEIMER DISEASE: CHOLINERGIC INVOLVEMENT AND DRUGS (continued)

cholinesterase inhibitors, such as donepezil, galantamine, and rivastigmine, are currently the most commonly used. Ongoing research is investigating other potential targets, such as enzymes responsible for synthesis or degradation of Aβ or τ protein, and other postulated mechanisms responsible for the etiology or progression of the disease.

Ischemic ←— **Stroke** —→ Hemorrhagic

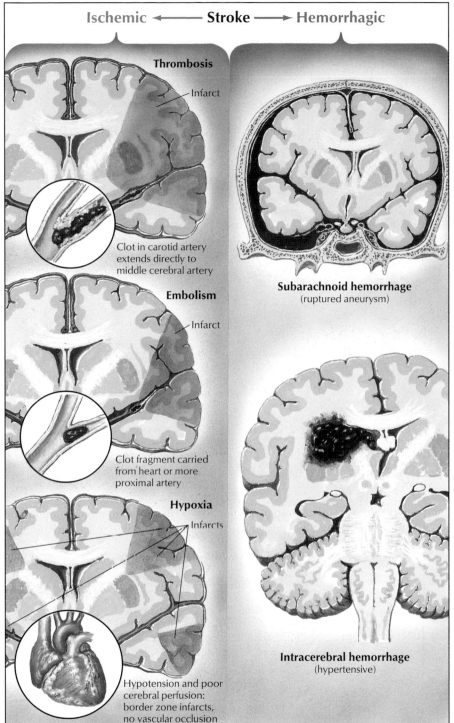

Thrombosis

Infarct

Clot in carotid artery extends directly to middle cerebral artery

Embolism

Infarct

Clot fragment carried from heart or more proximal artery

Hypoxia

Infarcts

Hypotension and poor cerebral perfusion: border zone infarcts, no vascular occlusion

Subarachnoid hemorrhage
(ruptured aneurysm)

Intracerebral hemorrhage
(hypertensive)

Thrombolysis

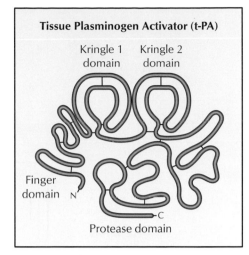

Tissue Plasminogen Activator (t-PA)

Kringle 1 domain   Kringle 2 domain

Finger domain   N

C

Protease domain

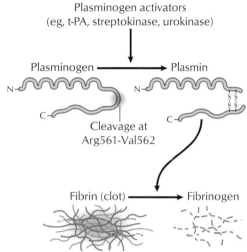

Plasminogen activators
(eg, t-PA, streptokinase, urokinase)

Plasminogen → Plasmin

N   N

C   C

Cleavage at
Arg561-Val562

Fibrin (clot) → Fibrinogen

J. Perkins
MS, MFA

FIGURE 3-23 STROKE: SYMPTOMS AND DRUG TREATMENT

Strokes are cerebrovascular accidents with CNS effects. Strokes can be categorized as ischemic (inadequate oxygen) or hemorrhagic (excess blood). Most ischemic strokes are caused by thrombi or emboli caused by cardiac or cerebrovascular disease, such as arteriosclerosis involving cerebral blood vessels. Early treatment intervention reduces subsequent neuronal damage and functional loss. The most common current drug therapies for ischemic stroke involve use of intravenous thrombolytic agents,

such as alteplase or reteplase (tissue plasminogen activators), anistreplase (prodrug: streptokinase plus recombinant human plasminogen), streptokinase, and urokinase (all plasminogen activators). The most important adverse effect of these drugs is bleeding (cerebral hemorrhage). Low-dose aspirin (COX-1 inhibitor) is given for stroke prevention. Hemorrhagic stroke requires anticoagulant or surgical intervention. Research efforts now focus on drugs that may limit the extent of CNS damage after stroke.

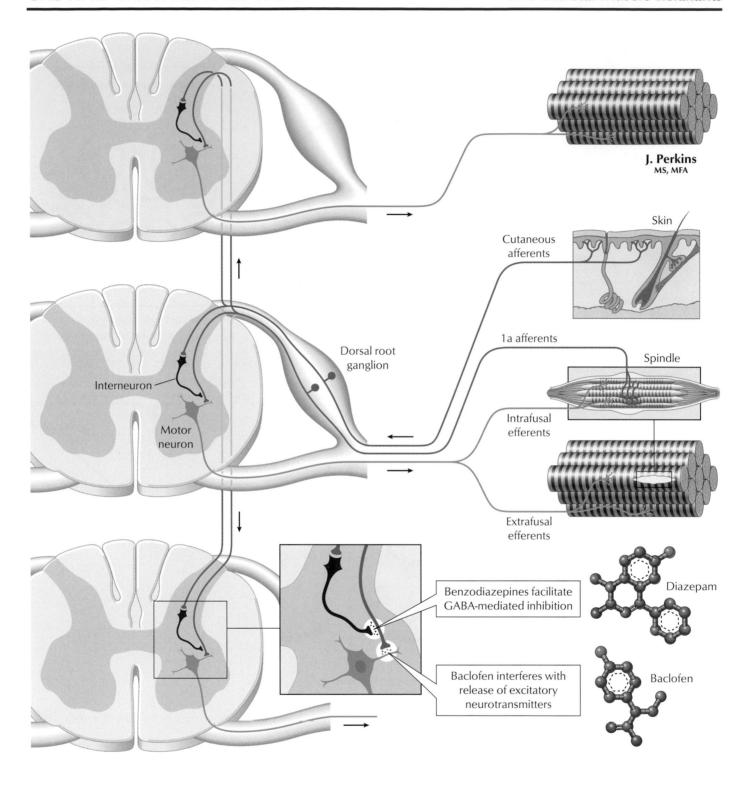

J. Perkins
MS, MFA

Skin

Cutaneous
afferents

1a afferents

Spindle

Dorsal root
ganglion

Interneuron

Intrafusal
efferents

Motor
neuron

Extrafusal
efferents

Benzodiazepines facilitate
GABA-mediated inhibition

Diazepam

Baclofen interferes with
release of excitatory
neurotransmitters

Baclofen

FIGURE 3-24 MOTOR NEURONS AND DRUGS

Skeletal muscle spasticity often results from neuronal, not muscle, deficits. The reflex arc involved in coordinated skeletal muscle action involves several neurons, including interneurons, in the spinal cord. These spinal polysynaptic reflex arcs are depressed by a number of drugs, including barbiturates. However, nonspecific depression of synapses is not desirable because normal muscle function can be disrupted. More specific agents, including CNS-acting drugs, are preferred. Benzodiazepines allosterically facilitate GABA-mediated Cl^- influx (Figure 3-9) throughout the CNS, including the spinal cord. They are used for muscle spasm of almost any cause but can also produce excess sedation. Baclofen is a $GABA_B$ receptor agonist that hyperpolarizes neurons by increasing K^+ conductance. Other CNS-acting antispasmodic agents include α_2-adrenoceptor agonists (eg, tizanidine), $GABA_A$ and $GABA_B$ receptor agonists, and the inhibitory amino acid Gly.

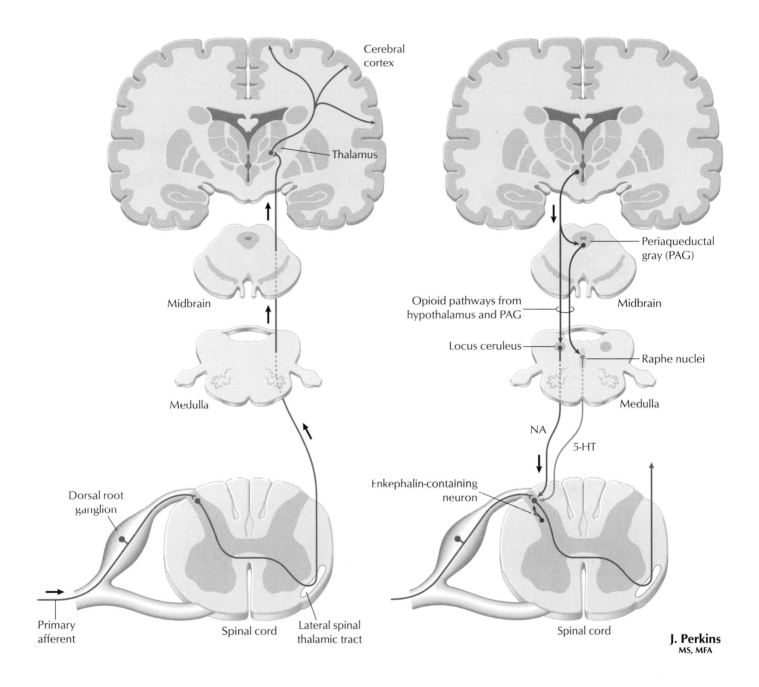

FIGURE 3-25 PAIN PATHWAYS

Tissue injury can lead to cellular changes involving release of chemicals (eg, histamine) that start or quicken neuronal impulses that are interpreted as pain. Many neuronal pathways transmit pain sensation. For example, pain from peripheral injury reaches the CNS via primary afferent neurons, whose cell bodies form the DRG. Disorders such as phantom limb pain may involve abnormal DRG structure or function. Primary afferents end mainly in the dorsal horn of the spinal cord. Secondary neurons cross the spinal cord and ascend in pathways to the thalamus, the cerebral cortex, and other sites. A descending system of opioid (endorphins, enkephalins), 5-HT (eg, from raphe nuclei), and noradrenergic (eg, from locus ceruleus) pathways can lessen afferent signals. Drugs that act at pathways mediating pain sensation or perception are local (eg, lidocaine) and general (eg, halothane) agents, opioids (eg, morphine), and nonopioids (eg, aspirin and acetaminophen).

Selected Local Anesthetics

Class	Drug	Relative Duration of Action	Class	Drug	Relative Duration of Action
Amides	Bupivacaine	Long	Esters	Benzocaine	Topical only
	Lidocaine	Medium		Cocaine	Medium
	Mepivacaine	Medium		Procaine	Short
	Prilocaine	Medium		Tetracaine	Long
	Ropivacaine	Long			

Voltage-Gated Na⁺ Channel

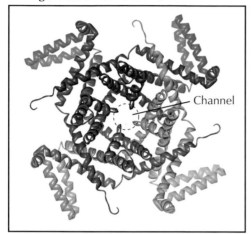

Extracellular ("top") view of Na⁺ channel

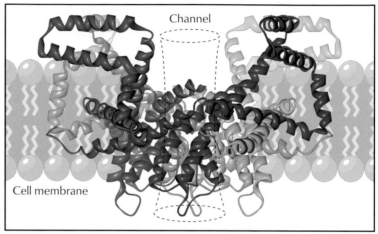

Side view of Na⁺ channel

Local Anesthetic Mechanism of Action

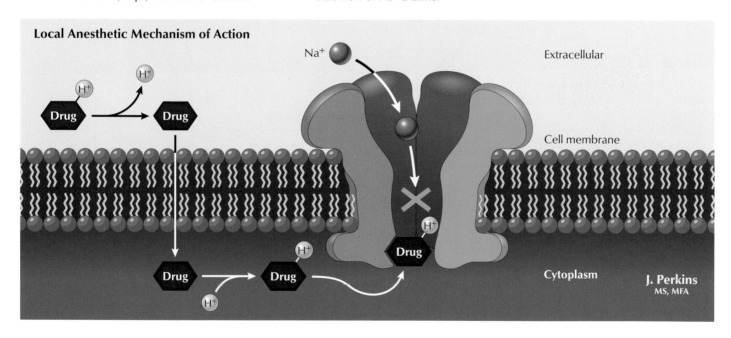

J. Perkins
MS, MFA

FIGURE 3-26 LOCAL ANESTHETICS: SPINAL AFFERENTS AND LOCAL ANESTHETIC MECHANISMS OF ACTION

Local anesthetics cause temporary loss of pain sensation without loss of consciousness by blocking conduction along sensory nerve fibers. Some selectivity for pain afferents is achieved partly by using the agent close to target neurons. All currently used drugs block voltage-dependent Na⁺ channels in excitable cells, which decreases the likelihood of an action potential. The target site of the drugs is on the cytoplasmic side of the neuron membrane, so drug molecules must pass through the membrane. They are both lipophilic and hydrophilic and are weak bases (amides or esters) that exist in equilibrium between ionized (hydrophilic) and nonionized (lipophilic) forms. The latter diffuse more readily through the membrane; the former diffuse more readily through cytoplasm. Esters are metabolized by plasma cholinesterases; amides are hydrolyzed in the liver. Because they act on all excitable cells, local anesthetics can cause toxicity, including fatal cardiovascular effects or seizures.

Selected General Anesthetics	
Drug Type and Name	**Mechanism of Action**

Inhalational
  Desflurane
  Enflurane
  Halothane
  Isoflurane
  Methoxyflurane
  Nitrous oxide
  Sevoflurane
	Not entirely known; postulated to directly activate the GABA$_A$ receptor, leading to enhanced influx of Cl$^-$ and hyperpolarization of neurons

Intravenous
  Barbiturates
    Methohexital
    Secobarbital
    Thiamylal
    Thiopental
	Facilitate inhibitory action of GABA at the GABA$_A$ receptor by increasing duration of Cl$^-$ channel opening

Benzodiazepines
    Alprazolam
    Clonazepam
    Flurazepam
    Midazolam
	Facilitate inhibitory action of GABA at the GABA$_A$ receptor by increasing frequency of Cl$^-$ channel opening

Opioids
    Alfentanil
    Fentanyl
    Morphine
    Remifentanil
	Agonists at opioid receptors widely distributed throughout the central nervous system

Phenol Propofol	Not known
Dissociative (anesthesia without loss of consciousness) Ketamine	Antagonist at the NMDA (*N*-methyl-D-aspartate) subtype of the excitatory amino acid glutamate receptor

Inhaled general anesthetics

Inspired gas mixture

Desflurane

Isoflurane

Δp

Alveoli

Venous blood

Arterial blood

Brain

Other tissues

Other tissues

Metabolism

J. Perkins
MS, MFA

Intravenous general anesthetics

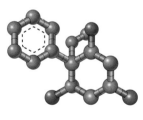

Phenobarbital
(a barbiturate)

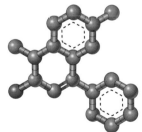

Diazepam
(a benzodiazepine)

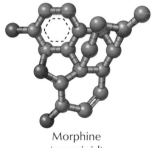

Morphine
(an opioid)

Propofol
(a phenol)

FIGURE 3-27 GENERAL ANESTHETICS: PROPERTIES

General anesthetics (inhalational and intravenous agents) have a rapid, smooth onset of action and clinically desirable rapid reversal of effect. Concentrations of inhalational agents in the body and the pharmacokinetics depend on the drugs' partial pressure in the lungs and solubility in blood and brain tissue. Induction of anesthesia is more rapid for drugs with high partial pressure in the lungs and high solubility in blood (eg, nitrous oxide, desflurane, sevoflurane). Onset of anesthesia is slowed when pulmonary blood flow is reduced. The site of drug action is the brain; the exact mechanism is unknown but may be related to lipid solubility and activation of GABA$_A$ receptors (enhanced Cl$^-$ influx, hyperpolarization of neurons). Elimination from brain and exhalation from lungs stop the effect of the drug. Redistribution to other tissues delays elimination and may increase occurrence of adverse effects. Intravenous agents include barbiturates, benzodiazepines, ketamine, opioids, and propofol.

Endorphin System

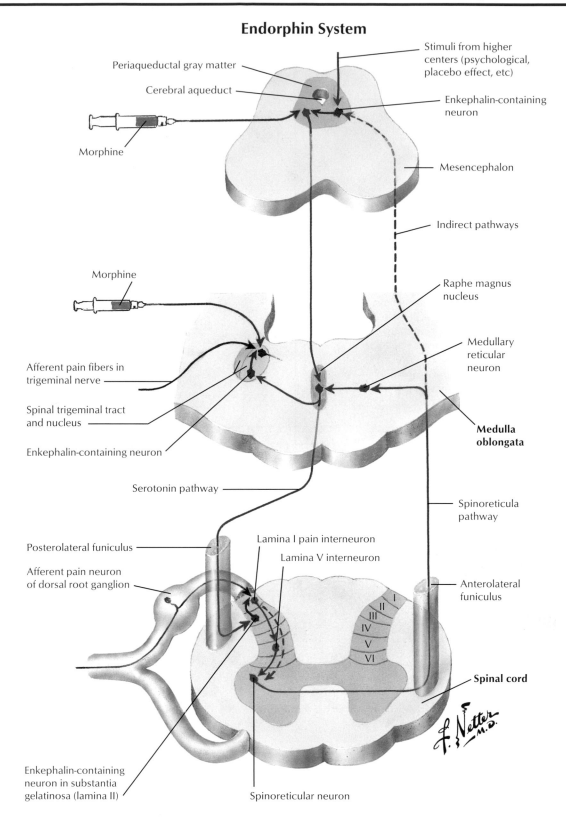

FIGURE 3-28 OPIOIDS: ENDOGENOUS OPIOID PATHWAY

Morphine and related compounds (opioids) mimic the effects of the endogenous opioid neurotransmitters—endorphins and enkephalins. Endogenous opioid receptors are located throughout the pathways that relay the pain signal from its source to higher CNS centers for processing, evaluation, and response (such as via the spinoreticular tract [see Figure 3-25]). Descending pathways, including endogenous opioids, NE, and 5-HT,

modulate the transmission of the incoming pain signal. These pathways can be activated subconsciously or consciously, which may account for a large analgesic placebo effect. Opioids alter the perception of pain. Such modulation of the affective component of pain can improve a patient's quality of life even in the presence of a continuing sensation of pain.

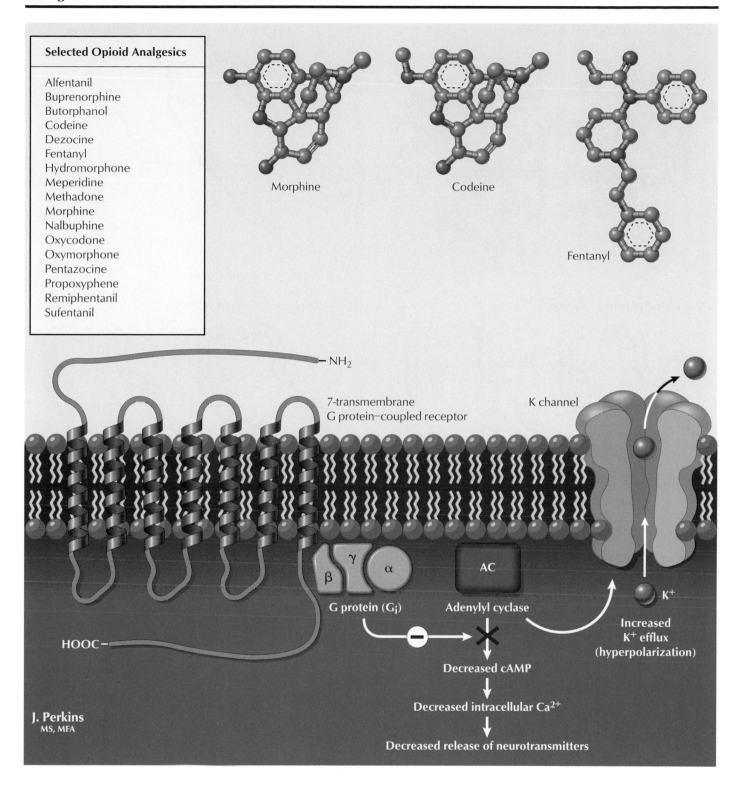

Selected Opioid Analgesics

Alfentanil
Buprenorphine
Butorphanol
Codeine
Dezocine
Fentanyl
Hydromorphone
Meperidine
Methadone
Morphine
Nalbuphine
Oxycodone
Oxymorphone
Pentazocine
Propoxyphene
Remiphentanil
Sufentanil

Morphine

Codeine

Fentanyl

NH$_2$

7-transmembrane
G protein–coupled receptor

K channel

γ

β   α

AC

HOOC—

G protein (G$_i$)

Adenylyl cyclase

K$^+$

Increased
K$^+$ efflux
(hyperpolarization)

Decreased cAMP

Decreased intracellular Ca^{2+}

J. Perkins
MS, MFA

Decreased release of neurotransmitters

FIGURE 3-29 OPIOIDS: RECEPTOR-TRANSDUCTION MECHANISMS

Opioids activate 7-transmembrane GPCRs located presynaptically and postsynaptically along pain transmission pathways. High densities of opioid receptors—known as μ, δ, and κ—are found in the dorsal horn of the spinal cord and higher CNS centers. Most currently used opioid analgesics act mainly at μ-opioid receptors. Opioids have an onset of action that depends on the route of administration and have well-known adverse effects, including constipation, respiratory depression, and abuse

potential. Cellular effects of these drugs involve enhancement of neuronal K$^+$ efflux (hyperpolarizes neurons and makes them less likely to respond to a pain stimulus) and inhibition of Ca^{2+} influx (decreases neurotransmitter release from neurons located along the pain transmission pathway). Brainstem opioid receptors mediate respiratory depression produced by opioid analgesics. Constipation results from activation of opioid receptors in the CNS and in the GI tract.

Cyclooxygenase (COX enzyme) dimer

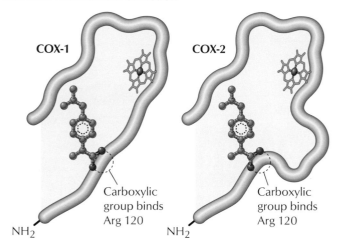

Heme group

Hydrophobic drug-binding channel

Endoplasmic reticulum

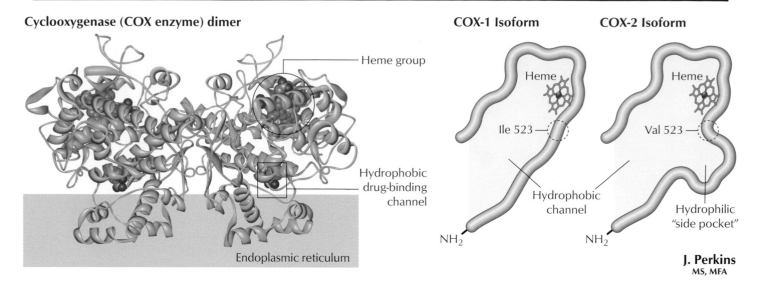

COX-1 Isoform   **COX-2 Isoform**

Heme   Heme

Ile 523   Val 523

Hydrophobic channel

Hydrophilic "side pocket"

NH_2 NH_2

J. Perkins
MS, MFA

NSAIDs: Mechanism of Action

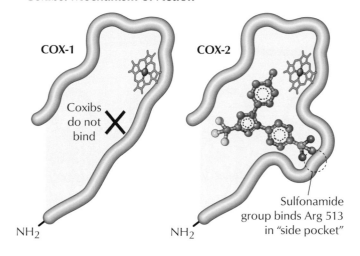

COX-1   COX-2

Carboxylic group binds Arg 120

Carboxylic group binds Arg 120

NH_2 NH_2

Coxibs: Mechanism of Action

COX-1   COX-2

Coxibs do not bind ✕

Sulfonamide group binds Arg 513 in "side pocket"

NH_2 NH_2

NSAIDs

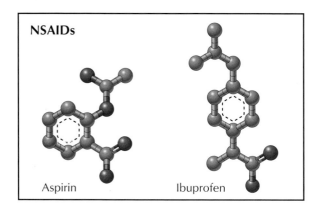

Aspirin   Ibuprofen

Coxibs

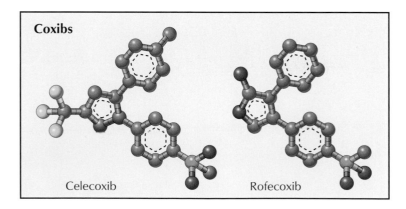

Celecoxib   Rofecoxib

FIGURE 3-30 NONOPIOIDS: NSAIDS, SELECTIVE CYCLOOXYGENASE-2 INHIBITORS, AND ACETAMINOPHEN

Nonsteroidal antiinflammatory drugs have good analgesic efficacy (but often less than that of opioids), relatively rapid onset, and adverse effects (eg, possibly fatal gastrointestinal bleeding and disturbed salt and water balance). All NSAID effects—analgesic, antiinflammatory, antipyretic, and antiplatelet—are thought to be due to decreased prostanoid biosynthesis via COX inhibition. Traditional NSAIDs inhibit both COX-1 and -2 isoforms, but newer COX-2 inhibitors are more selective. The

analgesic efficacy of selective COX-2 inhibitors (coxibs) is approximately equal to that of traditional NSAIDs, but the adverse effects of COX-2 inhibition have yet to be fully characterized and are somewhat controversial. The ability to selectively inhibit COX-2 has been related to the difference in amino acids at position 523 of COX-1 and COX-2: isoleucine in COX-1, valine in COX-2. The mechanism of action of acetaminophen is uncertain but is thought to be via CNS effects.

Aura Phase

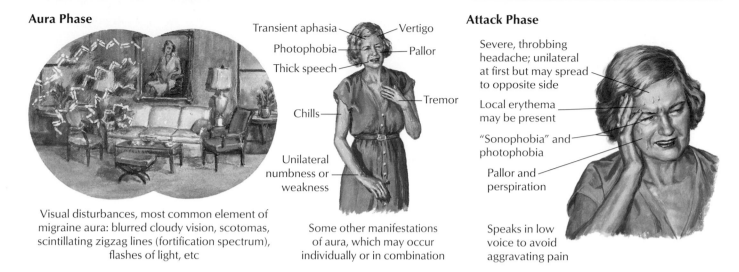

Visual disturbances, most common element of migraine aura: blurred cloudy vision, scotomas, scintillating zigzag lines (fortification spectrum), flashes of light, etc

Transient aphasia — Vertigo
Photophobia — Pallor
Thick speech
— Tremor
Chills
Unilateral numbness or weakness

Some other manifestations of aura, which may occur individually or in combination

Attack Phase

Severe, throbbing headache; unilateral at first but may spread to opposite side

Local erythema may be present

"Sonophobia" and photophobia

Pallor and perspiration

Speaks in low voice to avoid aggravating pain

Pathophysiology of Migraine

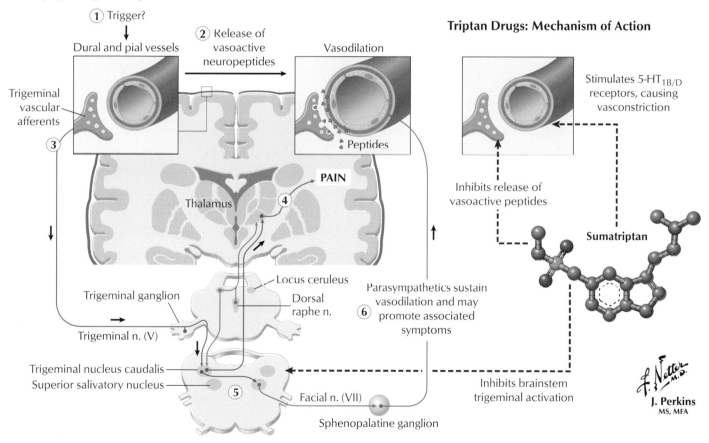

Triptan Drugs: Mechanism of Action

FIGURE 3-31 SUMATRIPTANS AND REUPTAKE INHIBITORS

Certain types of pain are sometimes successfully treated with drugs that are not analgesic for other types of pain. Two examples are sumatriptan and related compounds (triptans) and inhibitors of neuronal reuptake of NE or 5-HT. Triptans (eg, almo-, ele-, frova-, nara-, riza-, and sumatriptan) are often the first-line therapy for treatment of acute severe migraine attacks. Reuptake inhibitors (eg, tricyclics and more selective NF or 5-HT reuptake inhibitors) are used for some patients with migraine and for some patients experiencing neuropathic pain with hyperalgesia (increased sensitivity to painful stimuli) or allodynia (painful sensitivity to nonpainful stimuli). Neither the triptans nor the reuptake inhibitors are very effective against inflammatory or acute pain. Adverse cardiovascular effects can occur with the triptans, and numerous ANS effects can occur with the reuptake inhibitors.

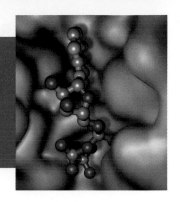

CHAPTER 4

DRUGS USED IN DISORDERS OF THE CARDIOVASCULAR SYSTEM

OVERVIEW

The heart and circulatory system are mechanical marvels that must provide continuous, efficient, and reliable operation while adapting to short- and long-term physiologic changes. As with other organ systems, evolutionary adaptations have resulted in a cardiovascular system that is designed to meet its multiple requirements.

Drugs that are used to treat cardiovascular disorders constitute one of the largest categories of prescription drugs used. Two factors suggest that the use of these drugs will continue to increase: an aging population and the increasing use of drugs as prevention against future cardiovascular disease. These 2 factors work synergistically: as preventive care increases the average lifespan, the population has a greater risk of cardiovascular disease, and as life expectancy increases, greater emphasis is placed on earlier preventive intervention.

Certain cardiovascular disorders, such as cardiac arrhythmias and congestive heart failure (CHF), produce symptoms that are readily apparent to the person affected and have consequences long known to necessitate treatment. Other conditions, however, do not produce obvious symptoms and have become recognized as health problems only as a result of epidemiologic studies in relatively recent years. For example, blood pressures that had been considered normal because they were average (the age-appropriate mean) are now widely considered to fall into the hypertension category and are routinely treated with medication. Even more recently, cholesterol levels that were once

deemed normal (or were even thought to be so insignificant that they went unmeasured) are now routinely treated with drugs.

For many years, the treatment of cardiovascular disorders primarily targeted the innervation of the heart and blood vessels by the 2 subclassifications of the ANS. Parasympathetic innervation of the heart is principally via the vagus nerve (cranial nerve X) and is mediated by the action of acetylcholine (ACh) at muscarinic cholinergic receptors. Sympathetic innervation of the heart is mediated principally by the action of norepinephrine (NE) on β adrenoceptors (more specifically, the β_1 subtype). The vasculature is controlled in a site-dependent manner by the parasympathetic subdivision mediated by ACh, which usually causes vasodilation, and by the sympathetic subclassification mediated by NE, which generally causes vasoconstriction. Hormones and local factors also contribute to overall vascular tone.

A major advance in treatment strategies for cardiovascular disorders occurred as a result of recognition of the significant contributions made by other neurotransmitter and hormone systems to normal and pathologic cardiovascular function. Targeting these systems, such as the renin-angiotensin system, has led to a broader variety of treatment options.

Cardiovascular drugs include some of the oldest medications, discovered by serendipity, and some of the newest, discovered by molecular modeling and screening technology. They include a wide variety of receptor agonists, receptor antagonists, and enzyme inhibitors.

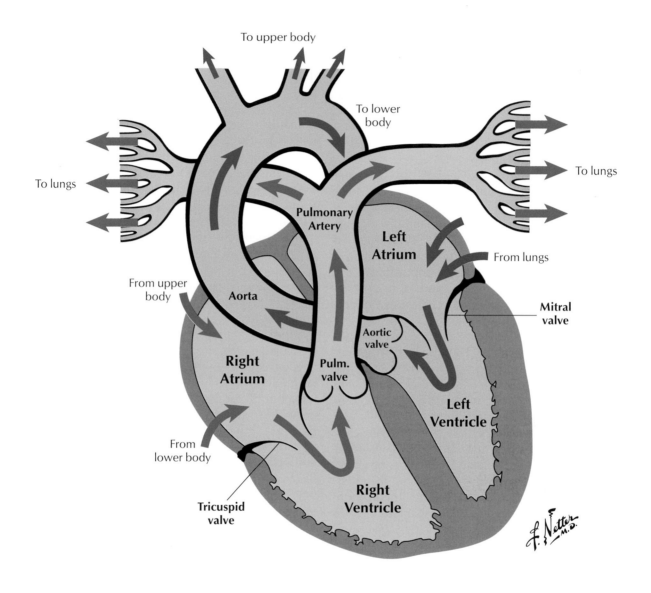

FIGURE 4-1 CARDIOVASCULAR FUNCTION: ANATOMY

The heart muscle pumps blood through the circulatory system. Each day, the heart beats 100,000 times and pumps 2000 gal of blood. The heart is composed of 4 chambers (divisions): the upper two, the right and left atria; the lower two, the right and left ventricles. Blood is pumped through the chambers, in only 1 direction, via 4 valves: the tricuspid, located between the right atrium and the right ventricle; the pulmonary, between the right ventricle and the pulmonary artery; the mitral, between the left atrium and the left ventricle; and the aortic, between the left ventricle and the aorta. Dark blood, low in oxygen, returns from body tissues through veins, enters the right atrium, and then flows to the right ventricle, the pulmonary artery, and the lungs, where it is oxygenated. Blood returns by pulmonary veins to the left atrium and goes through the mitral valve into the left ventricle, which pumps oxygen-rich, bright-red blood through the aortic valve into the aorta and then into the circulation.

Mechanism of Heart Adjustment to Body-Perfusion Requirements

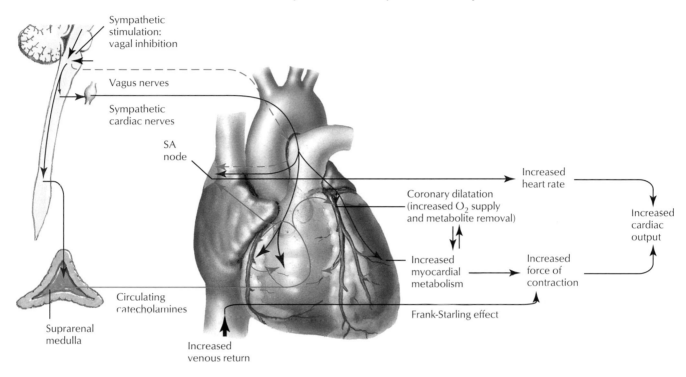

Effects of Resting Tension, Coronary Blood Flow, and Norepinephrine on Myocardial Contraction

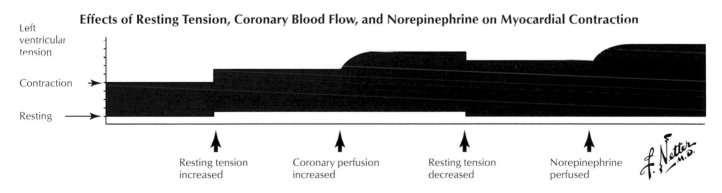

FIGURE 4-2 CARDIOVASCULAR FUNCTION: DEFINITION OF TERMS AND REGULATION

Cardiac output is the total blood volume pumped by ventricles per minute (heart rate × stroke volume). *Stroke volume* is the blood pumped by the left or right ventricle per beat; in a resting adult, it averages 60 to 80 mL of blood. *Systole* is the contraction phase of the cardiac cycle, when ventricles pump stroke volumes. *Diastole* is the resting phase of the cycle, which occurs between heartbeats. *End-diastolic volume* is the blood volume in each ventricle at the end of diastole: 120 mL at rest. *End-systolic*

volume is the blood volume in each ventricle after contraction: 50 mL at rest. To maintain equal flow through pulmonary and systemic circuits, the left and right ventricles maintain the same cardiac output. The resting cardiac output is 4.8 to 6.4 L/min. Cardiac output increases (20-85%) during intense exercise to transport more oxygen to muscles. This greater blood flow is caused by higher blood pressure and arteriolar vasodilation in muscles, which is due to smooth muscle relaxation.

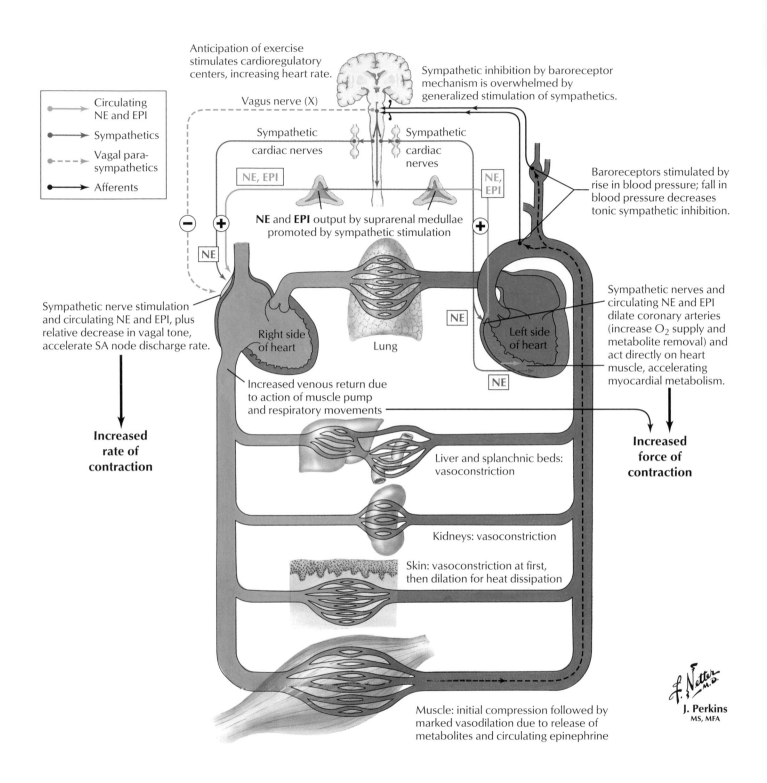

Anticipation of exercise stimulates cardioregulatory centers, increasing heart rate.

Sympathetic inhibition by baroreceptor mechanism is overwhelmed by generalized stimulation of sympathetics.

Vagus nerve (X)

Circulating NE and EPI

Sympathetics

Vagal para-sympathetics

Afferents

Sympathetic cardiac nerves

Sympathetic cardiac nerves

NE, EPI

NE, EPI

Baroreceptors stimulated by rise in blood pressure; fall in blood pressure decreases tonic sympathetic inhibition.

NE and EPI output by suprarenal medullae promoted by sympathetic stimulation

NE

Sympathetic nerve stimulation and circulating NE and EPI, plus relative decrease in vagal tone, accelerate SA node discharge rate.

Right side of heart

Lung

NE

Left side of heart

NE

Sympathetic nerves and circulating NE and EPI dilate coronary arteries (increase O_2 supply and metabolite removal) and act directly on heart muscle, accelerating myocardial metabolism.

Increased rate of contraction

Increased venous return due to action of muscle pump and respiratory movements

Increased force of contraction

Liver and splanchnic beds: vasoconstriction

Kidneys: vasoconstriction

Skin: vasoconstriction at first, then dilation for heat dissipation

J. Perkins
MS, MFA

Muscle: initial compression followed by marked vasodilation due to release of metabolites and circulating epinephrine

FIGURE 4-3 ROLE OF CATECHOLAMINES IN HEART FUNCTION

Norepinephrine and epinephrine (EPI), major catecholamine regulators of heart function, are released by the adrenal medulla after activation of preganglionic sympathetic nerves, which occurs during stress (eg, exercise, heart failure, pain). More EPI (85%) than NE (15%) is released. A second source of NE is that from sympathetic nerves, especially those innervating cardiac pacemaker cells. The sympathetic effects increase heart rate and contraction force by activating β_1 adrenoceptors; vasoconstriction in systemic arteries and veins by activating α-adrenoceptors; vasodilation in skeletal muscle at low concentrations by activating β_2 receptors; and vasoconstriction at high concentrations by activating α_1 receptors. The overall cardiovascular response is greater cardiac output plus a small mean arterial pressure change. EPI release has similar cardiac effects. Heart rate, first increased by NE, usually decreases because of baroceptor activation and vagal-mediated heart rate slowing.

Neural and Humoral Regulation of Cardiac Function

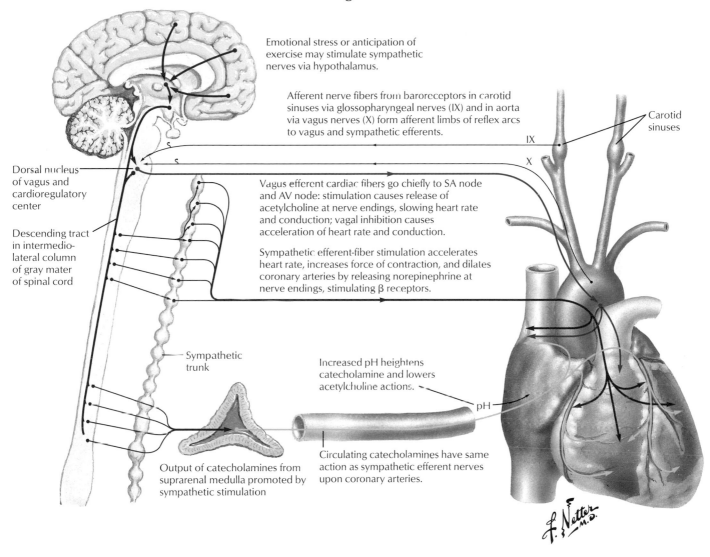

Emotional stress or anticipation of exercise may stimulate sympathetic nerves via hypothalamus.

Afferent nerve fibers from baroreceptors in carotid sinuses via glossopharyngeal nerves (IX) and in aorta via vagus nerves (X) form afferent limbs of reflex arcs to vagus and sympathetic efferents.

IX

X

Carotid sinuses

Dorsal nucleus of vagus and cardioregulatory center

Descending tract in intermediolateral column of gray mater of spinal cord

Vagus efferent cardiac fibers go chiefly to SA node and AV node: stimulation causes release of acetylcholine at nerve endings, slowing heart rate and conduction; vagal inhibition causes acceleration of heart rate and conduction.

Sympathetic efferent-fiber stimulation accelerates heart rate, increases force of contraction, and dilates coronary arteries by releasing norepinephrine at nerve endings, stimulating β receptors.

Sympathetic trunk

Increased pH heightens catecholamine and lowers acetylcholine actions.

pH

Output of catecholamines from suprarenal medulla promoted by sympathetic stimulation

Circulating catecholamines have same action as sympathetic efferent nerves upon coronary arteries.

FIGURE 4-4 SYMPATHETIC AND PARASYMPATHETIC REGULATION OF HEART FUNCTION

Sympathetic and parasympathetic systems innervate the heart and regulate function. Activation of the former increases heart rate and contraction force by increasing EPI and NE release. The latter system stimulates ACh release and reduces heart rate. The pacemaker cells of the SA node depolarize and promote atrial contraction. Ventricular contraction is due to impulses going from the AV node to the AV bundle to Purkinje fibers. Increased sympathetic drive activates β_1 receptors in the SA node and increases pacemaker cell depolarization rate, heart rate, and contraction strength. Parasympathetic impulses (through vagus nerves) reduce heart rate, AV node conduction, and contraction force. Increased ACh release and muscarinic M_2 receptor activation mediate these effects. M_2 receptor activation reduces cellular cAMP levels and increases K^+ conductance, which leads to pacemaker cell hyperpolarization. Reduced heart rate and contraction force result.

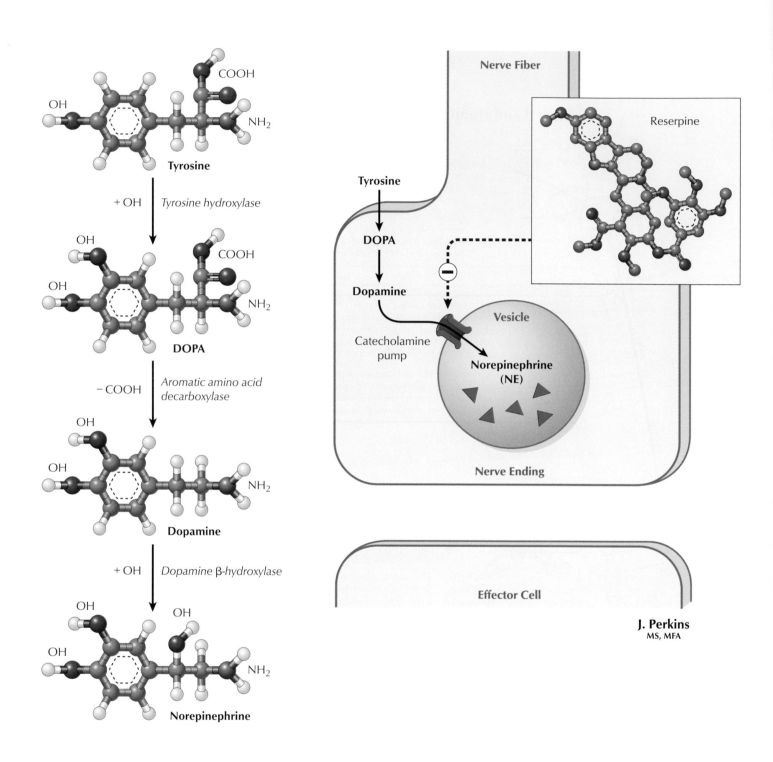

FIGURE 4-5 SYNTHESIS AND STORAGE OF CATECHOLAMINES

Norepinephrine synthesis starts with the amino acid tyrosine. Catecholaminergic nerves obtain it by active transport; tyrosine hydroxylase adds a hydroxyl group to form the catechol part of the molecule. Tyrosine hydroxylation is the rate-limiting step in catecholamine synthesis and is regulated by feedback inhibition. The product dihydroxyphenylalanine (dopa) is converted by aromatic amino acid decarboxylase into dopamine, one of 3 naturally occurring catecholamines. Dopamine enters synaptic vesicles via a catecholamine pump and is converted to NE by addition of a hydroxyl group. Synaptic vesicle catecholamine levels are much higher than surrounding cytosolic levels. Reserpine is a drug that inhibits the vesicular catecholamine pump, thus stopping vesicular catecholamine uptake and reducing catecholamine levels. The low cytosolic catecholamine level in nerves is maintained by the vesicular amine uptake pump and by mitochondrial monoamine oxidase, which degrades catecholamines.

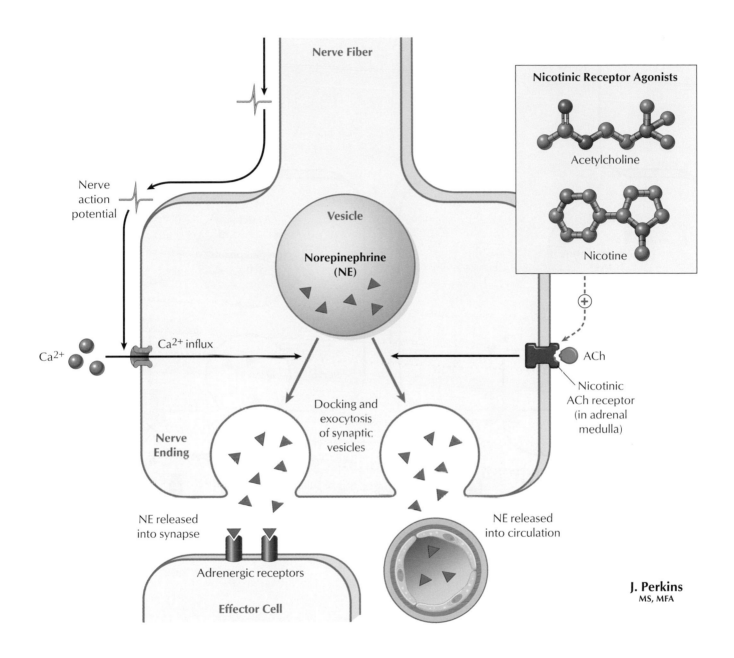

FIGURE 4-6 REGULATION OF NOREPINEPHRINE RELEASE

Vesicular release of NE depends on depolarization of the nerve terminal and the influx of Ca^{2+} ions. The influx of Ca^{2+} promotes the docking of synaptic vesicles at the plasma membrane and subsequent exocytosis of the vesicles. In the adrenal medulla, ACh acting as the neurotransmitter of the sympathetic ganglion acts on nicotinic receptors and promotes the release of catecholamines into the circulation. Certain drugs can also promote catecholamine release. Under certain experimental conditions, it is possible to mimic this nicotinic effect of ACh not only at the adrenal medulla, but at also at the sympathetic ganglia. Thus, activation of cholinergic receptors by nicotinic agonists evokes substantial catecholamine release from postganglionic neurons and the adrenal medulla.

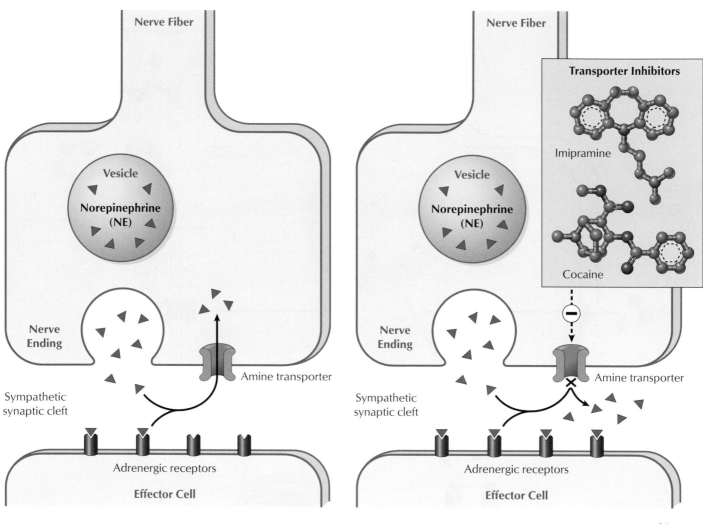

J. Perkins
MS, MFA

FIGURE 4-7 INACTIVATION OF NOREPINEPHRINE

The primary NE inactivation mechanism is reuptake via a plasma membrane amine transporter, the amine uptake pump. This transporter is a member of a family of membrane proteins that transport different transmitter substances across the plasma membrane of the nerve terminal. The amine uptake transporter is driven indirectly by a sodium gradient, is selective for NE and EPI, and is inhibited by cocaine and tricyclic antidepressants such as imipramine. NE uptake is a major mechanism for ending sympathetic nerve transmission. Inhibitors of the amine transporter potentiate responses to stimulation of the sympathetic nervous system or to injected compounds that are taken up by sympathetic nerve terminals. In a sympathetically innervated tissue, such as the heart, the major uptake of catecholamines is neuronal uptake.

Hypercholesterolemia
Cholesterol Synthesis and Metabolism

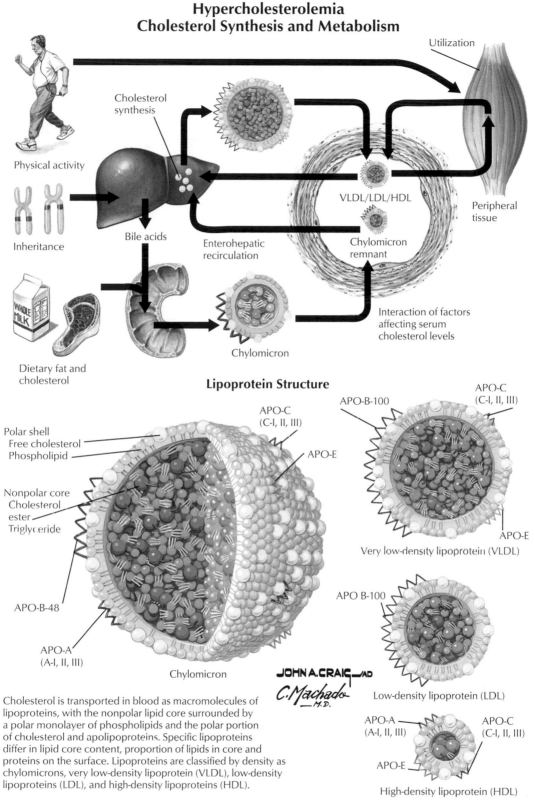

Cholesterol is transported in blood as macromolecules of lipoproteins, with the nonpolar lipid core surrounded by a polar monolayer of phospholipids and the polar portion of cholesterol and apolipoproteins. Specific lipoproteins differ in lipid core content, proportion of lipids in core and proteins on the surface. Lipoproteins are classified by density as chylomicrons, very low-density lipoprotein (VLDL), low-density lipoproteins (LDL), and high-density lipoproteins (HDL).

FIGURE 4-8 HYPERCHOLESTEROLEMIA: CAUSES

Cholesterol, a simple lipid found in cell membranes, is a precursor of steroids, bile acids, and vitamin D and a major part of atherosclerotic plaques. Most circulating blood cholesterol is synthesized from liver acetyl CoA and is excreted as bile salts. Only 25% of blood cholesterol is from the diet, but high-fat diets increase liver cholesterol production and blood cholesterol levels. HMG-CoA formation from HMG-CoA reductase, the rate-determining step in cholesterol synthesis, is regulated via feedback inhibition. When cholesterol uptake is low, the liver and small intestine increase cholesterol synthesis. The plaque-forming ability of cholesterol is related to LDLs, which promote plaque formation; HDLs remove cholesterol from arteries and transport it to the liver. HDLs remove cholesterol from plaques and slow atherosclerosis. Control of cholesterol and LDL levels is a major goal in heart disease therapy.

Hypercholesterolemia
General Management Measures
Dietary Management

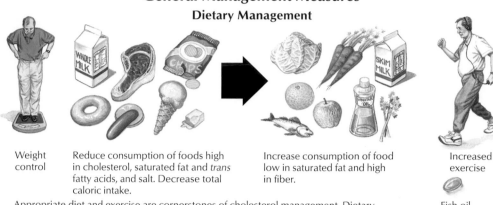

Weight control

Reduce consumption of foods high in cholesterol, saturated fat and *trans* fatty acids, and salt. Decrease total caloric intake.

Increase consumption of food low in saturated fat and high in fiber.

Increased exercise

Fish oil supplements

Appropriate diet and exercise are cornerstones of cholesterol management. Dietary counseling and reinforcement and a planned program of physical activity are recommended.

Actions of Lipid-Lowering Medications

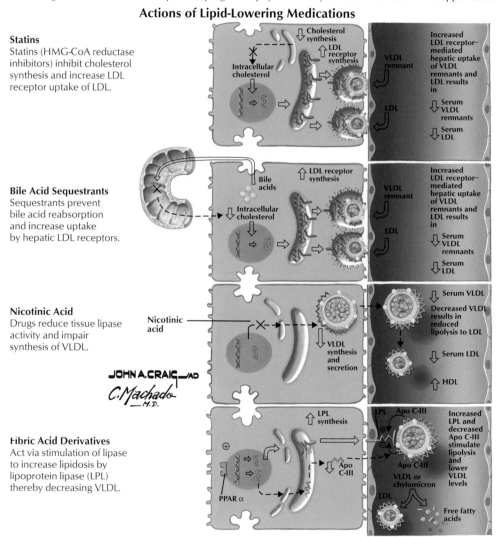

Statins
Statins (HMG-CoA reductase inhibitors) inhibit cholesterol synthesis and increase LDL receptor uptake of LDL.

Bile Acid Sequestrants
Sequestrants prevent bile acid reabsorption and increase uptake by hepatic LDL receptors.

Nicotinic Acid
Drugs reduce tissue lipase activity and impair synthesis of VLDL.

Fibric Acid Derivatives
Act via stimulation of lipase to increase lipidosis by lipoprotein lipase (LPL) thereby decreasing VLDL.

JOHN A. CRAIG ᴀᴅ
C. Machado ―ᴍ.ᴅ.

FIGURE 4-9 HYPERCHOLESTEROLEMIA: PHARMACOLOGIC THERAPY

Primary goals of therapy are lower LDL levels and higher HDL levels. The best drugs for such therapy are statins: lovastatin, fluvastatin, pravastatin, simvastatin, and atorvastatin. They interfere with the cholesterol production of the liver by blocking HMG-CoA synthesis, so the liver can better remove cholesterol from circulating blood. Statins lower LDL cholesterol by 60%; side effects can occur. Nicotinic acid (or niacin) lowers total and LDL cholesterol and raises HDL cholesterol levels, but it can be toxic because the therapeutic dose is 100-fold greater than the recommended daily allowance. Resins (eg, cholestyramine and colestipol) bind intestinal bile acids and prevent recycling through the liver. The liver needs cholesterol to make bile, so it increases uptake of cholesterol from blood. Fibric acid derivatives decrease triglyceride and increase HDL levels. Low doses of aspirin block platelet thromboxane A_2 synthesis, which leads to reduced platelet aggregation and blood viscosity.

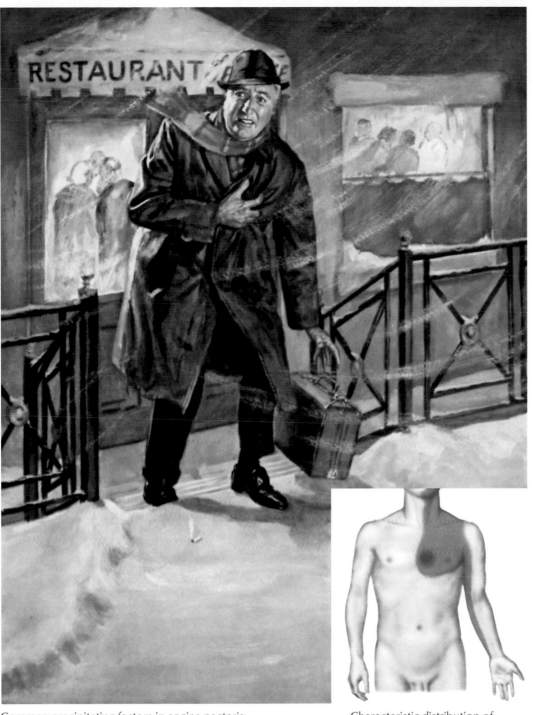

Common precipitating factors in angina pectoris: exertion, heavy meal, cold, smoking

Characteristic distribution of pain in angina pectoris

FIGURE 4-10 ANGINA OVERVIEW

Angina, or *angina pectoris*, is a gripping pain felt in the center of the chest that may move to the neck, jaw, and arms and is caused most often by exercise; emotion, eating, and cold weather are other causes. It occurs when the heart receives deficient oxygen because of blood vessel narrowing, which results mainly from aging and also from cigarette smoking, high cholesterol levels, obesity, and diabetes. The 3 types are stable angina (exertional or typical angina), caused by atherosclerosis, with treatment to reduce cardiac load and increase myocardial blood flow; vasospastic angina (variant or Prinzmetal angina), caused by severe coronary vessel contraction, with chest pain at rest and drugs aimed to stop vasospasm; and unstable angina (crescendo angina), in which pain occurs without stress. Nitrates and β blockers are used, as are calcium channel antagonists if the mechanism is vasospasm. Reducing platelet function and thrombotic episodes helps decrease mortality in unstable angina.

Nitrate Drugs

Drug	Duration of Action
"Short acting"	
Nitroglycerin, sublingual	10-30 minutes
Isosorbide dinitrate, sublingual	10-60 minutes
Amyl nitrate, inhalant	3-5 minutes
"Long acting"	
Nitroglycerin, oral sustained-action	6-8 hours
Nitroglycerin, 2% ointment	3-6 hours
Nitroglycerin, slow release, buccal	3-6 hours
Nitroglycerin, slow release, transdermal	8-10 hours
Isosorbide dinitrate, sublingual	1.5-2 hours
Isosorbide dinitrate, oral	4-6 hours
Isosorbide dinitrate, chewable	2-3 hours
Isosorbide mononitrate	6-10 hours

Side Effects

Headache, tachycardia (abnormal elevation in heart rate), orthostatic hypotension, facial flushing, and tolerance; contraindicated with sildenafil

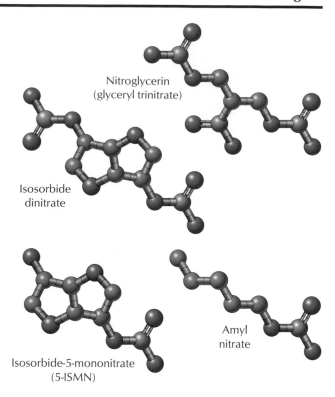

Nitroglycerin (glyceryl trinitrate)

Isosorbide dinitrate

Isosorbide-5-mononitrate (5-ISMN)

Amyl nitrate

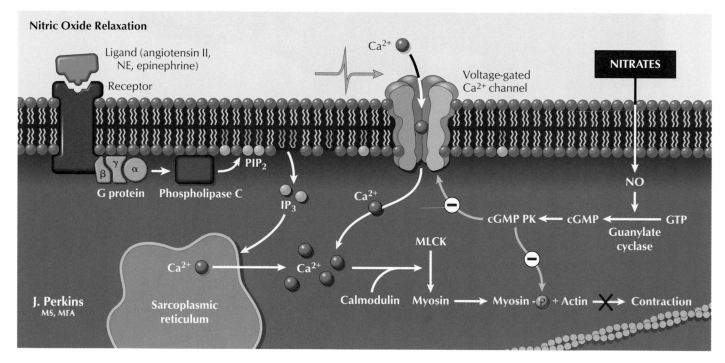

Nitric Oxide Relaxation

FIGURE 4-11 NITRATES FOR ANGINA TREATMENT: CLASSES, ADMINISTRATION ROUTES, PHARMACOLOGY, AND ADVERSE EFFECTS

Organic nitrates are known as *nitrovasodilators*. The most commonly used nitrates are GTN, isosorbide dinitrate, and 5-ISMN. Another group of agents, organic nitrites (eg, amyl nitrite, isobutyl nitrite), contain the nitrite functional group. The final class of drugs—NO-containing agents (nitroglycerin, nitroprusside)—are often classed as organic nitrates, although the chemical structure differs, because of similar pharmacologic effects. Oral GTN is completely absorbed but undergoes extensive first-pass metabolism in the liver; dinitrate metabolites likely produce the therapeutic effects. 5-ISMN avoids first-pass metabolism and is 100% available orally. Sublingual dosing relieves acute attacks, whereas long-acting drugs (oral, transdermal) with a slow onset of action are used for prolonged prophylaxis. Loss of nitrate efficacy caused by tolerance can be reversed by use of sulfhydryl-yielding agents such as *N*-acetylcysteine.

Atherogenesis: Unstable Plaque Formation

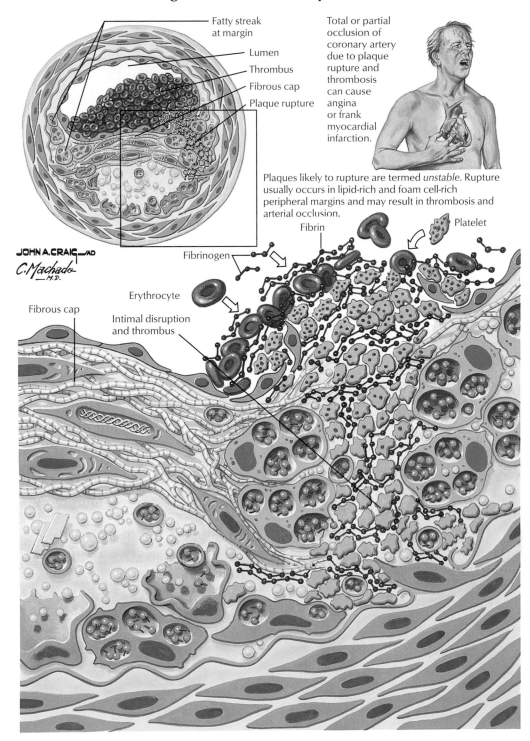

Fatty streak at margin

Lumen

Thrombus

Fibrous cap

Plaque rupture

Total or partial occlusion of coronary artery due to plaque rupture and thrombosis can cause angina or frank myocardial infarction.

Plaques likely to rupture are termed *unstable*. Rupture usually occurs in lipid-rich and foam cell-rich peripheral margins and may result in thrombosis and arterial occlusion.

Fibrin

Platelet

Fibrinogen

Erythrocyte

Fibrous cap

Intimal disruption and thrombus

JOHN A. CRAIG—MD

C. Machado —M.D.

FIGURE 4-12 NITROGLYCERIN IN ANGINA TREATMENT

Drugs that relax blood vessels, reduce the heart's workload, and increase the amount of oxygenated blood to the heart are used for angina. Drugs are given long-term to reduce the number of attacks, just before certain activities to prevent acute attacks, and during attacks to relieve pain and pressure. Nitroglycerin (short-acting, long-acting, or intravenous form) is indicated for angina, AMI, and CHF. By releasing NO, nitroglycerin promotes venous dilation, inhibits venous return and cardiac preload, reduces intraventricular work, dilates large coronary arteries, and reduces systemic vascular resistance. Adverse effects include hypotension and headache. Nitroglycerin is more effective than nitroprusside, a similar organic nitrate, in reducing venous return but is less effective in expanding arteries. Nitroglycerin should not be used with sildenafil because of possible marked hypotension; it also interferes with anticoagulant actions of heparin.

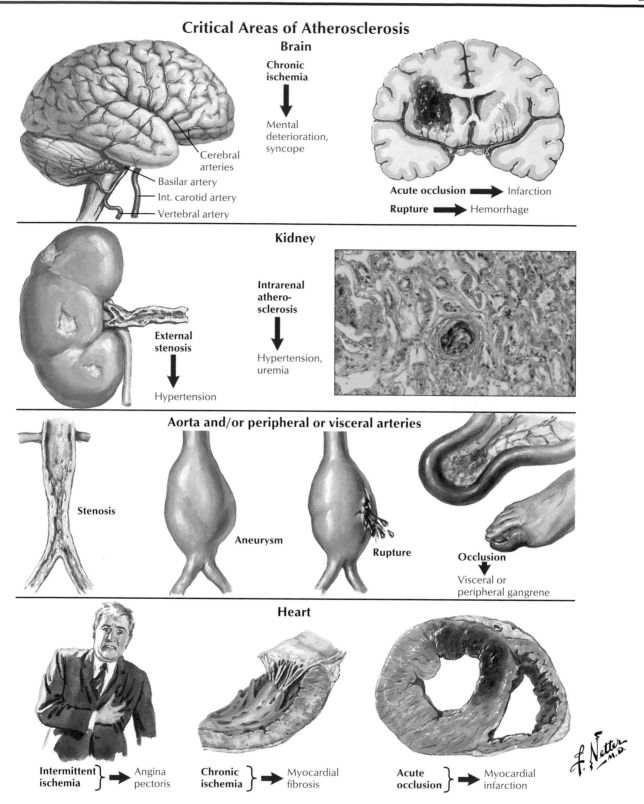

Critical Areas of Atherosclerosis

Brain

Chronic ischemia → Mental deterioration, syncope

Acute occlusion → Infarction

Rupture → Hemorrhage

Kidney

Intrarenal athero-sclerosis → Hypertension, uremia

External stenosis → Hypertension

Aorta and/or peripheral or visceral arteries

Stenosis

Aneurysm

Rupture

Occlusion → Visceral or peripheral gangrene

Heart

Intermittent ischemia → Angina pectoris

Chronic ischemia → Myocardial fibrosis

Acute occlusion → Myocardial infarction

FIGURE 4-13 NITROGLYCERIN: MECHANISM OF ACTION

Nitroglycerin produces vasodilation by releasing NO, which promotes blood vessel relaxation in cardiovascular and nervous systems. Drugs that release or induce NO release are important in treating hypertension, heart attacks, and other blood flow diseases. Heart attacks are caused by spasms or narrowing of blood vessels and occur when the blood cannot flow through the heart. NO relaxes the blood vessels and allows them to widen, thus increasing blood flow. NO released by nitroglycerin diffuses into cells and activates soluble guanylyl cyclase. This enzyme synthesizes the second messenger, cGMP, from GTP. cGMP modulates activity of protein kinase G, 2 cyclic nucleotide phosphodiesterases (PDE-2 and -3), and several ion channels. NO can also act through protein nitrosylation, interaction with transition metals, and direct modification of DNA. Thus, nitroglycerin promotes vasodilation and relief of the pressure associated with angina by activating the NO-cGMP pathway.

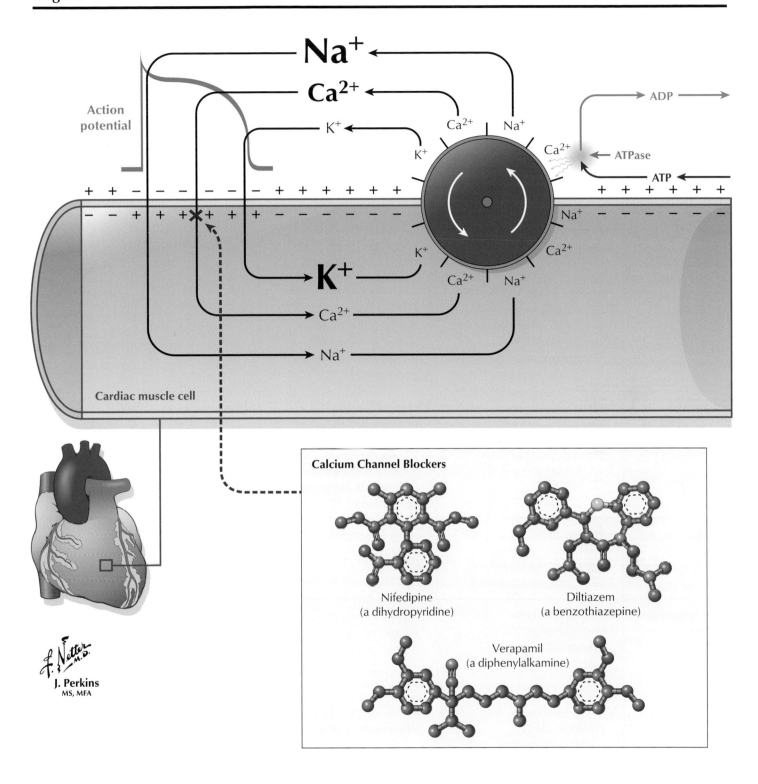

FIGURE 4-14   CALCIUM CHANNEL ANTAGONISTS

Calcium channel blockers (CCBs) reduce Ca^{2+} flow into heart cells by blocking L-type voltage-dependent calcium channels, which suppresses depolarization and reduces Ca^{2+}-dependent conduction in the heart. Ca^{2+} binds to calmodulin in smooth muscle and troponin in the heart and affects muscle contraction. CCBs block these processes, thus reducing contraction. Three classes of CCBs are dihydropyridines (nifedipine, nimodipine, nicardipine), phenylalkylamines (verapamil), and benzothiazepines (diltiazem).

Blockade of slow calcium channels by the latter 2 drugs can have negative inotropic effects and thus reduce SA or AV conduction rate. Results are negative inotropic (force of contraction), chronotropic (rate), and dromotropic (conduction) effects. CCBs reduce afterload (not preload), coronary vascular resistance, and workload; help with oxygen delivery; and increase coronary blood flow. Adverse effects include vasodilation, hypotension, cardiovascular events, GI bleeding, and cancer.

Summary of Pharmacologic Treatment of Patients
With Chronic Stable Angina

Medication	Dosage	Which Patients?	Effect on Cardiovascular Clinical End Points
Aspirin	80-325 mg qd	All patients with vascular disease	Decreases the risk of death, myocardial infarction, and stroke
Statin drugs	Varies depending on particular drug	If LDL >130; all patients who have extensive vascular disease. In patients with known CAD, LDL >100	Decreases the risk of death in patients who have had a prior myocardial infarction
ACE inhibitors	Varies depending on particular drug; initial dosage will depend on blood pressure	All patients with vascular disease (in particular, any patient with vascular disease and hypertension or diabetes)	In the HOPE trial, ramipril 10 mg/qd reduced the rate of death, MI, and stroke in patients with vascular disease
β Blockers	Begin at low dose (eg, metoprolol 6.25 or 12.5 mg bid) and titrate depending on heart rate and blood pressure	Patients with prior myocardial infarction or with cardiomyopathy (caution is needed when initiating β blockers in patients with congestive heart failure)	Decreases the risk of death in patients who have had a prior myocardial infarction and improves outcomes in patients with dilated cardiomyopathy
Nitrates	Sublingual or buccal spray can be used prn; longer acting oral and transdermal formulations are available	Patients with anginal symptoms	None
Calcium channel blockers	Varies depending on particular drug; initial dosage will depend on blood pressure and heart rate	Patients with anginal symptoms	No beneficial effect; nifedipine worsens survival in acute coronary syndromes; diltiazem worsens survival in left ventricular dysfunction
Warfarin	Varies depending on response; needs continual monitoring	Useful in selected patients with vascular disease	A meta-analysis demonstrates reduction in the risk of death, MI, or stroke if INR >2 and used with concurrent ASA; bleeding increased by 1.9-fold

FIGURE 4-15 DRUG SUMMARY FOR ANGINA

The aim of pharmacologic therapy for angina has changed from relieving symptoms to affecting survival. Drugs that improve survival and reduce the number of cardiovascular events include aspirin and statin drugs (HMG-CoA reductase inhibitors; eg, lovastatin); β blockers (eg, propranolol, metoprolol) reduce mortality in patients with previous myocardial infarction or left ventricular dysfunction. ACE inhibitors (eg, enalapril, captopril) are recommended when β blockers and diuretics are contraindicated, ineffective, or not tolerated. Nitrates (eg, nitroglycerin) and CCBs (eg, diltiazem) are used to treat symptoms without affecting survival. Warfarin can reduce the risk of serious cardiac events or death.

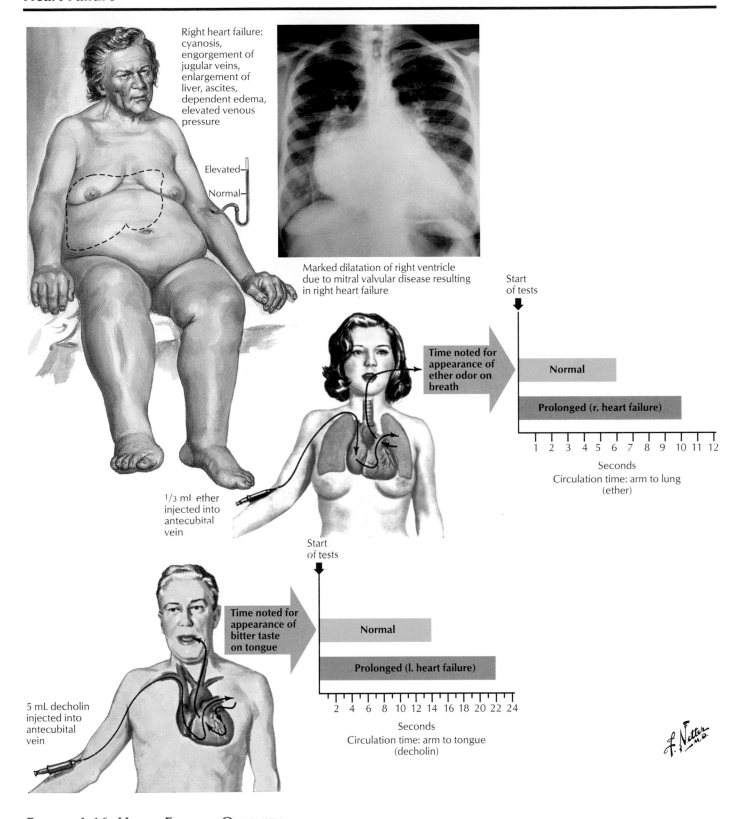

Right heart failure: cyanosis, engorgement of jugular veins, enlargement of liver, ascites, dependent edema, elevated venous pressure

Elevated—

Normal—

Marked dilatation of right ventricle due to mitral valvular disease resulting in right heart failure

Start of tests

Time noted for appearance of ether odor on breath

Normal

Prolonged (r. heart failure)

1 2 3 4 5 6 7 8 9 10 11 12
Seconds
Circulation time: arm to lung (ether)

1/3 ml ether injected into antecubital vein

Start of tests

Time noted for appearance of bitter taste on tongue

Normal

Prolonged (l. heart failure)

2 4 6 8 10 12 14 16 18 20 22 24
Seconds
Circulation time: arm to tongue (decholin)

5 mL decholin injected into antecubital vein

FIGURE 4-16 HEART FAILURE OVERVIEW

In heart failure, the most common cause of hospital stays of patients older than 65 years, the heart and circulation cannot meet peripheral metabolic demands while sustaining normal filling pressure. *Systolic failure* is the inability of the ventricle to empty normally; *diastolic dysfunction* is the inability of the ventricle to fill properly. Aging, smoking, obesity, fats, cholesterol, inactivity, viruses, and genetic defects promote heart failure; risk is also increased by hypertension and diabetes. Accumulation of fatty deposits in heart arteries leads to coronary artery disease. The normal heart tissue works harder because less blood is available. Previous myocardial infarctions cause oxygen and nutrient loss and heart damage. Abnormal heart valves that do not open or close completely during each heartbeat increase the workload. In COPD, abnormal lung function causes the heart to work harder to get oxygen to the body. Heart failure results when the workload is too great.

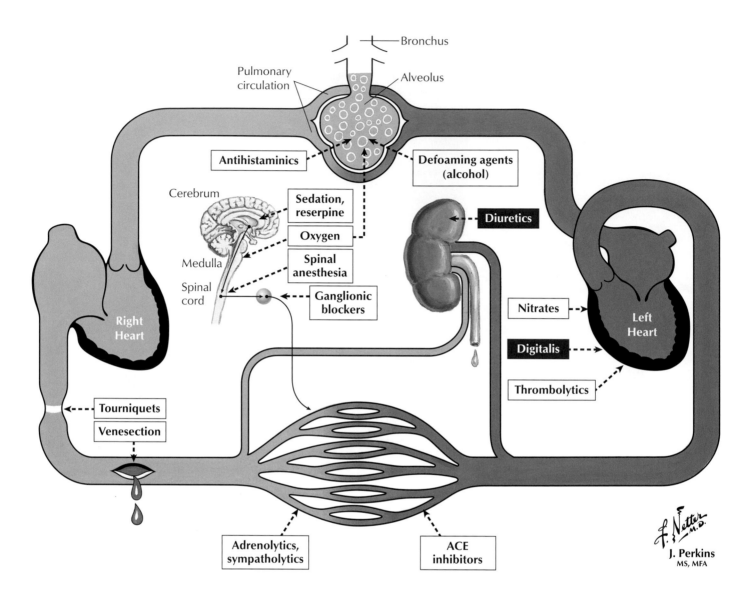

Digitalis (a glycoside)

--- Sugar

FIGURE 4-17 HEART FAILURE: TREATMENT

Heart failure caused by excessive workload is cured by treating the primary disease (eg, thyrotoxicosis); surgery can help that related to anatomical problems. Acute myocardial infarction (AMI) results when reduced blood supply to the heart, caused by thrombus, leads to insufficient cardiac oxygen supply. The most common forms of heart failure—caused by damaged heart muscle—are treated with drugs to improve quality of life and survival. Combinations of at least 2 drugs are usually given.

Diuretics reduce the amount of body fluid by decreasing salt and water retention. Glycosides increase heart contractility and contraction force by activating Na^+-K^+ pumps on heart cells. ACE inhibitors improve survival and slow the loss of heart-pumping activity by reducing blood pressure and workload. Organic nitrates are used when ACE inhibitors cannot be given. For AMI, thrombolytic drugs (eg, alteplase) or plasminogen activators produce plasmin and dissolve blood clots by digesting fibrin.

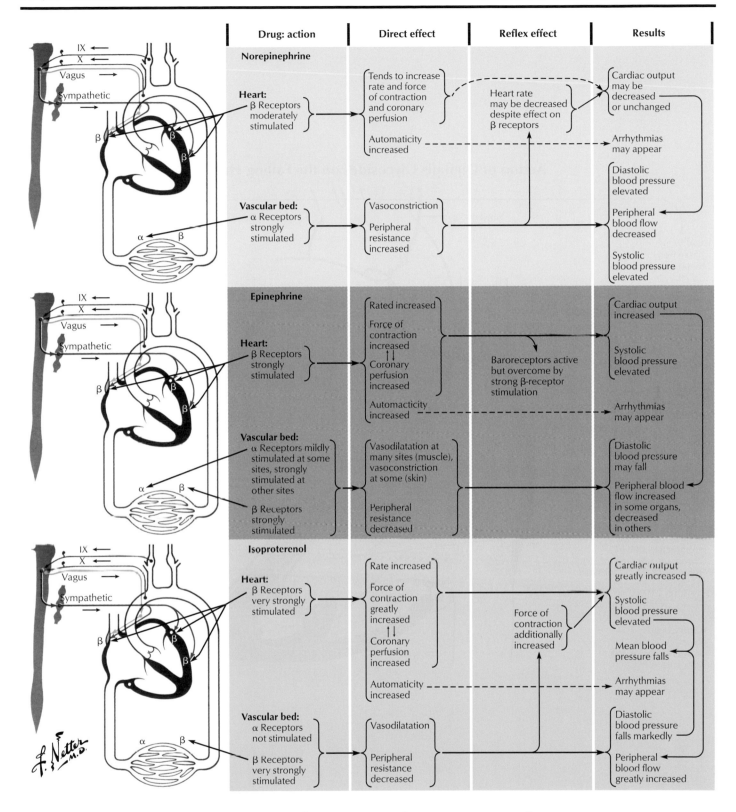

FIGURE 4-18 HEART FAILURE TREATMENT: β-ADRENERGIC STIMULATORS AND BLOCKERS

β-Receptor activation augments sympathetic output, which increases heart contraction and rate. β Blockers blunt these actions. They block β₁-receptor activation by NE and EPI, thus reducing heart contractility and heart rate. β Blockers such as propranolol are especially useful for exertional angina but are ineffective against vasospastic angina. They are used in combination with calcium channel antagonists (eg, dihydropyridines, verapamil, diltiazem), organic nitrates, or both to treat cardiac symptoms that are resistant to a single drug. Because dihydropyridines do not alter SA or AV nodal conduction, they do not enhance the adverse effect of propranolol. Triple therapy (coadministration of 3 drugs) is sometimes used. The decrease in preload by nitrates, afterload by CCBs, and heart rate by β blockers is effective for treatment of angina that is not controlled by 2 types of antianginal agents. Dihydropyridines, but not diltiazem and verapamil, can be used in such a combination.

Action of Digitalis Glycosides on the Failing Heart

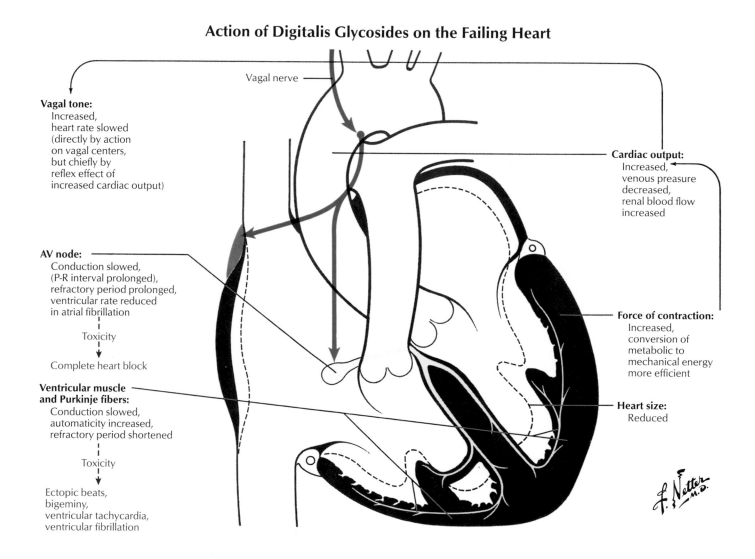

Vagal nerve

Vagal tone:
Increased,
heart rate slowed
(directly by action
on vagal centers,
but chiefly by
reflex effect of
increased cardiac output)

Cardiac output:
Increased,
venous preasure
decreased,
renal blood flow
increased

AV node:
Conduction slowed,
(P-R interval prolonged),
refractory period prolonged,
ventricular rate reduced
in atrial fibrillation

Toxicity

Complete heart block

Force of contraction:
Increased,
conversion of
metabolic to
mechanical energy
more efficient

**Ventricular muscle
and Purkinje fibers:**
Conduction slowed,
automaticity increased,
refractory period shortened

Toxicity

Ectopic beats,
bigeminy,
ventricular tachycardia,
ventricular fibrillation

Heart size:
Reduced

FIGURE 4-19 HEART FAILURE TREATMENT: CARDIAC GLYCOSIDES

Cardiac glycosides inhibit the Na^+,K^+-ATPase pump and increase intracellular Na^+, thus slowing the rate of the Na^+/Ca^{2+} exchanger and increasing intracellular Ca^{2+}. They are used in low-output heart failure with atrial arrhythmias. Digoxin is the most common digitalis preparation; digitoxin is used when a longer half-life is needed (7 days versus 1-2 days for digoxin). Improvement with digitalis depends on cardiac reserve; badly damaged hearts do not respond well. After digitalis restores heart function, its use is continued to prevent recurrence of heart failure. Digitalis may reduce the progression rate of heart damage in some patients, especially those in whom an increase in end-diastolic pressure and volume will occur. Digitalis reduces sympathetic tone by directly blunting the baroreceptor response. Because this drug has toxic effects, including ventricular tachyarrhythmias, GI distress, dizziness, and convulsions, its use by some patients should be avoided.

Winsor Sinus and Atrial Arrhythmias

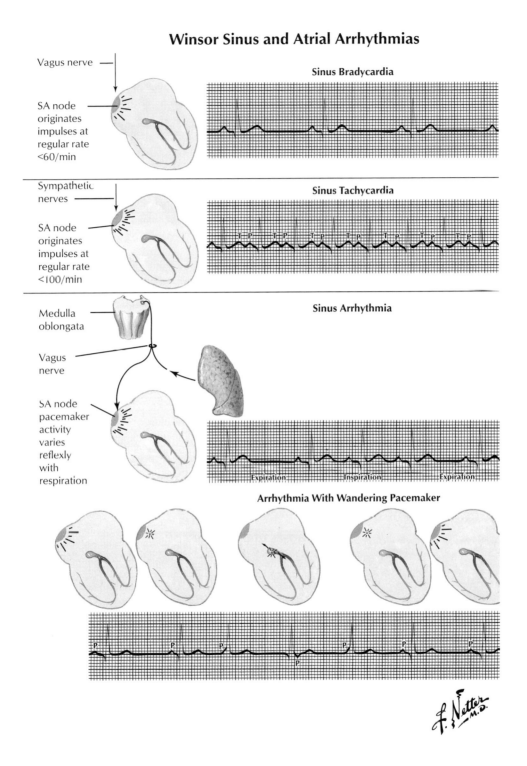

FIGURE 4-20 CARDIAC ARRHYTHMIAS: GENERAL

Arrhythmia is a disturbance of the heart rhythm. SA node malfunction usually triggers an abnormal electrical impulse rate. Because all heart tissue can start a beat, any part of the heart muscle can interrupt the electrical rhythm or take over as the heart's pacemaker to produce an abnormal beat and arrhythmia.

The term *sinus arrhythmia* is used when the changes are caused by spontaneous depolarization of SA node. The parasympathetic system normally slows the spontaneous discharge rate of the SA node from 100 beats/min to approximately 70 beats/min. Arrhythmias can range from entirely benign to immediately

Tachycardia, Fibrillation, and Atrial Flutter

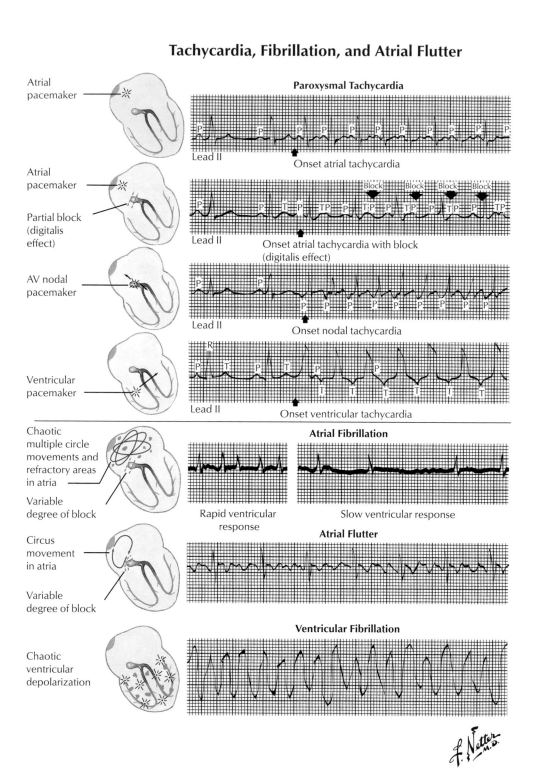

Paroxysmal Tachycardia

Atrial pacemaker

Lead II   Onset atrial tachycardia

Atrial pacemaker

Partial block (digitalis effect)

Lead II   Onset atrial tachycardia with block (digitalis effect)

AV nodal pacemaker

Lead II   Onset nodal tachycardia

Ventricular pacemaker

Lead II   Onset ventricular tachycardia

Atrial Fibrillation

Chaotic multiple circle movements and refractory areas in atria

Variable degree of block

Rapid ventricular response   Slow ventricular response

Atrial Flutter

Circus movement in atria

Variable degree of block

Ventricular Fibrillation

Chaotic ventricular depolarization

FIGURE 4-20 CARDIAC ARRHYTHMIAS: GENERAL (continued)

life-threatening. Most arrhythmias do not cause symptoms, but people may feel anxiety, lightheadedness, dizziness, fainting, heartbeat, and sensations of fluttering or pounding. Medical conditions (eg, anemia, fever, heart failure, electrolyte imbalance) may cause arrhythmias. Synchronized electrical shock (defibrillation), electronic pacemakers, and radiofrequency ablation are nondrug treatments.

Acute and Long-Term Management of Arrhythmias

Arrhythmia	Acute Care	Long-Term Management
Sinus tachycardia (>100 bpm)	Treat underlying cause	If inappropriate, β blocker/calcium channel blocker. Persistent, consider RFA of the superior portion of the sinus node.
Sinus bradycardia (<60 bpm)	If asymptomatic, no intervention. If symptomatic and severe (rates <40/min) with nonreversible cause, consider temporary pacing.	If asymptomatic, no intervention. If symptomatic and severe (rates <40/min) with nonreversible cause, consider permanent pacing.
Premature atrial complexes	If asymptomatic, no intervention. Check potassium, magnesium.	If asymptomatic, no intervention. Check potassium, magnesium. If symptomatic, consider β blocker.
Premature ventricular complexes	If asymptomatic, no intervention. Check potassium, magnesium.	Echo to assess LV and RV function, and LV wall thickness. Normal echo: no intervention. β Blocker for symptoms. Abnormal echo: Evaluate etiology and add β blocker.
Sinus node dysfunction	No intervention, unless unstable	Permanent pacemaker. Allows the use of β blocker in patients with tachybrady syndrome.
Prolonged PR interval	No intervention	No intervention unless symptomatic
Second-degree AV block Mobitz type 1 (Wenkebach)	No intervention, unless unstable	Symptomatic patient, consider permanent pacemaker
Mobitz type 2 AV block	No intervention, unless unstable	Permanent pacemaker
Complete heart block	Possible temporary pacemaker	Permanent pacemaker
Supraventricular tachycardia (SVT)	Control SVT with adenosine	
Wolff-Parkinson-White syndrome and concealed accessory pathway	Control SVT with adenosine	WPW with SVT needs EPS and RFA, because of risk of sudden death
Atrioventricular nodal reentrant tachycardia	Control SVT with adenosine, metoprolol, diltiazem	Consider EPS and RFA for recurrent episodes
Atrial tachycardia	Control SVT with metoprolol, diltiazem	Consider EPS and RFA for recurrent episodes

(continued)

FIGURE 4-21 CARDIAC ARRHYTHMIAS: TREATMENT _____

Several drug strategies are used to treat arrhythmias. Warfarin, an anticoagulant, is used for atrial fibrillation to prevent stroke-inducing blood clots. The most common adverse effect of warfarin is bleeding, from mild nosebleed to life-threatening hemorrhage. Antiarrhythmic drugs, such as amiodarone and sotalol, maintain the normal rhythm of the heart. Adverse effects include hypotension, AV block, various arrhythmias, and pulmonary toxicity (amiodarone) and bronchospasm (sotalol).

Acute and Long-Term Management of Arrhythmias (continued)

Arrhythmia	Acute Care	Long-Term Management
Atrial fibrillation	Rate control	Warfarin with INR 2.0 to 3.0 in all at-risk patients. Consider pharmacologic treatment and/or elective DC cardioversion
Paroxysmal	Rate control	Recurrent episodes need antiarrhythmic agent. Focal ablation for drug failures.
Persistent	Rate control	Cardioversion, addition of antiarrhythmic agent for recurrences. Focal ablation for drug failures.
Permanent	Rate control	Rate control. Unsuccessful AV node ablation and permanent pacemaker.
Atrial flutter	Rate control	RFA for recurrent episodes
Ventricular tachycardia	DC cardioversion if unstable or refractory to antiarrhythmic drugs	Echo to assess LV function. Ischemic evaluation ± revascularization. ICD placement. Normal echo, consider RVOT or LV VT and ablation.
Ventricular fibrillation	Emergent DC cardioversion	Rule out acute myocardial infarction. ICD placement in absence of acute myocardial infarction.
Nonsustained ventricular tachycardia (3 to 30 beats)	Rate control	Low ejection fraction, need electrophysiology study. If positive, needs ICD.
Left ventricular dysfunction	Primary prevention of sudden cardiac death	Previous myocardial infarction, LV ejection fraction <30% require, ICD placement
Hypertrophic cardiomyopathy	Treat as for arrhythmia	EPS for any ventricular tachycardia. If positive, needs IC.
Long QT syndrome	Resuscitate as for arrhythmia	β Blocker/permanent pacemaker at 85 bpm/ICD
Brugada syndrome	Resuscitate as for arrhythmia	ICD placement. Asymptomatic and abnormal EKG, EPS ± ICD.

AV indicates atrioventricular; DC, direct current; EPS, electrophysiology study; ICD, implantable cardioverter defibrillator; INR, International Normalized Ratio; LV, left ventricular; RFA, radiofrequency ablation; RV, right ventricular; RVOT, right ventricular outflow tract; VT, ventricular tachycardia; WPW, Wolff-Parkinson-White syndrome.

FIGURE 4-21 CARDIAC ARRHYTHMIAS: TREATMENT (continued)

β Blockers, such as acebutolol, esmolol, and propranolol, limit stimulating effects of EPI and NE on the heart, thus slowing the heart rate in atrial fibrillation. The selective β blockers have fewer central adverse effects than nonselective β blockers, such as propanolol. CCBs, such as verapamil and diltiazem, slow the heart rate and suppress tachycardia, although they can worsen ventricular tachycardia.

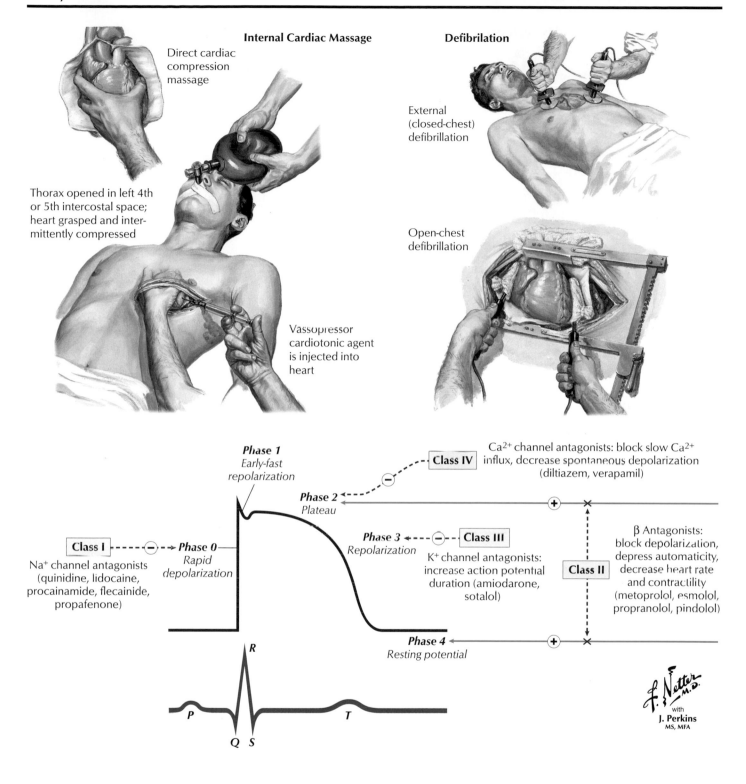

Internal Cardiac Massage

Direct cardiac compression massage

Thorax opened in left 4th or 5th intercostal space; heart grasped and intermittently compressed

Vassopressor cardiotonic agent is injected into heart

Defibrilation

External (closed-chest) defibrillation

Open-chest defibrillation

Phase 1
Early-fast repolarization

Ca^{2+} channel antagonists: block slow Ca^{2+} influx, decrease spontaneous depolarization (diltiazem, verapamil)

Class IV

⊖

Phase 2
Plateau

⊕

Class I

⊖

Phase 0
Rapid depolarization

Na$^+$ channel antagonists (quinidine, lidocaine, procainamide, flecainide, propafenone)

Phase 3 ⊖ **Class III**
Repolarization

K$^+$ channel antagonists: increase action potential duration (amiodarone, sotalol)

Class II

β Antagonists: block depolarization, depress automaticity, decrease heart rate and contractility (metoprolol, esmolol, propranolol, pindolol)

Phase 4
Resting potential

⊕

R

P   T

Q S

J. Perkins
MS, MFA

FIGURE 4-22 CARDIAC ARRHYTHMIAS: DRUG CLASSIFICATION

The standard classification was based on the 4 types of action of these drugs. Class I drugs block voltage-gated sodium channels and are classified into 3 subgroups on the basis of effects on phase 0 depolarization and repolarization: IA drugs have moderate potency at blocking the sodium channel and usually prolong repolarization (increase QRS). IB drugs are the least potent sodium channel blockers, do not alter action potential duration, and shorten repolarization. IC drugs are the most potent sodium channel–blocking agents but have little effect on repolarization (increase PR). Class II drugs act indirectly on electrophysiologic parameters by blocking β adrenoceptors (increase PR). Class III drugs prolong repolarization (increase refractoriness), with little effect on depolarization rate (QT). Class IV drugs are relatively selective AV nodal CCBs, primarily L-type channels (increase PR). In addition to these drug classes, cardiac glycosides act on arrhythmias.

Hypertension as Risk Factor for Cardiovascular Disease*

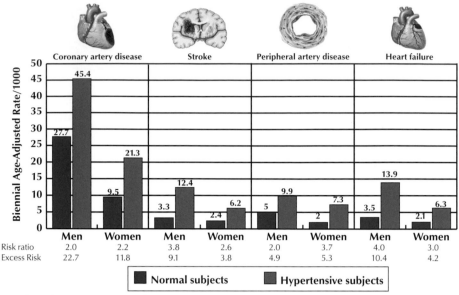

	Coronary artery disease		Stroke		Peripheral artery disease		Heart failure	
	Men	Women	Men	Women	Men	Women	Men	Women
Normal subjects	27.7	9.5	3.3	2.4	5	2	3.5	2.1
Hypertensive subjects	45.4	21.3	12.4	6.2	9.9	7.3	13.9	6.3
Risk ratio	2.0	2.2	3.8	2.6	2.0	3.7	4.0	3.0
Excess Risk	22.7	11.8	9.1	3.8	4.9	5.3	10.4	4.2

Biennial Age-Adjusted Rate/1000

■ Normal subjects   ■ Hypertensive subjects

* According to hypertensive status in subjects 35-64 years of age from the Framingham Study at 36-year follow-up. Adapted from Kannel WB. Blood pressure as a cardiovascular risk factor: prevention and treatment. *JAMA.* 1996;275:1571-1576.

Level of blood pressure is associated with cardiovascular events in a continuous, graded, and apparently independent fashion.†

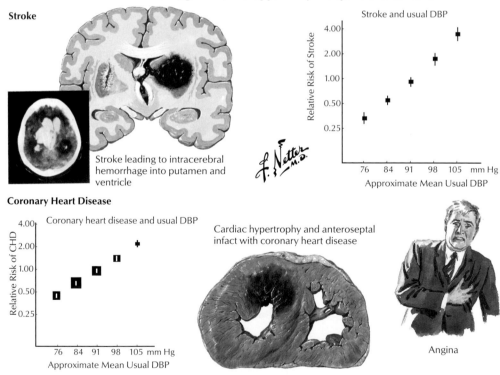

Stroke

Stroke leading to intracerebral hemorrhage into putamen and ventricle

Stroke and usual DBP

Relative Risk of Stroke — Approximate Mean Usual DBP — 76 84 91 98 105 mm Hg

Coronary Heart Disease

Coronary heart disease and usual DBP

Relative Risk of CHD — Approximate Mean Usual DBP — 76 84 91 98 105 mm Hg

Cardiac hypertrophy and anteroseptal infact with coronary heart disease

Angina

† Relative risk of stroke and coronary heart disease as a function of usual diastolic pressure in 420,000 individuals 25 years or older with a mean follow-up period of 10 years. Adapted from MacMahon S, Peto R, Cutter S, et al. Blood pressure, stroke, and coronary heart disease: part one. *Lancet.* 1990;335:765-767.

FIGURE 4-23 HYPERTENSION OVERVIEW

Nearly 25% of adults have hypertension (high blood pressure)—increased arterial blood pressure that stays abnormally high for a long period. The heart pumps blood from the left atrium into the arteries. The blood flow exerts a force against arterial walls. This force, or blood pressure, is a measure of how much work is required by the heart to push blood through the arteries. The 2 numbers used to indicate blood pressure correspond to systole and diastole (eg, 120/80 mm Hg). The systolic (top) number

reflects pressure of blood against arterial walls that results from contraction of the heart. The diastolic number (bottom) reflects arterial blood pressure while the heart is filling and resting between beats. *High blood pressure* in adults is defined as a consistently increased blood pressure of 140/90 mm Hg or greater. Hypertension is called the "silent killer" because it causes serious complications without obvious symptoms. Some signs are headaches, dizziness, and blurred vision.

Causes of Hypertension

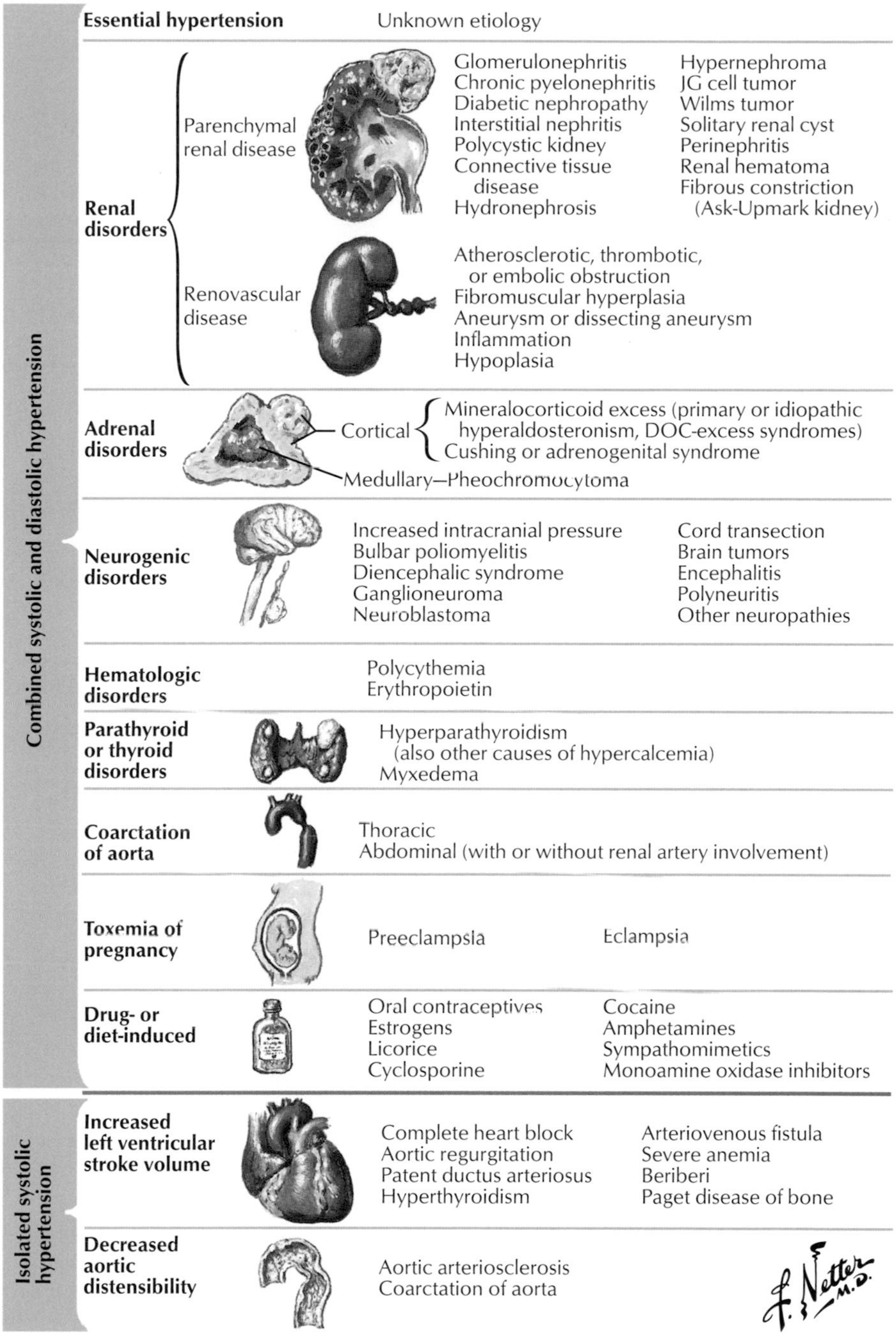

Choice of Antihypertensive Agent Based on Coexistent Illnesses

Indications for specific drugs	
Diabetes mellitus	ACE inhibitor or ARB
Congestive heart failure	ACE inhibitor or ARB, β blocker, diuretic
Myocardial infarction	ACE inhibitor, β blocker
Chronic coronary artery disease	ACE inhibitor, β blocker
Renal insufficiency	ACE inhibitor, ARB
Contraindications to specific drugs	
Pregnancy	ACE inhibitors, ARB
Renal insufficiency*	Potassium-sparing agents
Peripheral vascular disease	β Blockers
Gout*	Diuretics
Depression*	β Blockers, central α agonists
Reactive airway disease	β Blockers
2nd- or 3rd-degree heart block	β Blockers, non-dihydropyridine calcium antagonists
Hepatic insufficiency	Labetalol, methyldopa

*Relative contraindications.

Essential hypertension — Unknown etiology

Combined systolic and diastolic hypertension

Renal disorders

Parenchymal renal disease:
Glomerulonephritis
Chronic pyelonephritis
Diabetic nephropathy
Interstitial nephritis
Polycystic kidney
Connective tissue disease
Hydronephrosis
Hypernephroma
JG cell tumor
Wilms tumor
Solitary renal cyst
Perinephritis
Renal hematoma
Fibrous constriction (Ask-Upmark kidney)

Renovascular disease:
Atherosclerotic, thrombotic, or embolic obstruction
Fibromuscular hyperplasia
Aneurysm or dissecting aneurysm
Inflammation
Hypoplasia

Adrenal disorders
Cortical:
Mineralocorticoid excess (primary or idiopathic hyperaldosteronism, DOC-excess syndromes)
Cushing or adrenogenital syndrome
Medullary—Pheochromocytoma

Neurogenic disorders
Increased intracranial pressure
Bulbar poliomyelitis
Diencephalic syndrome
Ganglioneuroma
Neuroblastoma
Cord transection
Brain tumors
Encephalitis
Polyneuritis
Other neuropathies

Hematologic disorders
Polycythemia
Erythropoietin

Parathyroid or thyroid disorders
Hyperparathyroidism (also other causes of hypercalcemia)
Myxedema

Coarctation of aorta
Thoracic
Abdominal (with or without renal artery involvement)

Toxemia of pregnancy
Preeclampsia   Eclampsia

Drug- or diet-induced
Oral contraceptives
Estrogens
Licorice
Cyclosporine
Cocaine
Amphetamines
Sympathomimetics
Monoamine oxidase inhibitors

Isolated systolic hypertension

Increased left ventricular stroke volume
Complete heart block
Aortic regurgitation
Patent ductus arteriosus
Hyperthyroidism
Arteriovenous fistula
Severe anemia
Beriberi
Paget disease of bone

Decreased aortic distensibility
Aortic arteriosclerosis
Coarctation of aorta

F. Netter, M.D.

FIGURE 4-24 HYPERTENSION: CAUSES

Hypertension is classed as primary (essential) or secondary. The former cannot be directly related to a cause and constitutes 90% of hypertension cases. The latter occurs in less than 10% of hypertensive patients and is caused by liver and kidney disease, adrenal hormone overproduction, pregnancy, and sleep disorders as well as corticosteroids (eg, prednisone, cortisone), NSAIDs (eg, aspirin, ibuprofen), alcohol, nicotine, and caffeine. The renin-angiotensin system regulates all aspects of blood pressure control. ACE converts angiotensin I (AI) into angiotensin II (AII). Circulating AII increases sympathetic drive, constricts vascular smooth muscle, reduces bradykinin levels, and increases salt and water retention, all of which increase blood pressure and cardiac preload and afterload.

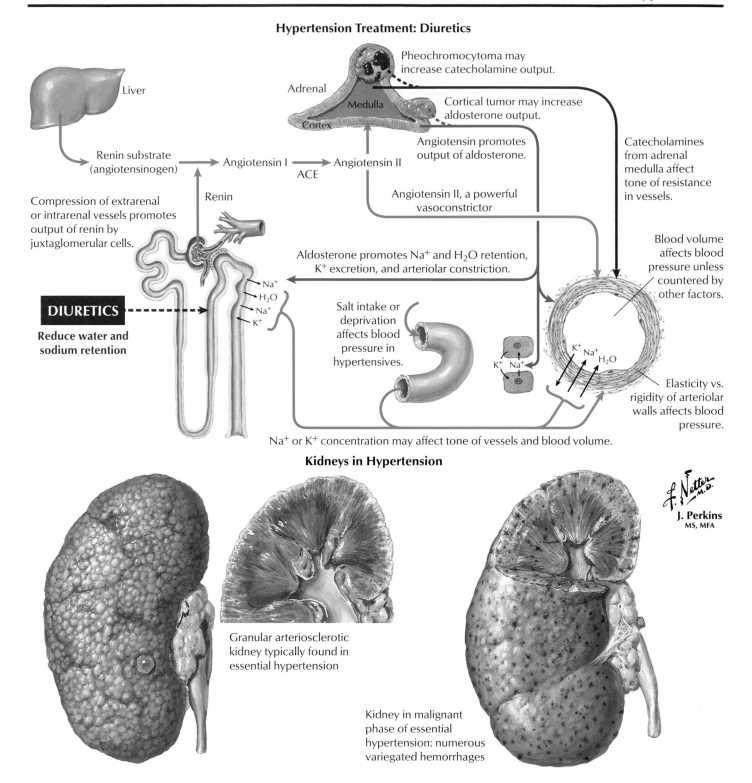

Hypertension Treatment: Diuretics

Liver

Pheochromocytoma may increase catecholamine output.

Adrenal

Medulla

Cortex

Cortical tumor may increase aldosterone output.

Renin substrate (angiotensinogen) → Angiotensin I →(ACE)→ Angiotensin II

Angiotensin promotes output of aldosterone.

Catecholamines from adrenal medulla affect tone of resistance in vessels.

Compression of extrarenal or intrarenal vessels promotes output of renin by juxtaglomerular cells.

Renin

Angiotensin II, a powerful vasoconstrictor

Aldosterone promotes Na^+ and H_2O retention, K^+ excretion, and arteriolar constriction.

Blood volume affects blood pressure unless countered by other factors.

Na^+
H_2O
Na^+
K^+

DIURETICS

Reduce water and sodium retention

Salt intake or deprivation affects blood pressure in hypertensives.

K^+ Na^+

K^+ Na^+ H_2O

Elasticity vs. rigidity of arteriolar walls affects blood pressure.

Na^+ or K^+ concentration may affect tone of vessels and blood volume.

Kidneys in Hypertension

J. Netter M.D.
J. Perkins
MS, MFA

Granular arteriosclerotic kidney typically found in essential hypertension

Kidney in malignant phase of essential hypertension: numerous variegated hemorrhages

FIGURE 4-25 HYPERTENSION TREATMENT: DIURETICS

The goal for most patients is to decrease blood pressure to less than 140 mm Hg systolic and less than 90 mm Hg diastolic. Drug therapy involves 4 major drug classes: diuretics, ACE inhibitors, CCBs, and β blockers (used with drugs of another class). Diuretics have been the major antihypertensive drugs for decades and are still thought to be the best therapy for African-American and elderly patients and the best agents for preventing stroke. Diuretics also minimize blood clotting and reduce osteoporosis in the elderly. Three major types of diuretics are used. Thiazides (eg, chlorothiazide, chlorthalidone) are taken alone for moderate hypertension or used in combination with other drug types. Loop diuretics (eg, furosemide, bumetanide) block Na^+ transport in the kidney. Their onset of action and potency are greater than those of thiazides. Potassium-sparing agents (eg, amiloride, spironolactone) increase potassium retention by kidneys and increase K^+ levels in the body.

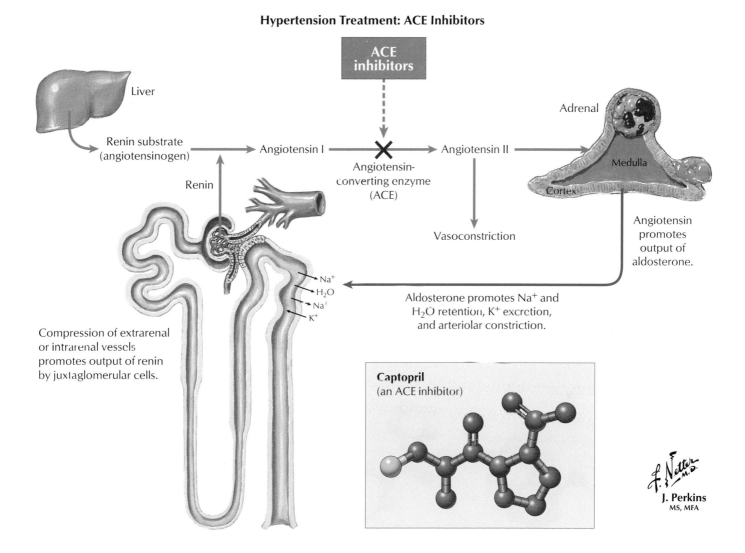

Hypertension Treatment: ACE Inhibitors

ACE inhibitors

Liver

Renin substrate (angiotensinogen)

Renin

Angiotensin I

Angiotensin-converting enzyme (ACE)

Angiotensin II

Vasoconstriction

Adrenal

Medulla

Cortex

Angiotensin promotes output of aldosterone.

Na⁺
H₂O
Na⁺
K⁺

Aldosterone promotes Na⁺ and H₂O retention, K⁺ excretion, and arteriolar constriction.

Compression of extrarenal or intrarenal vessels promotes output of renin by juxtaglomerular cells.

Captopril
(an ACE inhibitor)

J. Perkins
MS, MFA

FIGURE 4-26 HYPERTENSION TREATMENT: ANGIOTENSIN-CONVERTING ENZYME INHIBITORS

Angiotensin-converting enzyme converts the inactive form of angiotensin (AI) to the active AII. AII causes arterial vasoconstriction and increases blood pressure. Blocking ACE with inhibitors (eg, captopril, enalapril) inhibits AII formation, which reduces blood pressure, enhances the pumping efficiency of the heart, and improves cardiac output in heart failure patients. ACE inhibitors also slow progression of kidney disease, especially in diabetic patients. These agents are thus the best drugs for high blood pressure in cases that also involve chronic kidney failure in diabetic and nondiabetic patients, CHF, and heart attack, which damage heart muscle. Using only ACE inhibitors allows 60% of white patients to control hypertension; black patients need higher doses and use with a diuretic. AII receptor antagonists are new drugs that decrease blood pressure by blocking AII from binding to receptors in vascular smooth muscle. Most adverse effects are mild; renal failure and fetal/neonatal morbidity may occur.

Hypertension Treatment: β and α Blockers

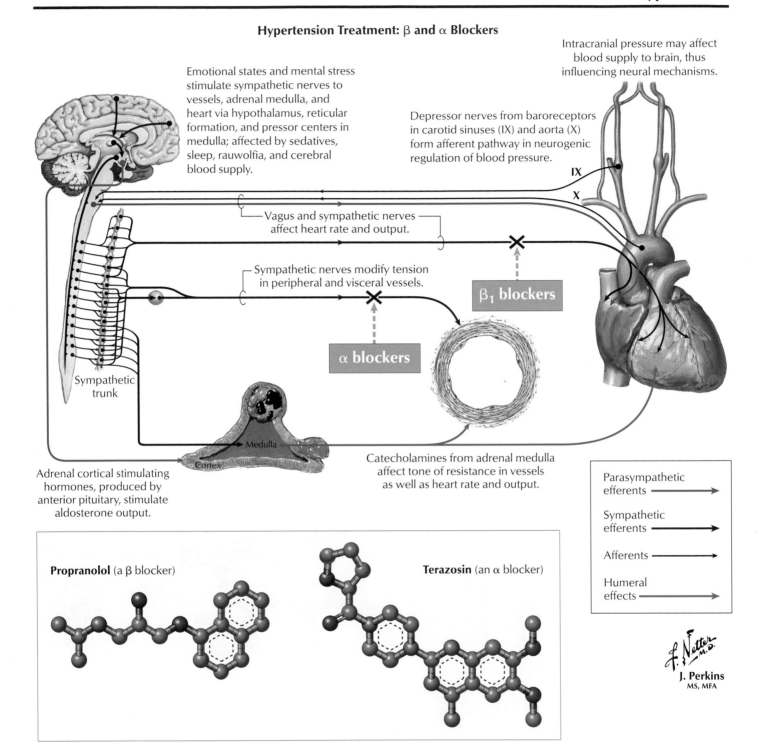

Emotional states and mental stress stimulate sympathetic nerves to vessels, adrenal medulla, and heart via hypothalamus, reticular formation, and pressor centers in medulla; affected by sedatives, sleep, rauwolfia, and cerebral blood supply.

Intracranial pressure may affect blood supply to brain, thus influencing neural mechanisms.

Depressor nerves from baroreceptors in carotid sinuses (IX) and aorta (X) form afferent pathway in neurogenic regulation of blood pressure.

IX

X

Vagus and sympathetic nerves affect heart rate and output.

Sympathetic nerves modify tension in peripheral and visceral vessels.

β₁ blockers

α blockers

Sympathetic trunk

Medulla

Cortex

Adrenal cortical stimulating hormones, produced by anterior pituitary, stimulate aldosterone output.

Catecholamines from adrenal medulla affect tone of resistance in vessels as well as heart rate and output.

Parasympathetic efferents ⟶
Sympathetic efferents ⟶
Afferents ⟶
Humeral effects ⟶

Propranolol (a β blocker)

Terazosin (an α blocker)

J. Netter M.D.

J. Perkins
MS, MFA

FIGURE 4-27 HYPERTENSION TREATMENT: β AND α BLOCKERS

β Blockers decrease cardiac output and blood pressure by reducing the frequency of spontaneous depolarizations in pacemaker cells. They prevent activation of β adrenoceptors by NE and EPI and block increased sympathetic effects on the heart. β Blockers are prescribed in combination with other antihypertensive agents to treat hypertension. They are excellent for patients with angina but should be avoided by patients with bradycardia (low heart rate), asthma, and chronic bronchitis. Main β blockers include propranolol, atenolol, acebutolol, metoprolol, pindolol, and nadolol. Side effects are fatigue, insomnia, nightmares, impotence, GI disorders, and limb cooling. α-Adrenergic antagonists (terazosin, doxazosin) decrease blood pressure by blocking sympathetic effects on α receptors in smooth muscle of peripheral arteries. These agents increase the risk of heart attack and stroke and are not the drugs of first choice for treating hypertension.

Hypertension Treatment: Minoxidil

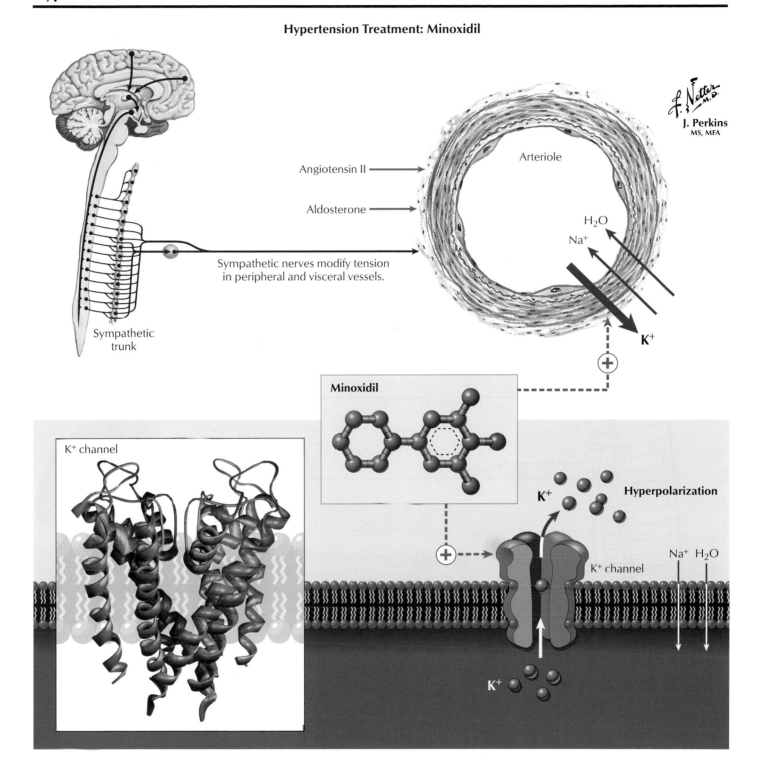

J. Netter
J. Perkins
MS, MFA

Angiotensin II

Arteriole

Aldosterone

H_2O

Na^+

Sympathetic nerves modify tension in peripheral and visceral vessels.

K^+

Sympathetic trunk

Minoxidil

K^+

Hyperpolarization

K^+ channel

K^+

K^+ channel

Na^+ H_2O

K^+

FIGURE 4-28 HYPERTENSION TREATMENT: MINOXIDIL

Minoxidil given orally is the most potent of the drugs that decrease blood pressure by dilating peripheral arteries. Topical minoxidil has garnered much attention for its ability to increase hair growth in men and women. Minoxidil, unlike α and β blockers, does not work through the peripheral sympathetic nervous system. Instead, it is a muscle relaxant that directly activates K^+ channels in smooth muscle cells of the peripheral arteries. This effect increases K^+ permeability and enhances K^+ efflux, which causes hyperpolarization of the cell membrane and an overall reduction in blood pressure. Blood flow to the skin, skeletal muscle, and heart increases. This drug is used only in patients who do not respond to other antihypertensive agents. It is used in combination with β blockers or clonidine to reduce heart rate and is contraindicated during pregnancy. The most common adverse effects are fluid and salt retention and hair growth on the face, back, arms, and legs.

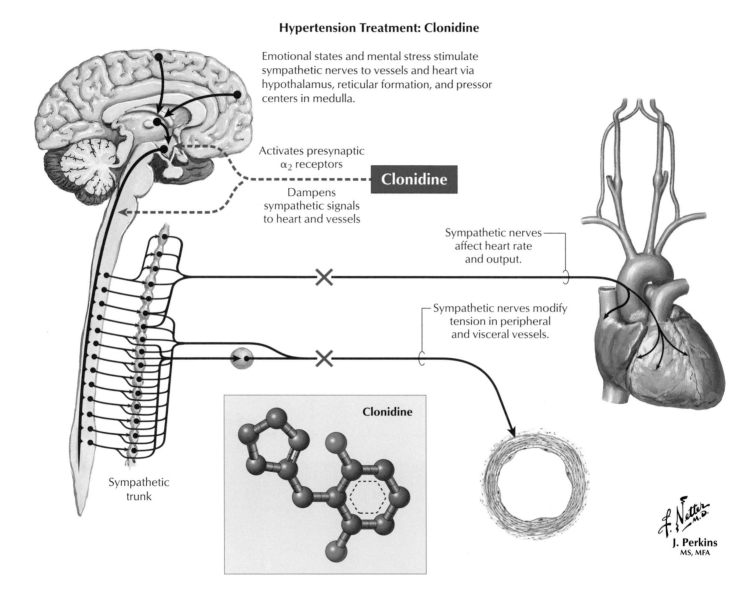

Hypertension Treatment: Clonidine

Emotional states and mental stress stimulate sympathetic nerves to vessels and heart via hypothalamus, reticular formation, and pressor centers in medulla.

Activates presynaptic α₂ receptors

Clonidine

Dampens sympathetic signals to heart and vessels

Sympathetic nerves affect heart rate and output.

Sympathetic nerves modify tension in peripheral and visceral vessels.

Sympathetic trunk

Clonidine

J. Perkins
MS, MFA

FIGURE 4-29 HYPERTENSION TREATMENT: CLONIDINE

Clonidine, an oral and topical drug, slows heart rate and reduces blood pressure. By stimulating adrenoceptors in the brain, it dampens signals that start in the CNS and are transmitted to the body by the sympathetic nervous system. Clonidine acts on the central sympathetic control center and is called a *central α agonist*. It reduces sympathetic drive from the brain and peripheral arterial resistance, which results in lower blood pressure via vasodilation. Clonidine is used only when other drugs have been unsuccessful. Adverse effects are dry mouth and fatigue. Clonidine can lead to bradycardia, so it should not be used with β blockers and calcium channel antagonists, which decrease heart rate. Clonidine also increases sedation caused by narcotic pain relievers, barbiturates, and alcohol. Abnormal heart rhythms can occur with clonidine plus verapamil. Also, cocaine, pseudoephedrine, phenylephrine, and amphetamine counteract the antihypertensive actions of clonidine.

The diagnosis of hypertension for all adults is based on the finding of systolic blood pressure of over 140 mm Hg with diastolic blood pressure of over 90 mm Hg, after 2 or more readings. Each reading must be performed after the person has been sitting for 3 minutes. A single reading with systolic blood pressure of over 210 mm Hg or diastolic blood pressure of over 120 mm Hg is consistent with hypertension.

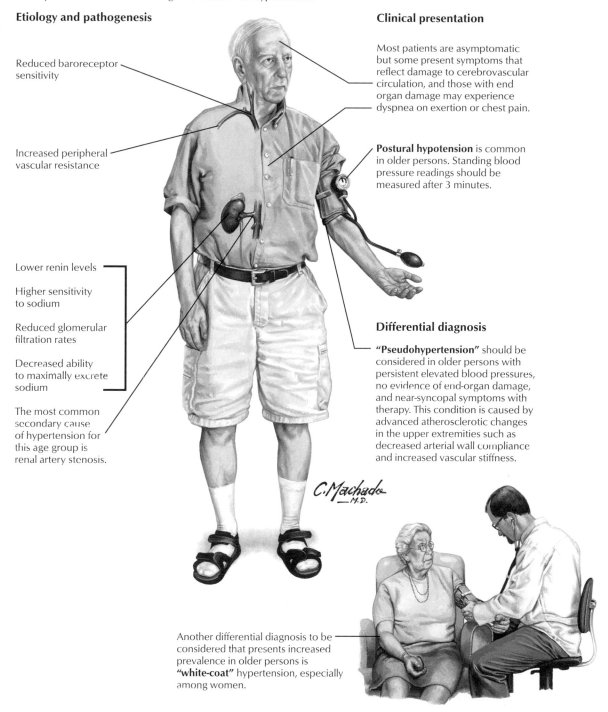

Etiology and pathogenesis

Reduced baroreceptor sensitivity

Increased peripheral vascular resistance

Lower renin levels

Higher sensitivity to sodium

Reduced glomerular filtration rates

Decreased ability to maximally excrete sodium

The most common secondary cause of hypertension for this age group is renal artery stenosis.

Clinical presentation

Most patients are asymptomatic but some present symptoms that reflect damage to cerebrovascular circulation, and those with end organ damage may experience dyspnea on exertion or chest pain.

Postural hypotension is common in older persons. Standing blood pressure readings should be measured after 3 minutes.

Differential diagnosis

"Pseudohypertension" should be considered in older persons with persistent elevated blood pressures, no evidence of end-organ damage, and near-syncopal symptoms with therapy. This condition is caused by advanced atherosclerotic changes in the upper extremities such as decreased arterial wall compliance and increased vascular stiffness.

Another differential diagnosis to be considered that presents increased prevalence in older persons is **"white-coat"** hypertension, especially among women.

FIGURE 4-30 HYPERTENSION IN ELDERLY PATIENTS

Older patients present a challenge in both drug selection and dosage adjustment to control blood pressure. One major concern is impaired drug-metabolizing ability, so toxic actions of agents must be considered. Diuretics are safe, effective, and well tolerated, but high doses can induce effects such as hypokalemia (low blood K⁺ levels) and hyperglycemia (high blood glucose levels). Thiazides expel water from the body, which makes them useful for reducing edema caused by heart, liver, or kidney disorders. Potassium supplements or potassium-sparing agents can help to counter the K⁺ loss. Drugs other than diuretics can be given, but they are usually more costly and less effective. β Blockers are less effective than diuretics in preventing stroke, and CCBs have side effects such as postural hypotension, ankle swelling, and upset stomach. ACE inhibitors and AII antagonists relieve hypertension but should not be given to patients with renal or carotid artery stenosis.

Pheochromocytoma

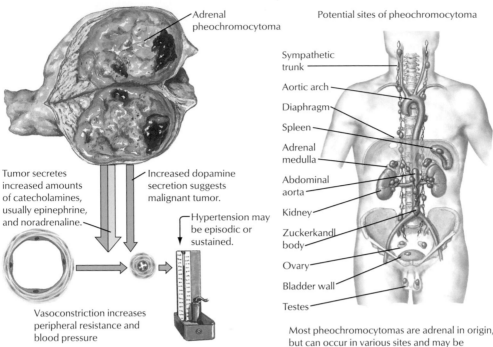

Adrenal pheochromocytoma

Tumor secretes increased amounts of catecholamines, usually epinephrine, and noradrenaline.

Increased dopamine secretion suggests malignant tumor.

Hypertension may be episodic or sustained.

Vasoconstriction increases peripheral resistance and blood pressure

Pheochromocytoma is a chromaffin cell tumor secreting excessive catecholamines resulting in increased peripheral vascular resistance and hypertension.

Potential sites of pheochromocytoma

Sympathetic trunk
Aortic arch
Diaphragm
Spleen
Adrenal medulla
Abdominal aorta
Kidney
Zuckerkandl body
Ovary
Bladder wall
Testes

Most pheochromocytomas are adrenal in origin, but can occur in various sites and may be associated with multiple endocrine neoplasia (men) syndromes. Most are sporadic, but some are hereditary.

Clinical Features of Pheochromocytoma

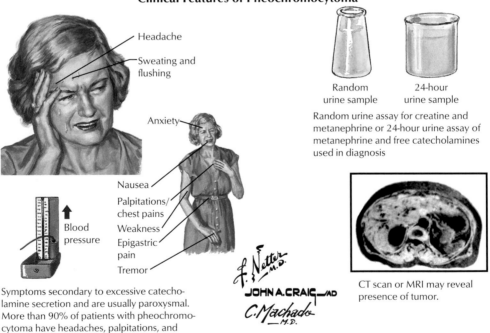

Headache

Sweating and flushing

Anxiety

Nausea
Palpitations/ chest pains
Weakness
Epigastric pain
Tremor

Blood pressure

Random urine sample

24-hour urine sample

Random urine assay for creatine and metanephrine or 24-hour urine assay of metanephrine and free catecholamines used in diagnosis

CT scan or MRI may reveal presence of tumor.

Symptoms secondary to excessive catecholamine secretion and are usually paroxysmal. More than 90% of patients with pheochromocytoma have headaches, palpitations, and sweating alone or in combination.

FIGURE 4-31 PHEOCHROMOCYTOMA-INDUCED HYPERTENSION

Pheochromocytoma is a rare tumor that arises from adrenal gland tissue. The tumor increases production of EPI and NE, thus increasing the level of catecholamines in blood, increasing sympathetic effects on cardiac cells and peripheral blood vessels, and increasing blood pressure and heart rate. Sweating, headache, anxiety, and fright often occur. Pheochromocytomas are normally benign, but they may be associated with malignant tumors in endocrine glands. Surgical removal of the tumor is usually needed to abolish the high catecholamine levels, increased sympathetic activity, hypertension, and cardiac dysfunction. However, before surgery and in cases in which surgery is not possible, drugs such as α and β blockers are used to block effects of the catecholamines. In cases of dangerous hypertension, organic nitrates such as nitroprusside or phentolamine are routinely given intravenously.

Cushing Syndrome/Mineralocorticoid Hypertension

Causes of Cushing syndrome

Clinical features

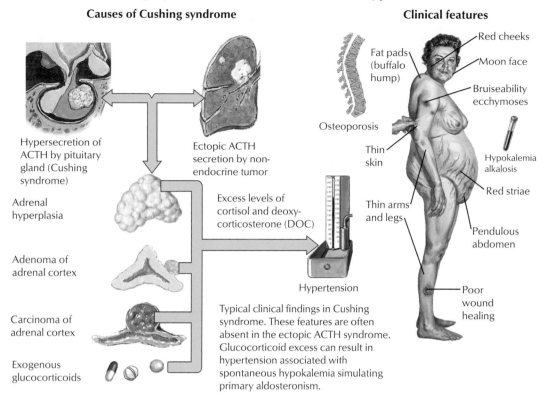

Hypersecretion of ACTH by pituitary gland (Cushing syndrome)

Ectopic ACTH secretion by non-endocrine tumor

Adrenal hyperplasia

Excess levels of cortisol and deoxy-corticosterone (DOC)

Adenoma of adrenal cortex

Carcinoma of adrenal cortex

Exogenous glucocorticoids

Hypertension

Typical clinical findings in Cushing syndrome. These features are often absent in the ectopic ACTH syndrome. Glucocorticoid excess can result in hypertension associated with spontaneous hypokalemia simulating primary aldosteronism.

Fat pads (buffalo hump)

Osteoporosis

Thin skin

Thin arms and legs

Red cheeks

Moon face

Bruiseability ecchymoses

Hypokalemia alkalosis

Red striae

Pendulous abdomen

Poor wound healing

Possible Mechanisms of Hypertension Associated With Glucocorticoid Excess

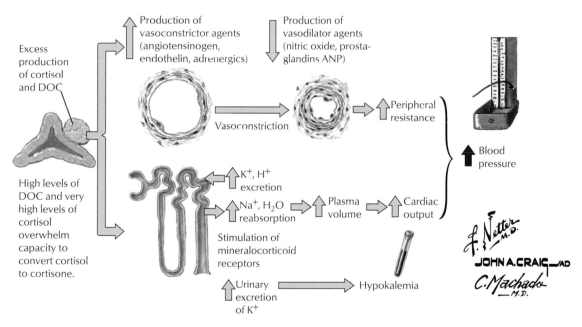

Excess production of cortisol and DOC

Production of vasoconstrictor agents (angiotensinogen, endothelin, adrenergics)

Production of vasodilator agents (nitric oxide, prosta-glandins ANP)

Vasoconstriction

Peripheral resistance

Blood pressure

High levels of DOC and very high levels of cortisol overwhelm capacity to convert cortisol to cortisone.

K^+, H^+ excretion

Na^+, H_2O reabsorption

Plasma volume

Cardiac output

Stimulation of mineralocorticoid receptors

Urinary excretion of K^+

Hypokalemia

FIGURE 4-32 HYPERTENSION IN CUSHING SYNDROME

Cushing syndrome, or hypercortisolism, results from excessive cortisol production and is caused when adrenal glands overproduce cortisol or after prolonged corticosteroid use. The unique features of this syndrome are a fatty hump between the shoulders, a rounded face, and pink-to-purple striations on the skin. The syndrome can cause hypertension, diabetes, and bone loss. Therapy aims to decrease cortisol levels. If corticosteroid use is the cause, decreasing the dose may eliminate the syndrome while still controlling asthma, arthritis, and associated conditions. If a tumor causes the syndrome, total surgical removal or radiation therapy is preferred. When surgery and radiation do not normalize cortisol levels, therapy with drugs, most commonly ketoconazole and mitotane, can impede cortisol synthesis. They are taken orally. Antihypertensive agents can control the headache and high blood pressure that accompany Cushing syndrome, but they are not used to treat other conditions induced by the syndrome.

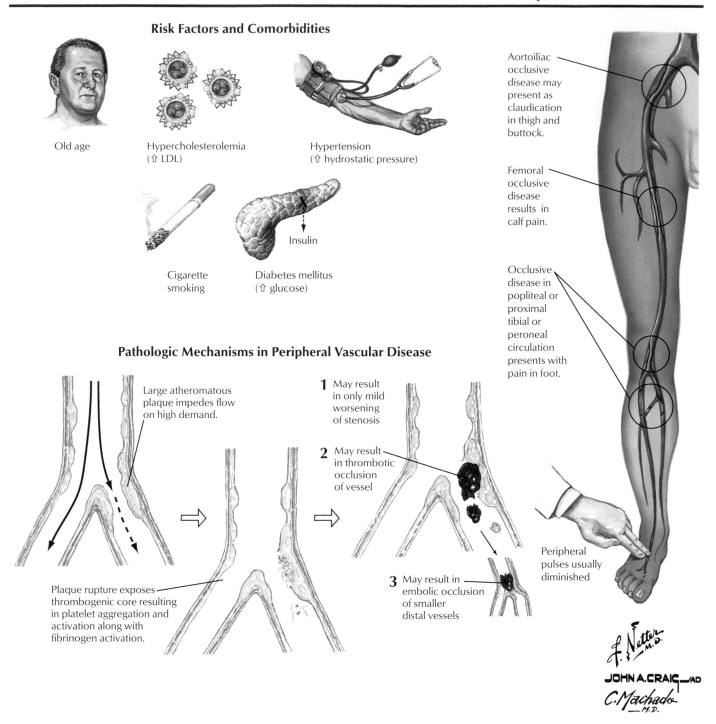

Risk Factors and Comorbidities

Old age

Hypercholesterolemia
(⇧ LDL)

Hypertension
(⇧ hydrostatic pressure)

Insulin

Cigarette
smoking

Diabetes mellitus
(⇧ glucose)

Aortoiliac occlusive disease may present as claudication in thigh and buttock.

Femoral occlusive disease results in calf pain.

Occlusive disease in popliteal or proximal tibial or peroneal circulation presents with pain in foot.

Pathologic Mechanisms in Peripheral Vascular Disease

Large atheromatous plaque impedes flow on high demand.

Plaque rupture exposes thrombogenic core resulting in platelet aggregation and activation along with fibrinogen activation.

1 May result in only mild worsening of stenosis

2 May result in thrombotic occlusion of vessel

3 May result in embolic occlusion of smaller distal vessels

Peripheral pulses usually diminished

FIGURE 4-33 PERIPHERAL VASCULAR DISEASE

Peripheral vascular disease can cause loss of limb or life and is characterized by chronic progression of symptoms such as intermittent claudication (leg pain produced by atherosclerosis) and sores that do not heal. Insufficient tissue perfusion resulting from atherosclerosis and compounded by emboli is the primary cause. Coronary artery disease, myocardial infarction, atrial fibrillation, stroke, and renal failure are additional causes. Risk factors are hyperlipidemia, smoking, diabetes, hyperviscosity, and autoimmune disorders. Conventional treatment includes antiplatelet (platelet-inhibiting) drugs (aspirin, dipyridamole, ticlopidine) and cholesterol-decreasing drugs (niacin, lovastatin, pravastatin), which are often used in combination with anticlaudication medications (cilostazol, pentoxifylline). Operations to restore blood supply or revascularization procedures (ie, angioplasty, atherectomy, stent placement, and bypass) are reserved for patients with progressive symptoms.

CHAPTER 5

DRUGS USED IN DISORDERS OF THE ENDOCRINE SYSTEM

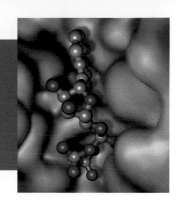

OVERVIEW

The endocrine system has often been viewed as more complex than other physiologic systems, primarily because the target organ is usually located relatively far from the site of release of the chemical mediator of the signal. However, it is now recognized that the signaling mechanisms—which use enzymes, neurochemical transmitters, hormones, and receptors—are similar (aside from distance) to those of other systems. Hence, the basic pharmacologic principles of therapy are the same. Some of the major applications of these drugs include treatment of hypothalamic and pituitary disorders, thyroid dysfunctions, disorders involving adrenal corticosteroids, and diabetes.

Hypopituitarism may be partial or complete and may result from hypothalamic disease (leading to deficiency of hypothalamic-releasing hormones) or intrinsic pituitary disease (causing pituitary hormone deficiency). Hypopituitarism may affect any of these pituitary hormones: thyrotropin, growth hormone (GH), luteinizing hormone, follicle-stimulating hormone, and corticotropin (ACTH). In targeting one of these hormones, therapy for GH deficiency aims to restore normal body composition, as well as, in children, to promote linear growth. Therapy for acromegaly, caused by excessive GH secretion, includes surgery and/or radiation, or use of a GH inhibitor.

Hypothyroidism can result from either thyroid or hypothalamic dysfunction. The treatment of choice is hormone substitution by using a synthetic hormone. Hyperthyroidism (thyrotoxicosis) is characterized by increased metabolism, and the primary treatment options include surgery, radioactive iodine, or drugs that inhibit the formation of thyroid hormones, such as by blocking the utilization of iodine.

The principal functions of glucocorticoids involve regulation of carbohydrate metabolism and a variety of other physiologic actions. Synthetic corticosteroids (eg, hydrocortisone, prednisone, and dexamethasone) are widely used as therapeutic agents in treatment of cancer and autoimmune or inflammatory-type disorders. Pharmacologic treatment is also available for insufficient adrenal function, which is manifested as Addison disease, and excess glucocorticoid exposure, which results in Cushing syndrome.

Diabetes mellitus (DM) is a syndrome caused by a relative or absolute deficiency of insulin, with hyperglycemia being the hallmark medical finding. DM can occur as either an early onset form (type 1) or a gradual-onset form (type 2). In the former, insulin-producing β cells of the pancreas are destroyed or insufficiently active, and patients require lifelong treatment with exogenous insulin. In type 2 DM, adequate control of disease may be achieved by means of diet and exercise; if these methods fail, patients take oral hypoglycemic agents, which cause lower plasma glucose levels, improve insulin resistance, and reduce long-term complications (macrovascular and microvascular problems such as neuropathy, nephropathy, and retinopathy). Insulin is the sole treatment for type 1 DM and is sometimes also used for type 2 DM. For type 2 DM, drugs include sulfonylureas, which stimulate insulin secretion from pancreatic β cells; metformin, a biguanide that decreases blood glucose levels by reducing hepatic glucose production and glycogen metabolism in the liver and improving insulin resistance; meglitinides, which increase insulin secretion from pancreatic β cells; α-glucosidase inhibitors, which delay carbohydrate digestion and glucose absorption; and thiazolidinedione (TZD) derivatives (eg, rosiglitazone and pioglitazone), which reduce insulin resistance.

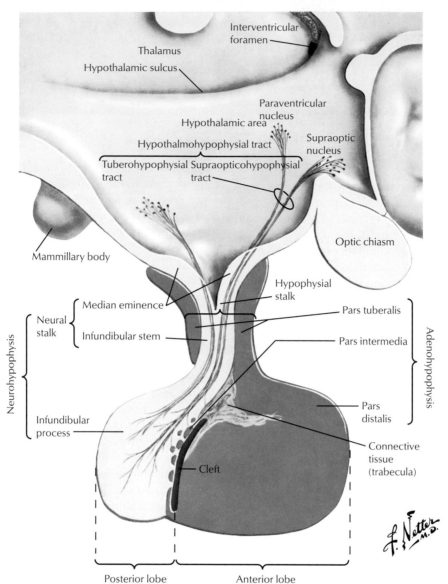

Hypothalamic Hormones	Pituitary Hormones	Target Organ	Specific Hormone
Somatostatin (−) GHRH (growth hormone-releasing hormone) (+)	GH (growth hormone; somatotropin)	Liver	Somatomedins, IGFs
CRH (corticotropin-releasing hormone)	ACTH (corticotropin)	Adrenal cortex	Glucocorticoids, mineralocorticoids, androgens
TRH (thyrotropin-releasing hormone)	TSH (thyroid-stimulating hormone, or thyrotropin)	Thyroid	Thyroxine, triiodothyronine
GnRH (gonadotropin-releasing hormone)	FSH (follicle-stimulating hormone)	Gonads	Estrogen
	LH (luteinizing hormone)	Gonads	Progesterone, testosterone

FIGURE 5-1 REGULATION OF HYPOTHALAMIC AND PITUITARY HORMONES

The hypothalamus and pituitary control a complex neuroendocrine system that governs metabolism, growth, and reproduction. The hypothalamus produces both inhibitory and releasing neuropeptides and hormones, which reach the pituitary via a hypophysial portal system. Hypothalamic hormones trigger release of anterior pituitary hormones, which are sent to target organs where they induce hormone synthesis. Most of these endocrine-organ systems function via negative feedback, eg,

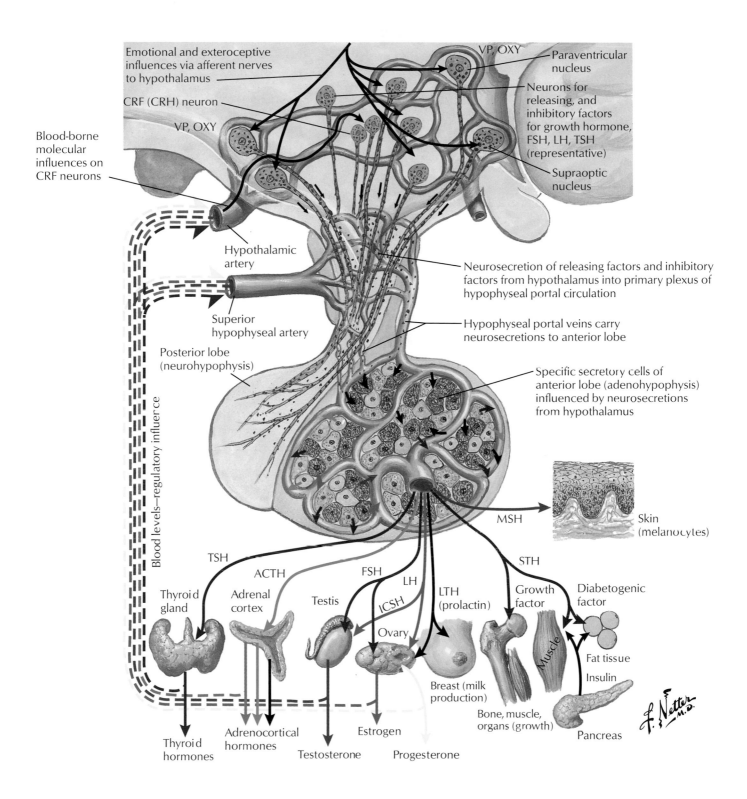

Emotional and exteroceptive influences via afferent nerves to hypothalamus

VP, OXY

Paraventricular nucleus

CRF (CRH) neuron

VP, OXY

Neurons for releasing, and inhibitory factors for growth hormone, FSH, LH, TSH (representative)

Blood-borne molecular influences on CRF neurons

Supraoptic nucleus

Hypothalamic artery

Neurosecretion of releasing factors and inhibitory factors from hypothalamus into primary plexus of hypophyseal portal circulation

Superior hypophyseal artery

Hypophyseal portal veins carry neurosecretions to anterior lobe

Posterior lobe (neurohypophysis)

Specific secretory cells of anterior lobe (adenohypophysis) influenced by neurosecretions from hypothalamus

Blood levels—regulatory influence

MSH

Skin (melanocytes)

TSH

ACTH

FSH

LH

LTH (prolactin)

STH

ICSH

Growth factor

Diabetogenic factor

Thyroid gland

Adrenal cortex

Testis

Ovary

Breast (milk production)

Muscle

Fat tissue

Insulin

Bone, muscle, organs (growth)

Pancreas

Thyroid hormones

Adrenocortical hormones

Testosterone

Estrogen

Progesterone

FIGURE 5-1 REGULATION OF HYPOTHALAMIC AND PITUITARY HORMONES (continued)

hypothalamic CRH stimulates pituitary ACTH secretion, which stimulates adrenal cortisol secretion, which in turn inhibits CRH and ACTH secretion. Hypothalamic and pituitary hormones are used as tools in stimulation tests to diagnose hypofunctioning or hyperfunctioning endocrine states. For example, ACTH and CRH, which target the adrenal cortex, aid adrenal insufficiency diagnosis. Pituitary hormones are also used as replacement therapy for deficiencies such as hypopituitarism.

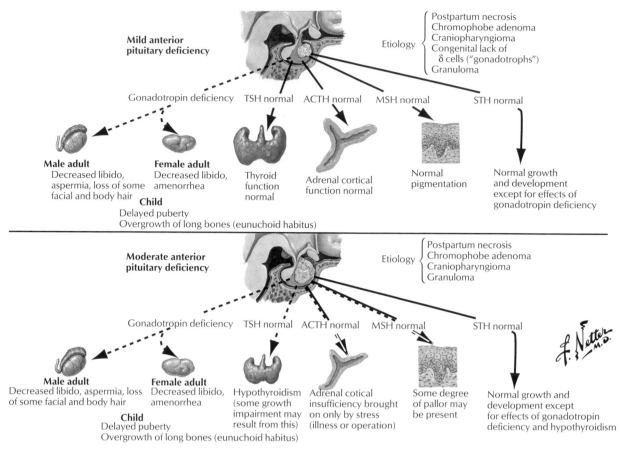

Deficient Hormone	Manifestations
ACTH	Fatigue, weakness, headache, anorexia, weight loss, nausea, vomiting, abdominal pain, altered mental activity occur. Women with long-standing adrenal insufficiency often have loss of axillary and pubic hair. Hyponatremia may occur as a result of increased vasopressin secretion, but serum potassium concentration is usually normal because adrenal aldosterone production does not depend on ACTH. In contrast, both hyponatremia and hyperkalemia are common in patients with primary adrenal insufficiency. Normochromic, normocytic anemia and eosinophilia may also occur.
Thyrotropin	Fatigue, weakness, inability to lose weight (or weight gain), puffiness, constipation, and cold intolerance occur. Impaired memory or altered mental activity is characteristic of severe hypothyroidism. Physical examination may reveal bradycardia, periorbital puffiness, and delayed relaxation of tendon reflexes. Other findings include mild hyponatremia and normochromic, normocytic anemia.
Luteinizing hormone and FSH (produced by the same pituitary cell type)	Men with hypogonadism have decreased libido and erectile dysfunction. Diminished facial and body hair, fine facial wrinkles, gynecomastia, and soft testes are characteristic of long-standing hypogonadism. Women of reproductive age with gonadotropin deficiency have alterations in menstrual function ranging from regular but anovulatory cycles to oligomenorrhea or amenorrhea. Other symptoms of ovarian failure include hot flashes, decreased libido, vaginal dryness, and dyspareunia. Pubic and axillary hair is present unless there is concomitant adrenal failure.
Growth hormone	In adults, deficiency manifests as lack of vigor, decreased tolerance of exercise, and decreased social functioning. Children present with short stature and low growth velocity for age and pubertal stage.

FIGURE 5-2 HYPOPITUITARISM

Hypopituitarism may be partial or complete and may result from hypothalamic disease (leading to deficiency of hypothalamic-releasing hormones) or intrinsic pituitary disease (causing pituitary hormone deficiency). Patients may present with, for example, adrenal insufficiency or hypothyroidism. Clinical signs depend on the degree and rapidity of onset of the deficiency. For example, basal cortisol secretion is normal in partial ACTH deficiency, but during an illness, adrenal insufficiency may occur. In complete

ACTH deficiency, cortisol secretion is always subnormal. Diagnosis of complete deficiency is relatively easy: most patients have symptoms, and serum levels of target-organ hormone (eg, cortisol, thyroxine, and testosterone in men) and pituitary hormone (eg, ACTH, thyrotropin, and luteinizing hormone, respectively) are low. Causes of hypopituitarism include pituitary tumor (most common); hypothalamic tumor or cyst; infiltrative, vascular, and other disorders; and pituitary or cranial radiotherapy.

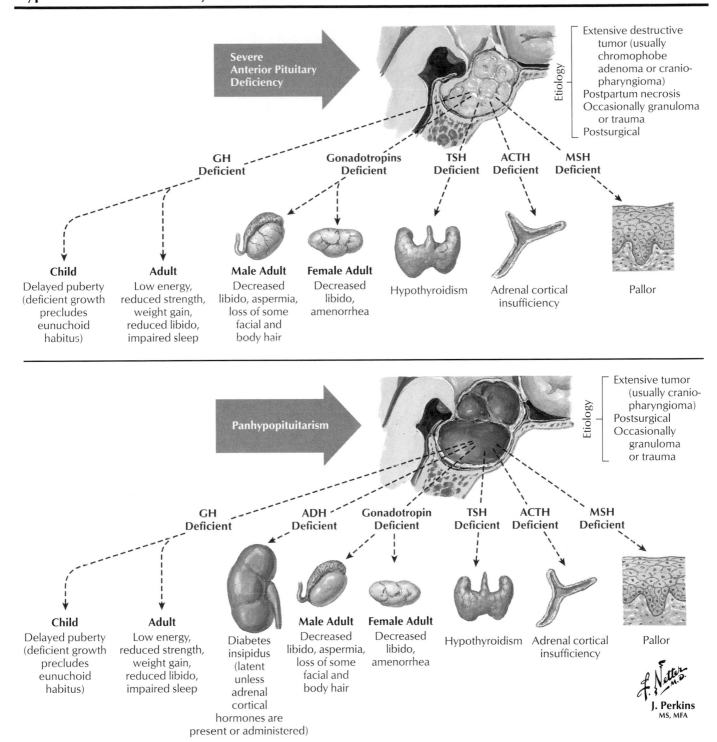

FIGURE 5-3 GROWTH HORMONE DEFICIENCY AND TREATMENT

Growth hormone promotes linear growth by regulating endocrine and paracrine production of IGF-1. Besides disruption in growth, GH deficiency also causes increased subcutaneous visceral fat and reduced muscle mass, bone density, and exercise performance. Children have short stature and low growth velocity for age and pubertal stage. Adults, who usually have had pituitary tumors or head trauma, show low energy, reduced strength, weight gain, anxiety, reduced libido, and impaired sleep. GH therapy goals differ in children and adults. In adults, they are to improve conditioning and strength, restore normal body composition, and improve quality of life. In children, therapy promotes linear growth and restores body composition. Synthetic GH is effective for children with GH deficiency as long as epiphyses are not closed. Side effects include edema, muscle and joint pain, benign intracranial hypertension, hair loss, hypothyroidism, hypoglycemia or hyperglycemia, and the more serious risk of cancer.

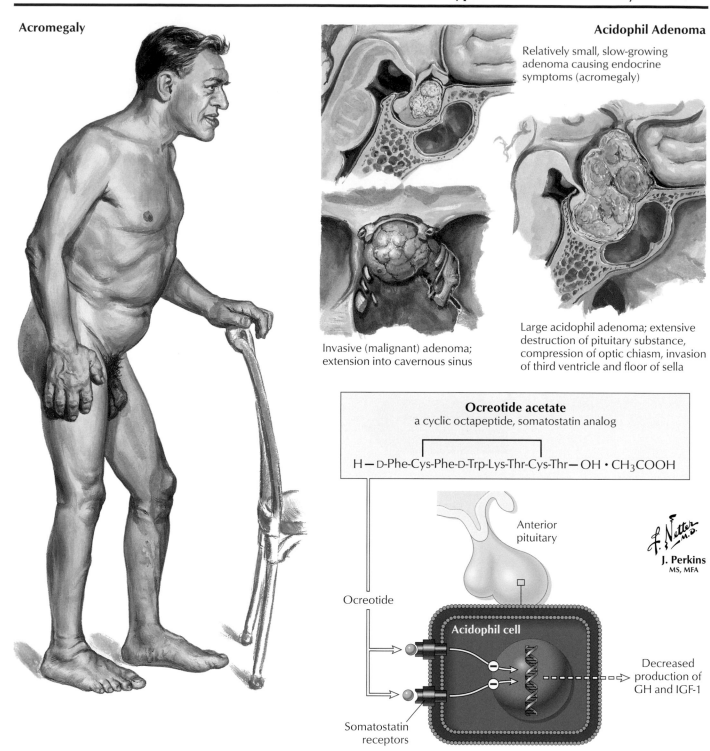

Acromegaly

Acidophil Adenoma

Relatively small, slow-growing adenoma causing endocrine symptoms (acromegaly)

Invasive (malignant) adenoma; extension into cavernous sinus

Large acidophil adenoma; extensive destruction of pituitary substance, compression of optic chiasm, invasion of third ventricle and floor of sella

Ocreotide acetate
a cyclic octapeptide, somatostatin analog

$$H - \text{D-Phe-Cys-Phe-D-Trp-Lys-Thr-Cys-Thr} - OH \cdot CH_3COOH$$

Anterior pituitary

Ocreotide

Acidophil cell

Somatostatin receptors

Decreased production of GH and IGF-1

J. Netter M.D.
J. Perkins
MS, MFA

FIGURE 5-4 GROWTH HORMONE EXCESS (ACROMEGALY) AND TREATMENT

Acromegaly is a disfiguring hormonal disorder caused by excessive GH secretion from a pituitary tumor. Signs of acromegaly include coarse facial features and enlarged hands, feet, tongue, and internal organs (which lead to heart disease, hypertension, diabetes, arthralgias). Therapy includes surgical removal of the tumor and/or radiation, or subcutaneous use of octreotide, a GH inhibitor, available in a long-acting depot form. Octreotide effects mimic those of the natural hormone somatostatin (inhibition of GH and IGF-1 levels; suppression of the response of luteinizing hormone to gonadotropin-releasing hormone). By normalizing levels of GH and IGF-1—both markers for acromegaly—octreotide controls clinical signs and symptoms. Common adverse effects are gastrointestinal; the more serious effects include cardiac arrhythmias, hypoglycemia or hyperglycemia, suppression of thyrotropin, pancreatitis, and biliary tract abnormalities.

Anatomy of the Thyroid and Parathyroid Glands

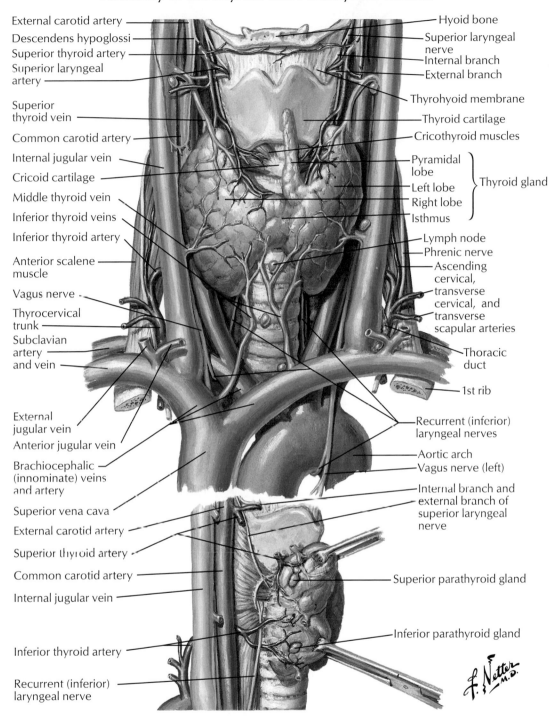

External carotid artery
Descendens hypoglossi
Superior thyroid artery
Superior laryngeal artery

Superior thyroid vein

Common carotid artery

Internal jugular vein

Cricoid cartilage

Middle thyroid vein

Inferior thyroid veins

Inferior thyroid artery

Anterior scalene muscle

Vagus nerve

Thyrocervical trunk

Subclavian artery and vein

External jugular vein

Anterior jugular vein

Brachiocephalic (innominate) veins and artery

Superior vena cava

External carotid artery

Superior thyroid artery

Common carotid artery

Internal jugular vein

Inferior thyroid artery

Recurrent (inferior) laryngeal nerve

Hyoid bone
Superior laryngeal nerve
Internal branch
External branch
Thyrohyoid membrane
Thyroid cartilage
Cricothyroid muscles
Pyramidal lobe
Left lobe   Thyroid gland
Right lobe
Isthmus
Lymph node
Phrenic nerve
Ascending cervical, transverse cervical, and transverse scapular arteries
Thoracic duct
1st rib
Recurrent (inferior) laryngeal nerves
Aortic arch
Vagus nerve (left)
Internal branch and external branch of superior laryngeal nerve
Superior parathyroid gland
Inferior parathyroid gland

FIGURE 5-5 THYROID HORMONES

The thyroid gland is responsible for regulating normal growth and development by maintaining a level of metabolism in body tissues that is optimal for normal function. The thyroid synthesizes, stores, and releases 2 major, metabolically active hormones: triiodothyronine (T_3) and thyroxine (T_4). T_3, the active form of the thyroid hormone, is 4 times more potent than T_4, but its serum concentration is lower. Approximately 80% of the gland's total daily production of T_3 results from conversion of T_4

to T_3 through deiodination of T_4. T_3 and T_4 exist in either free (active) or protein-bound (inactive) forms. More than 99% of circulating T_4 is bound to plasma proteins, so only a small fraction exists in free form. As a result, T_4 is metabolized very slowly and has a long half-life (7 days). T_3 is less bound to plasma proteins and thus undergoes faster metabolism and has a shorter half-life (1.5 days).

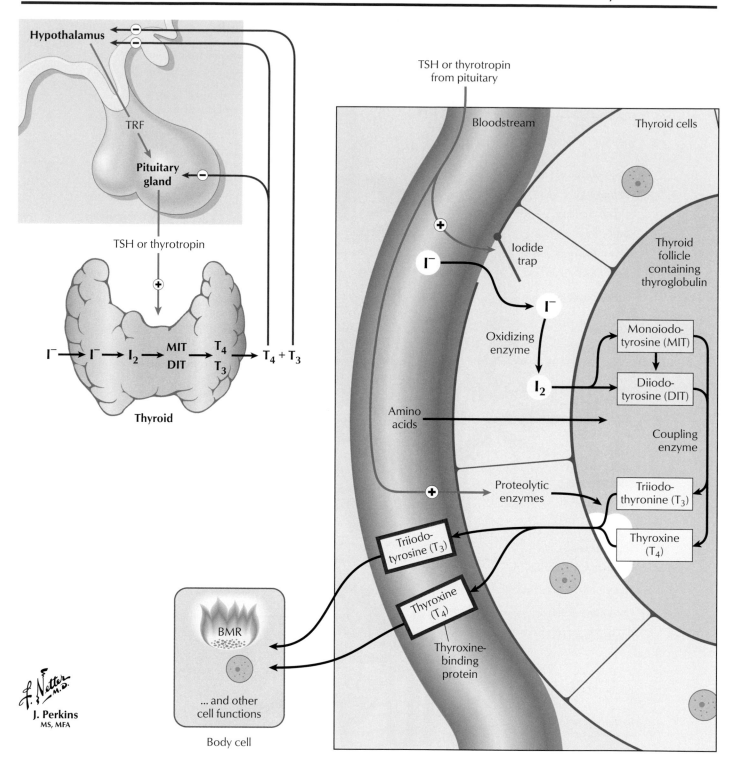

FIGURE 5-6 THYROID HORMONES: SYNTHESIS, RELEASE, AND REGULATION

Thyroid hormones are synthesized and stored as amino acid residues of thyroglobulin. Major steps in synthesis and release include thyroid uptake of iodide, oxidation of iodide and iodination of tyrosyl groups of thyroglobulin, coupling iodotyrosine residues to produce iodothyronines, proteolysis of thyroglobulin, release of T_4 and T_3 into blood, and conversion of T_4 to T_3 in peripheral tissues and the thyroid. Hormone synthesis and release are controlled by a negative feedback mechanism (thyroid; hypothalamic-pituitary axis; autoregulation of iodide uptake). Low circulating hormone levels trigger hypothalamic release of thyrotropin-releasing factor (TRF), which induces pituitary secretion of thyrotropin (thyroid-stimulating hormone, TSH). Increasing TSH levels stimulate thyroid iodide uptake and hormone synthesis. Circulating hormones halt TRF and TSH secretion. The thyroid also regulates its own iodine uptake to protect against excess hormone production if extra iodide is ingested.

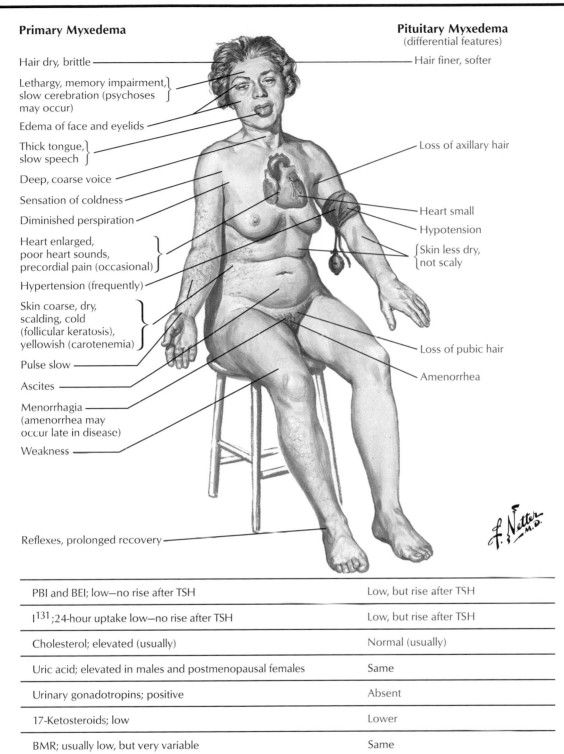

Primary Myxedema

- Hair dry, brittle
- Lethargy, memory impairment, slow cerebration (psychoses may occur)
- Edema of face and eyelids
- Thick tongue, slow speech
- Deep, coarse voice
- Sensation of coldness
- Diminished perspiration
- Heart enlarged, poor heart sounds, precordial pain (occasional)
- Hypertension (frequently)
- Skin coarse, dry, scalding, cold (follicular keratosis), yellowish (carotenemia)
- Pulse slow
- Ascites
- Menorrhagia (amenorrhea may occur late in disease)
- Weakness
- Reflexes, prolonged recovery

Pituitary Myxedema
(differential features)

- Hair finer, softer
- Loss of axillary hair
- Heart small
- Hypotension
- Skin less dry, not scaly
- Loss of pubic hair
- Amenorrhea

Primary Myxedema	Pituitary Myxedema
PBI and BEI; low—no rise after TSH	Low, but rise after TSH
I^{131};24-hour uptake low—no rise after TSH	Low, but rise after TSH
Cholesterol; elevated (usually)	Normal (usually)
Uric acid; elevated in males and postmenopausal females	Same
Urinary gonadotropins; positive	Absent
17-Ketosteroids; low	Lower
BMR; usually low, but very variable	Same

FIGURE 5-7 HYPOTHYROIDISM

Hypothyroidism, a syndrome that results from a deficiency of thyroid hormones, can be caused by either primary (thyroid gland) or secondary (hypothalamic pituitary) dysfunction. The most common cause of primary hypothyroidism is Hashimoto thyroiditis, an autoimmune disorder in which unsuppressed T lymphocytes produce excessive amounts of antibodies that destroy thyroid cells. Certain drugs, such as lithium, nitroprusside, iodides, and sulfonylureas, can also induce hypothyroidism. The condition is usually more prevalent in females and persons older than 60 years. It typically presents with symptoms of "slowing down" (eg, weight gain, fatigue, sluggishness, cold intolerance, constipation, muscle aches). Goiter may be present. Patients with end-stage hypothyroidism or myxedema coma may experience hypothermia, confusion, stupor or coma, carbon dioxide retention, hyponatremia, and ileus. Laboratory findings include increased TSH and low free T_4 levels.

Medications and Conditions Affecting Levothyroxine	
Drug or Condition	**Effect**
Resin binders (eg, cholestyramine, colestipol)	Decrease T_4 absorption
Aluminum-containing products	Decrease T_4 absorption
Iron sulfate	Decrease T_4 absorption
Calcium carbonate	Decrease T_4 absorption
Sertraline and possibly other selective serotinin reuptake inhibitors	Increase T_4 elimination
Enzyme inducers (eg, carbamazapine, phenytoin, rifampin, phenobarbital)	Increase metabolism and clearance of T_4
Pregnancy	Increase demand for T_4
Age	Decrease clearance of T_4
Malabsorption (eg, diarrhea)	Decrease T_4 absorption

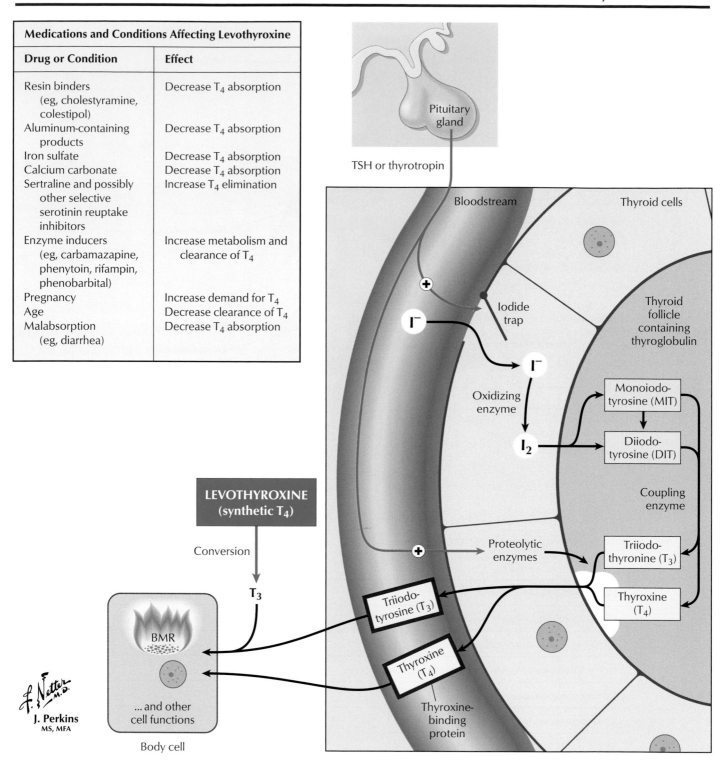

J. Perkins
MS, MFA

FIGURE 5-8 HYPOTHYROIDISM: TREATMENT OF CHOICE

The principal treatment goal for hypothyroidism is to achieve a euthyroid state with thyroid replacement therapy. The preparation of choice is levothyroxine, a synthetic T_4 formulation with advantages including stability, uniform potency, relatively low cost, once-daily dosing, and lack of foreign proteins. Levothyroxine may have innate metabolic activity, but most of its activity is due to its conversion to T_3. Patients should notice improvement in typical symptoms of hypothyroidism after 3 to 4 weeks of treatment. Toxicity is directly related to T_4 levels and manifests as nervousness, tachycardia, heat intolerance, and weight loss. Levothyroxine is available in various brands and generics, which may not be bioequivalent, so only 1 product should be used throughout treatment.

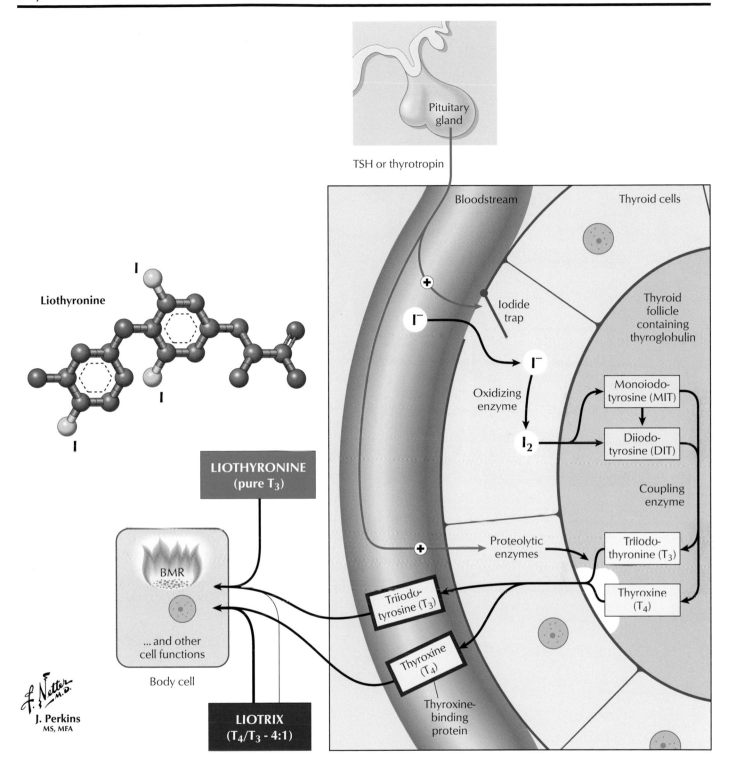

FIGURE 5-9 LIOTHYRONINE AND T₄/T₃ COMBINATIONS

Liothyronine is a pure T_3 preparation that is not recommended for routine thyroid replacement. After oral ingestion, T_3 is absorbed more rapidly than T_4, which may produce supraphysiologic plasma T_3 levels, which can lead to thyrotoxicosis. Also, free T_4 levels remain low during T_3 administration and, if misinterpreted, could lead to incorrect use of more hormone. Therefore, T_3 levels must be monitored. Other disadvantages are the need for multiple doses, higher expense, and greater potential for cardiotoxicity. T_3 is therefore not better than T_4, which is converted to T_3 anyway. However, T_3 is recommended for acute severe myxedema. Liotrix (a stable synthetic) and desiccated thyroid contain T_4 plus T_3. Liotrix uses a physiologic ratio of $4:1$ but has the same problems as T_3 and is more expensive. Desiccated thyroid, derived mostly from pork, is not recommended: product potency and composition vary and can result in toxic effects, including allergic reactions to animal protein.

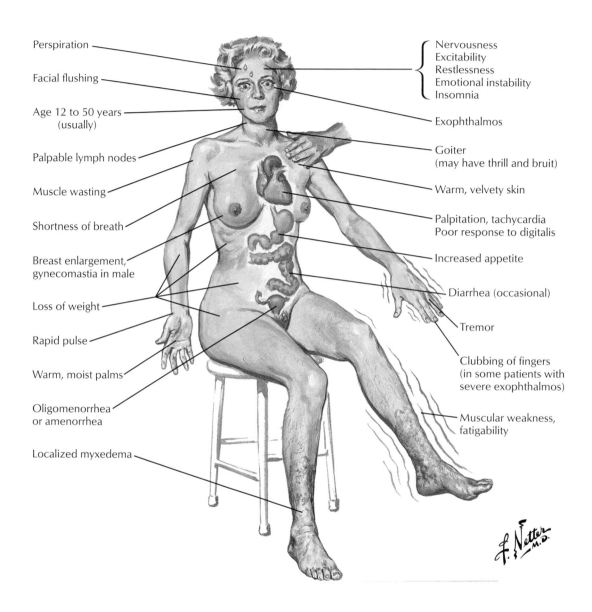

Perspiration

Facial flushing

Age 12 to 50 years
(usually)

Palpable lymph nodes

Muscle wasting

Shortness of breath

Breast enlargement,
gynecomastia in male

Loss of weight

Rapid pulse

Warm, moist palms

Oligomenorrhea
or amenorrhea

Localized myxedema

Nervousness
Excitability
Restlessness
Emotional instability
Insomnia

Exophthalmos

Goiter
(may have thrill and bruit)

Warm, velvety skin

Palpitation, tachycardia
Poor response to digitalis

Increased appetite

Diarrhea (occasional)

Tremor

Clubbing of fingers
(in some patients with
severe exophthalmos)

Muscular weakness,
fatigability

FIGURE 5-10 HYPERTHYROIDISM

Hyperthyroidism, or thyrotoxicosis, is due to excessive thyroid hormone production and is characterized by increased metabolism in all body tissues. The most common cause of hyperthyroidism is Graves disease, an autoimmune disorder in which an abnormal thyroid receptor binds to the TSH receptor and causes uncontrolled thyroid hormone production. Drugs such as amiodarone, iodides, and lithium can also cause hyperthyroidism. Like hypothyroidism, hyperthyroidism occurs more often in females than in males. Symptoms include goiter, exophthalmos, nervousness, heat intolerance, palpitations, weight loss, insomnia, and new or worsening cardiac findings (atrial fibrillation, angina). Untreated hyperthyroidism can progress to thyroid storm, a possibly fatal state with acute onset of high fever, exaggerated thyrotoxicosis symptoms, cardiovascular collapse, and shock. Laboratory findings include high serum levels of free T_4, undetectable TSH levels, or both.

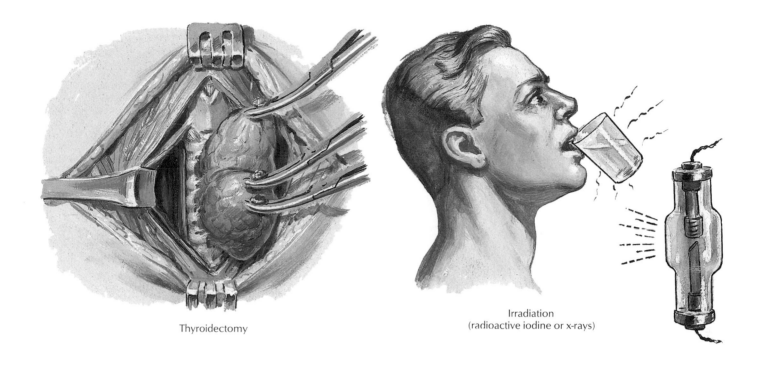

Thyroidectomy

Irradiation
(radioactive iodine or x-rays)

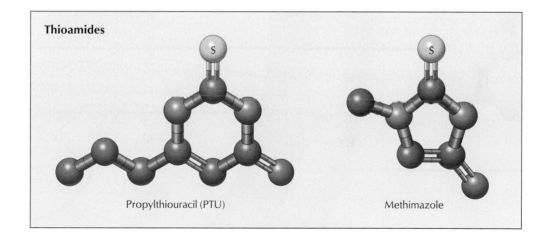

Thioamides

S

S

Propylthiouracil (PTU)

Methimazole

J. Perkins
MS, MFA

FIGURE 5-11 HYPERTHYROIDISM: TREATMENT

Primary treatment options for patients with hyperthyroidism include thioamides, radioactive iodine (RAI), and surgery. Adjuncts to primary therapies include adrenergic antagonists and iodides. Surgery (subtotal or total thyroidectomy) is considered the treatment of choice in cases of suspected malignancy, esophageal obstruction, respiratory difficulties, presence of large goiter, or contraindications to other treatments. Of the pharmacologic options, thioamides (propylthiouracil, or PTU, and methimazole) are the preferred agents for children, pregnant women, and young adults with uncomplicated Graves disease. The agents can be used as long-term therapy or as short-term therapy to reduce thyroid hormone levels before RAI or surgery.

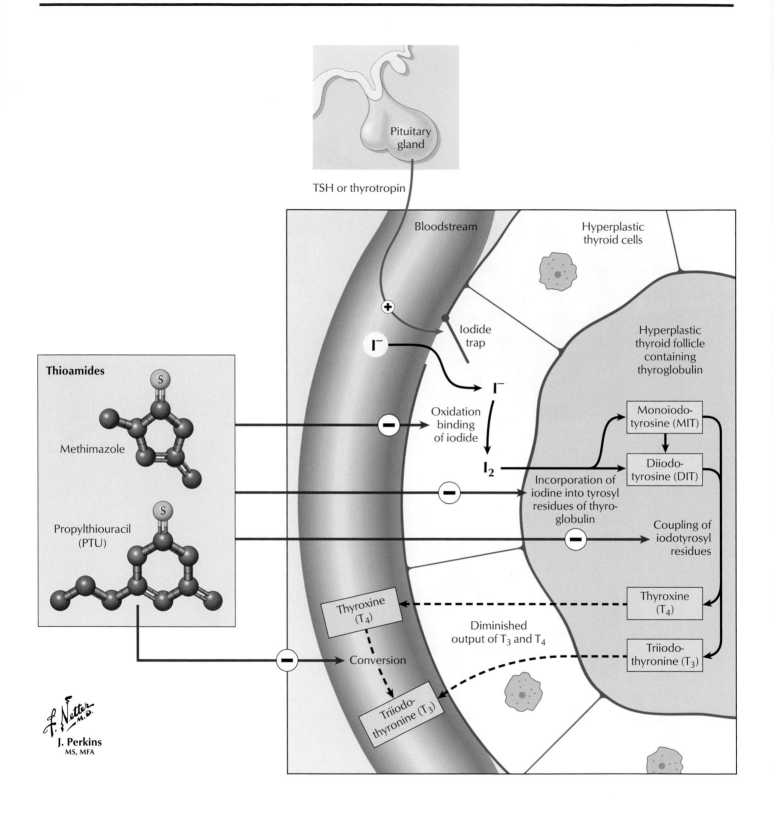

FIGURE 5-12 THIOAMIDES

Thioamides inhibit formation of thyroid hormones by interfering with incorporation of iodine into tyrosyl residues of thyroglobulin and inhibiting coupling of iodotyrosyl residues to form iodothyronines. Thioamides also block the oxidative binding of iodide because they are iodinated and degraded within the thyroid gland, which diverts oxidized iodide away from thyroglobulin. PTU, but not methimazole, inhibits peripheral deiodination of T_4 to T_3, which causes a more rapid decline in T_3 levels in patients with thyroid storm. Methimazole is 10 times more potent than PTU, but both drugs are equally effective if given in equipotent dosages. Methimazole can be given once daily, whereas PTU must be given every 6 to 8 hours. PTU is preferred for pregnant women. A clinical response is usually seen after 6 to 8 weeks of therapy with thioamides. The duration of therapy is usually 12 to 18 months.

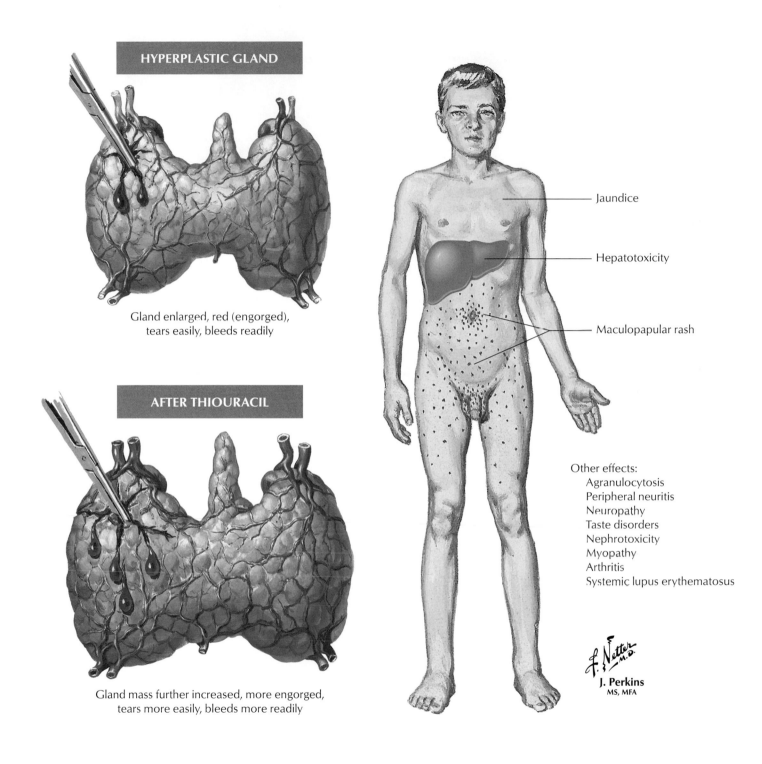

HYPERPLASTIC GLAND

Gland enlarged, red (engorged),
tears easily, bleeds readily

AFTER THIOURACIL

Gland mass further increased, more engorged,
tears more easily, bleeds more readily

Jaundice

Hepatotoxicity

Maculopapular rash

Other effects:
  Agranulocytosis
  Peripheral neuritis
  Neuropathy
  Taste disorders
  Nephrotoxicity
  Myopathy
  Arthritis
  Systemic lupus erythematosus

J. Perkins
MS, MFA

FIGURE 5-13 THIOAMIDES: ADVERSE EFFECTS

A pruritic maculopapular rash, without other systemic symptoms, is the most common adverse effect of thioamides. In mild cases, the rash resolves despite therapy, or another thioamide can be used (minimal cross-sensitivity exists). If systemic symptoms (eg, fever, arthralgias) occur, thioamide therapy should be stopped. Hepatotoxicity involves hepatocellular damage (with PTU) and obstructive jaundice (with methimazole). Liver function test (LFT) results should be watched if a history of liver disease or risk for hepatitis exists. Agranulocytosis (leukopenia with much lower polymorphonuclear leukocyte numbers) is the most serious adverse effect. Onset of symptoms (fever, malaise, sore throat) is quite sudden; high methimazole doses may lead to greater risk. If this disorder is diagnosed, thioamide administration should be stopped, and the patient should be monitored for infection. Other serious effects include peripheral neuritis, neuropathy, taste disorders, nephrotoxicity, myopathy, arthritis, and systemic lupus erythematosus.

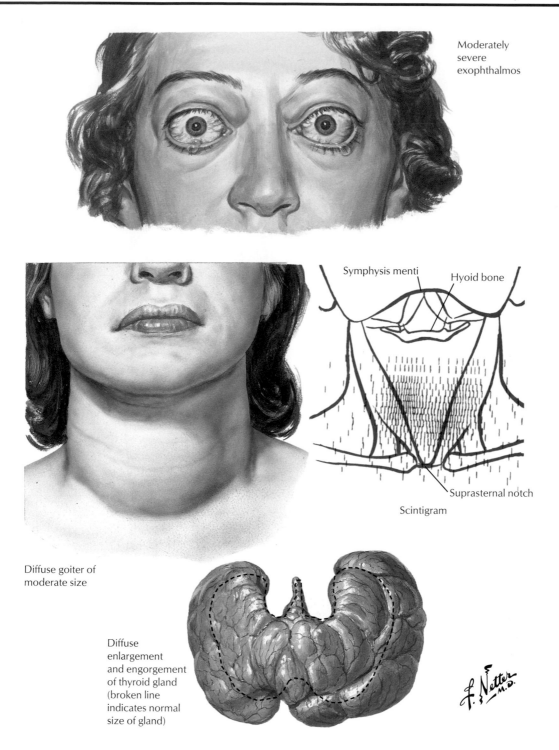

Moderately severe exophthalmos

Symphysis menti

Hyoid bone

Suprasternal notch

Scintigram

Diffuse goiter of moderate size

Diffuse enlargement and engorgement of thyroid gland (broken line indicates normal size of gland)

FIGURE 5-14 RADIOACTIVE IODINE

Radioactive iodine is used for postadolescent patients, patients with Graves ophthalmopathy or history of thyroid surgery, poor surgical candidates, and those who do not respond to thio-amides. It is the treatment of choice in older patients with heart disease and those with toxic multinodular goiter. The maximal effects of RAI do not occur for 3 to 4 months. [131]I, used most often, is rapidly trapped by the thyroid; β particles act mostly on parenchymal thyroid cells, with minimal damage to adjacent tissues. Effects of radiation depend on dosage, with larger doses causing cytotoxicity. Proper RAI doses can destroy the gland without injuring nearby tissues. The major adverse effect of RAI is hypothyroidism. Post-RAI hyperthyroidism, caused by hormones leaking from damaged thyroid, can occur but is minimized by use of thioamides or β blockers before RAI (depletes the gland of hormones). Immediate adverse effects include mild thyroid pain and hair thinning; long-term effects include carcinogenesis and genetic damage.

Hyperplastic Gland

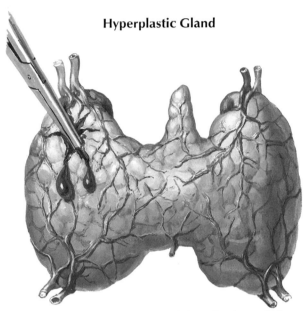

Gland enlarged, red (engorged);
tears easily, bleeds readily

After Thiouracil Plus Iodide (Itrumil)

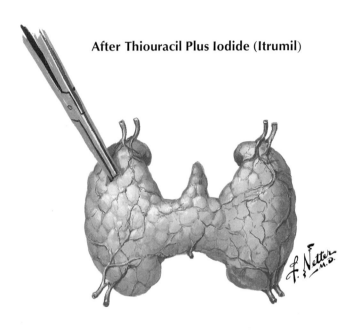

Gland reduced in size, pale and firm;
does not tear or bleed so readily

FIGURE 5-15 IODIDE

Iodide (ie, Lugol solution: 5% iodine and 10% potassium iodide) is the oldest known remedy for symptomatic relief of hyperthyroidism, and, before the advent of pharmacologic therapy, it was the sole treatment available. Today, iodide therapy has been mostly replaced by thioamides and β blockers. Iodides act by blocking organification of iodine, inhibiting release of thyroid hormones, and decreasing gland size and vascularity. Iodides act rapidly and produce symptomatic relief after 2 to 7 days. They are thus useful in patients with thyroid storm and those awaiting relief from thioamide therapy. Iodides are also routinely given, preferably with thioamides, 10 to 14 days before surgery to facilitate removal of the gland by reducing its size and vascularity. Iodide cannot be given before RAI because it can block retention of RAI by the gland. Major adverse effects of iodide include hypersensitivity reactions and the risk of hypothyroidism or worsening of hyperthyroidism.

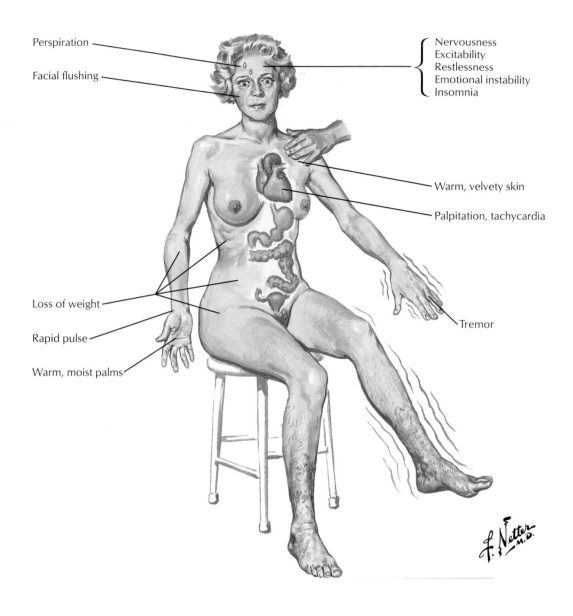

Perspiration

Facial flushing

Nervousness
Excitability
Restlessness
Emotional instability
Insomnia

Warm, velvety skin

Palpitation, tachycardia

Loss of weight

Rapid pulse

Warm, moist palms

Tremor

FIGURE 5-16 ADRENERGIC ANTAGONISTS

Many signs and symptoms of hyperthyroidism are mediated through the sympathetic nervous system, so it seems logical to use adrenergic antagonists for symptomatic relief because these agents block the effects of thyroid hormones on catecholamines. Adrenergic antagonists do not affect the underlying disease process, so they are not used as primary therapy, but they are quite useful in providing rapid symptomatic relief before thioamides, RAI, or surgery can take effect. They can also be used as adjuncts to thioamides and RAI for neonatal thyrotoxicosis, thyrotoxicosis in pregnancy, and thyroid storm. The β blocker propranolol, which reduces conversion of T_4 to T_3, is the most widely used adrenergic antagonist; it relieves palpitations, tachycardia, anxiety, sweating, tremor, and neuromuscular manifestations of hyperthyroidism. The calcium channel blocker diltiazem may be useful when propranolol should be avoided (eg, patients with asthma, CHF, diabetes).

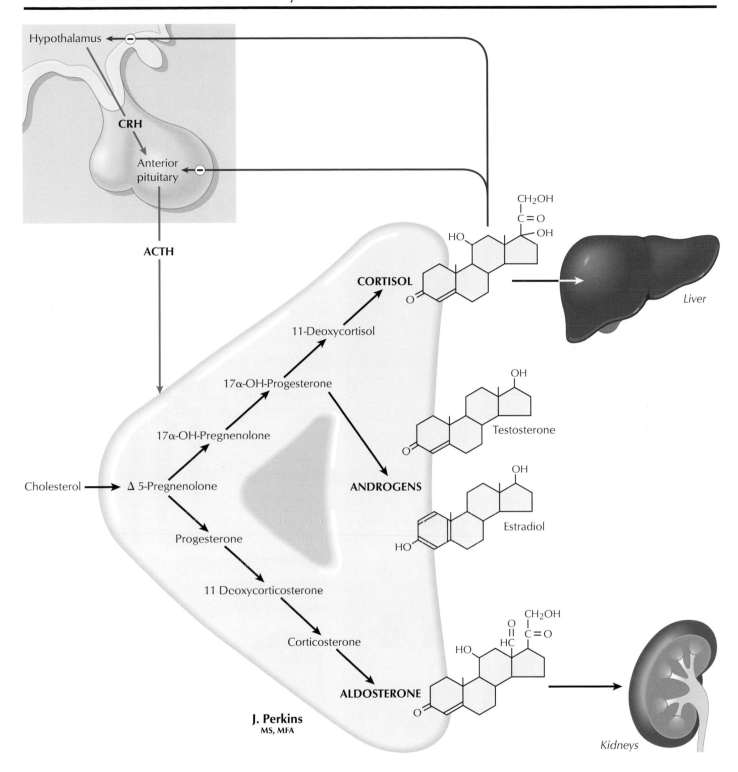

FIGURE 5-17 REGULATION OF ADRENAL HORMONES

The 2 adrenal glands in the human body are responsible for producing mineralocorticoids (eg, aldosterone), which regulate fluid and electrolyte balance, and glucocorticoids (eg, cortisol), which are essential for carbohydrate metabolism. Aldosterone production is mediated primarily by the renin-angiotensin system; cortisol production is regulated by a feedback mechanism involving the hypothalamic-pituitary-adrenal (HPA) axis. First, the hypothalamus releases CRH in response to various stimuli including neurotransmitters, vasopressin, and catecholamines. CRH stimulates the anterior pituitary to release ACTH, which then stimulates the adrenal cortex to produce cortisol. As serum cortisol levels increase, synthesis and secretion of CRH and ACTH decrease via a negative feedback loop.

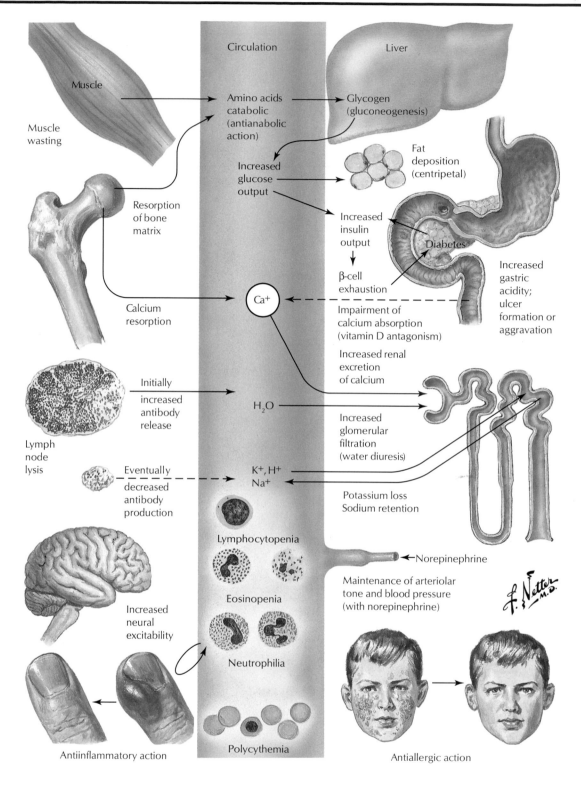

FIGURE 5-18 MINERALOCORTICOIDS AND GLUCOCORTICOIDS

Mineralocorticoids enhance reabsorption of sodium and water from the distal tubule of the kidney and increase urinary potassium and hydrogen ion excretion. The principal function of glucocorticoids involves regulation of carbohydrate metabolism, but they are also involved in other physiologic actions, including gluconeogenesis, glucose utilization, lipid and bone metabolism, fluid and electrolyte homeostasis, alteration of levels of various immune cells, alleviation of the inflammatory response, and participation in neuropsychiatric functions. As a result of these functions—most notably immunosuppressive and antiinflammatory actions (a direct result of immunosuppressive effects)—glucocorticoids are widely used in treatment of cancer and autoimmune and inflammatory disorders such as asthma, inflammatory bowel disease, arthritis, and allergies.

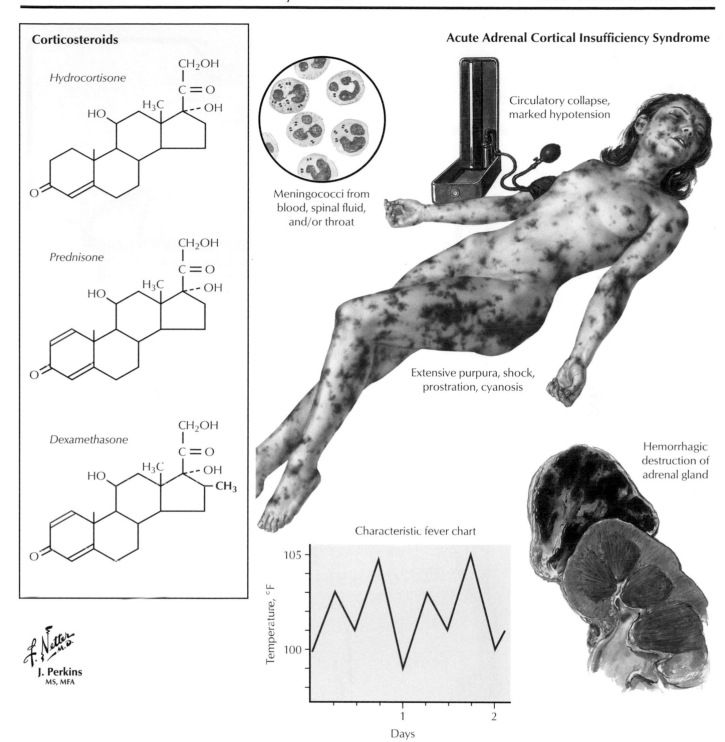

Corticosteroids

Hydrocortisone

Prednisone

Dexamethasone

J. Perkins
MS, MFA

Acute Adrenal Cortical Insufficiency Syndrome

Meningococci from blood, spinal fluid, and/or throat

Circulatory collapse, marked hypotension

Extensive purpura, shock, prostration, cyanosis

Hemorrhagic destruction of adrenal gland

Characteristic fever chart

FIGURE 5-19 CORTICOSTEROIDS

Therapeutic corticosteroids (eg, hydrocortisone, prednisone, dexamethasone), with different mineralocorticoid and glucocorticoid activities, are antiinflammatory and immunosuppressive via inhibiting immune cells. This reduces formation, release, and activity of inflammation mediators (eg, cytokines, histamine, prostaglandins, leukotrienes). Short-term therapy adverse effects include insomnia, euphoria, and increased appetite, and long-term therapy effects include osteoporosis, hypertension, edema, hyperglycemia, and Cushing-like syndrome. Long-term drug use can suppress the HPA axis, and abrupt stopping of therapy can cause the possibly fatal acute adrenal insufficiency syndrome. Slow dosage tapering allows the HPA axis to begin functioning. To reduce systemic absorption and side effects, drugs can be given topically or by inhalation or nasal spray, intraarticular injection, or rectal suppository. Alternate-day and lowest effective dosing may limit side effects and adrenal atrophy.

149

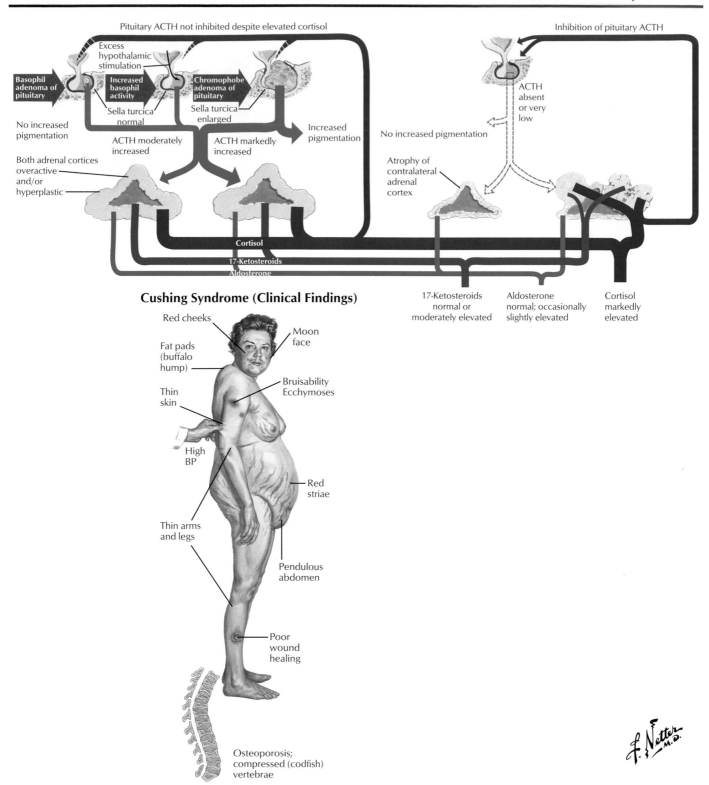

Cushing Syndrome (Clinical Findings)

FIGURE 5-20 CUSHING SYNDROME

Cushing syndrome is a group of clinical symptoms that result from prolonged exposure to excess glucocorticoids. The condition may be caused by exogenous factors, such as long-term corticosteroid use, or it may be of endogenous origin. The latter may be due to either excess ACTH secretion (ACTH dependent) or autonomous cortisol hypersecretion (ACTH independent). Conditions such as adrenocortical adenomas and carcinomas as well as ectopic ACTH and CRH syndromes are responsible for

the endogenous syndrome. Clinical manifestations affect multiple organ systems and depend on the degree and duration of hypercortisolism. The most common sign is progressive obesity, which is seen in the face, neck, trunk, and abdomen. Facial fat accumulation produces a moon-face appearance, and an enlarged dorsocervical fat pad produces a buffalo hump. Other symptoms include weakness, muscle wasting, reduced arm muscle mass, osteoporosis, and cardiovascular and metabolic complications.

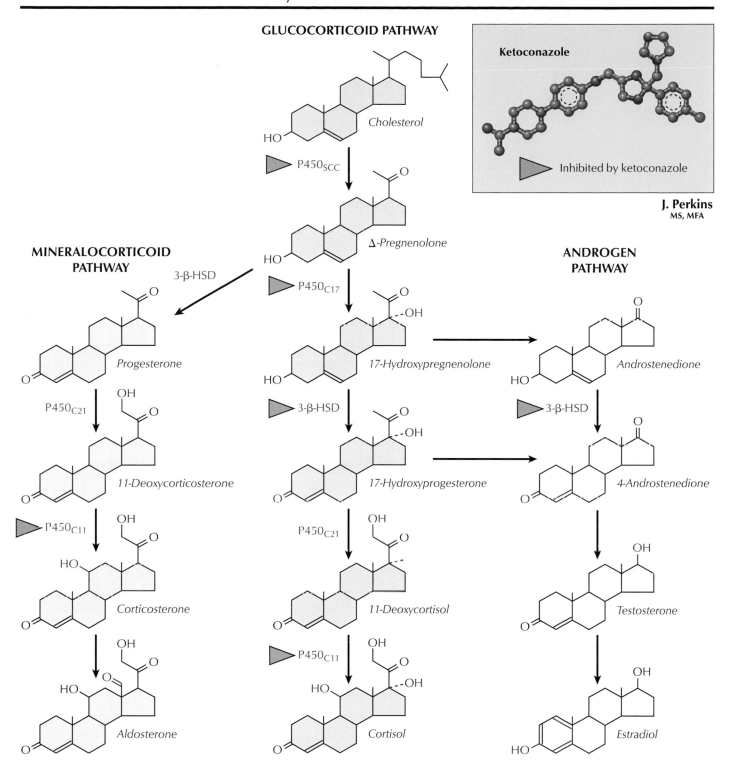

GLUCOCORTICOID PATHWAY

Cholesterol

P450$_{SCC}$

Δ-Pregnenolone

MINERALOCORTICOID PATHWAY

3-β-HSD

P450$_{C17}$

Progesterone

17-Hydroxypregnenolone

ANDROGEN PATHWAY

Androstenedione

P450$_{C21}$

3-β-HSD

3-β-HSD

11-Deoxycorticosterone

17-Hydroxyprogesterone

4-Androstenedione

P450$_{C11}$

Corticosterone

P450$_{C21}$

11-Deoxycortisol

Testosterone

P450$_{C11}$

Aldosterone

Cortisol

Estradiol

Ketoconazole

▷ Inhibited by ketoconazole

J. Perkins
MS, MFA

FIGURE 5-21 KETOCONAZOLE

Therapy for exogenous Cushing syndrome consists of minimizing exposure to glucocorticoids or ACTH. For the endogenous syndrome, therapy aims to reduce cortisol production in preparing patients for surgery or to maintain normal plasma cortisol levels until full effects of surgery or radiation are felt. The antifungal agent ketoconazole is used to treat paraneoplastic Cushing syndrome secondary to ectopic ACTH production. The agent is highly effective in decreasing cortisol by inhibiting adrenocortical cytochrome P-450–dependent enzymes. These enzymes catalyze formation of cortisol precursors such as pregnenolone as well as metabolizing drugs. Because ketoconazole inhibits the latter effect, it can increase levels of many hepatically metabolized agents such as cyclosporine, warfarin, digoxin, and phenytoin. Side effects include blood dyscrasias, headache, dizziness, fatigue, gynecomastia, GI symptoms, and rash. Patients respond to therapy after 4 to 6 weeks.

GLUCOCORTICOID PATHWAY

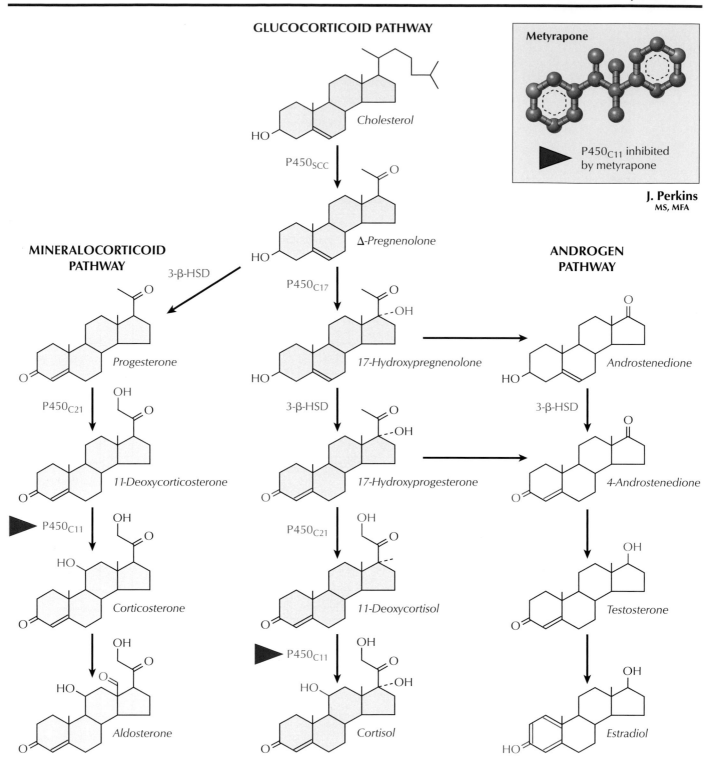

FIGURE 5-22 METYRAPONE

Metyrapone is used to treat Cushing syndrome when dose-limiting side effects occur with ketoconazole, and it can be used in combination with other agents. The agent can also be used as a test for adrenal function. Metyrapone reduces cortisol production by inhibiting 11-β-hydroxylation, the final step in glucocorticoid synthesis. This process leads to accumulation of

adrenal androgens and the potent mineralocorticoid 11-deoxycorticosterone. Resultant adverse effects include water retention, hirsutism, GI disturbances, and dizziness. Dose reduction can limit these adverse effects. Metyrapone may take up to 4 months to produce a response.

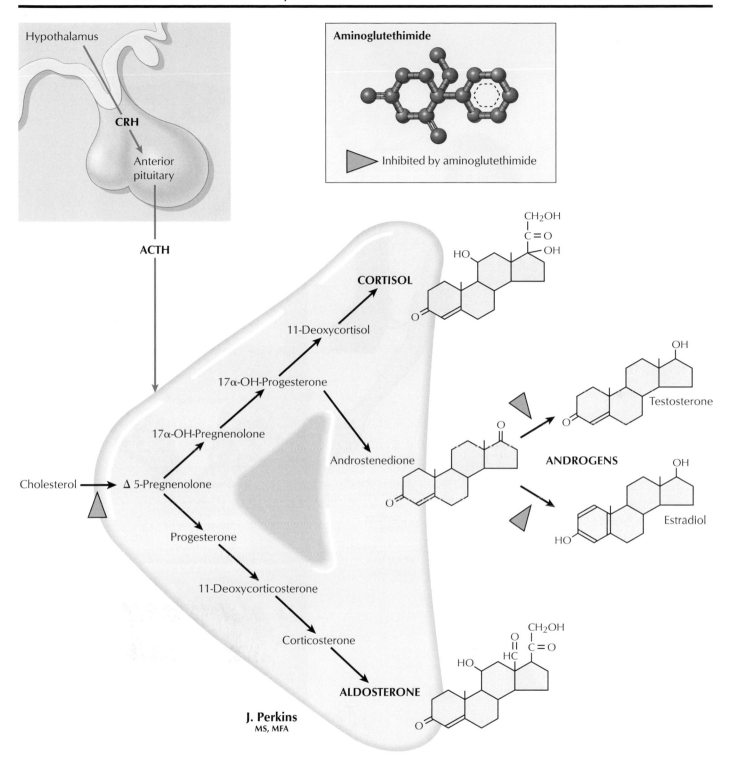

Hypothalamus

CRH

Anterior pituitary

ACTH

Aminoglutethimide

▷ Inhibited by aminoglutethimide

CORTISOL

11-Deoxycortisol

17α-OH-Progesterone

17α-OH-Pregnenolone

Androstenedione

Cholesterol → Δ 5-Pregnenolone

Testosterone

ANDROGENS

Estradiol

Progesterone

11-Deoxycorticosterone

Corticosterone

ALDOSTERONE

J. Perkins
MS, MFA

FIGURE 5-23 AMINOGLUTETHIMIDE

Aminoglutethimide is used primarily for Cushing syndrome secondary to adrenal hyperplasia, ectopic ACTH production, or adrenal carcinoma. The drug seems most useful when given after pituitary irradiation or in combination with metyrapone. Aminoglutethimide partially inhibits conversion of cholesterol to pregnenolone in the adrenal glands and blocks conversion of androstenedione (prehormone produced in the adrenals) to estrone and estradiol in peripheral tissues. This inhibition interrupts production of cortisol, aldosterone, and estrogens. A reflex increase in ACTH results, which partly or completely overcomes the blockade, but this reflex can be prevented by replacement amounts of hydrocortisone, but not dexamethasone, given concomitantly. Adverse effects include headache, sedation, dizziness, nausea, anorexia, rash, blood dyscrasias, tachycardia, and hypertension. This drug may take up to 4 months to produce a response.

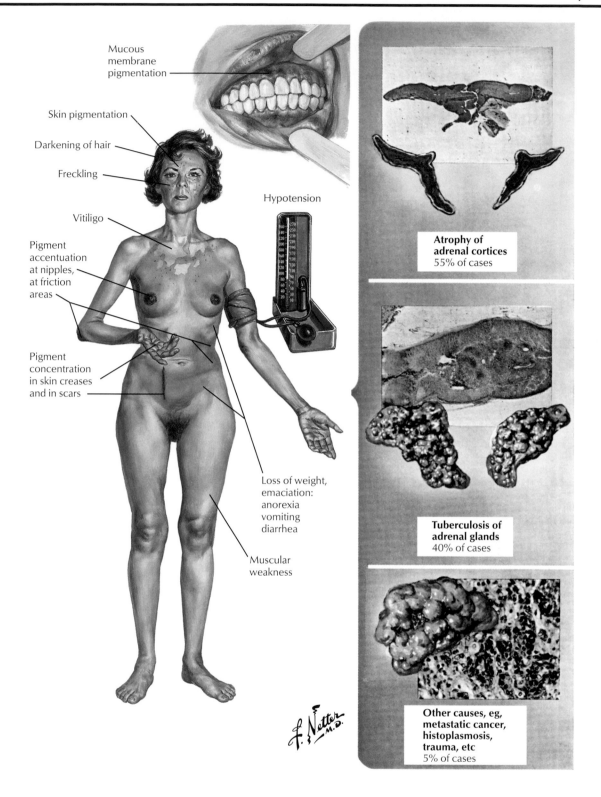

Mucous membrane pigmentation

Skin pigmentation

Darkening of hair

Freckling

Vitiligo

Pigment accentuation at nipples, at friction areas

Pigment concentration in skin creases and in scars

Hypotension

Loss of weight, emaciation: anorexia vomiting diarrhea

Muscular weakness

Atrophy of adrenal cortices 55% of cases

Tuberculosis of adrenal glands 40% of cases

Other causes, eg, metastatic cancer, histoplasmosis, trauma, etc 5% of cases

FIGURE 5-24 ADDISON DISEASE, OR PRIMARY ADRENAL INSUFFICIENCY

Addison disease is due to autoimmune-mediated destruction of adrenal cortex, mycobacterial infection, adrenal metastases, or use of certain drugs. Symptoms, caused by reduced production of glucocorticoids, mineralocorticoids, and sex hormones, range from vague feelings of illness to acute syncope and mental status changes. Biochemical abnormalities (eg, hyponatremia, hyperkalemia) usually exist. The life-threatening adrenal crisis, which occurs in cases of undiagnosed adrenal insufficiency and

untreated stress, mimics septic shock and presents with severe anorexia, dehydration, and hypotension; IV fluids and high-dose IV glucocorticoids are used for therapy. Chronic disease is managed with a glucocorticoid (hydrocortisone) plus a mineralocorticoid (fludrocortisone), with dosage tailored to avoid Cushing syndrome or inadequate therapy. Patients should be monitored for fludrocortisone side effects (eg, electrolyte changes, hypertension, edema, and hyperglycemia).

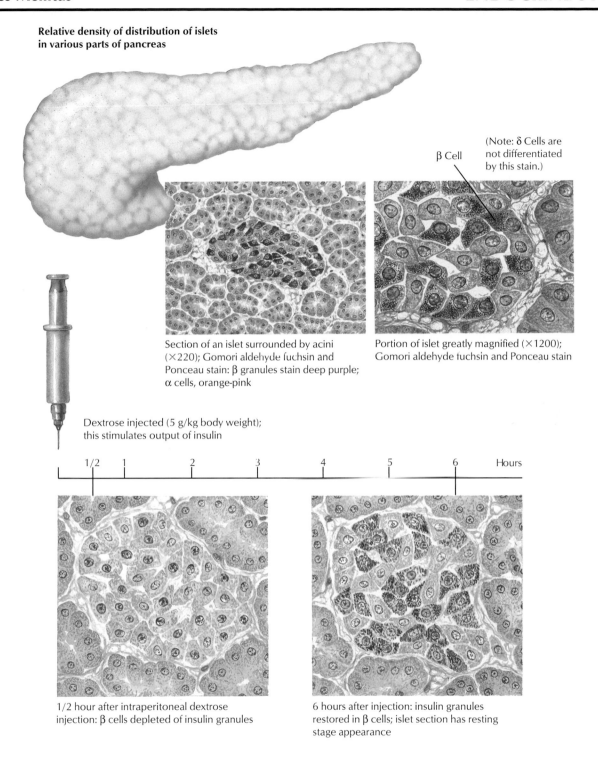

Relative density of distribution of islets in various parts of pancreas

(Note: δ Cells are not differentiated by this stain.)

β Cell

Section of an islet surrounded by acini (×220); Gomori aldehyde fuchsin and Ponceau stain: β granules stain deep purple; α cells, orange-pink

Portion of islet greatly magnified (×1200); Gomori aldehyde fuchsin and Ponceau stain

Dextrose injected (5 g/kg body weight); this stimulates output of insulin

1/2   1   2   3   4   5   6   Hours

1/2 hour after intraperitoneal dextrose injection: β cells depleted of insulin granules

6 hours after injection: insulin granules restored in β cells; islet section has resting stage appearance

FIGURE 5-25 THE PANCREAS AND INSULIN PRODUCTION

The pancreas is the principal organ involved in production and secretion of hormones that maintain normal blood glucose levels, or euglycemia. The pancreatic β cells of the islets of Langerhans produce, store, and secrete insulin. The pancreas first produces a parent protein called *preproinsulin*, which is then cleaved to form the smaller compound proinsulin. Proinsulin is then cleaved to form insulin and peptide C. The pancreas also produces glucagon, a hormone that increases blood glucose levels, and somatostatin, a hormone that inhibits both insulin and glucagon secretion. Ingestion of carbohydrates prompts an increase in the release of insulin and a concomitant decrease in plasma glucagon levels. Glucagon is released in response to low blood glucose levels and protein ingestion. It stimulates insulin secretion, which in turn inhibits glucagon release in a negative feedback loop.

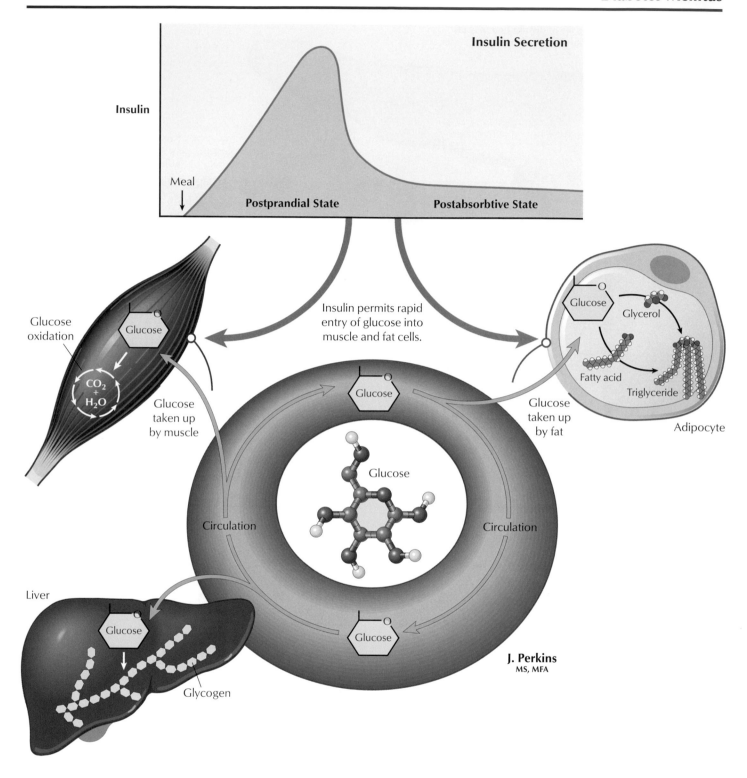

FIGURE 5-26 INSULIN SECRETION

Insulin secretion is a highly regulated process that varies throughout the day. In a postprandial setting (after a meal), a burst of insulin secretion normally occurs in response to a transient increase in the plasma glucose level. In a postabsorptive period, the pancreas reduces insulin secretion, which maintains low basal levels of circulating insulin. Insulin is the key to the body's use of glucose. It promotes the uptake of glucose, fatty acids, and amino acids, and it facilitates their conversion to forms used for storage in most tissues. The important metabolic sites that are sensitive to insulin include the liver, where glycogen (the main carbohydrate reserve, which is easily converted to glucose) is synthesized, stored, and broken down; skeletal muscle, where glucose oxidation produces energy; and adipose tissue, where glucose is converted to fatty acids, glycerol phosphate, and triglycerides.

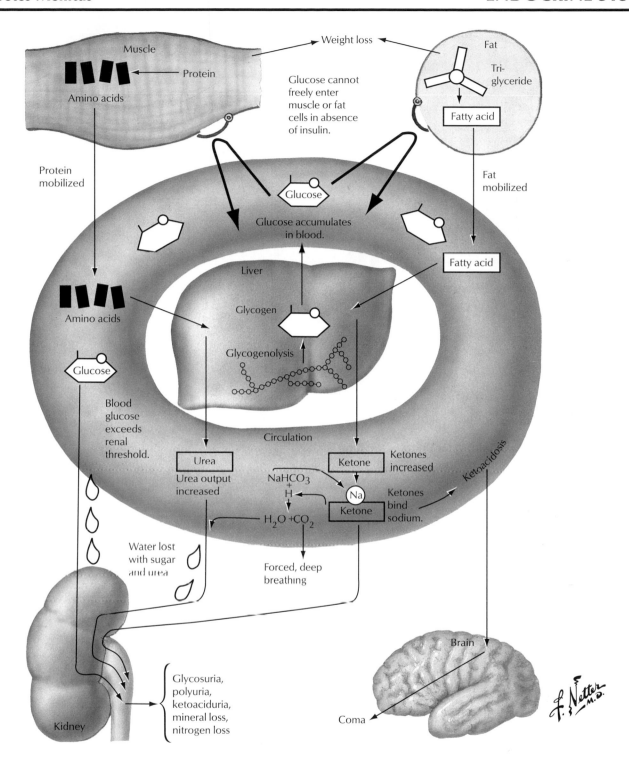

FIGURE 5-27 LACK OF INSULIN

Without insulin, glucose is not transported across cell membranes, which leads to a cascade of metabolic events. The body reacts by inducing gluconeogenesis (the liver converts glycogen to glucose). To produce energy, skeletal muscle converts its structural proteins to amino acids, which are carried to the liver, where they are converted to glucose. Resultant excess glucose, still not being used by cells, leads to hyperglycemia. Insulin deficiency increases fat catabolism: free fatty acids are broken down into keto acids to increase energy sources. Kidneys eliminate keto acids, which produces ketonuria and ketonemia. Keto acids also reduce blood pH, which can result in ketoacidoses, coma, and death. Diabetes is caused by a relative or absolute lack of insulin, with hyperglycemia being the hallmark medical finding. Once thought of as 1 disease, diabetes is now believed to be a chronic heterogeneous group of disorders that result from pathologic processes that depend on diabetes type.

Microvascular and Macrovascular Complications

Diabetic retinopathy
Diabetic retinopathy can be easily detected during a dilated eye exam and is the leading cause of blindness among adults in the United States. Visual loss can be prevented with early recognition and treatment of retinopathy.

Cerebrovascular disease
The high incidence of vascular complications among patients with diabetes is related not only to blood glucose elevations, but also to the frequent association of dyslipidemia, hypertension, a procoagulant state, and the tendency to form unstable plaques in the arterial wall.

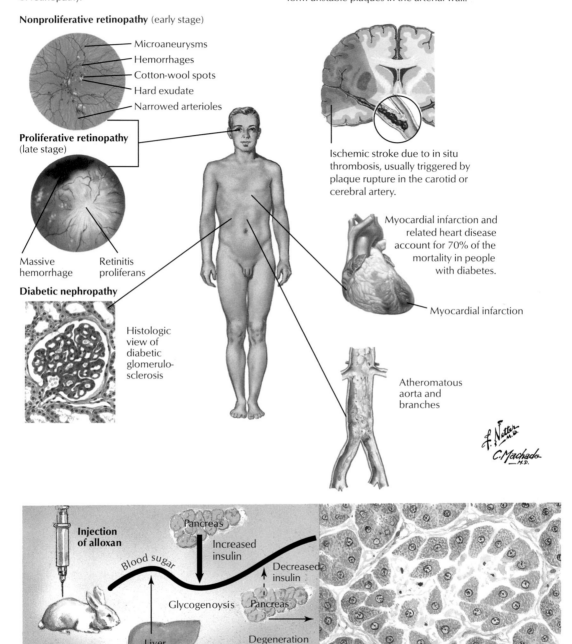

Nonproliferative retinopathy (early stage)

- Microaneurysms
- Hemorrhages
- Cotton-wool spots
- Hard exudate
- Narrowed arterioles

Proliferative retinopathy (late stage)

Massive hemorrhage   Retinitis proliferans

Diabetic nephropathy

Histologic view of diabetic glomerulosclerosis

Ischemic stroke due to in situ thrombosis, usually triggered by plaque rupture in the carotid or cerebral artery.

Myocardial infarction and related heart disease account for 70% of the mortality in people with diabetes.

Myocardial infarction

Atheromatous aorta and branches

Injection of alloxan

Blood sugar

Pancreas — Increased insulin

Decreased insulin

Pancreas

Glycogenoysis

Liver

Degeneration of β cells

FIGURE 5-28 TYPE 1 DIABETES MELLITUS

In type 1 DM, the insulin-producing β cells of the pancreas are destroyed by either intrinsic genetic factors or extrinsic factors such as viruses or chemical toxins. In one theory that involves an autoimmune-mediated mechanism, predisposed patients react abnormally to environmental triggers by producing antibodies that are directed against β cells. Insulin secretion is impaired early in the disease and eventually stops. Type 1 DM usually develops abruptly during childhood or adolescence and usually presents with polydipsia, polyuria, and polyphagia. Ketoacidosis is more likely to occur in type 1 than in type 2 DM. Patients require lifelong treatment with exogenous insulin to control blood glucose levels and prevent short- and long-term macrovascular and microvascular complications such as nephropathy, neuropathy, retinopathy, and cardiovascular disease. Oral hypoglycemic agents are ineffective in patients with type 1 DM because functioning β cells are required.

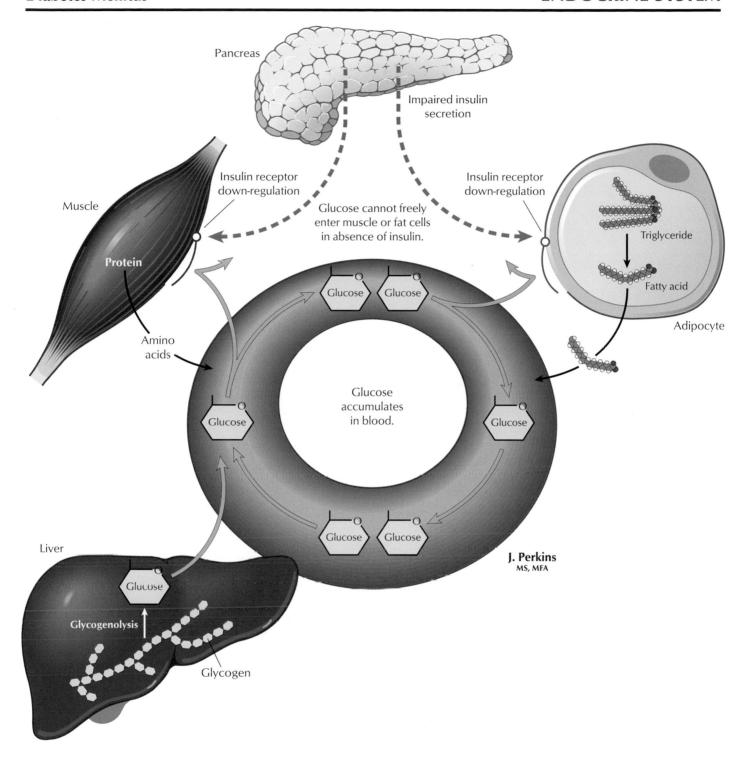

FIGURE 5-29 TYPE 2 DIABETES MELLITUS

Central defects in type 2 DM are decreased insulin secretion and insulin resistance. Before diabetes is diagnosed, patients, often obese, have hyperinsulinemia caused by excess dietary carbohydrates. The pancreas malfunctions and fails to supply high insulin demands. This impaired secretion is complicated by insulin resistance: insulin cannot decrease plasma glucose levels through suppression of hepatic glucose production and stimulation of glucose use in skeletal muscle and adipose tissue. Resistance develops in several possible ways, eg, chronic hyperinsulinemia causes insulin receptor down-regulation, which leads to defects in insulin binding and postreceptor insulin signaling pathways. Unlike type 1 DM, type 2 DM has a more gradual onset, may not present with symptoms, and usually occurs in overweight patients older than 35 years. Oral hypoglycemic agents decrease plasma glucose levels, improve insulin resistance, and reduce long-term complications. Many patients need insulin therapy.

Oral Antihyperlipidemic Agents

Drug	Interactions	Contraindications
Sulfonylureas (first generation) Acetohexamide Chlorpropamide Tolazamide Tolbutamide	Numerous interactions with drugs that alter hepatic metabolism or urinary excretion (eg, chloramphenicol, cimetidine, warfarin, salicylates, certain sulfonamide antibiotics), especially with chlorpropamide and tolbutamide	Type 1 DM, pregnancy or breast feeding, severe hepatic or renal dysfunctions, severe acute comorbidities or surgery
Sulfonylureas (second generation) Glimepiride Glipizide Glyburide	Less likely to have drug interactions than first-generation agents	
α-Glucosidase inhibitors Acarbose Miglitol	Absorption possibly reduced by charcoal and digestive enzymes; possibly reduced digoxin, propranolol, and ranitidine levels	Malabsorption, inflammatory bowel disease, intestinal obstruction
Biguanide Metformin	Effect potentiated by alcohol and cimetidine; acute renal failure possibly caused by iodinated materials; metformin-induced lactic acidosis	Renal failure (creatinine clearance >1.4 mg/dL in females, >1.5 mg/dL in males), hepatic disease, congestive heart failure requiring drug treatment, history of lactic acidosis, alcoholism, imminent surgery, before and 48 hours after parenteral contrast studies
Meglitinides Repaglinide Nateglinide	Effect of repaglinide possibly reduced by drugs that induce cytochrome P-450 enzyme system (antiepileptics, rifampin)	Type 1 DM
Thiazolidinediones Pioglitazone Rosiglitazone	Metabolism of pioglitazone inhibited by drugs metabolized by cytochrome enzymes, such as ketoconazole; plasma concentrations of oral contraceptives reduced by pioglitazone	Type 1 DM, preexisting liver disease, severe congestive heart failure, premenopausal anovulatory women (TZDs may cause resumption of ovulation and unpredicted, possibly unwanted, pregnancy), drugs metabolized by cytochrome enzymes

Matching Pharmacology to Pathophysiology

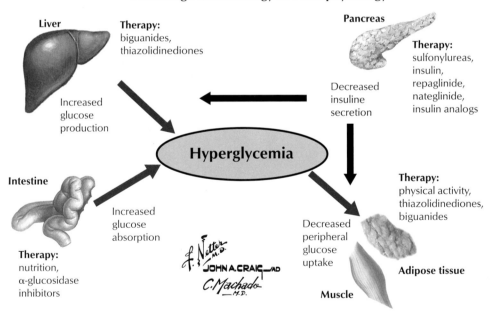

FIGURE 5-30 INSULIN THERAPY

Insulin is the sole therapy for type 1 DM. It is also used (combination therapy or monotherapy) in type 2 DM poorly controlled with diet and oral agents. Exogenous insulin stimulates carbohydrate metabolism and helps with transfer of glucose into cardiac and skeletal muscle and adipose tissue. Insulin also aids in conversion of glucose to glycogen, stimulates lipogenesis and protein synthesis, and reduces serum potassium and magnesium levels. Insulin, a protein, is degraded in the GI system if used orally, so it is given subcutaneously, or, in emergencies, intravenously. Absorption of an insulin product may vary in a patient from one injection to the next, absorption being affected by site of injection, temperature, physical activity, and dose. Insulin preparations differ in dose, onset, duration, and sources of origin, including biosynthetic and semisynthetic human (therapeutically equal), human insulin (least antigenic and most soluble), and beef and pork (replaced by human).

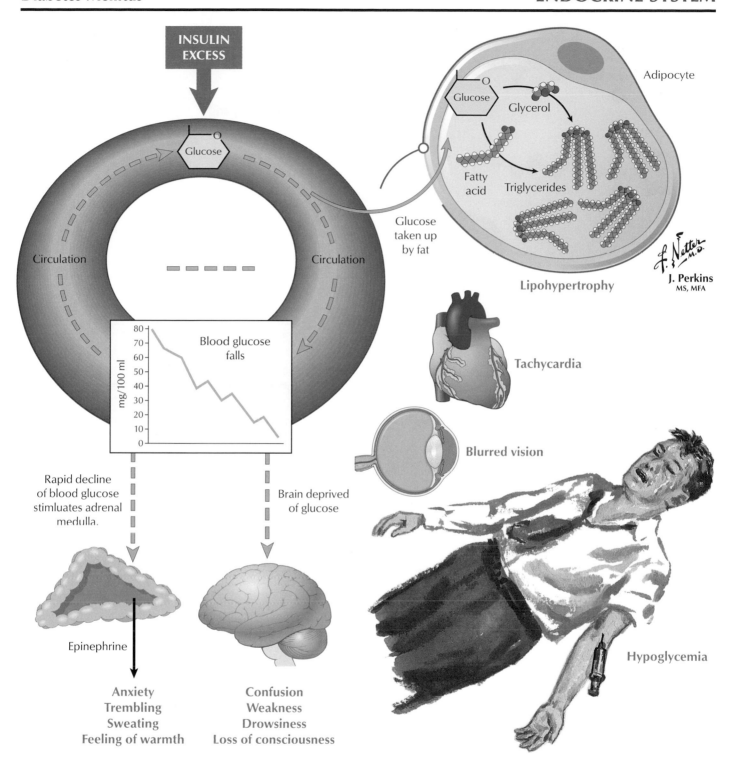

FIGURE 5-31 REACTIONS TO INSULIN: HYPOGLYCEMIA AND ADIPOSE TISSUE CHANGES

Major predisposing factors to hypoglycemia, the most common and serious adverse reaction to insulin, include inadequate food intake, poor timing of injections, exercise, and use of hypoglycemic drugs. Symptoms are autonomic (eg, sweating, trembling, feeling of warmth) or neuroglycopenic (eg, confusion, weakness, drowsiness). Hunger, tachycardia, blurred vision, and loss of consciousness also occur. Elderly patients with neuropathy, patients with long-standing diabetes (>10 years), and patients taking β blockers can have blunted symptoms. Use of sugar packets, candy, or pure glucose products can help with hypoglycemia. Unconscious patients must be injected with glucagon or IV glucose or dextrose. Insulin injection may also cause lipohypertrophy, which occurs in patients who use only 1 site rather than rotating sites. Rotating sites solves the problem. Lipoatrophy, an immunologic reaction to insulin, is treated by changing to human insulin and injecting it into the affected area.

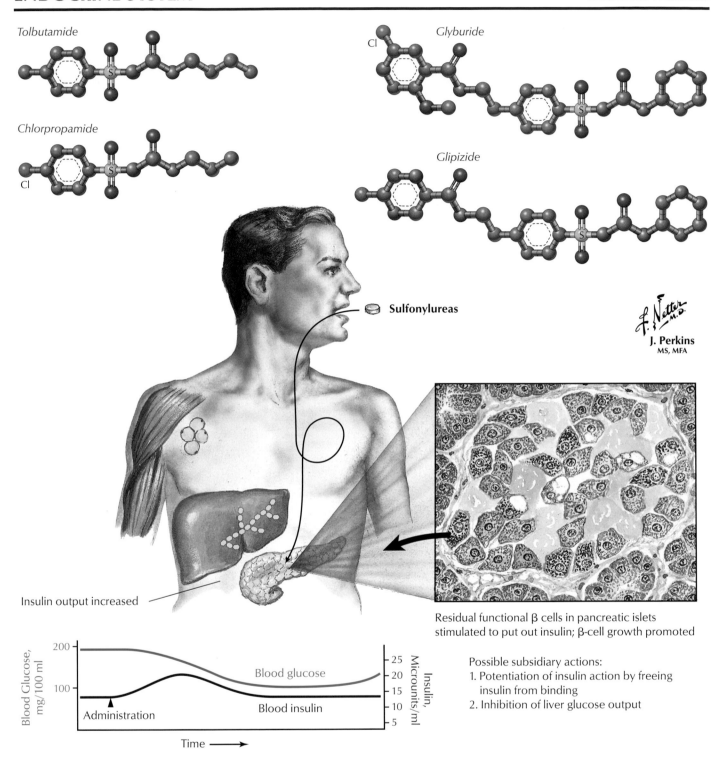

Tolbutamide

Chlorpropamide

Glyburide

Glipizide

Sulfonylureas

J. Perkins
MS, MFA

Insulin output increased

Residual functional β cells in pancreatic islets stimulated to put out insulin; β-cell growth promoted

Possible subsidiary actions:
1. Potentiation of insulin action by freeing insulin from binding
2. Inhibition of liver glucose output

Blood Glucose, mg/100 ml

200

100

Administration

Blood glucose

Blood insulin

Insulin, Microunits/ml

25
20
15
10
5

Time

FIGURE 5-32 SULFONYLUREAS

Sulfonylureas, the historical mainstay of therapy in type 2 DM, used as monotherapy or with insulin or other oral agents, act mainly by stimulating insulin secretion from pancreatic β cells, enhancing β-cell sensitivity to glucose, and reducing glucagon release. They work only if β cells are functioning. Older drugs (eg, chlorpropamide, tolbutamide) have been replaced by new agents (eg, glimepiride, glipizide, glyburide), with greater potency, fewer drug interactions, and better pharmacokinetic profiles. If glucose control fails with long-term sulfonylurea use, other agents may be added instead of increasing sulfonylurea doses. Sulfonylureas are best for patients diagnosed after the age of 40 years or when disease duration is less than 5 years, body weight is nearly ideal, and fasting glucose levels are less than 180 mg/dL. Main adverse effects are hypoglycemia and weight gain; others are GI-related effects, allergic reactions, hepatotoxicity, hypothyroidism, and disulfiram reaction (chlorpropamide).

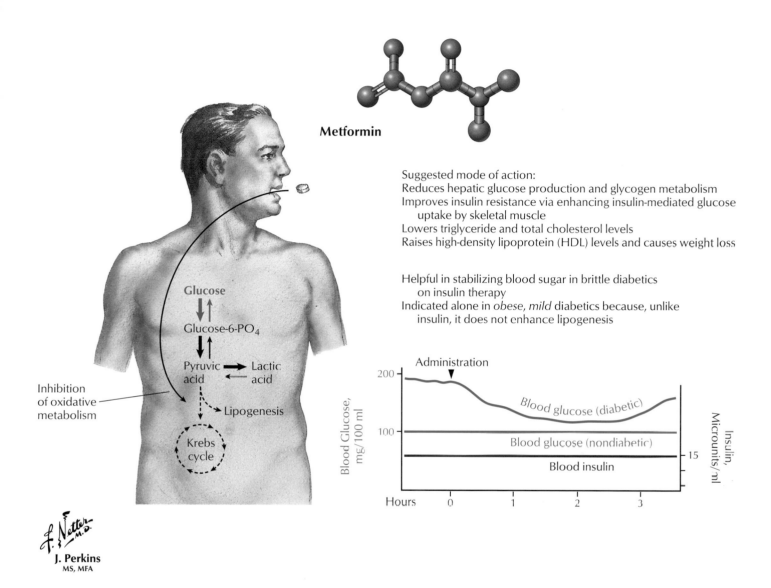

Metformin

Suggested mode of action:
Reduces hepatic glucose production and glycogen metabolism
Improves insulin resistance via enhancing insulin-mediated glucose
    uptake by skeletal muscle
Lowers triglyceride and total cholesterol levels
Raises high-density lipoprotein (HDL) levels and causes weight loss

Helpful in stabilizing blood sugar in brittle diabetics
    on insulin therapy
Indicated alone in *obese, mild* diabetics because, unlike
    insulin, it does not enhance lipogenesis

Glucose

Glucose-6-PO$_4$

Pyruvic → Lactic
acid ← acid

Inhibition
of oxidative → → Lipogenesis
metabolism

Krebs
cycle

Administration

Blood Glucose, mg/100 ml

200

100

Blood glucose (diabetic)

Blood glucose (nondiabetic)

15

Blood insulin

Insulin, Microunits/ml

Hours   0   1   2   3

J. Perkins
MS, MFA

FIGURE 5-33 BIGUANIDES

Metformin, the only biguanide available in the United States, is used as initial monotherapy or with insulin or other oral drugs in patients with type 2 DM who have secondary failure to sulfonyl-urea monotherapy (initial response but then failed glucose control with long-term use). Metformin decreases blood glucose levels by reducing hepatic glucose production and glycogen metabolism and improving insulin resistance via enhancing insulin-mediated glucose uptake. It decreases triglyceride and total cholesterol levels, increases HDL levels, and causes weight loss and is ideal for overweight hyperlipidemic patients. Hypo-glycemia occurs only when metformin is used with insulin or hypoglycemic drugs. Adverse effects are GI related and, of greatest concern, the rare lactic acidosis, caused by inhibited conversion of lactate to glucose and greater lactate production, which mostly affects patients with renal, hepatic, or cardiovascular disorders.

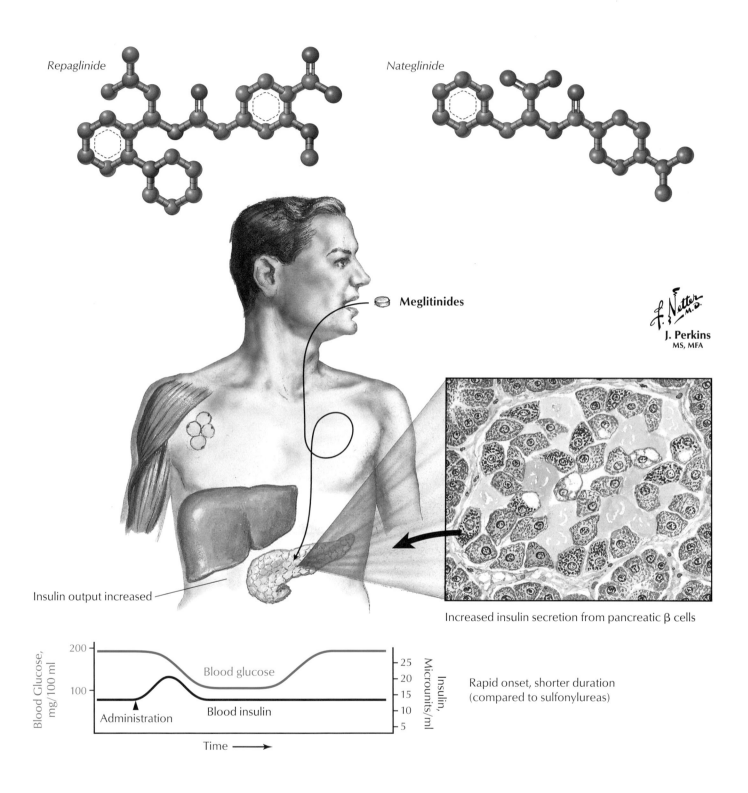

Repaglinide

Nateglinide

Meglitinides

J. Perkins
MS, MFA

Insulin output increased

Increased insulin secretion from pancreatic β cells

Rapid onset, shorter duration (compared to sulfonylureas)

Blood glucose

Blood insulin

Administration

Time ⟶

FIGURE 5-34 MEGLITINIDES

Meglitinides (repaglinide and nateglinide) are approved as monotherapy or in combination with metformin or TZDs in patients with type 2 DM. Similar to sulfonylureas, meglitinides cause an increase in insulin secretion from pancreatic β cells. Unlike sulfonylureas, meglitinides have a rapid onset and a shorter duration, which necessitates dosing within 30 minutes of each meal. These agents are especially useful for patients who have

difficulty controlling postprandial hyperglycemia. The efficacy of meglitinides in producing reductions in glycosylated hemoglobin concentration (HbA_{1c}) and the fasting plasma glucose (FPG) level is comparable to that of sulfonylureas and metformin (reduces HbA_{1c} by 1.5-2% and FPG level by 50-70 mg/dL). Adverse effects include mild hypoglycemia (particularly if administration is not followed with food) and weight gain.

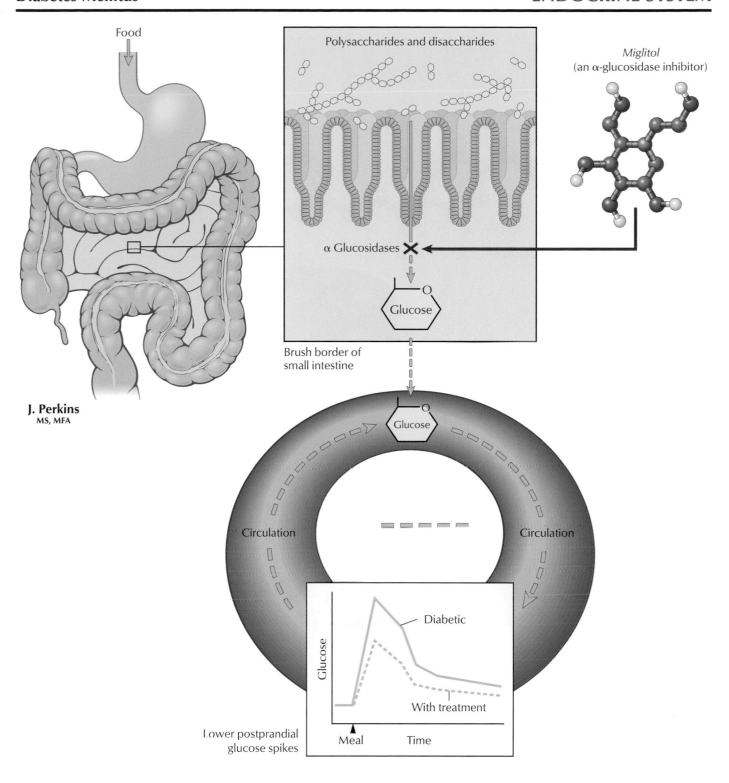

Food

Polysaccharides and disaccharides

Miglitol
(an α-glucosidase inhibitor)

α Glucosidases

Glucose

Brush border of
small intestine

J. Perkins
MS, MFA

Glucose

Circulation

Circulation

Diabetic

Glucose

With treatment

Meal   Time

Lower postprandial
glucose spikes

FIGURE 5-35 α-GLUCOSIDASE INHIBITORS

α-Glucosidase inhibitors (acarbose, miglitol) can be used singly or with insulin or other oral drugs for type 2 DM. These drugs inhibit glucosidases in the small intestine brush border that break down (hydrolyze) complex polysaccharides and sucrose into absorbable monosaccharides. The rate of carbohydrate digestion and glucose absorption is thus delayed, which leads to lower postprandial glucose spikes (by 25-50 mg/dL). These drugs work best in patients with postprandial hyperglycemia and when taken with a meal containing complex carbohydrates. The drugs decrease FPG slightly (20-30 mg/dL) and HbA$_{1c}$ levels by 0.5% to 1.0%. Adverse effects are GI related (flatulence, diarrhea, abdominal pain), which result from fermentation of unabsorbed carbohydrates in the small intestine and are lessened by slow dose titration. Used with insulin or other oral drugs, they can cause hypoglycemia. Hepatic trans-aminase levels can increase (acarbose), so LFT results must be watched.

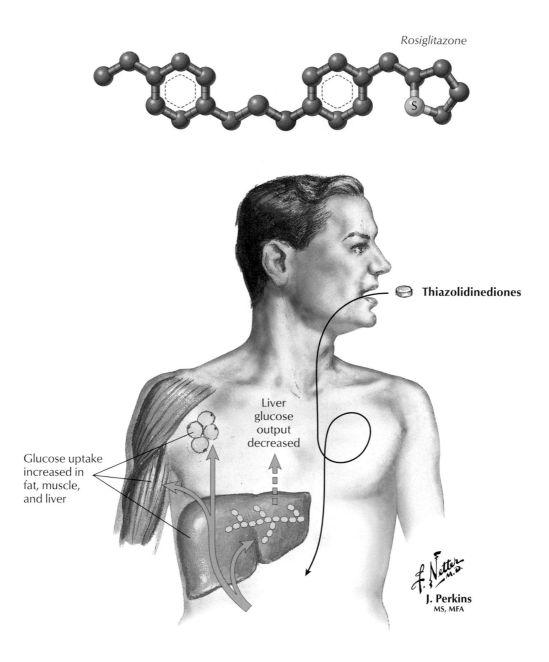

Rosiglitazone

Thiazolidinediones

Liver
glucose
output
decreased

Glucose uptake
increased in
fat, muscle,
and liver

J. Perkins
MS, MFA

FIGURE 5-36 THIAZOLIDINEDIONES

Thiazolidinediones (rosiglitazone and pioglitazone) are a relatively new class of antihyperglycemic agents that can be used as monotherapy or in combination with insulin or other oral agents in patients with type 2 DM. TZDs reduce hyperglycemia and hyperinsulinemia by decreasing insulin resistance (via enhancement of insulin-mediated glucose uptake) at peripheral sites and in the liver, which results in increased insulin-dependent glucose disposal and decreased hepatic glucose output. These effects are accomplished by selective binding at the peroxisome PPAR-g, which is found in adipose tissue, skeletal muscle, and liver. Receptor activation modulates transcription of several insulin-responsive genes that control glucose and lipid metabolism.

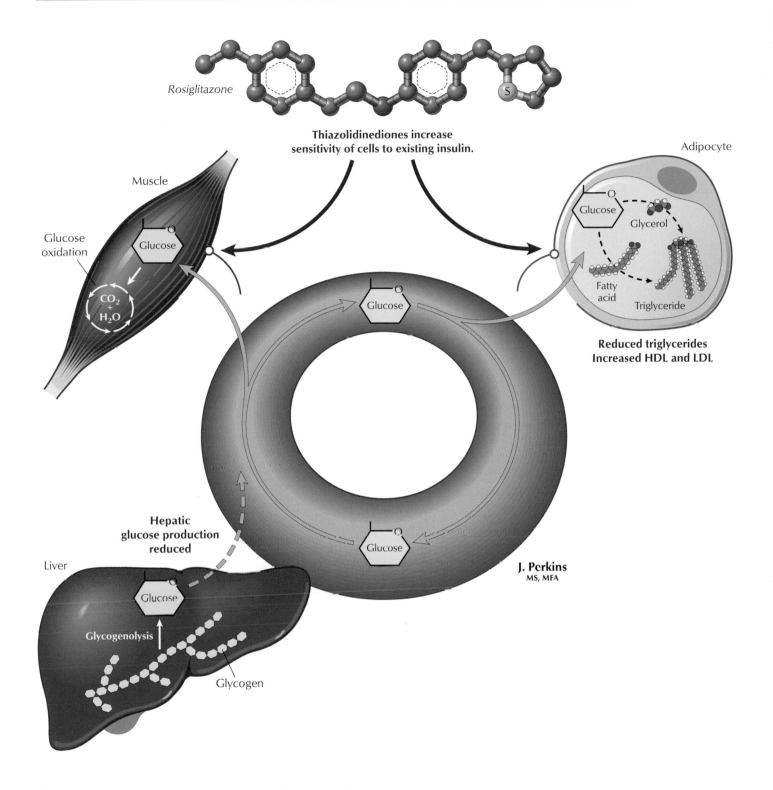

Rosiglitazone

**Thiazolidinediones increase
sensitivity of cells to existing insulin.**

Adipocyte

Muscle

Glucose
oxidation

CO_2
+
H_2O

Glucose

Glycerol

Fatty
acid

Triglyceride

**Reduced triglycerides
Increased HDL and LDL**

Glucose

Glucose

**Hepatic
glucose production
reduced**

Glucose

Liver

J. Perkins
MS, MFA

Glucose

Glycogenolysis

Glycogen

FIGURE 5-37 THIAZOLIDINEDIONES: CLINICAL RATIONALE AND ADVERSE EFFECTS

Thiazolidinedione pharmacology is based on suggestions that patients with type 2 DM already have too much insulin. The liver, however, is resistant to that insulin and therefore continues to produce large amounts of glucose. Instead of stimulating the pancreas to produce more insulin, sensitivity to existing insulin should be increased to slow hepatic glucose production. TZD effects on HbA_{1c} and FPG fall between those of acarbose and the sulfonylureas and metformin. TZDs plus insulin enhance glycemic control and decrease insulin needs. TZDs also reduce

triglyceride levels and increase HDL, but they also increase LDL levels. The first TZD (troglitazone) was withdrawn after causing hepatotoxicity. The 2 drugs now used have not had hepatotoxic effects, but LFTs should be checked before and during TZD therapy. TZDs also cause hematologic effects (reduced hemoglobin, hematocrit, neutrophils), hypoglycemia (when used with other drugs), and edema (thus should be used with care in congestive heart failure).

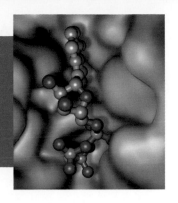

CHAPTER 6

DRUGS USED IN DISORDERS OF THE GASTROINTESTINAL SYSTEM

OVERVIEW

The *gastrointestinal (GI) tract* is an epithelium-lined muscular tube that runs from the mouth to the anus. The major functions of the GI system are food digestion, nutrient absorption, and delivery of nutrients to the blood for distribution. Other functions are excretion of waste and secretion of hormones into the blood for delivery to distal targets. The GI system has an important role in fluid and electrolyte balance. It is the normal route for water and salt intake and a potential source of fluid and electrolyte loss. During digestion, a large volume of digestive secretions is added to the ingested, chewed, and swallowed food. Nearly all of this combined mixture must be reabsorbed to avoid major disturbances in fluid-electrolyte and acid-base balance. The small intestine provides a large surface area for the absorption of nutrients and drugs. Substances are moved through the GI tract by peristalsis. Abnormally fast or slow peristalsis can disrupt absorption of nutrients, drugs, and water—the origin of most GI dysfunctions, including constipation, diarrhea, peptic ulcer disease, gastroesophageal reflux disease (GERD), and emesis.

Laxatives are used for constipation. Laxatives cause emptying of the colon and defecation by stimulating peristalsis or by adding more bulk or water to the feces. Opioids (diphenoxylate and loperamide) are the most effective drugs for controlling diarrhea. Diarrhea is also treated with antiinflammatory drugs such as the nonsteroidal antiinflammatory drugs (NSAIDs) aspirin and indomethacin. Bismuth compounds are used for simple diarrhea.

Peptic ulcer disease is caused by an erosion of the mucosal layer of the stomach or proximal small intestine (duodenum). *Helicobacter pylori* infection is the most common cause. GERD is a similar disorder that occurs in the esophagus and is treated with similar medications. Peptic ulcer disease is best treated by a combination of lifestyle changes and drugs. Histamine H_2-receptor antagonists are the first-line drugs for peptic ulcers. These blockers reduce stomach acidity without producing adverse effects. Proton pump inhibitors (PPIs) are effective at reducing gastric acid secretion by blocking H^+,K^+-ATPase, an enzyme expressed by stomach parietal cells. PPIs are therapeutically effective but usually must be discontinued because of an adverse effect profile. Antacids neutralize stomach acid and blunt reflux disease symptoms. They are the first-line drugs for GERD.

Several drugs are available to treat nausea, vomiting, and motion sickness. These agents include histamine antagonists, corticosteroids, phenothiazines, benzodiazepines, and serotonin receptor antagonists.

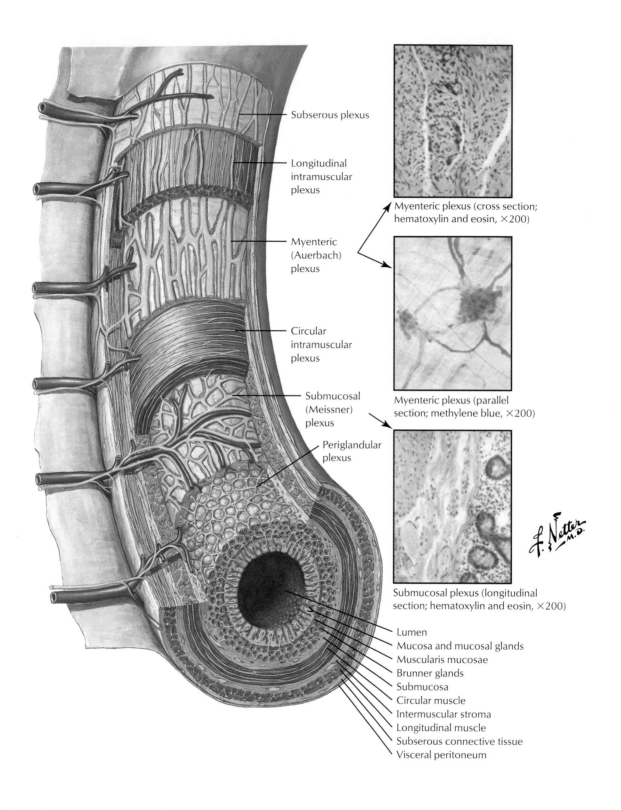

Subserous plexus

Longitudinal intramuscular plexus

Myenteric (Auerbach) plexus

Circular intramuscular plexus

Submucosal (Meissner) plexus

Periglandular plexus

Myenteric plexus (cross section; hematoxylin and eosin, ×200)

Myenteric plexus (parallel section; methylene blue, ×200)

Submucosal plexus (longitudinal section; hematoxylin and eosin, ×200)

Lumen
Mucosa and mucosal glands
Muscularis mucosae
Brunner glands
Submucosa
Circular muscle
Intermuscular stroma
Longitudinal muscle
Subserous connective tissue
Visceral peritoneum

FIGURE 6-1 ENTERIC NERVOUS SYSTEM

The nervous system exerts a profound influence on all digestive processes (motility, ion transport associated with secretion and absorption, and blood flow). Some of this control emanates from connections between the digestive system and the CNS, but just as important, the digestive system is endowed with its own, local nervous system, referred to as the *enteric* or *intrinsic nervous system*. Principal components of the enteric nervous system are 2 networks or plexuses of neurons, both of which are embedded in the wall of the digestive tract and extend from the esophagus to the anus. The myenteric (Auerbach) plexus is located between the longitudinal and circular layers of muscle in the tunica muscularis and controls primarily digestive tract motility. The submucosal (Meissner) plexus regulates GI blood flow and epithelial cell function by monitoring luminal contents.

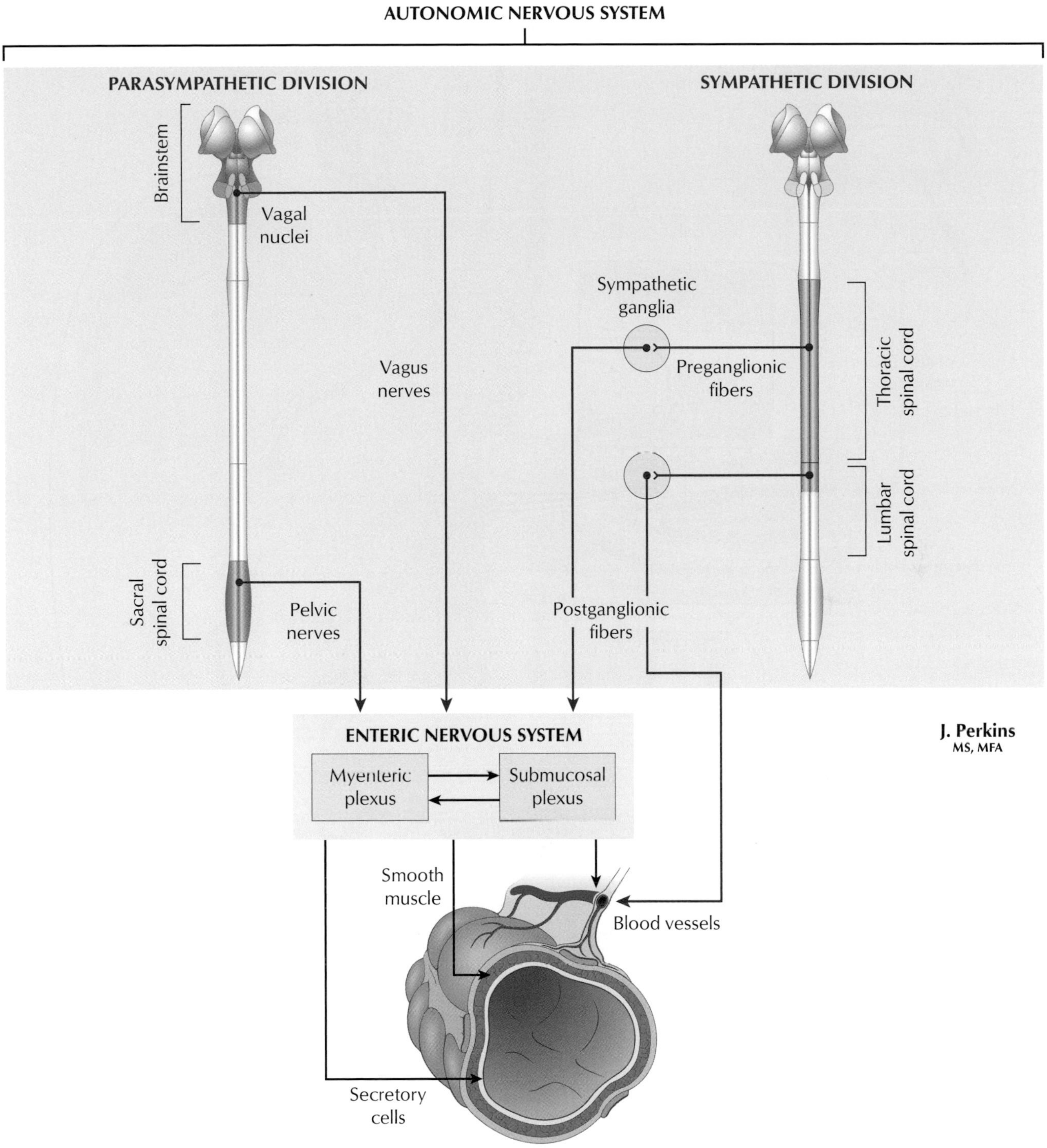

AUTONOMIC NERVOUS SYSTEM

PARASYMPATHETIC DIVISION

Brainstem

Vagal
nuclei

Vagus
nerves

Sacral
spinal cord

Pelvic
nerves

SYMPATHETIC DIVISION

Sympathetic
ganglia

Preganglionic
fibers

Thoracic
spinal cord

Lumbar
spinal cord

Postganglionic
fibers

J. Perkins
MS, MFA

ENTERIC NERVOUS SYSTEM

Myenteric
plexus

Submucosal
plexus

Smooth
muscle

Blood vessels

Secretory
cells

FIGURE 6-2 INTEGRATION OF THE AUTONOMIC AND ENTERIC NERVOUS SYSTEMS

The enteric plexuses contain 3 types of neurons, most of which are multipolar. Motor neurons control GI motility, secretion, and absorption. They act directly on smooth muscle, secretory cells (parietal, chief, mucous, pancreatic exocrine cells), and GI endocrine cells. Sensory neurons receive information from sensory receptors in the mucosa and muscle. They respond to mechanical, thermal, osmotic, and chemical stimuli. Chemoreceptors are sensitive to pH, glucose, and amino acids. Sensory receptors in muscle respond to stretch and tension. Interneurons integrate information from sensory neurons and transmit it to enteric motor neurons. Enteric neurons secrete ACh and norepinephrine. Neurons that secrete ACh are excitatory and stimulate smooth muscle contraction, increase intestinal secretions, release enteric hormones, and relax (dilate) blood vessels. Norepinephrine, released from extrinsic sympathetic neurons, is inhibitory and opposes biologic actions of ACh.

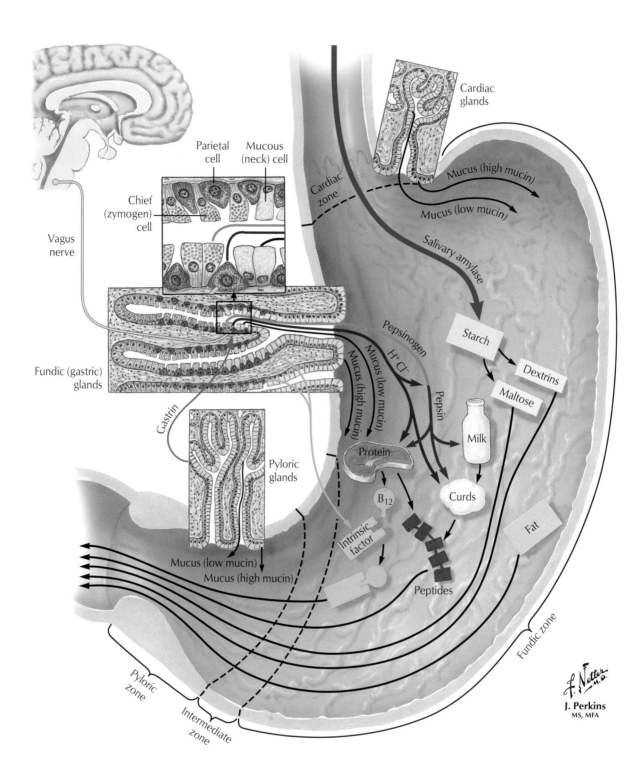

FIGURE 6-3 GASTROINTESTINAL MOTILITY

The digestive tube shows 2 basic motility patterns: propulsion, the movement of food along the tube so that food can be catabolized and absorbed, and peristalsis, the major type of propulsive motility, seen especially in the esophagus and small intestine. A ring of muscle contraction appears on the oral side of a food bolus and moves toward the anus, so the luminal contents are forced in that direction. As the ring moves, the muscle on the other side of the distended area relaxes for smooth passage of the

Factors Affecting Gastric Emptying

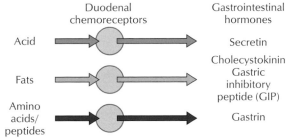
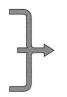
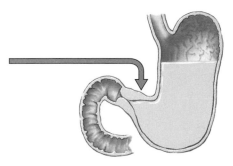

Duodenal stimuli elicit hormonal inhibition of gastric emptying.

Sequence of Gastric Motility

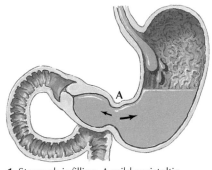

1. Stomach is filling. A mild peristaltic wave (A) has started in antrum and is passing toward pylorus. Gastric contents are churned and largely pushed back into body of stomach.

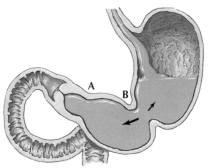

2. Wave (A) fading out as pylorus fails to open. A stronger wave (B) is originating at incisure and is again squeezing gastric contents in both directions.

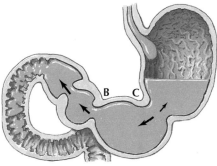

3. Pylorus opens as wave (B) approaches it. Duodenal bulb is filled, and some contents pass into second portion of duodenum. Wave (C) starting just above incisure.

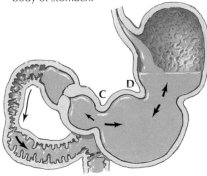

4. Pylorus again closed. Wave (C) fails to evacuate contents. Wave (D) starts higher on body of stomach. Duodenal bulb may contract or may remain filled as peristaltic wave originating just beyond it empties second portion.

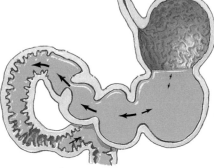

5. Peristaltic waves are now originating higher on body of stomach. Gastric contents are evacuated intermittently. Contents of duodenal bulb area pushed passively into second portion as more gastric contents emerge.

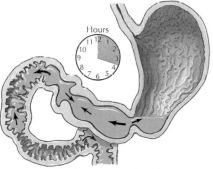
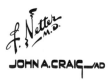

6. 3 to 4 hours later, stomach is almost empty. Small peristaltic wave empties duodenal bulb with some reflux into stomach. Reverse and antegrade peristalsis present in duodenum.

f. Netter, M.D.

JOHN A.CRAIG—AD

FIGURE 6-3 GASTROINTESTINAL MOTILITY (continued)

bolus. Mixing ensures that ingested materials are exposed to digestive enzymes and properly absorbed. In the absence of mixing, food is not in contact with epithelial cells that absorb nutrients. Segmentation contractions are a common type of mixing motility seen especially in the small intestine; segmental rings of contraction break down and mix food. Alternating contraction and relaxation of longitudinal muscle in the gut wall also provides effective mixing of its contents.

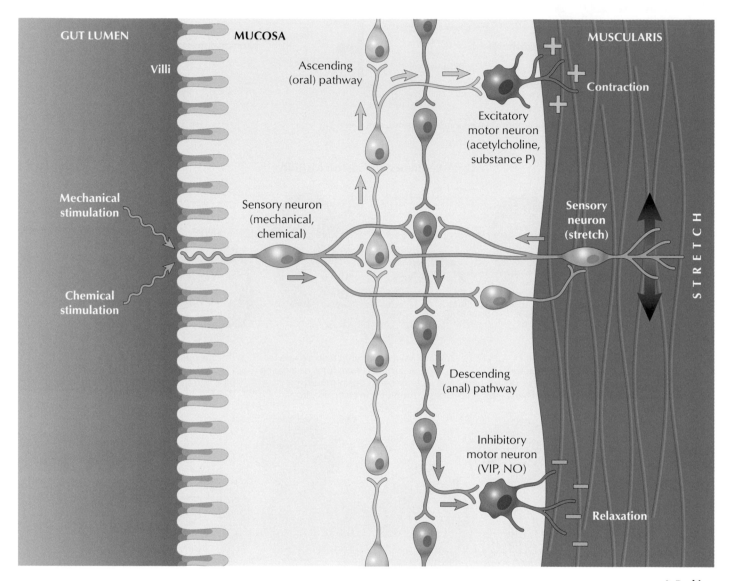

J. Perkins
MS, MFA

FIGURE 6-4 CONTROL OF PERISTALSIS

Food in the intestinal lumen causes smooth muscle contraction above the bolus and relaxation below, so that a peristaltic wave moves food down the intestine from the mouth to the anus. The enteric nervous system controls peristalsis and can work separately from the CNS, but digestion needs enteric nervous system and CNS coordination. Parasympathetic and sympathetic neurons connect the CNS and digestive tract, which allows sensory information to be sent to the CNS, as well as CNS regulation of

GI function and relay of non-GI system signals. Sympathetic stimulation inhibits GI secretion and motor activity and causes GI sphincter and blood vessel contraction. Parasympathetic stimulation increases GI secretion and motor activity and causes GI sphincter and blood vessel dilation. Important peristaltic reflexes are the gastrocolic, in which stomach distension causes colonic exodus, and the enterogastric, in which small intestine distension or irritation reduces stomach secretion and motor activity.

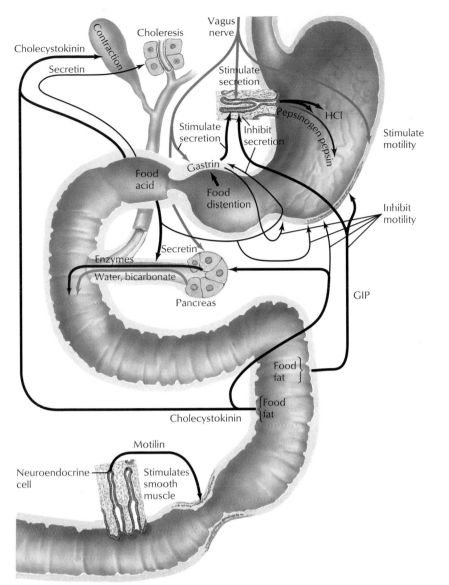

LEGEND

Thick line indicates primary action ━━━━━

Thin line indicates secondary action ───

Hormone	Neuroendocrine Cell Type and Location	Stimulus for Secretion	Primary Action	Other Actions
Gastrin	**G cell** Stomach, duodenum	Vagus, distention, amino acids	Stimulate HCl secretion	Inhibit gastric emptying
Secretin	**S cell** Duodenum	Acid	Stimulate pancreatic ductal cell H_2O and HCO_3^- secretion	Inhibit gastric secretion, inhibit gastric motility, and stimulate bile duct secretion of H_2O and HCO_3^-
Cholecystokinin	**I cell** Duodenum, jejunum	Fat, vagus	Stimulate enzyme secretion by pancreatic acinar cells and contract the gallbladder	Inhibit gastric motility
GIP	**K cell** Duodenum, jejunum	Fat	Inhibit gastric secretion and motility	Stimulate insulin secretion
Motilin	**M cell** Duodenum, jejunum		Increase motility and initiate the MMC	

FIGURE 6-5 HORMONES OF THE GASTROINTESTINAL TRACT

The endocrine system regulates GI function by secreting hormones. Hormones are chemical messengers secreted into blood that modify the physiology of target cells. Digestive function is affected by hormones produced in many endocrine glands, but the greatest control is exerted by hormones produced within the GI tract. The GI tract is the largest endocrine organ in the body, and the endocrine cells within it are referred to collectively as the *enteric endocrine system*. Three of the best-studied enteric hormones are gastrin, cholecystokinin (CCK), and secretin. Gastrin is secreted from the stomach and plays an important role in control of gastric acid secretion. CCK is a small intestinal hormone that stimulates secretion of pancreatic enzymes and bile. Secretin is a hormone secreted from small intestinal epithelial cells that stimulates secretion of bicarbonate-rich fluids from the pancreas and liver.

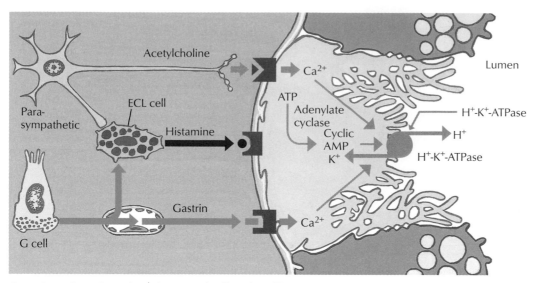

Secretions of gastric acid (H⁺) by parietal cell mediated by neurocrine, paracrine, and endocrine mechanisms. Medical or surgical blockade of these mechanisms affords therapeutic options.

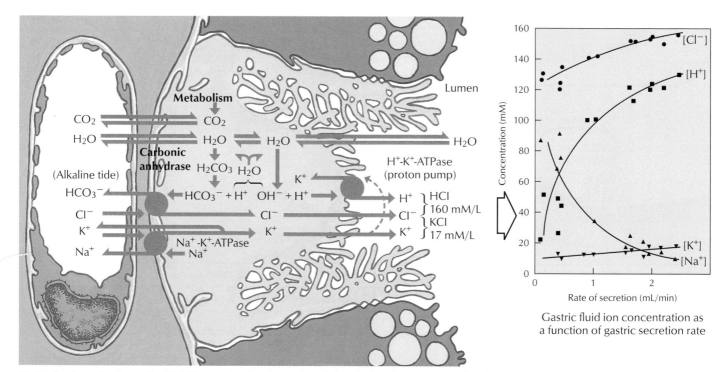

Parietal cell mechanisms of acid (H⁺) secretion involve series of chemical exchanges across basal membrane, with final active exchange of H⁺ for K⁺ mediated across apical (secretory) membrane by H⁺-K⁺-ATPase (proton pump).

Gastric fluid ion concentration as a function of gastric secretion rate

JOHN A. CRAIG—AD

FIGURE 6-6 PARIETAL CELL FUNCTION REGULATION

The stomach's parietal cells secrete approximately 2 L of acid a day as hydrochloric acid. This acid eradicates bacteria, aids in digestion by solubilizing food, and maintains optimal pH (1.8-3.2) for the function of pepsin, a digestive enzyme. H⁺,K⁺-ATPase (the proton pump) is expressed on parietal cell apical membranes and uses energy from ATP hydrolysis to pump hydrogen ions into the lumen in exchange for potassium ions. Three regulatory molecules stimulate acid secretion—ACh, histamine,

gastrin—and one inhibits acid secretion—somatostatin. ACh increases acid secretion by stimulating muscarinic (M_1) receptors. Histamine, a paracrine hormone released from enterochromaffin-like cells, stimulates acid secretion by activating H_2 receptors. Gastrin, a hormone released by G cells (endocrine cells in gastric epithelium), increases acid release by activating gastric receptors. Somatostatin is also secreted by gastric endocrine cells and, with prostaglandins, opposes the stimulatory actions of gastrin.

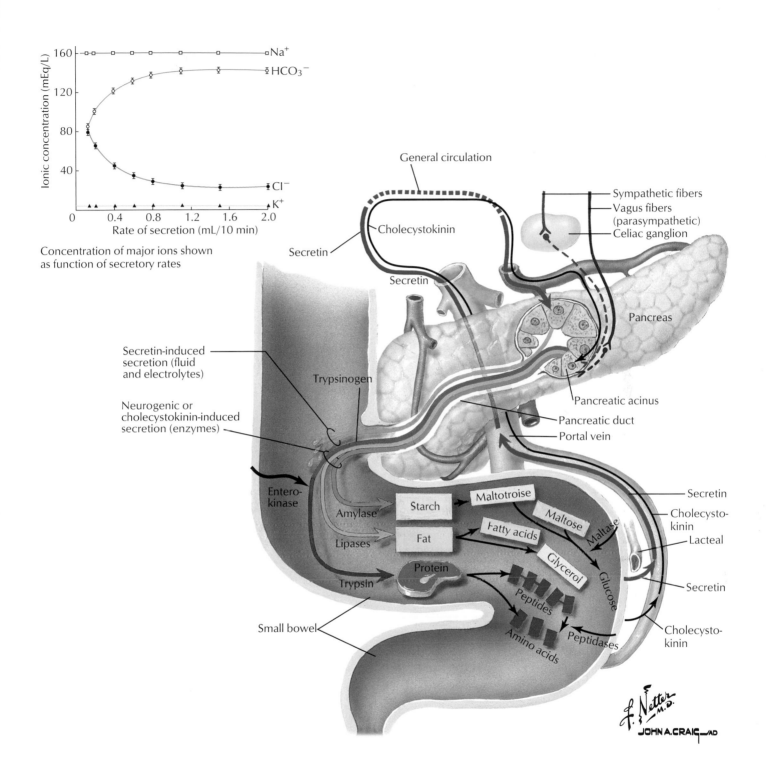

FIGURE 6-7 PANCREATIC SECRETION

Exocrine pancreas secretion is under neural and endocrine control. Pancreatic secretions, the major mechanism for neutralizing gastric acid in the small intestine, are stimulated by food entering the stomach and chyme entering the small intestine. The vagus nerve innervates the pancreas (and the stomach) and applies a low-level stimulus for secretion in anticipation of a meal. The most important stimuli for pancreatic secretion come from 3 enteric nervous system hormones. CCK is synthesized and secreted by duodenal endocrine cells in response to partly digested proteins and fats in the small intestine. CCK is released into blood and binds to receptors on pancreatic acinar cells, which induces digestive enzyme secretion. Secretin, secreted in response to acid in the duodenum, stimulates pancreatic secretion of water and bicarbonate. Gastrin, like CCK, is secreted by the stomach and stimulates acid secretion by parietal cells and digestive enzyme secretion by pancreatic acinar cells.

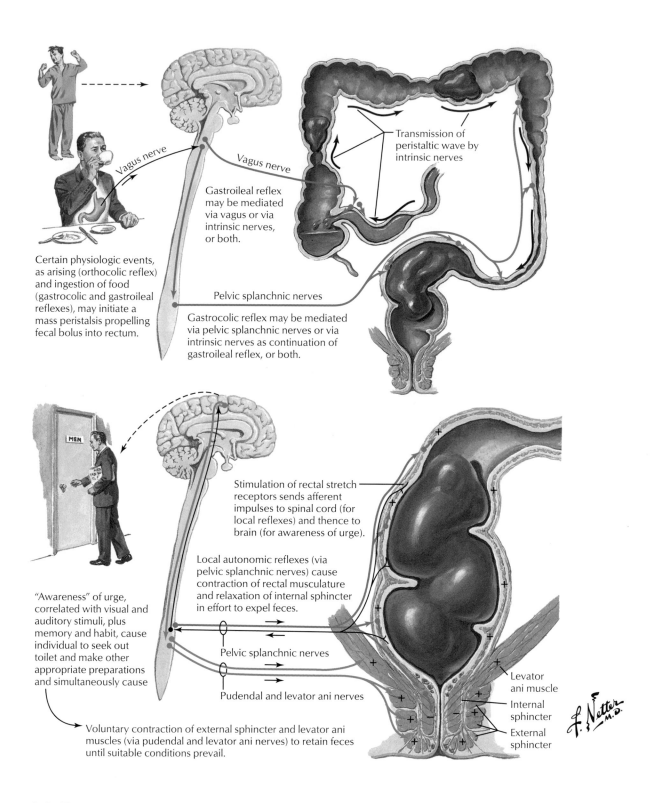

FIGURE 6-8 DEFECATION

Defecation (passing of feces through the rectum and anus) occurs via relaxation of the involuntary and voluntary internal anal sphincter and heeding the rectosphincteric reflex; it is prevented by external anal sphincter contraction. The rectum filling with fecal material causes the urge to defecate. When the external anal sphincter relaxes, rectal smooth muscle contracts to force feces out. The presence of food in the stomach increases colon motility. A rapid parasympathetic response (stimulated GI motility by depolarizing smooth muscle cells) is initiated; CCK and gastrin mediate a slower hormonal response. Disorders of large intestine motility may be caused by emotional factors via the extrinsic autonomic nervous system; IBS, a disorder worsened by stress, causes constipation or diarrhea. Megacolon (Hirschsprung disease), the absence of the colon enteric nervous system, causes intestinal contents near the constriction to accumulate and severe constipation.

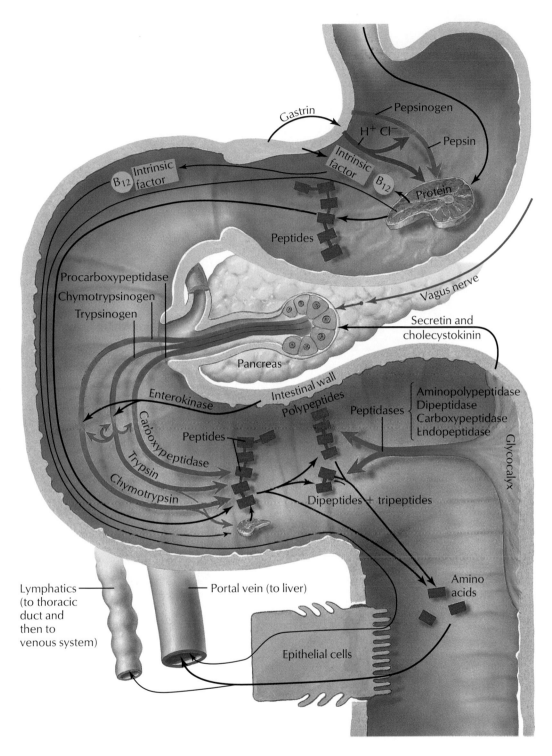

Labels on figure: Gastrin · Pepsinogen · H⁺ Cl⁻ · Pepsin · Intrinsic factor · B₁₂ · Protein · Intrinsic factor B₁₂ · Peptides · Procarboxypeptidase · Chymotrypsinogen · Trypsinogen · Vagus nerve · Secretin and cholecystokinin · Pancreas · Enterokinase · Intestinal wall · Polypeptides · Aminopolypeptidase · Dipeptidase · Carboxypeptidase · Endopeptidase · Peptidases · Peptides · Carboxypeptidase · Trypsin · Chymotrypsin · Dipeptides + tripeptides · Glycocalyx · Amino acids · Lymphatics (to thoracic duct and then to venous system) · Portal vein (to liver) · Epithelial cells

H^+ Cl^- ... B_{12}

FIGURE 6-9 PROTEIN DIGESTION

Proteolytic enzymes are packaged in vesicles in an inactive form and are thus protected against the harsh pH conditions of the GI tract. *Pepsin* is a stomach enzyme derived from pepsinogen that is active at low pH. Pepsin cleaves the peptide bond between acidic (aspartic or glutamic acid) and aromatic (phenylalanine, tyrosine) amino acids. This endonuclease catabolizes proteins into smaller peptides. *Trypsin* is a pancreatic enzyme derived from trypsinogen that is active at slightly basic pH. Trypsin hydrolyzes peptide bonds adjacent to the basic amino acids lysine and arginine, thus hydrolyzing proteins into smaller peptides. Other endopeptidases, such as chymotrypsin and enterokinase, digest proteins into multiple amino acid fragments. *Pancreatic carboxypeptidase* is an exopeptidase that hydrolyzes dipeptides at the carboxyl end. *Small intestine aminopeptidase* is an exopeptidase that hydrolyzes dipeptides from the amino end. Finally, *dipeptidase* liberates free amino acids.

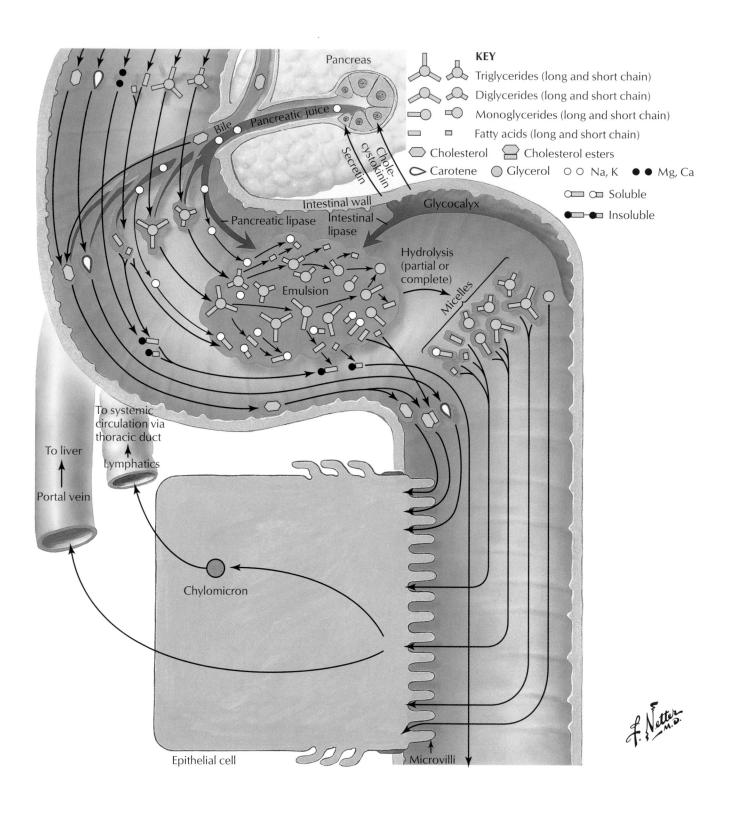

KEY

Triglycerides (long and short chain)
Diglycerides (long and short chain)
Monoglycerides (long and short chain)
Fatty acids (long and short chain)
Cholesterol   Cholesterol esters
Carotene   Glycerol   Na, K   Mg, Ca
Soluble
Insoluble

FIGURE 6-10 FAT DIGESTION

Fat digestion and absorption depend on bile, which, secreted by the liver and released into the gut by the action of CCK on the gallbladder, acts as an emulsifier to break up fat globules to aid digestion. Pancreatic lipase is a water-soluble enzyme and thus acts only on fat globule surfaces (hydrolyzes neutral fats to give free fatty acids and 2-monoglycerides). The detergent action of bile salts, especially lecithin, is needed to disperse fat into small globules for efficient lipase action. Bile also forms micelles—aggregates of free fatty acids, monoglycerides, and bile—which help transport water-insoluble fatty acids. Micelles take fat digestion products away from the digestion site to be absorbed by enterocytes. These products thus do not inhibit lipases (negative feedback). Poor fat absorption causes excess fat in stools, or steatorrhea. Stools are bulky, pale, and odiferous.

Diarrhea

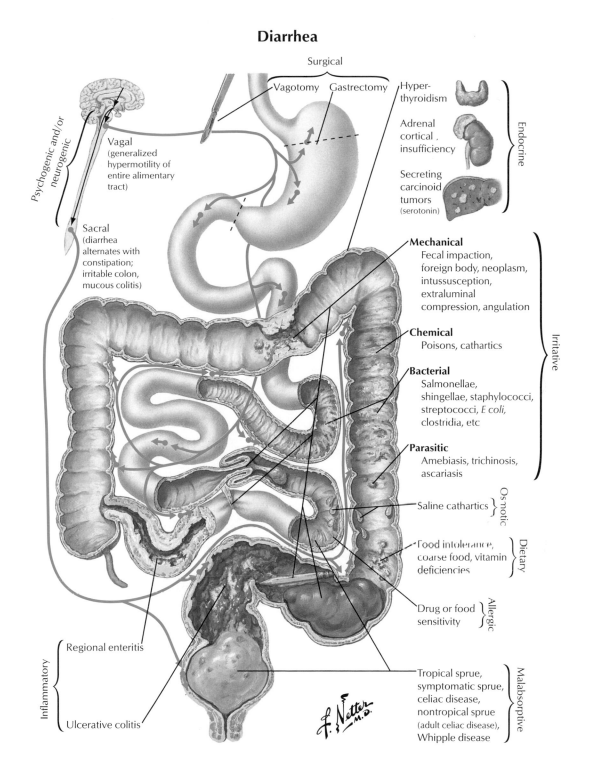

FIGURE 6-11 COLONIC MOTILITY AND TREATMENT OF DIARRHEA

Motility patterns in the colonic lumen include peristalsis, which propels luminal contents toward the rectum, and those that extend contact of the luminal contents with absorptive epithelial cells. Prolonging contact facilitates absorption of fluid from the feces. Processes that promote propulsive patterns produce diarrhea. *Diarrhea* is defined as loose, watery stools that occur at least 3 times per day. Bacterial infections, viral infections, adverse food reactions, parasites, and functional bowel disorders can lead to diarrhea. Because dehydration is caused by diarrhea, treatments include rehydration with electrolytes (eg, broths, soup, potassium supplements) or slowing motility with loperamide, bismuth subsalicylate, or kaolin pectin suspension. Most types of diarrhea are caused by viruses, so antibiotics are usually ineffective. Raspberry or blueberry leaves are sometimes taken with tea to alleviate some symptoms.

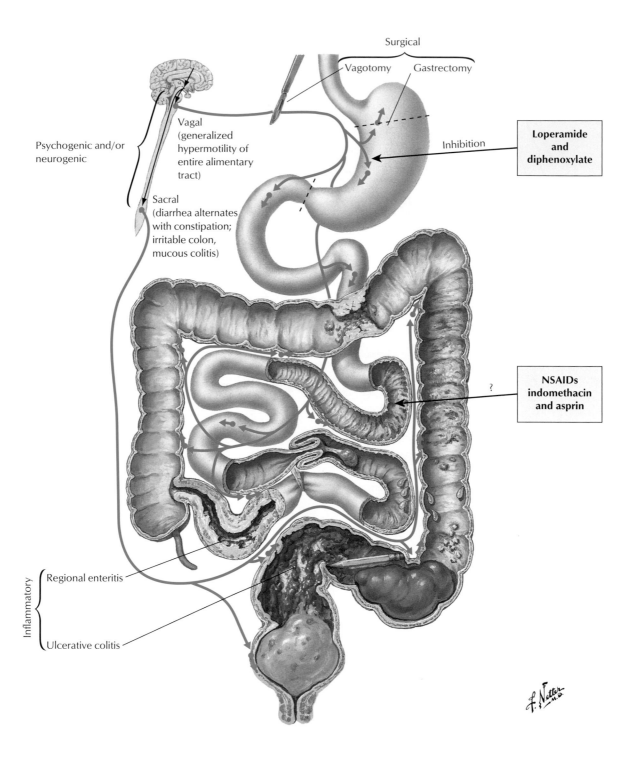

Surgical

Vagotomy Gastrectomy

Psychogenic and/or neurogenic

Vagal (generalized hypermotility of entire alimentary tract)

Inhibition

Loperamide and diphenoxylate

Sacral (diarrhea alternates with constipation; irritable colon, mucous colitis)

NSAIDs indomethacin and asprin

Inflammatory — Regional enteritis

Ulcerative colitis

FIGURE 6-12 ANTIDIARRHEAL DRUGS AND THEIR ADVERSE EFFECTS

Other antidiarrheal drugs include agents that inhibit motility and modify fluid and electrolyte transport, such as NSAIDs. Loperamide and diphenoxylate (meperidine derivatives) are 2 antimotility drugs that reduce peristalsis by activating presynaptic opioid receptors in the GI tract and decreasing acetylcholine release. Adverse effects include dizziness, drowsiness, and stomach cramping; the use of these drugs is contraindicated in children. NSAIDs such as indomethacin and aspirin are thought to relieve diarrhea by blocking COX-1 and inhibiting prostaglandin synthesis. The most common adverse effects of aspirin are bleeding, respiratory depression, hypersensitivity reactions, hepatitis (particularly children), and salicylate toxicity.

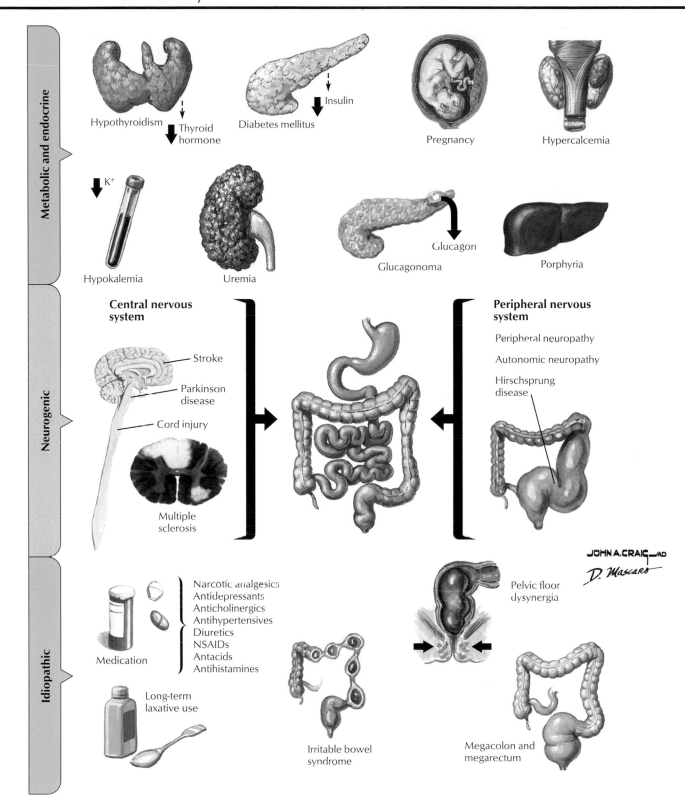

Central nervous system

Peripheral nervous system

FIGURE 6-13 CAUSES OF CONSTIPATION

Constipation, one of the most common GI problems in the United States, refers to passage of small amounts of hard and dry stools. Bowel movements occur fewer than 3 times a week. Women (especially pregnant) and older adults (older than 65 years) report constipation most often. Under normal conditions, the colon absorbs water as food passes through it and waste products (stool) form. Stool becomes solid because most of the water is absorbed. The hard and dry stools occur when the colon absorbs too much water or the colon's muscle contractions are slow. Common symptoms are lethargy, feeling bloated, and painful bowel movements. Causes can be metabolic and endocrine; neurogenic (involving the CNS or PNS); and idiopathic. These causes include a lack of dietary fiber, inadequate hydration, lack of exercise, IBS, changes in life routines (pregnancy, travel), aging, laxative abuse, ignoring urges to have a bowel movement, stroke, colonic disease, and intestinal disease.

Diagnosis and Management of Constipation

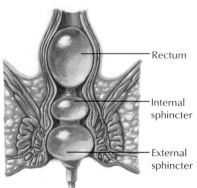

3-balloon manometer inserted in rectum.

- Rectum
- Internal sphincter
- External sphincter

Anorectal manometry

Normal   Hirschsprung disease

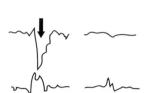

Balloon expulsion test

Normal   Abnormal (dysynergia)

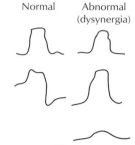

In normal circumstances, balloon distention should cause transient relaxation of internal sphincter.

Expulsion should cause increase in rectal pressure and decrease in baseline pressure.

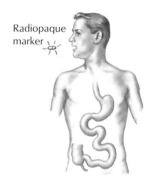

Radiopaque marker

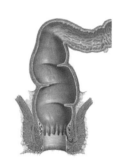

Radiopaque paste introduced into rectum. Fluoroscopic monitored digestion provides information on anorectal angle, pelvic floor descent, rectocele, intussusception, and rectal prolapse.

Patient ingests radiopaque markers followed by abdominal x-rays obtained several days after ingestion. Number of retained markers utilized to determine colonic transit time.

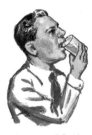

Increased fluid intake

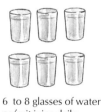

6 to 8 glasses of water or fruit juice daily

Whole Wheat Bread   Brown Rice

Adequate fiber intake (may be supplemented with psyllium)

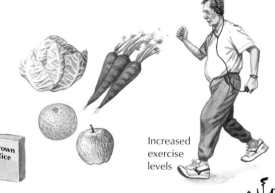

Increased exercise levels

FIGURE 6-14 TREATMENT OF CONSTIPATION

Treatments for constipation include aluminum- and calcium-containing antacids, calcium channel blockers (antihypertensives), iron supplements, diuretics, and antidepressants. Bulk-forming laxatives (fiber supplements) are considered the safest but can interfere with absorption of some drugs. They are taken with water and absorb water in the intestine and to make the stool softer. Stimulant laxatives cause rhythmic muscle contractions in the intestines. Because phenolphthalein, an ingredi-ent in some stimulants, may increase the risk of cancer, the US FDA proposed a ban on over-the-counter products containing phenolphthalein. Thus, safer ingredients replaced phenolphthalein in most laxatives. Stool softeners provide moisture to the stool, prevent dehydration, and are used after childbirth and surgery. Lubricants (mineral oil) add oil to the stool, which allows the stool to move through the intestine more easily. Saline laxatives draw water into the colon for easier passage of stool.

Irritable Bowel Syndrome

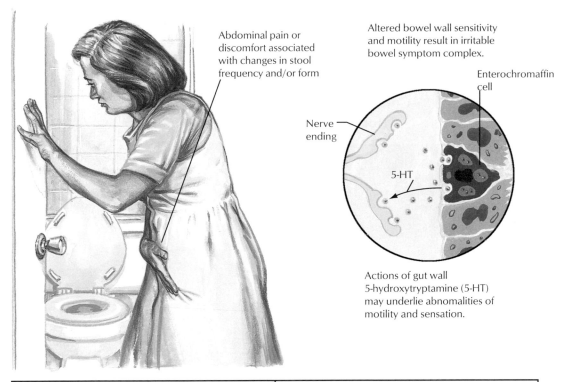

Abdominal pain or discomfort associated with changes in stool frequency and/or form

Altered bowel wall sensitivity and motility result in irritable bowel symptom complex.

Enterochromaffin cell

Nerve ending

5-HT

Actions of gut wall 5-hydroxytryptamine (5-HT) may underlie abnomalities of motility and sensation.

Rome II diagnostic criteria* for irritable bowel syndrome 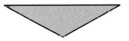	Symptoms not essential for the diagnosis, but if present increase the confidence in the diagnosis and help to identify subgroups of IBS 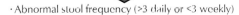
12 weeks[†] or more in the past 12 months of abdominal discomfort or pain that has 2 of 3 features: a. Relieved with defecation b. Onset associated with change in frequency of stool c. Onset associated with change in form (appearance) of stool * In the absence of structural or metabolic abnormalities to explain the symptoms [†] The 12 weeks need not be consecutive	· Abnormal stool frequency (>3 daily or <3 weekly) · Abnormal stool form (lumpy/hard or loose/watery stool) >1/4 of defecations · Abnormal stool passage (straining, urgency, or feeling of incomplete evacuation) >1/4 of defecations · Passage of mucus >1/4 of defecations · Bloating or feeling of abdominal distension >1/4 of days

JOHN A. CRAIG—AD
C. Machado—M.D.
D. Mascaro

FIGURE 6-15 TREATMENT OF IRRITABLE BOWEL SYNDROME

Irritable bowel syndrome, a functional disorder that mainly affects the bowel, causes cramping, bloating, gas, diarrhea, and constipation. Other names for IBS are *spastic colon*, *mucous colitis*, *spastic colitis*, and *nervous stomach*. IBS is caused by disturbed interaction of the intestines, brain, and ANS that alters bowel motility (motor function) or sensory function. Added dietary fiber may relieve constipation and diarrhea but can lead to worsened bloating and distension. Less flatulence may occur

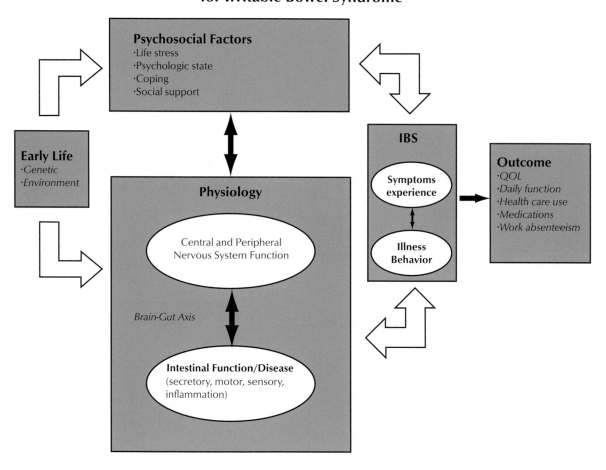

Conceptual (Biopsychosocial) Model for Irritable Bowel Syndrome

Psychosocial Factors
·Life stress
·Psychologic state
·Coping
·Social support

Early Life
·Genetic
·Environment

Physiology

Central and Peripheral Nervous System Function

Brain-Gut Axis

Intestinal Function/Disease
(secretory, motor, sensory, inflammation)

IBS

Symptoms experience

Illness Behavior

Outcome
·*QOL*
·*Daily function*
·*Health care use*
·*Medications*
·*Work absenteeism*

FIGURE 6-15 TREATMENT OF IRRITABLE BOWEL SYNDROME (continued)

with polycarbophil agents than psyllium ones. Peripheral narcotic opiate antagonists (trimebutine and fedotozine), serotonin antagonists (tegaserod), and muscarinic antagonists (zamifenacin) are being studied. Trimebutine, with equal affinity for μ-, δ-, and κ-opioid receptors, stimulates small intestine transit but inhibits colonic motility. Serotonin blockers inhibit intestinal motility; muscarinic blockers inhibit colonic motility and GI secretion. CCK and calcium channel antagonists may also be useful.

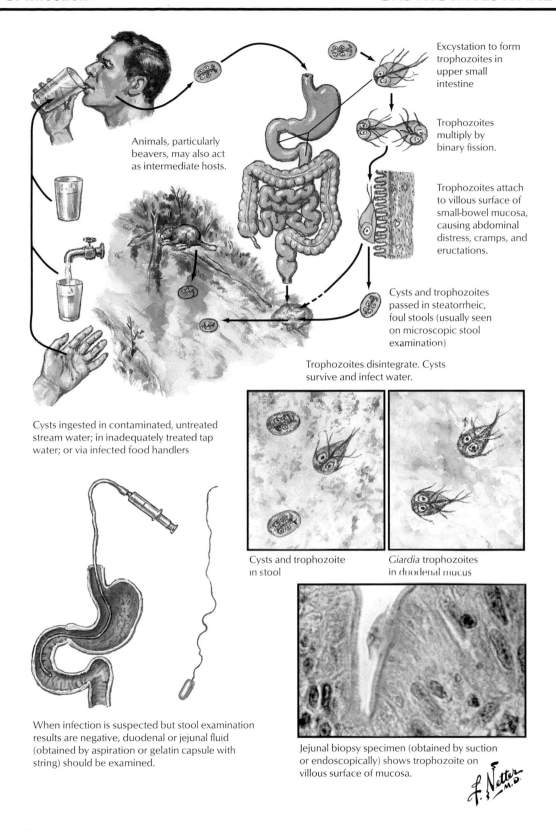

Excystation to form trophozoites in upper small intestine

Trophozoites multiply by binary fission.

Trophozoites attach to villous surface of small-bowel mucosa, causing abdominal distress, cramps, and eructations.

Animals, particularly beavers, may also act as intermediate hosts.

Cysts and trophozoites passed in steatorrheic, foul stools (usually seen on microscopic stool examination)

Trophozoites disintegrate. Cysts survive and infect water.

Cysts ingested in contaminated, untreated stream water; in inadequately treated tap water; or via infected food handlers

Cysts and trophozoite in stool

Giardia trophozoites in duodenal mucus

When infection is suspected but stool examination results are negative, duodenal or jejunal fluid (obtained by aspiration or gelatin capsule with string) should be examined.

Jejunal biopsy specimen (obtained by suction or endoscopically) shows trophozoite on villous surface of mucosa.

FIGURE 6-16 GIARDIASIS

Giardiasis is the most frequent cause of nonbacterial diarrhea in North America. Human giardiasis may involve diarrhea within 1 week after ingestion of the cyst, which is the environmental survival form and infective stage of the organism. Illness normally lasts for 1 to 2 weeks, but cases of chronic infections have lasted months to years. Chronic cases, both those with defined immune deficiencies and those without, are difficult to treat. The disease mechanism is unknown, with some investigators reporting that the organism produces a toxin but others not being able to confirm existence of the toxin. Metronidazole is normally quite effective in terminating infections. Antibiotics such as albendazole, metronidazole, and furazolidone are often prescribed to treat giardiasis; paromomycin may be considered for pregnant women.

Etiology and Pathogenesis of *Helicobacter pylori*

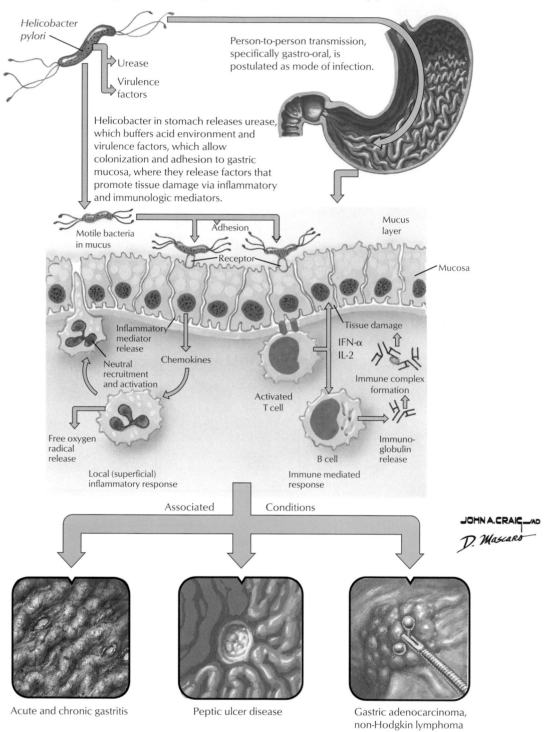

FIGURE 6-17 *HELICOBACTER PYLORI* INFECTION OVERVIEW

Helicobacter pylori, a spiral bacterium found in the gastric mucous layer or adherent to the epithelial lining of the stomach, causes more than 90% of duodenal ulcers and up to 80% of gastric ulcers. Approximately 66% of the world's population is infected with *H pylori*. It causes chronic persistent and atrophic gastritis in adults and children. Before *H pylori* was discovered in 1982, spicy food, acid, stress, and lifestyle were considered major causes of ulcers. Most patients had long-term pharmaco-therapy with histamine antagonists (H_2 blockers) and PPIs. These drugs relieve ulcer-related symptoms and gastric mucosal inflammation but do not eradicate the infection. When acid suppression is removed, the majority of *H pylori*–induced ulcers recur. Chronic infection with *H pylori* weakens natural defenses of the stomach lining against acid. Agents that eradicate *H pylori* (antimicrobials), neutralize stomach acid (antacids), and reduce stomach acid output (H_2 blockers, PPIs) are used.

Diagnosis and Management of *Helicobacter pylori*

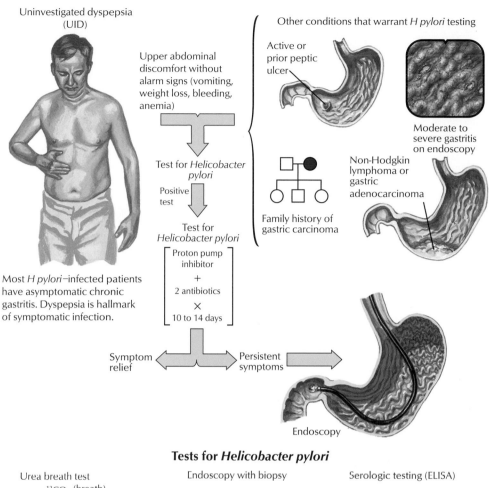

Tests for *Helicobacter pylori*

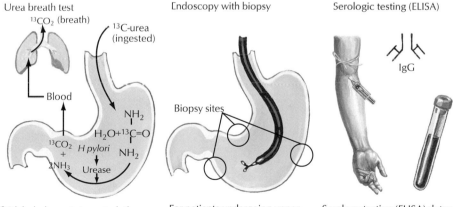

Urea breath test

$^{13}CO_2$ (breath)
^{13}C-urea (ingested)

Blood

$H_2O+^{13}C=O$
NH_2
NH_2
$^{13}CO_2$ + *H pylori*
$2NH_3$ Urease

^{13}C-labeled urea is ingested; if *H pylori* is present it provides "urease," which splits off the labeled CO_2, which is passed into circulation and expired in breath (active infection).

Endoscopy with biopsy

Biopsy sites

For patients undergoing upper endoscopy, biopsy samples submitted for histology or rapid urea testing (RUT) histology is gold standard (active infection).

Serologic testing (ELISA)

IgG

Serology testing (ELISA) detects IgG antibodies and documents past or current infection, but not eradication.

JOHN A.CRAIG—MD
D. Mascaro

FIGURE 6-18 TREATMENT OF *HELICOBACTER PYLORI* INFECTION

Antibiotics can eliminate the infection in most patients, with resolution of mucosal inflammation and minimal ulcer recurrence. *H pylori* is difficult to eradicate from the stomach because the organism can develop antibiotic resistance. Antibiotics are usually coadministered with a PPI and/or bismuth-containing compounds, which have anti–*H pylori* effects. Therapy for *H pylori* infection consists of 2 weeks of 1 or 2 antibiotics, such as amoxicillin, tetracycline (not for children younger than 12 years),

metronidazole, orclarithromycin, plus ranitidine bismuth citrate, bismuth subsalicylate, or a PPI. Acid suppression by an H_2 antagonist or PPI in conjunction with antibiotics alleviates ulcer-related symptoms (eg, abdominal pain, nausea), heals gastric mucosal inflammation, and enhances efficacy of antibiotics against *H pylori* at the gastric mucosal surface. Common combinations are a PPI, amoxicillin, and clarithromycin or a PPI, metronidazole, tetracycline, and bismuth subsalicylate.

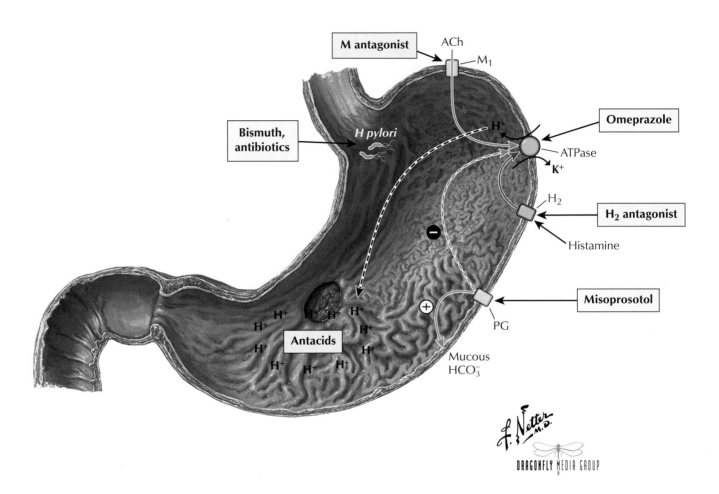

FIGURE 6-19 PEPTIC ULCER TREATMENT

Antacids, PPIs, H_2 blockers, muscarinic antagonists (M_1 blockers), and misoprostol (prostaglandin E_2 derivative) are commonly used. PPIs (eg, omeprazole) bind irreversibly to and inactivate the H^+,K^+-ATPase pump, which blocks acid secretion until more pumps are synthesized. Antacids neutralize 90% of gastric acid at a pH of 3.3. Histamine stimulates acid secretion by activating H_2 receptors, so drugs that block H_2 receptors (eg, cimetidine, ranitidine) reduce acid levels. Common side effects are allergic reactions, interference with phase 1 oxidation (hepatic cytochrome P-450 system), and impotence (especially with cimetidine). Misoprostol stimulates mucous secretion, which protects GI endothelial cells from high acid levels. The cytoprotective sucralfate (sucrose-sulfate-aluminum hydroxide) stimulates bicarbonate, mucus, and prostaglandin secretion. ACh activates M_1 receptors to stimulate acid release; M_1 blockers (eg, hyoscyamine) block this action and reduce GI acid levels.

Complications of Peptic Reflux (Esophagitis and Stricture)

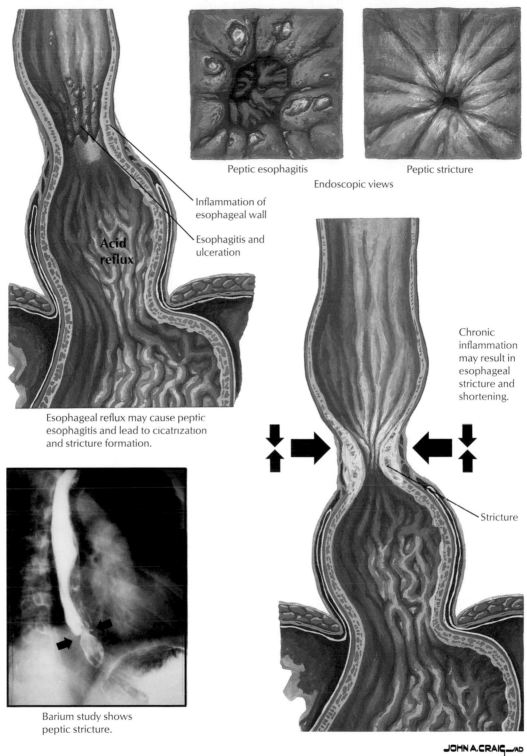

Peptic esophagitis

Peptic stricture

Endoscopic views

Inflammation of
esophageal wall

Esophagitis and
ulceration

Acid
reflux

Esophageal reflux may cause peptic
esophagitis and lead to cicatrization
and stricture formation.

Chronic
inflammation
may result in
esophageal
stricture and
shortening.

Stricture

Barium study shows
peptic stricture.

JOHN A. CRAIG—AD

FIGURE 6-20 GASTROESOPHAGEAL REFLUX DISEASE OVERVIEW

In GERD, stomach acids move back into the esophagus, an action called reflux. The esophagus moves swallowed food into the stomach via peristalsis. Reflux occurs when these muscles fail to prevent acid from moving backward. Starch, fat, and protein in food are broken down by hydrochloric acid and enzymes (pepsin). The mucous lining of the stomach protects it from acid and enzymes, but the esophageal lining offers only weak resistance to these substances. GERD symptoms are usually short-lived and infrequent, but GERD is chronic in approximately 20% of cases. Esophagitis occurs when acid causes irritation or inflammation; extensive esophageal damage and injury lead to erosive esophagitis. GERD symptoms can occur with no signs of esophageal inflammation or injury (nonerosive esophageal reflux disease, or NERD), but patients have some GERD symptoms (burning sensations behind the breastbone). Nerves near the endothelial lining are exposed to acid, and pain results.

Symptoms and Medical Management of Sliding Esophageal Hiatus Hernia

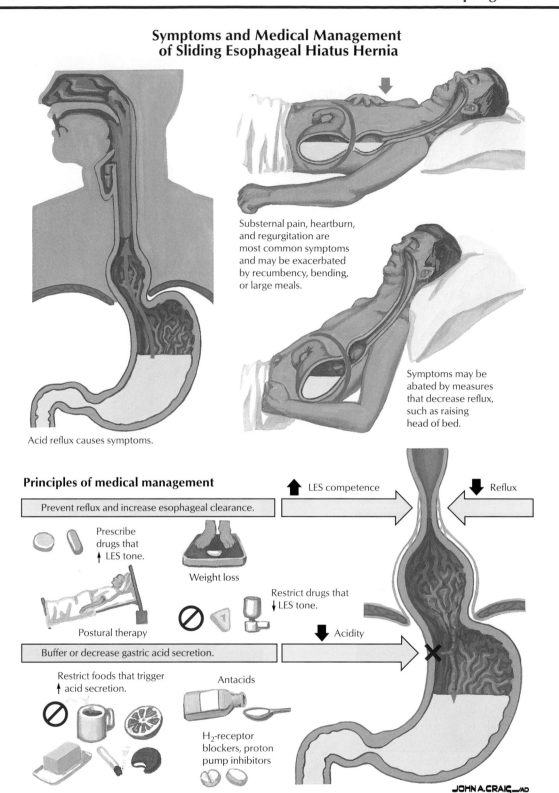

Substernal pain, heartburn, and regurgitation are most common symptoms and may be exacerbated by recumbency, bending, or large meals.

Symptoms may be abated by measures that decrease reflux, such as raising head of bed.

Acid reflux causes symptoms.

Principles of medical management

Prevent reflux and increase esophageal clearance.

LES competence

Reflux

Prescribe drugs that ↑ LES tone.

Weight loss

Restrict drugs that ↓ LES tone.

Postural therapy

Acidity

Buffer or decrease gastric acid secretion.

Restrict foods that trigger ↑ acid secretion.

Antacids

H₂-receptor blockers, proton pump inhibitors

JOHN A.CRAIG—AD

FIGURE 6-21 GASTROESOPHAGEAL REFLUX DISEASE TREATMENT

Proton pump inhibitors reduce acid reflux using by blocking the expulsion of hydrogen ions by proton pumps. The standard agent used has been omeprazole. Newer oral PPIs include lansoprazole, esomeprazole, and rabeprazole, but they do not cure the condition. Even when drugs relieve symptoms completely, the condition usually recurs within months after the drugs are discontinued. Chronic cases require treatment for life. Celecoxib, rofecoxib, and valdecoxib, the COX-2 inhibitors, reduce inflammation and pain in a manner similar to that of aspirin and ibuprofen. Unlike aspirin, however, these COX-2 drugs block the activity of COX-2, which alters the activity of COX-1. This action is important because COX-1 is constitutive (unvarying gene expression regardless of molecular conditions), whereas COX-2 is inducible (variable and dependent on molecular conditions such as inflammation or infection). It is hoped that these COX-2 blockers will cause fewer peptic ulcers and bleeding compared with aspirin.

Acute Pancreatitis

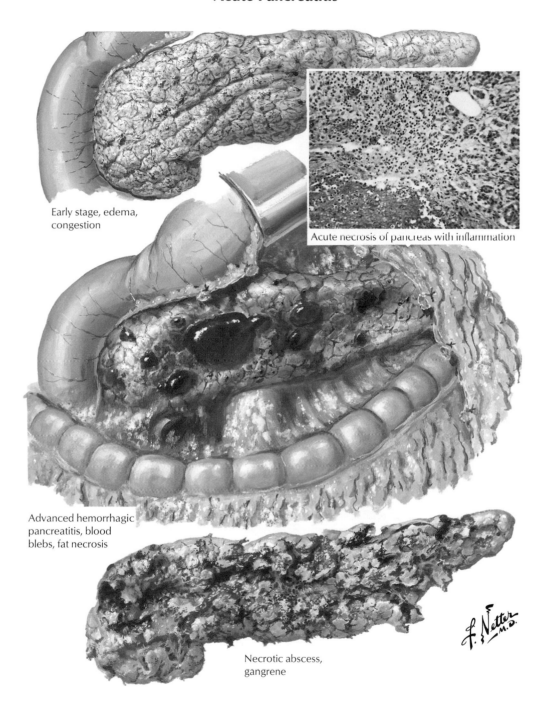

Early stage, edema, congestion

Acute necrosis of pancreas with inflammation

Advanced hemorrhagic pancreatitis, blood blebs, fat necrosis

Necrotic abscess, gangrene

FIGURE 6-22 TREATMENT OF PANCREATITIS

Pancreatitis is acute or chronic inflammation of the pancreas, which secretes digestive enzymes into the small intestine (for fat, protein, and carbohydrate digestion) and insulin and glucagon into the blood (for glucose regulation). *Acute pancreatitis* is sudden and brief and caused by gallstones or excessive alcohol consumption. Dyspnea and hypoxia are common. Treatment of acute pancreatitis includes use of IV fluids, oxygen, antibiotics (eg, imipenem-cilastatin), or surgery. *Chronic pancreatitis*, which

Chronic (Relapsing) Pancreatitis

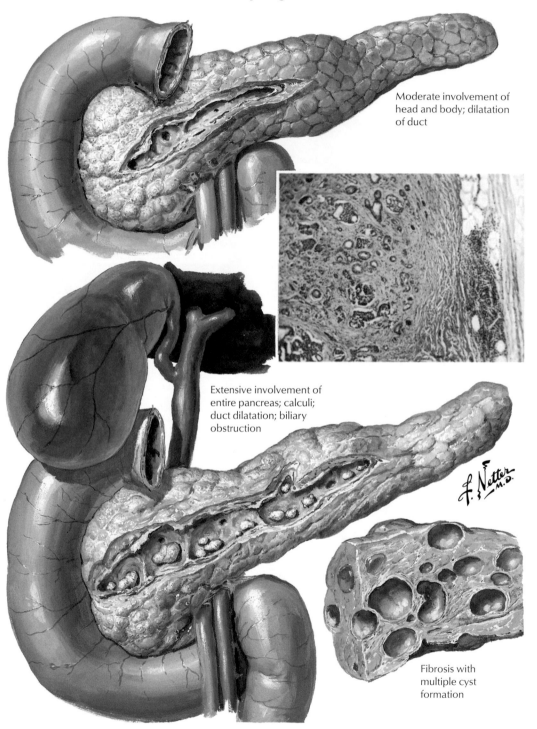

Moderate involvement of head and body; dilatation of duct

Extensive involvement of entire pancreas; calculi; duct dilatation; biliary obstruction

Fibrosis with multiple cyst formation

FIGURE 6-22 TREATMENT OF PANCREATITIS (continued)

may develop if pancreatic injury continues, is caused by digestive enzymes attacking and destroying pancreatic tissue. Prolonged alcohol abuse is a common cause, but the chronic form may occur after only 1 acute attack, especially if a patient has damaged pancreatic ducts, cystic fibrosis, hypercalcemia, or hyperlipidemia. Chronic pancreatitis therapy includes use of antiinflammatory agents, a high-carbohydrate diet, a low-fat diet, and protease pancreatic enzyme supplements.

Cholelithiasis
Pathologic Features, Choledocholithiasis

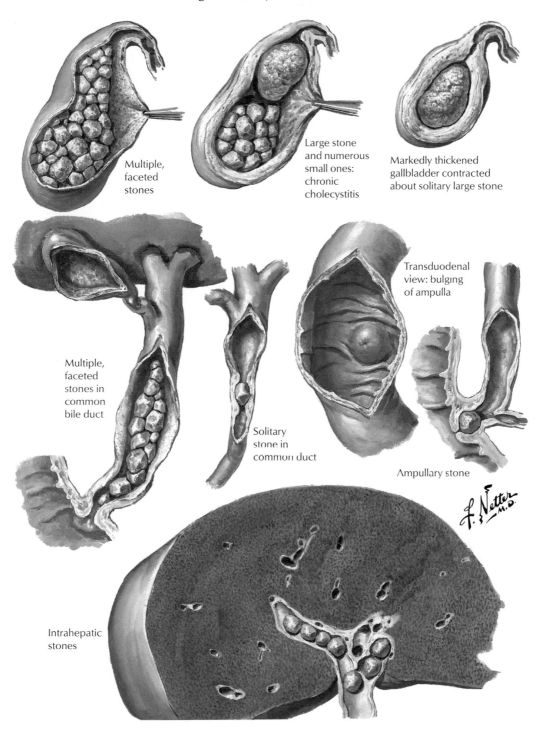

Multiple, faceted stones

Large stone and numerous small ones: chronic cholecystitis

Markedly thickened gallbladder contracted about solitary large stone

Multiple, faceted stones in common bile duct

Solitary stone in common duct

Transduodenal view: bulging of ampulla

Ampullary stone

Intrahepatic stones

FIGURE 6-23 PATHOLOGIC FEATURES OF GALLSTONES

Gallstones develop in the gallbladder from crystals of cholesterol or bilirubin. Stones can be too small to be seen with the eye (biliary sludge) or can be the size of golf balls. There may be 1 or hundreds of stones. The presence of gallstones is called *cholelithiasis*. Obstruction by gallstones of the cystic duct (that leads from the gallbladder to the common bile duct) causes pain (biliary colic), infection, and inflammation (cholecystitis). Gallstone disease affects 10% to 15% of the US population, but only 1% to 3% report symptoms in a given year. Women, particularly during pregnancy, are at increased risk because estrogen stimulates the liver to remove more cholesterol from blood and divert it into bile. Avoidance of fatty meals or nonsurgical approaches are used only in special situations (when a serious medical condition prevents surgery and for cholesterol stones). Stones usually recur after nonsurgical intervention.

Pathogenesis of Gallstones

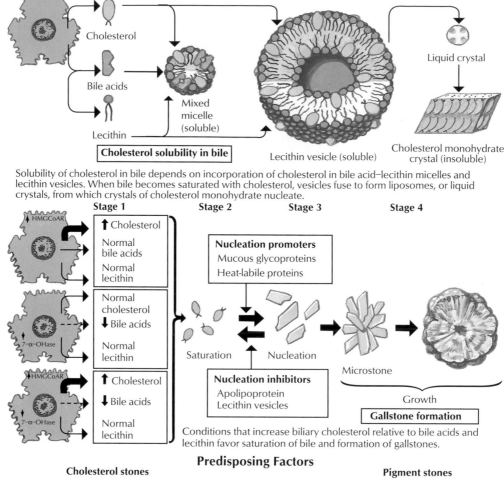

Cholesterol solubility in bile

Solubility of cholesterol in bile depends on incorporation of cholesterol in bile acid–lecithin micelles and lecithin vesicles. When bile becomes saturated with cholesterol, vesicles fuse to form liposomes, or liquid crystals, from which crystals of cholesterol monohydrate nucleate.

Conditions that increase biliary cholesterol relative to bile acids and lecithin favor saturation of bile and formation of gallstones.

Predisposing Factors

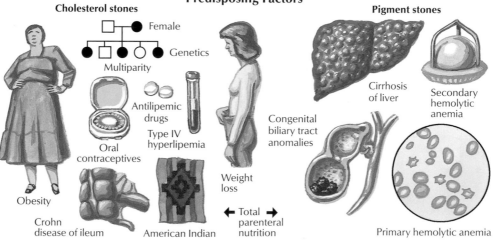

FIGURE 6-24 GALLSTONE PATHOGENESIS AND TREATMENT

Using drugs synthesized from bile acid to dissolve gallstones is known as *oral dissolution therapy*. Ursodiol and chenodiol work best for small cholesterol stones. Months of treatment may be necessary before all the stones dissolve. Both drugs cause mild diarrhea, and chenodiol may increase blood cholesterol levels and increase the activity of transaminase, a hepatic enzyme. *Contact dissolution therapy* is an experimental procedure that involves injecting a drug directly into the gallbladder to dissolve stones. The drug *methyl-tert*-butyl ether can dissolve some stones in 1 to 3 days, but it must be used carefully because it is a flammable and toxic anesthetic. *Extracorporeal shock wave lithotripsy* (ESWL) is the use of shock waves to disintegrate stones into tiny pieces that can pass through bile ducts without causing blockage. Attacks of biliary colic (intense pain) are common after treatment, and the success rate of ESWL is unknown.

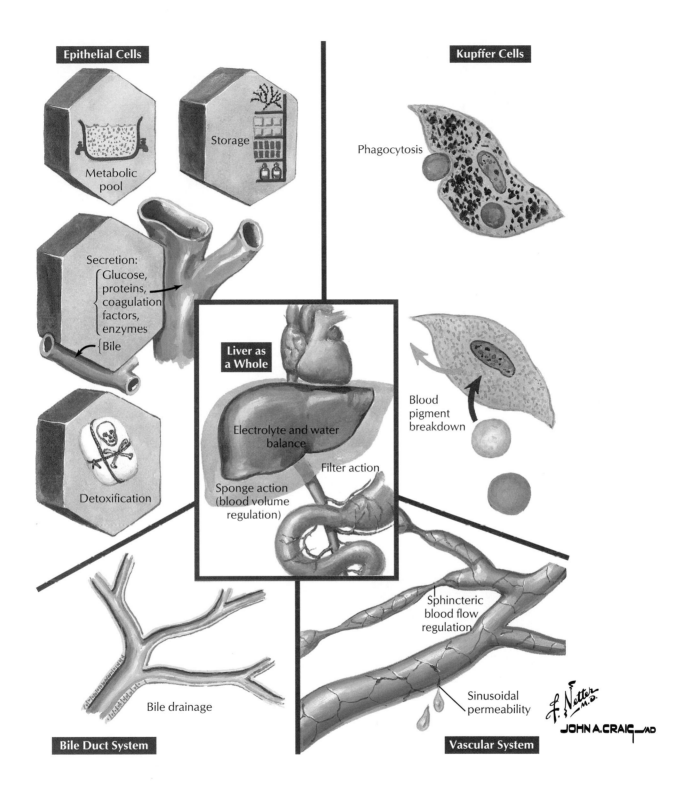

Epithelial Cells

Metabolic pool

Storage

Secretion:
{ Glucose, proteins, coagulation factors, enzymes
{ Bile

Detoxification

Kupffer Cells

Phagocytosis

Blood pigment breakdown

Liver as a Whole

Electrolyte and water balance

Filter action

Sponge action (blood volume regulation)

Sphincteric blood flow regulation

Sinusoidal permeability

Bile Duct System

Bile drainage

Vascular System

FIGURE 6-25 LIVER FUNCTION

The liver creates, regulates, stores, and secretes substances used by the GI system, bile being the major digestive chemical synthesized. During a meal, bile is secreted by liver cells and moves through the hepatic duct system into the small intestine, where it is used to break down fat molecules. Between meals, the gallbladder stores bile. Bile serves as a waste disposal system for toxins removed from blood by the liver. The liver plays a major role in regulation of blood glucose. The liver also synthesizes, dissolves, and stores amino acids, protein, and fat, and it stores several important vitamins (B_{12} and A). The liver disposes of cellular waste and decomposes toxic substances such as alcohol, with disposal occurring via the bile. Because the liver clears toxins, hepatocytes are organized for optimal contact with sinusoids (leading to and from blood vessels) and bile ducts. The liver is unique in that it can regenerate, but this capacity can be exceeded by extensive damage.

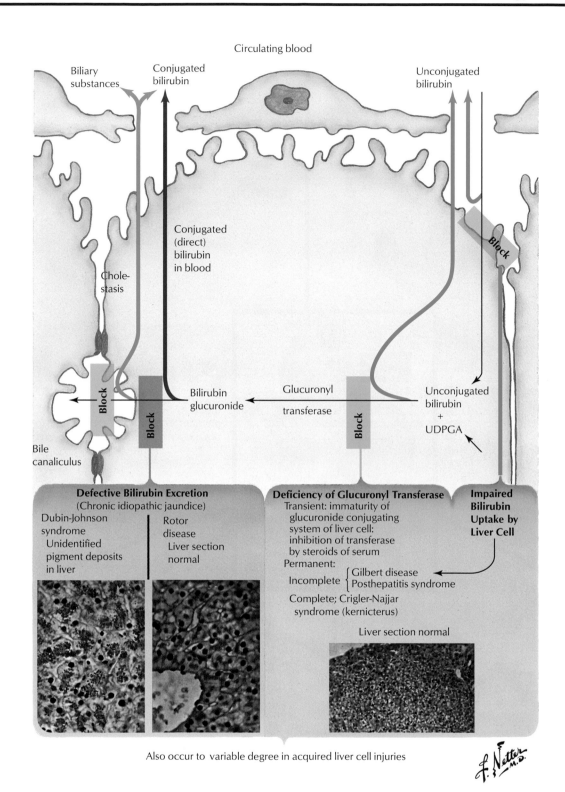

Circulating blood

FIGURE 6-26 BILIRUBIN PRODUCTION AND EXCRETION

Specific hepatic cells produce bilirubin (unconjugated or indirect), a degradation product of hemoglobin. Hepatocytes sequester bilirubin, conjugate it with glucuronic acid, and excrete it into bile. Intestinal bacteria convert conjugated (direct) bilirubin into urobilinogen, which is returned to the liver and bile or excreted by kidneys. Bilirubin assay is used to determine liver (jaundice) or gallbladder dysfunction. Jaundice occurs, as a result of liver disease or bile duct blockage, when red blood cells are broken down too fast for the liver to process. Syndromes related to bilirubin include Crigler-Najjar type II, which causes increased indirect bilirubin levels. These patients live into old age and are not at risk for kernicterus (brain damage). Patients with Gilbert syndrome, a benign disorder with no increase in mortality or morbidity, usually have no complications from hyperbilirubinemia. Phenobarbital is used for high bilirubin levels and is thought to act by enzyme induction.

Septal Cirrhosis

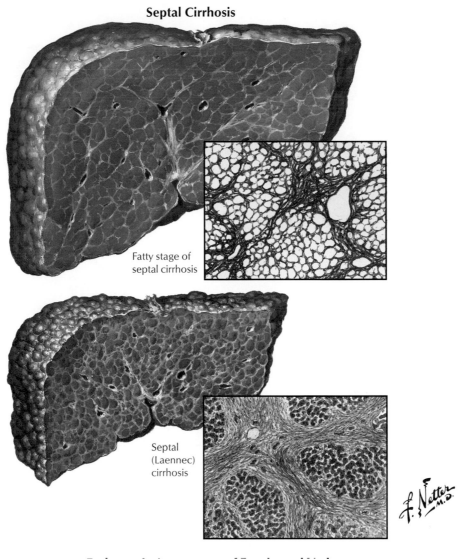

Fatty stage of
septal cirrhosis

Septal
(Laennec)
cirrhosis

**Endoscopic Appearance of Esophageal Varices
With Evidence of Recent Hemorrhage**

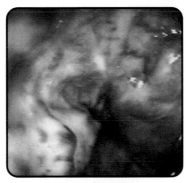 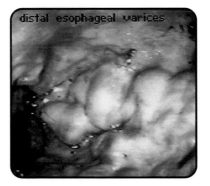

distal esophageal varices

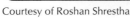
Courtesy of Roshan Shrestha

FIGURE 6-27 CIRRHOSIS

In cirrhosis, widespread nodules in the liver combined with fibrosis distort normal liver architecture, which interferes with blood flow through the organ. Cirrhosis can also lead to inability of the liver to perform biochemical functions. The most common cause is alcoholic liver disease. Others are chronic viral hepatitis B, C, and D; chronic autoimmune hepatitis; inherited metabolic diseases (hemochromatosis, Wilson disease); bile duct diseases; chronic congestive heart failure; parasitic infections (schistosomi-asis); and long-term exposure to toxins or drugs. Cirrhosis is irreversible, but treatment of underlying liver disease may slow its progression. Cessation of alcohol intake stops progress of alcoholic cirrhosis. Stopping a hepatotoxic drug or removal of an environmental toxin also halts disease progression. Interferon is used to treat viral hepatitis B and C; prednisone and azathioprine are used to treat autoimmune hepatitis. Drugs such as ursodiol may help in primary biliary cirrhosis.

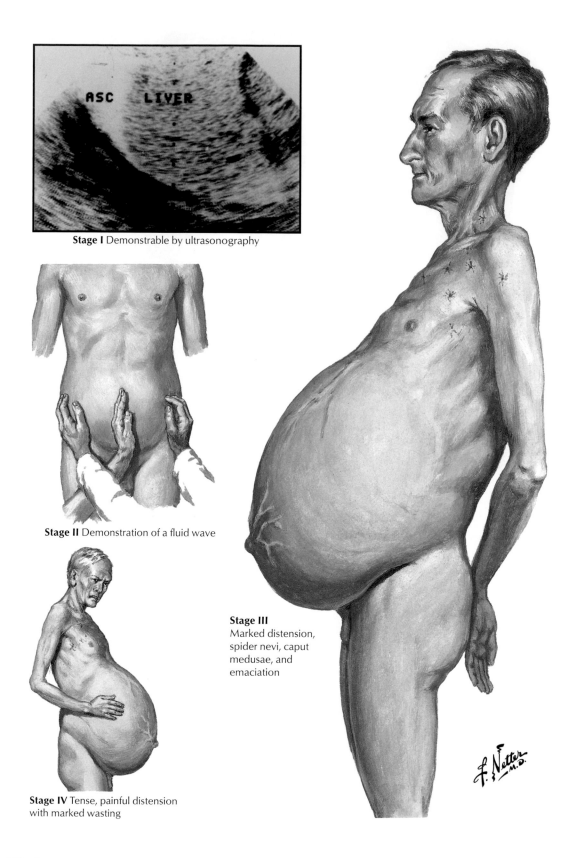

Stage I Demonstrable by ultrasonography

Stage II Demonstration of a fluid wave

Stage III
Marked distension,
spider nevi, caput
medusae, and
emaciation

Stage IV Tense, painful distension
with marked wasting

FIGURE 6-28 ASCITES

Ascites, the abnormal accumulation of fluid within the abdominal cavity, has a wide range of causes (cancer and kidney, heart, and pancreatic disease) but most often develops as a result of liver disease. The underlying disorder requires treatment (eg, bed rest to improve kidney function and decreased sodium and fluid intake to reduce blood volume). Diuretics used include potassium-sparing agents such as spironolactone, amiloride, and triamterene. Spironolactone blocks aldosterone receptors in

Pathophysiology of Ascites Formation

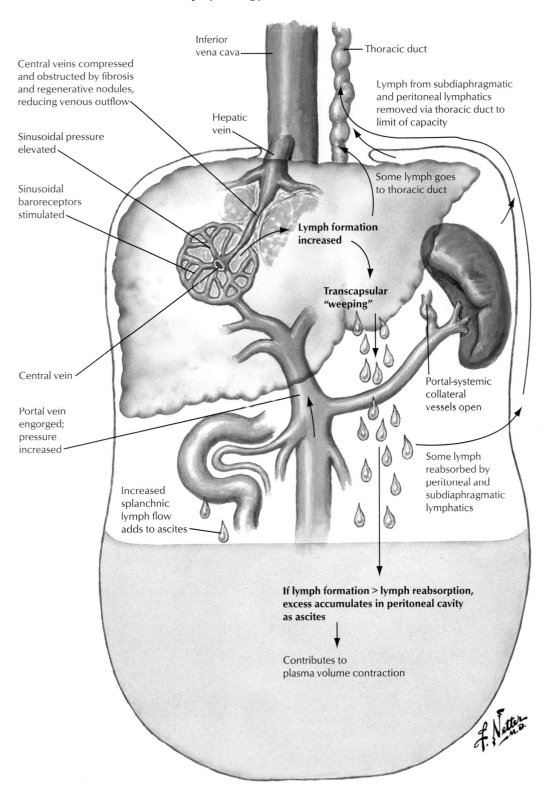

Central veins compressed and obstructed by fibrosis and regenerative nodules, reducing venous outflow

Sinusoidal pressure elevated

Sinusoidal baroreceptors stimulated

Central vein

Portal vein engorged; pressure increased

Increased splanchnic lymph flow adds to ascites

Inferior vena cava

Hepatic vein

Thoracic duct

Lymph from subdiaphragmatic and peritoneal lymphatics removed via thoracic duct to limit of capacity

Some lymph goes to thoracic duct

Lymph formation increased

Transcapsular "weeping"

Portal-systemic collateral vessels open

Some lymph reabsorbed by peritoneal and subdiaphragmatic lymphatics

If lymph formation > lymph reabsorption, excess accumulates in peritoneal cavity as ascites

Contributes to plasma volume contraction

FIGURE 6-28 ASCITES (continued)

collecting ducts of kidneys, thus stopping aldosterone-evoked sodium reabsorption and potassium loss. Triamterene and amiloride indirectly antagonize actions of aldosterone by blocking sodium channels and preventing sodium reabsorption. Stronger diuretics such as loop diuretics (eg, bumetanide, furosemide, torsemide) and thiazides (eg, hydrochlorothiazide) may be used if potassium-sparing agents are ineffective but can cause hypokalemia, hypovolemia (and shock), and hyperuricemia (and gout).

201

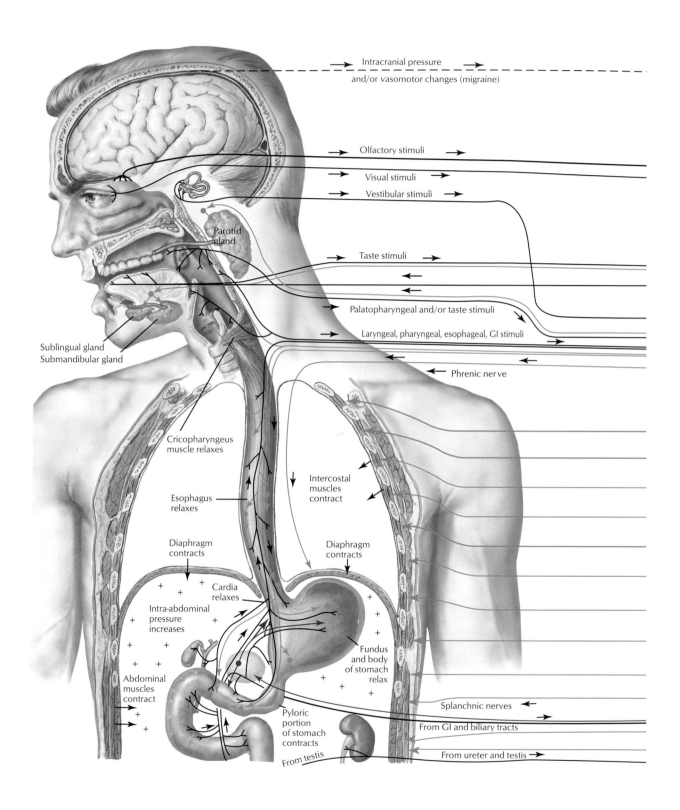

Intracranial pressure and/or vasomotor changes (migraine)

Olfactory stimuli

Visual stimuli

Vestibular stimuli

Parotid gland

Taste stimuli

Palatopharyngeal and/or taste stimuli

Laryngeal, pharyngeal, esophageal, GI stimuli

Sublingual gland
Submandibular gland

Phrenic nerve

Cricopharyngeus muscle relaxes

Intercostal muscles contract

Esophagus relaxes

Diaphragm contracts

Diaphragm contracts

Cardia relaxes

Intra-abdominal pressure increases

Fundus and body of stomach relax

Abdominal muscles contract

Splanchnic nerves

Pyloric portion of stomach contracts

From GI and biliary tracts

From testis

From ureter and testis

FIGURE 6-29 PHYSIOLOGY OF EMESIS

Emesis is expulsion of undigested food through the mouth. Nausea, the state preceding vomiting, is the sensation of needing to vomit. Emesis is caused by allergy, food, anticancer drugs (eg, cisplatin), hepatitis, stress, and pregnancy. Central neural vomiting regulation is located in the medulla. The chemoreceptor trigger zone (CTZ), in the area postrema on the floor of ventricle IV, is quite sensitive to chemicals. The blood-brain barrier is poorly developed in the CTZ (accessible to emetic agents in

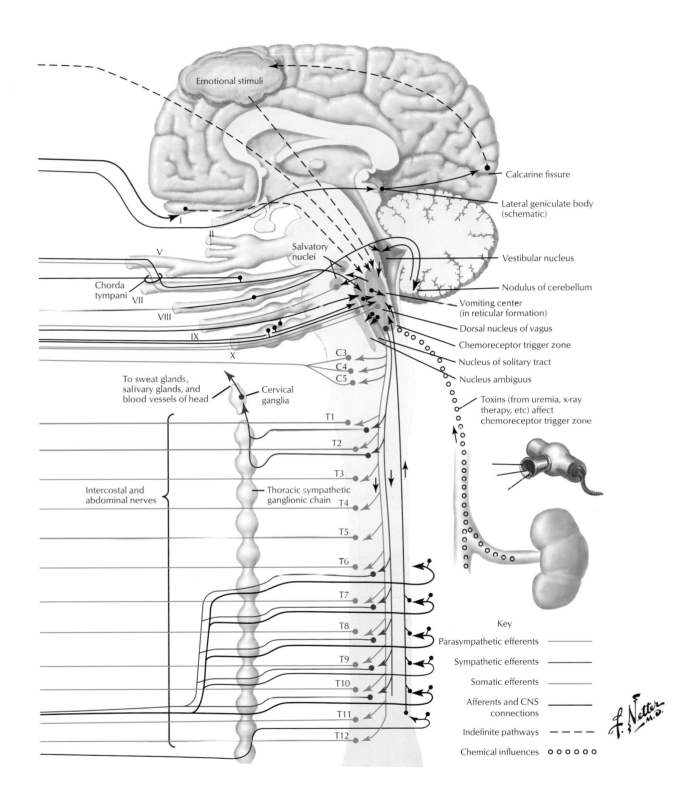

FIGURE 6-29 PHYSIOLOGY OF EMESIS (continued)

circulation). The vomiting center (VC) integrates the emetic response and is located in the dorsolateral border of the medullar reticular formation (includes the nucleus tractus solitarius, parvicellular reticular formation, and visceral and somatic motor nuclei). The VC gets excitatory inputs from nerve endings of vagal sensory fibers in the GI tract, vestibular nuclei, higher centers in the cortex (for vomiting induced by disgust), the CTZ, and intracranial pressure receptors.

Emesis

Vomiting induced by the emetic syrup of ipecac is occasionally recommended for pediatric ingestions, being managed at home, in consultation with the poison center. It no longer has a role in the hospital management of poisonings.

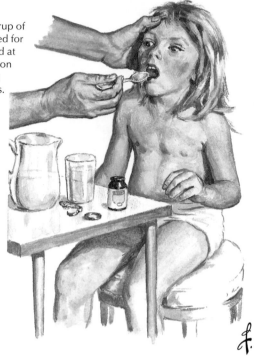

Receptors, Transmitters, and Drugs Involved in Mediating Vomiting

Structures	Receptors	Agonists	Antagonists
Area postrema	D_2	Apomorphine L-Dopa	Antidopaminergic drugs
CTZ			
Vestibular nuclei	M, H_1	Cholinomimetics	Dimenhydrinate
Nucleus tractus solitarius		Histamine	Atropine
Vomiting center	M	Cholinomimetics (eg, physostigmine)	Atropine
Vagal sensory nerve endings	$5\text{-}HT_3$	Serotonin	Ondansetron Granisetron

FIGURE 6-30 ANTIEMETICS

There are several classes of antiemetic drugs. H_1 antagonists (eg, dimenhydrinate, clizines, diphenhydramine, hydroxyzine) block H_1 receptors in the midbrain to relieve histamine-induced emesis. Most H_1 blockers have additional anticholinergic action, and adverse effects include drowsiness and loss of coordination. The newer histamine blockers are not useful because they cannot penetrate the blood-brain barrier. Dopamine antagonists (eg, metoclopramide, domperidone, chlorpromazine, droperidol) are usually used as antipsychotic drugs but can suppress emesis by blocking D_2 receptors in the area postrema and CTZ. Benzodiazepines (eg, diazepam, lorazepam) are useful for anticipatory nausea and vomiting before cancer therapy. They are also used for vestibular disorders (vertigo, dizziness, nystagmus). Muscarinic receptor antagonists have also been used (scopolamine is no longer available). These drugs relieve emesis by blocking M_1 receptors in vestibular nuclei.

CHAPTER 7

DRUGS USED IN DISORDERS OF THE RESPIRATORY SYSTEM

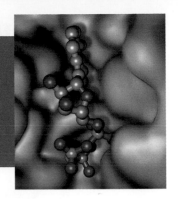

OVERVIEW

Respiration comprises the sequence of events that result in exchange of oxygen and carbon dioxide between the atmosphere and the body's cells. The major structural components of the respiratory system are the nasal cavity, larynx, pharynx, trachea, and lungs. The lungs contain the bronchi, which branch into smaller passages called *bronchioles* and end as pulmonary alveoli. The respiratory system serves 4 major functions: (1) gas exchange (oxygen and carbon dioxide); (2) sound production, or vocalization, caused by passage of air over the vocal cords; (3) coughing; and (4) abdominal compression during urination, defecation, and parturition (childbirth).

Cellular respiration requires inspiration of oxygen and elimination (via expiration) of excess carbon dioxide, the poisonous waste product of this process. Gas exchange supports cellular respiration by constantly supplying oxygen and removing carbon dioxide. Inspiration occurs when contraction of respiratory muscles produces an expansion of lung volume, decrease in alveolar pressure, and influx of air (oxygen) into lungs. Expiration compresses the lungs and increases alveolar pressure, thus pushing carbon dioxide–rich gas out of the lungs. Every 3 to 5 seconds, nerve impulses stimulate the breathing process, or ventilation, which moves air through a series of passages into and out of the lungs, after which an exchange of gases occurs between the lungs and the blood (called *external respiration*). Blood transports the gases to and from cells in tissues. Exchange of gases between the blood and cells is called *internal respiration*. Finally, cells use oxygen for specific functions: cellular metabolism, or cellular respiration.

The process of cellular respiration is compromised by diseases of the respiratory system. Common respiratory diseases include asthma, chronic obstructive pulmonary disease (COPD, which includes emphysema and chronic bronchitis), acute bronchitis, dyspnea (difficult breathing), and pneumonia. Drugs for treating the respiratory system are used primarily to open bronchial tubes, either by reversing effects of histamines (which are released by the body when exposed to substances that cause allergic reactions) or by relaxing muscle bundles surrounding bronchial tubes.

Asthma, which involves constriction of pulmonary passages and secretion of excess mucus, is characterized by dyspnea, coughing, and wheezing and can be precipitated by triggers such as allergens, cold air, viral infections, bacterial infections, and exercise. Anti-IgE antibodies, mast cell degranulation blockers, smooth muscle relaxants, and antiinflammatory agents are major drug classes used for asthma.

Emphysema results from the breakdown of alveolar walls, which leads to reduced alveolar surface area and impaired cellular respiration and gas exchange. Acute bronchitis results from inflammation of bronchial passages and has causes similar to those of asthma. Chronic bronchitis is characterized by persistent production of excess mucus in bronchial tubes. Cough, shortness of breath, and lung damage are typical of chronic bronchitis. Medications for COPD include short-acting b2 agonists and bronchodilators.

Pneumonia is an acute lung inflammation that results in collapse of lung tissue and can be treated with antibiotics only when the cause is bacterial.

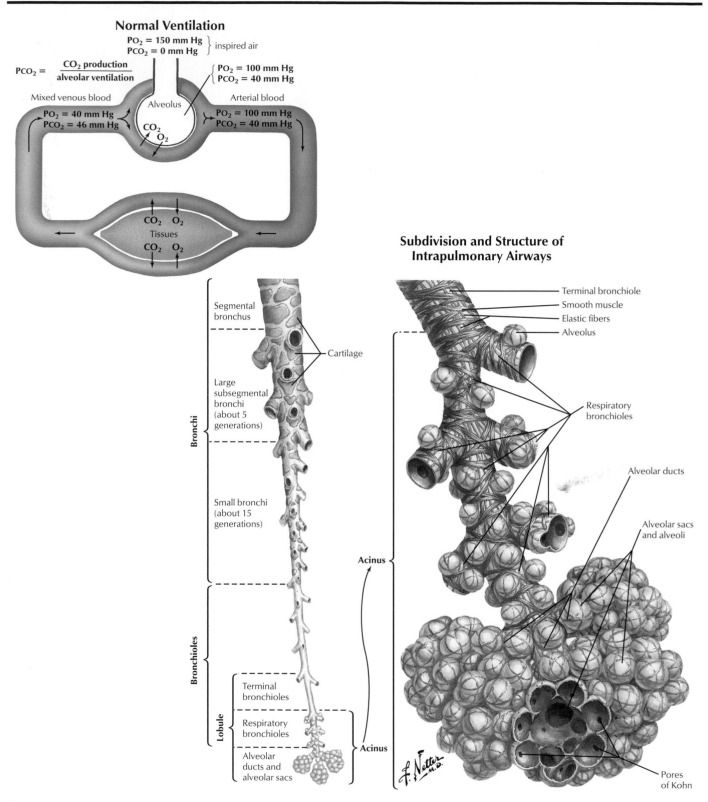

Normal Ventilation

$PO_2 = 150$ mm Hg
$PCO_2 = 0$ mm Hg } inspired air

$PCO_2 = \dfrac{CO_2 \text{ production}}{\text{alveolar ventilation}}$

{ $PO_2 = 100$ mm Hg
$PCO_2 = 40$ mm Hg

Alveolus

Mixed venous blood

$PO_2 = 40$ mm Hg
$PCO_2 = 46$ mm Hg

CO_2
O_2

Arterial blood

$PO_2 = 100$ mm Hg
$PCO_2 = 40$ mm Hg

$CO_2 \quad O_2$
Tissues
$CO_2 \quad O_2$

Subdivision and Structure of Intrapulmonary Airways

Terminal bronchiole
Smooth muscle
Elastic fibers
Alveolus

Segmental bronchus

Cartilage

Respiratory bronchioles

Large subsegmental bronchi (about 5 generations)

Alveolar ducts

Bronchi

Small bronchi (about 15 generations)

Alveolar sacs and alveoli

Acinus

Bronchioles

Terminal bronchioles

Lobule

Respiratory bronchioles

Acinus

Alveolar ducts and alveolar sacs

Pores of Kohn

FIGURE 7-1 RESPIRATION OVERVIEW

Respiration means ventilation, or breathing. The 2 phases of breathing are inspiration (inhalation) and expiration (exhalation). Primary functions of the respiratory system are to provide oxygen to tissues and to expel carbon dioxide from the body. Respiration is classified into 3 functional categories: external respiration, exchange of gas between the atmosphere and blood; internal respiration, exchange of gas between the blood and cells; and cellular respiration, the process whereby cells use oxygen and convert energy into useful forms. The major waste product of cellular respiration, carbon dioxide, diffuses from cells into blood, in which it is transported to the lungs and expelled during expiration. Secondary functions of the respiratory system are sound production, coughing, sneezing, and abdominal compression during urination, defecation, and parturition. Pharmacologic intervention becomes necessary when the respiratory system functions improperly.

Sites of Pathologic Disturbances in Control of Breathing

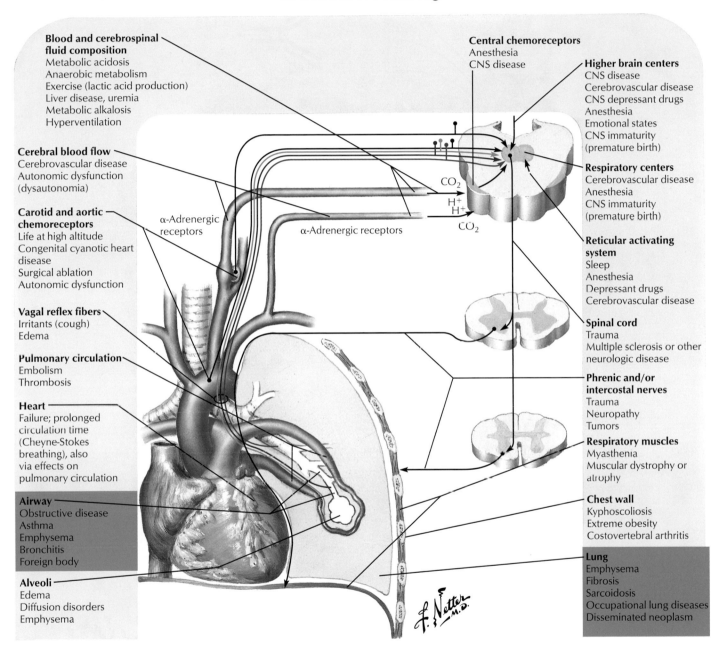

Blood and cerebrospinal fluid composition
Metabolic acidosis
Anaerobic metabolism
Exercise (lactic acid production)
Liver disease, uremia
Metabolic alkalosis
Hyperventilation

Cerebral blood flow
Cerebrovascular disease
Autonomic dysfunction (dysautonomia)

Carotid and aortic chemoreceptors
Life at high altitude
Congenital cyanotic heart disease
Surgical ablation
Autonomic dysfunction

Vagal reflex fibers
Irritants (cough)
Edema

Pulmonary circulation
Embolism
Thrombosis

Heart
Failure; prolonged circulation time (Cheyne-Stokes breathing), also via effects on pulmonary circulation

Airway
Obstructive disease
Asthma
Emphysema
Bronchitis
Foreign body

Alveoli
Edema
Diffusion disorders
Emphysema

α-Adrenergic receptors

α-Adrenergic receptors

CO_2
H^+
H^+
CO_2

Central chemoreceptors
Anesthesia
CNS disease

Higher brain centers
CNS disease
Cerebrovascular disease
CNS depressant drugs
Anesthesia
Emotional states
CNS immaturity (premature birth)

Respiratory centers
Cerebrovascular disease
Anesthesia
CNS immaturity (premature birth)

Reticular activating system
Sleep
Anesthesia
Depressant drugs
Cerebrovascular disease

Spinal cord
Trauma
Multiple sclerosis or other neurologic disease

Phrenic and/or intercostal nerves
Trauma
Neuropathy
Tumors

Respiratory muscles
Myasthenia
Muscular dystrophy or atrophy

Chest wall
Kyphoscoliosis
Extreme obesity
Costovertebral arthritis

Lung
Emphysema
Fibrosis
Sarcoidosis
Occupational lung diseases
Disseminated neoplasm

FIGURE 7-2 RESPIRATORY DISEASES

The most common respiratory disorders are asthma, cough, COPD (emphysema; chronic bronchitis), and pneumonia. Less common disorders are hyperventilation (excessive inspiration and expiration); apnea (temporary breathing cessation that may follow hyperventilation); and rhinitis (nasal mucosa inflammation). Drugs used for these conditions are normally given by inhalation (metered-dose or nebulized inhaler) or by oral means. Inhalation is preferred because of direct drug delivery to lungs,

avoidance of first-pass metabolism by the liver and intestine, and minimization of adverse effects. Certain drugs used to treat asthma (eg, theophylline, albuterol, terbutaline) can be given orally. Parenteral dosing (intravascular, subcutaneous, or intramuscular) may be needed, especially when rapid onset of action is critical or drug absorption from the GI tract is poor; it controls the dose delivered, but adverse effects can result.

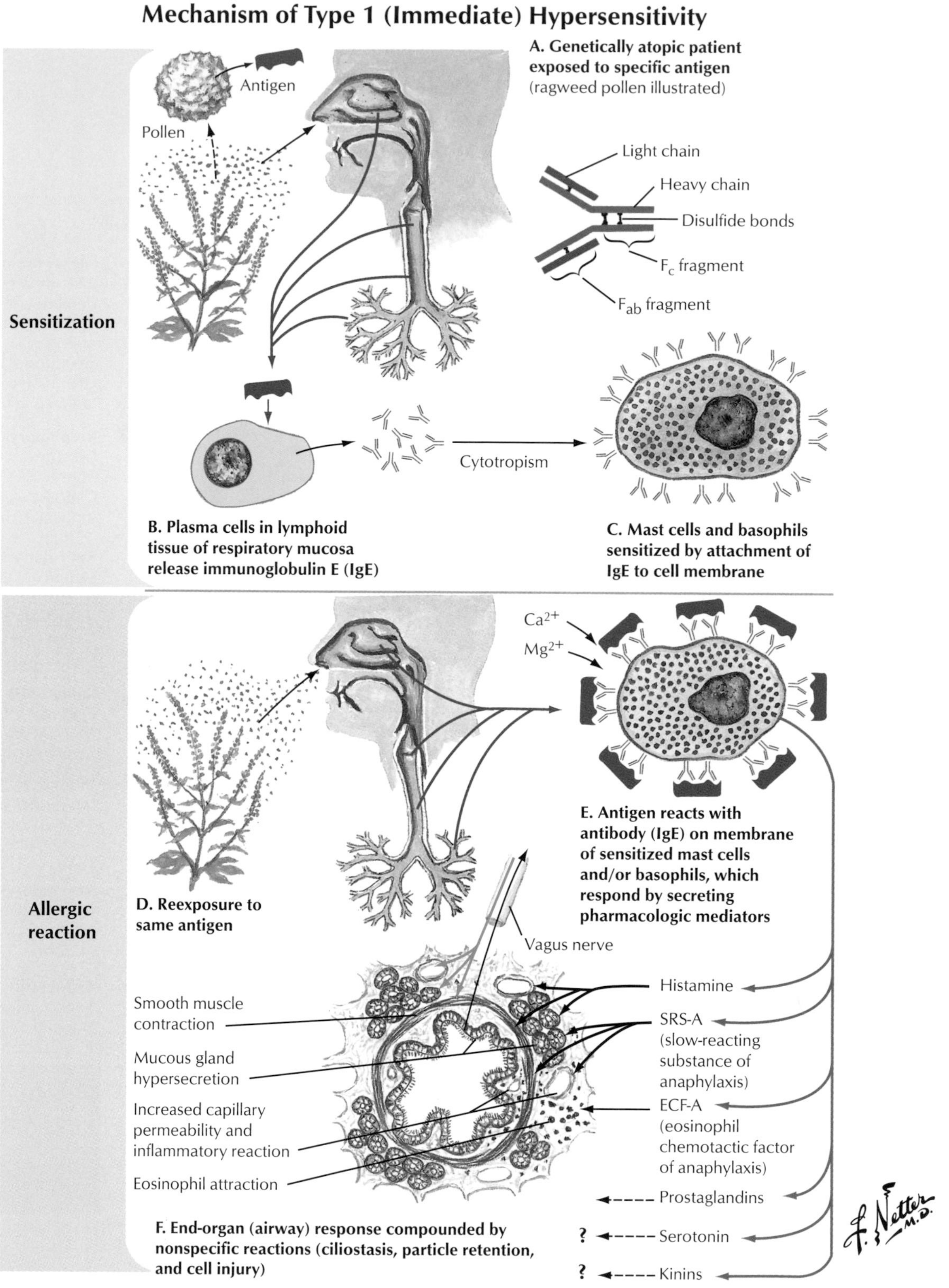

Mechanism of Type 1 (Immediate) Hypersensitivity

Sensitization

Pollen

Antigen

A. Genetically atopic patient exposed to specific antigen
(ragweed pollen illustrated)

Light chain
Heavy chain
Disulfide bonds
F_c fragment
F_{ab} fragment

Cytotropism

B. Plasma cells in lymphoid tissue of respiratory mucosa release immunoglobulin E (IgE)

C. Mast cells and basophils sensitized by attachment of IgE to cell membrane

Allergic reaction

Ca^{2+}
Mg^{2+}

D. Reexposure to same antigen

Vagus nerve

E. Antigen reacts with antibody (IgE) on membrane of sensitized mast cells and/or basophils, which respond by secreting pharmacologic mediators

Smooth muscle contraction

Mucous gland hypersecretion

Increased capillary permeability and inflammatory reaction

Eosinophil attraction

Histamine

SRS-A (slow-reacting substance of anaphylaxis)

ECF-A (eosinophil chemotactic factor of anaphylaxis)

Prostaglandins

? Serotonin

? Kinins

F. End-organ (airway) response compounded by nonspecific reactions (ciliostasis, particle retention, and cell injury)

F. Netter M.D.

FIGURE 7-3 ALLERGY

The term *allergy*, from the Greek *allos* (altered state) and *ergon* (reactivity), was first used to describe patients who had reactions caused by the effect of external factors, or allergens, on the body's immune system. It is often defined as hypersensitive reactions of the immune system to substances (allergens) that are usually innocuous in most people, such as food, animal dander, pollen, bee stings, mold, ragweed, and drugs. The allergic person's immune system recognizes something as foreign and mounts a specific reaction to identify the allergen and destroy it via inflammation. Thus, a sensitivity to a material that causes a symptom is allergic only if it has an identifiable mechanism. This distinction between allergic and nonallergic disorders is important because it determines evaluation and treatment. Treatment of an allergy as if it were nonallergic will fail and vice versa. In asthma, allergens increase sensitivity of bronchial smooth muscle, thereby creating an allergic state.

Leukocytes

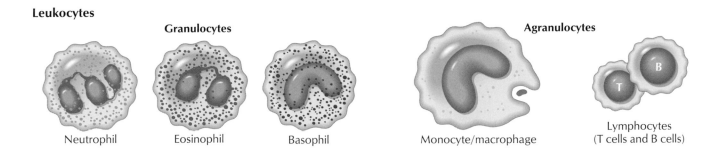

Granulocytes

Neutrophil   Eosinophil   Basophil

Agranulocytes

Monocyte/macrophage   Lymphocytes
(T cells and B cells)

Leukocytes in the Asthmatic Response

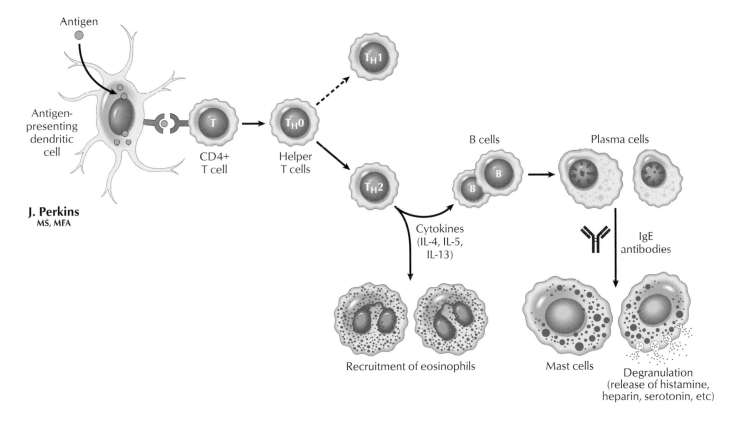

Antigen

Antigen-
presenting
dendritic
cell

CD4+
T cell

Helper
T cells

T_H1

T_H2

B cells

Plasma cells

J. Perkins
MS, MFA

Cytokines
(IL-4, IL-5,
IL-13)

IgE
antibodies

Recruitment of eosinophils   Mast cells   Degranulation
(release of histamine,
heparin, serotonin, etc)

FIGURE 7-4 LEUKOCYTE FUNCTION

Humans have a special immune system to combat infectious and toxic agents (eg, bacteria and viruses). Major cells involved in defense against foreign substances are leukocytes, or white blood cells. Like all blood cells, they are synthesized in bone marrow. Leukocytes can be classified into 2 basic classes: granular, which store mediators in granules, and mononuclear or agranular, which have no granules. Three types of granular leukocytes exist: neutrophils, eosinophils, and basophils. Eosinophils, which

phagocytize antigen-antibody complexes (antigen-IgE complexes that initiate an asthmatic reaction), and basophils, which release heparin (clotting), serotonin (clotting), and histamine (immune reaction), play primary roles in asthma. Agranular cells are monocytes, which phagocytize foreign particles, and lymphocytes, which play a critical role in the delayed asthmatic response. T cells (a subtype of lymphocytes) synthesize cytokines; B cells (another subtype) synthesize IgE antibodies.

General Management Principles for Allergic Rhinitis

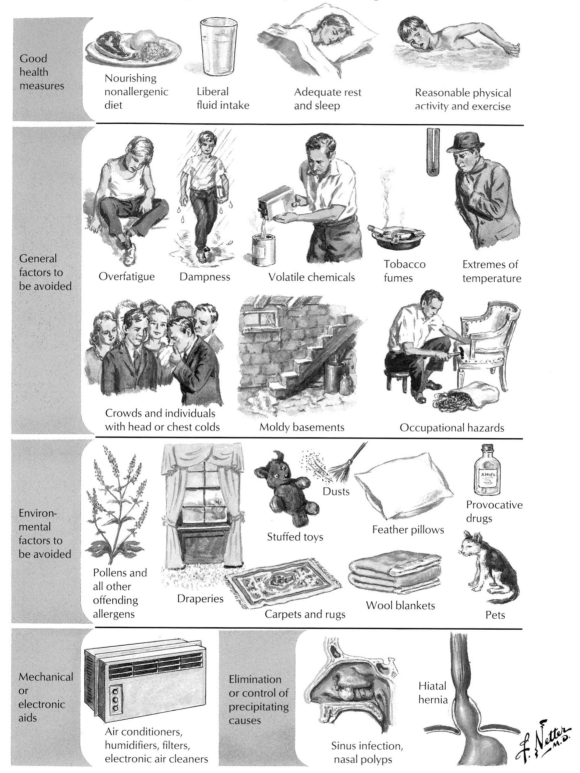

Good health measures
- Nourishing nonallergenic diet
- Liberal fluid intake
- Adequate rest and sleep
- Reasonable physical activity and exercise

General factors to be avoided
- Overfatigue
- Dampness
- Volatile chemicals
- Tobacco fumes
- Extremes of temperature
- Crowds and individuals with head or chest colds
- Moldy basements
- Occupational hazards

Environmental factors to be avoided
- Pollens and all other offending allergens
- Draperies
- Stuffed toys
- Dusts
- Feather pillows
- Provocative drugs
- Carpets and rugs
- Wool blankets
- Pets

Mechanical or electronic aids
- Air conditioners, humidifiers, filters, electronic air cleaners

Elimination or control of precipitating causes
- Sinus infection, nasal polyps
- Hiatal hernia

FIGURE 7-5 ALLERGIC RHINITIS

Allergic rhinitis (hay fever), an inflammation or irritation of the mucous membranes lining the nose, is initiated when allergens cause the body to defend itself by producing antibodies. The allergen-antibody combination prompts histamine release and the allergic response. Symptoms are sneezing, stuffy or runny nose, itchy eyes, noisy breathing, chronic fatigue, poor appetite, and nausea. The seasonal disorder is caused by pollen and normally wanes during winter; the perennial disorder occurs year-round and is caused by indoor allergens (eg, animal dander, mold spores, dust mites). Treatments are antihistamines (treatment of choice; blocks histamine action but can cause drowsiness), decongestants (relieve nasal stuffiness but can increase histamine release and worsen congestion), corticosteroids (desensitize cellular response to histamine and minimize the allergic reaction), and cromolyn sodium (inhibits histamine release, which reduces or stops the allergic response).

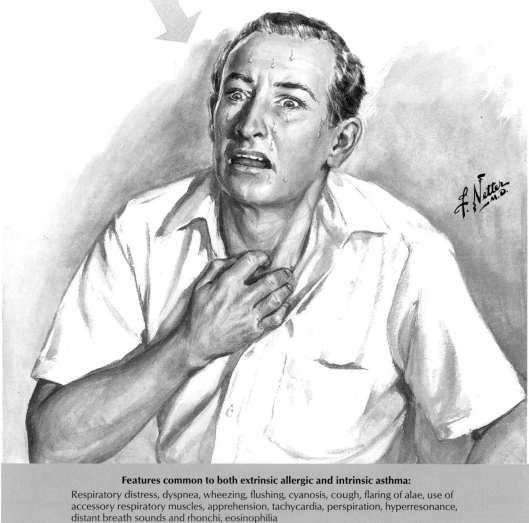

Instrinsic Asthma: Clinical Features

Adult patient: age 35 or over

Family history usually negative

Attacks related to infections, exercise, other stimuli

Skin tests usually negative

No history of eczema in childhood

Unfavorable response to hyposensitization

Not IgE associated

Attacks more fulminant; prognosis poorer; condition may become chronic; death may occur

Features common to both extrinsic allergic and intrinsic asthma:
Respiratory distress, dyspnea, wheezing, flushing, cyanosis, cough, flaring of alae, use of accessory respiratory muscles, apprehension, tachycardia, perspiration, hyperresonance, distant breath sounds and rhonchi, eosinophilia

FIGURE 7-7 EXTRINSIC AND INTRINSIC ASTHMA (continued)

from mast cells. Bronchoconstriction and vascular leakage result. Other substances (eg, cytokines) mediate the late response (IgE release). Corticosteroids reduce bronchial responses by inhibiting cytokine production. In some asthmatic patients who are not hypersensitive to antigens, infections and nonantigenic stimuli can evoke symptoms. Intrinsic asthma develops later in life, has unclear causes, is associated with a worse prognosis, and is less responsive to treatment than extrinsic asthma.

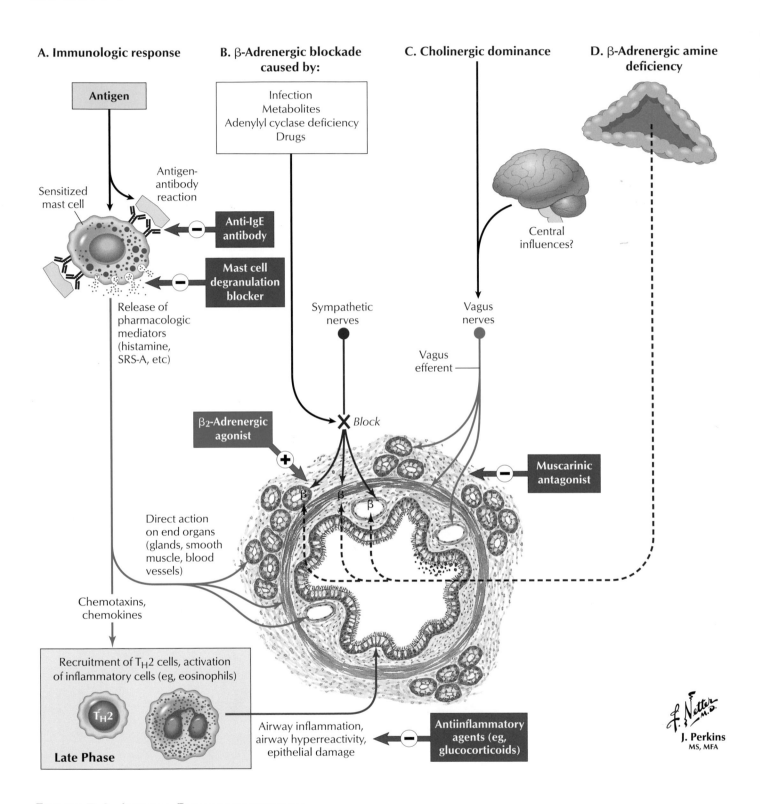

A. Immunologic response

Antigen

Sensitized mast cell

Antigen-antibody reaction

Anti-IgE antibody

Mast cell degranulation blocker

Release of pharmacologic mediators (histamine, SRS-A, etc)

Chemotaxins, chemokines

Recruitment of T$_H$2 cells, activation of inflammatory cells (eg, eosinophils)

T$_H$2

Late Phase

B. β-Adrenergic blockade caused by:

Infection
Metabolites
Adenylyl cyclase deficiency
Drugs

Sympathetic nerves

β$_2$-Adrenergic agonist

Direct action on end organs (glands, smooth muscle, blood vessels)

Block

β   β   β

C. Cholinergic dominance

Central influences?

Vagus nerves

Vagus efferent

Muscarinic antagonist

D. β-Adrenergic amine deficiency

Airway inflammation, airway hyperreactivity, epithelial damage

Antiinflammatory agents (eg, glucocorticoids)

J. Perkins
MS, MFA

FIGURE 7-8 ASTHMA PHARMACOTHERAPY

When exposure to allergens cannot be avoided, drug therapy is needed, the major goals being to reverse asthmatic symptoms and prevent recurrent episodes by disrupting actions of endogenous agents that worsen bronchospasm and inflammation. Major classes of drugs for asthma are anti-IgE antibodies, blockers of mast cell degranulation, smooth muscle relaxants, and antiinflammatory agents. Bronchodilators were the first and most effective treatment, but a better approach is prophylactic use of

antiinflammatory agents to control bronchial inflammation. With these agents, patients with asthma are rarely hospitalized, seriously ill, or in need of emergency treatment. Patients can control their disease, and this therapy is much less expensive than previous emergency management. Now, antiinflammatory agents are the first-line therapy for patients who have more than occasional symptoms. Bronchodilators are still used but only when antiinflammatory therapy is inadequate, and then in smaller amounts.

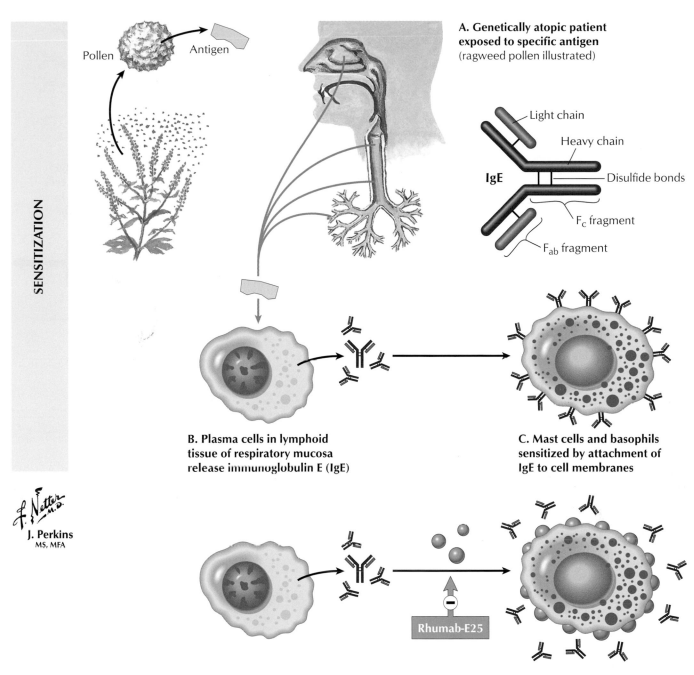

Pollen

Antigen

A. Genetically atopic patient exposed to specific antigen
(ragweed pollen illustrated)

SENSITIZATION

Light chain

Heavy chain

IgE

Disulfide bonds

F_c fragment

F_{ab} fragment

J. Perkins
MS, MFA

B. Plasma cells in lymphoid tissue of respiratory mucosa release immunoglobulin E (IgE)

C. Mast cells and basophils sensitized by attachment of IgE to cell membranes

Rhumab-E25

Rhumab-E25 (anti-IgE) prevents binding of IgE to mast cells

FIGURE 7-9 ANTI-IgE ANTIBODIES

One of the more novel therapies is use of anti-IgE antibodies. In theory, drugs acting as anti-IgE antibodies would prevent IgE binding to mast cell surfaces. This action would reduce formation of activated antigen-IgE complexes and suppress release of mediators that induce immediate bronchoconstriction in the early phase. That is, mediators such as histamine, prostaglandins, and leukotrienes would be unable to cause sneezing, wheezing, itching, and coughing. The most notable anti-IgE antibody, Rhumab-E25, is a recombinant humanized monoclonal antibody to IgE. By binding to circulating IgE in the blood, Rhumab-E25 blocks release of inflammatory mediators by keeping IgE from binding to mast cells. This antibody, administered by parenteral injection, is currently in phase III clinical trials for seasonal allergic rhinitis and allergic asthma.

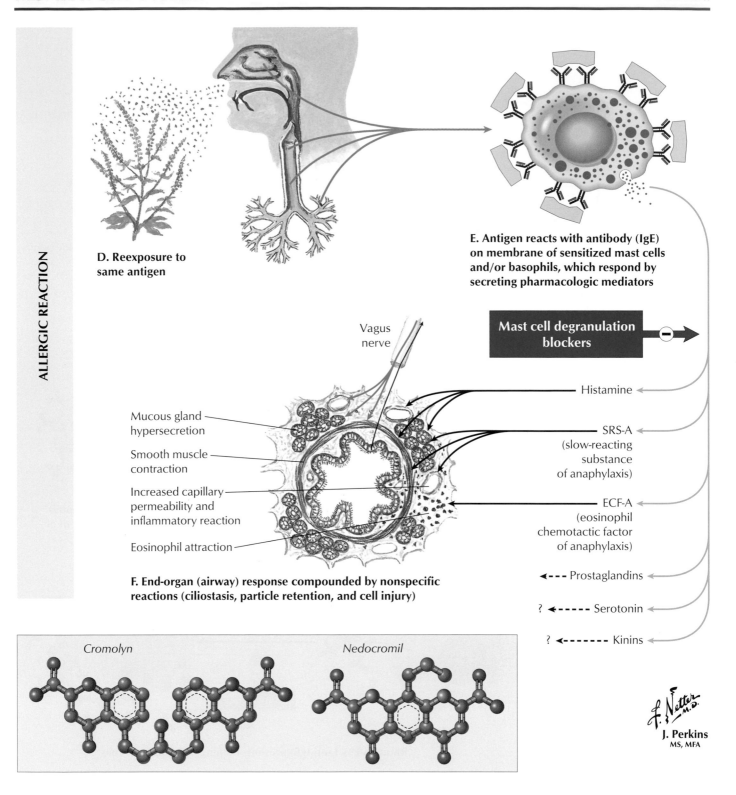

ALLERGIC REACTION

D. Reexposure to same antigen

E. Antigen reacts with antibody (IgE) on membrane of sensitized mast cells and/or basophils, which respond by secreting pharmacologic mediators

Mast cell degranulation blockers

Vagus nerve

Mucous gland hypersecretion

Smooth muscle contraction

Increased capillary permeability and inflammatory reaction

Eosinophil attraction

F. End-organ (airway) response compounded by nonspecific reactions (ciliostasis, particle retention, and cell injury)

Histamine

SRS-A (slow-reacting substance of anaphylaxis)

ECF-A (eosinophil chemotactic factor of anaphylaxis)

◄--- Prostaglandins

? ◄----- Serotonin

? ◄------- Kinins

Cromolyn

Nedocromil

J. Perkins
MS, MFA

FIGURE 7-10 MAST CELL DEGRANULATION BLOCKERS

Cromolyn and nedocromil block mast cell degranulation by suppressing release of mediators of immediate bronchoconstriction (early response) and reducing eosinophil recruitment causing airway inflammation. Neither drug directly alters smooth muscle tone or reverses bronchospasm. Both drugs, usually inhaled as aerosols, can be used for intrinsic (antigen-induced) or extrinsic (non–antigen-induced) asthma. Nedocromil enhances corticosteroid effects and is more potent than cromolyn in patients with extrinsic asthma (especially exercise induced); even when given after reexposure to antigen, it blocks delayed inflammation. Both drugs are poorly absorbed, so adverse effects (eg, chest tightness, cough) are restricted to deposition site. Cromolyn is preferred for young patients. Both drugs alter Cl^- channel function, which (1) on airway neurons underlies cough inhibition, (2) on mast cells delays antigen-evoked bronchoconstriction, and (3) on eosinophils prevents inflammatory responses to antigens.

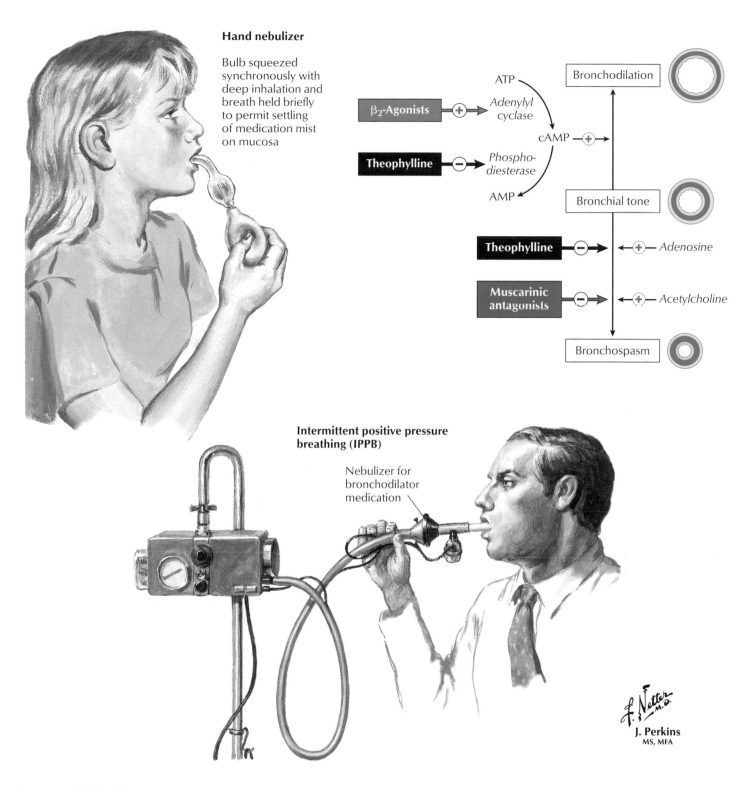

Hand nebulizer

Bulb squeezed synchronously with deep inhalation and breath held briefly to permit settling of medication mist on mucosa

ATP

β₂-Agonists (+) Adenylyl cyclase

cAMP (+) → Bronchodilation

Theophylline (−) Phospho-diesterase

AMP → Bronchial tone

Theophylline (−) → (+) ← Adenosine

Muscarinic antagonists (−) → (+) ← Acetylcholine

Bronchospasm

Intermittent positive pressure breathing (IPPB)

Nebulizer for bronchodilator medication

J. Perkins
MS, MFA

FIGURE 7-11 BRONCHODILATORS

Drugs that expand pulmonary airways (bronchi)—bronchodilators—block the early response by inhibiting immediate bronchoconstriction. Some agents, especially theophylline and β₂-adrenergic agonists, inhibit late response inflammation. These drugs are usually used when a persistent cough and bronchial constriction are present. In addition to relaxing smooth muscles and reducing airway reactivity, bronchodilators reduce coughing, wheezing, and shortness of breath. Agents are usually given via inhalation, but some can be given orally or parenterally (intravenous, intramuscular, or subcutaneous route). Most drugs have a rapid onset of action (within minutes), but the effect usually wanes in 5 to 7 hours. Some agents, especially theophylline, inhibit the delayed response to antigen. The most common bronchodilators are methylxanthines (eg, theophylline, caffeine), β-adrenergic agonists (eg, isoproterenol, albuterol, epinephrine), and cholinergic antagonists (eg, atropine, tiotropium).

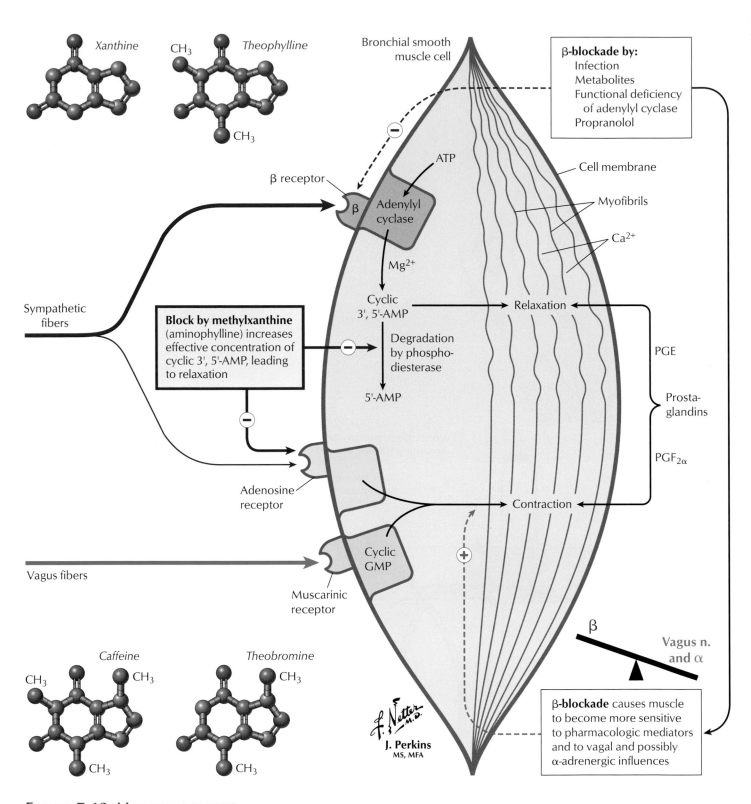

FIGURE 7-12 METHYLXANTHINES

The methylxanthines theophylline, caffeine, and theobromine, found in cola, tea, and coffee, are bronchodilators that reduce bronchial smooth muscle activity, most likely by increasing intracellular cAMP levels. Signal molecules (eg, transmitters, drugs) activate GPCRs on airway smooth muscle cells and increase the conversion rate of ATP to cAMP. Increased cAMP levels relax bronchial muscle and reduce airway reactivity. Phosphodiesterase stops cAMP effects and reduces cAMP levels by catalyzing hydrolysis of cAMP to AMP. Methylxanthines may prevent cAMP hydrolysis. Or, theophylline may block cell surface receptor effects of adenosine, which may induce bronchoconstriction and inflammation. These drugs may also be antiinflammatory. Theophylline, the most widely prescribed and of low cost, comes as short-acting tablets and syrups, sustained-release capsules and tablets, and intravenous doses. The synthetic dyphylline may help patients who are unable to use theophylline.

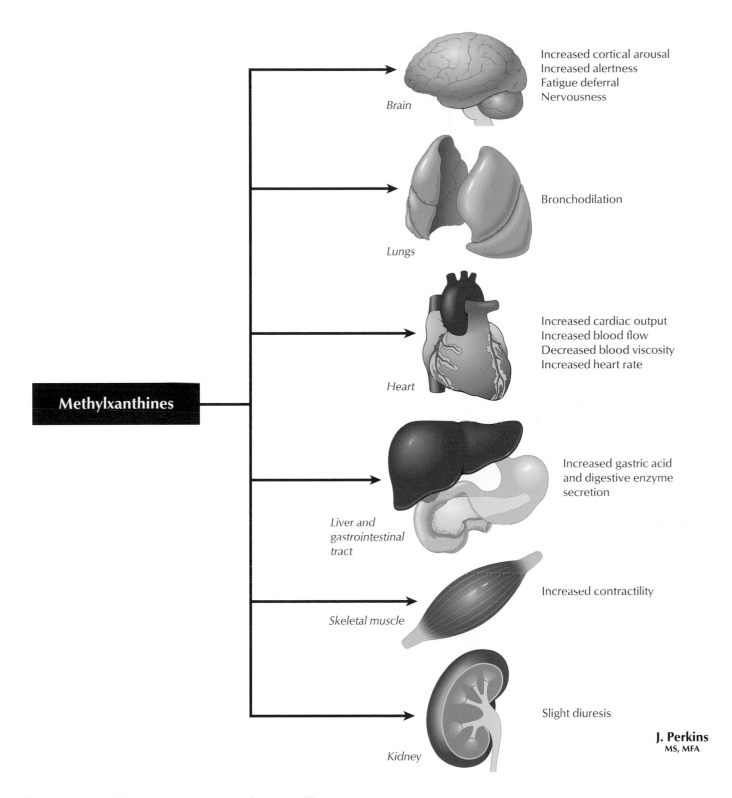

Brain — Increased cortical arousal
Increased alertness
Fatigue deferral
Nervousness

Lungs — Bronchodilation

Heart — Increased cardiac output
Increased blood flow
Decreased blood viscosity
Increased heart rate

Liver and gastrointestinal tract — Increased gastric acid and digestive enzyme secretion

Skeletal muscle — Increased contractility

Kidney — Slight diuresis

Methylxanthines

J. Perkins
MS, MFA

FIGURE 7-13 METHYLXANTHINES: ADVERSE EFFECTS

Methylxanthine doses must be closely watched. Low doses have little effect, if any, whereas high doses can affect the central nervous, cardiovascular, skeletal muscle, GI, and renal systems. Theophylline is most selective at smooth muscle; caffeine induces the most marked CNS effects. Even at low to moderate doses, these drugs enhance cortical arousal and alertness and defer fatigue. In hypersensitive patients, insomnia and nervousness may occur. Methylxanthines reduce blood viscosity, increase blood flow, increase cardiac output, and induce tachycardia in healthy subjects. In sensitive persons, cardiac arrhythmias are common. These drugs strengthen contractions of isolated skeletal muscles in vitro and improve contractility and reverse fatigue of the diaphragm in patients with COPD, which accounts for their usefulness in COPD. Although methylxanthines enhance gastric acid and digestive enzyme secretion in the GI tract and induce a slight diuresis, these effects are minor.

Catecholamine Action on α and β Receptors of Heart and Bronchial Tree

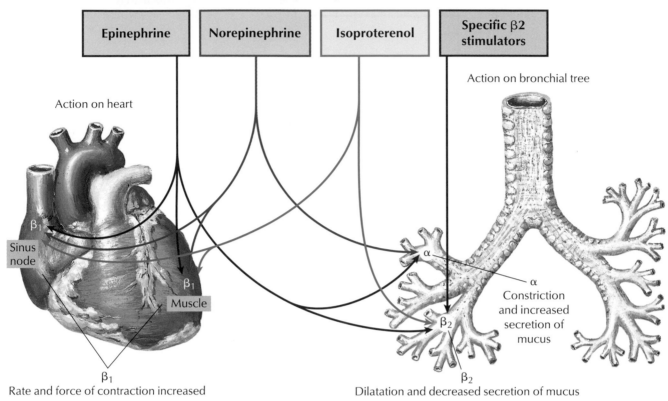

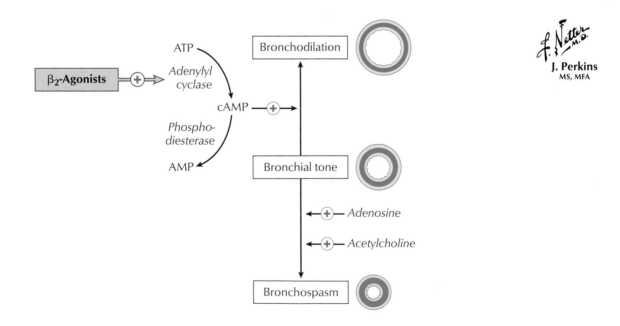

FIGURE 7-14 β-ADRENERGIC AGONISTS

Another class of drugs that enhance sympathetic discharge, β-adrenergic agonists, is used to relieve a sudden asthma attack or block exercise-induced asthma. These drugs relax bronchial smooth muscle, inhibit mediator release, increase transport of mucus, and alter composition of mucus by stimulating β adrenoceptors. Bronchodilation is mediated by β_2 adrenoceptors that are located on smooth muscle cells in human airways.

Nonselective β-adrenoceptor agonists (eg, epinephrine, ephedrine, isoproterenol) stimulate all β adrenoceptors (β_1 and β_2 classes). These nonselective actions often produce adverse effects, particularly in the CNS and cardiovascular system. Selective drugs that activate only β_2 receptors (eg, albuterol, terbutaline, salmeterol) are the most commonly prescribed sympathomimetic agents.

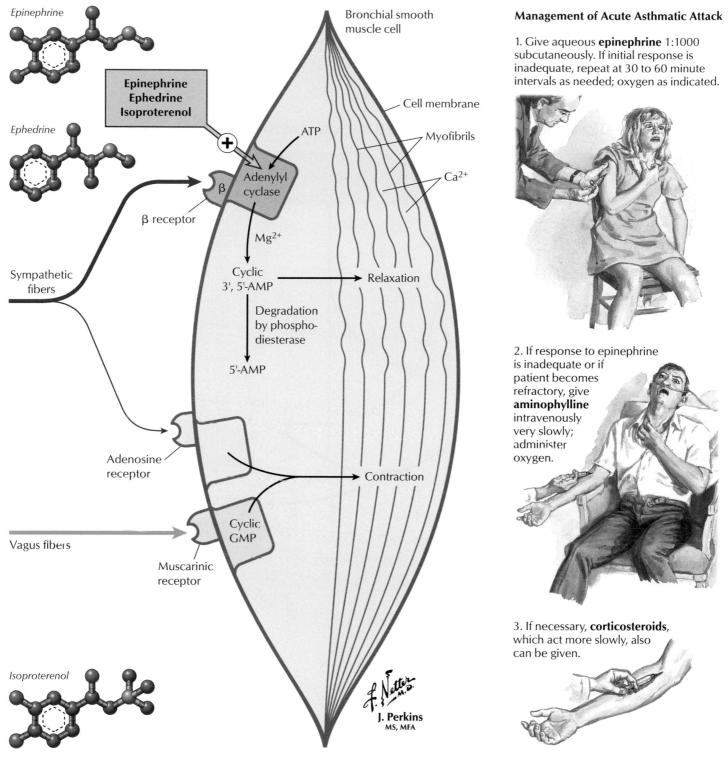

Epinephrine

Ephedrine

**Epinephrine
Ephedrine
Isoproterenol**

Isoproterenol

Bronchial smooth
muscle cell

ATP

Cell membrane

Myofibrils

Ca²⁺

β

Adenylyl
cyclase

β receptor

Sympathetic
fibers

Mg²⁺

Cyclic
3', 5'-AMP

Relaxation

Degradation
by phospho-
diesterase

5'-AMP

Adenosine
receptor

Contraction

Cyclic
GMP

Vagus fibers

Muscarinic
receptor

J. Netter M.D.

J. Perkins
MS, MFA

Management of Acute Asthmatic Attack

1. Give aqueous **epinephrine** 1:1000
subcutaneously. If initial response is
inadequate, repeat at 30 to 60 minute
intervals as needed; oxygen as indicated.

2. If response to epinephrine
is inadequate or if
patient becomes
refractory, give
aminophylline
intravenously
very slowly;
administer
oxygen.

3. If necessary, **corticosteroids**,
which act more slowly, also
can be given.

FIGURE 7-15 NONSELECTIVE β-ADRENERGIC AGONISTS

Agents that activate both β₁ and β₂ adrenoceptors have long
been used to treat asthma. These drugs are potent, rapidly acting
bronchodilators, but their stimulation of the cardiac system is a
serious drawback. The major agents are epinephrine, ephedrine,
and isoproterenol. Epinephrine is either inhaled or given subcutaneously and is the active agent in many over-the-counter preparations. Maximal bronchodilation is achieved 15 minutes after
injection and lasts approximately 90 minutes. Because this drug
stimulates cardiac output, increases heart rate, and exacerbates

angina, physicians rarely prescribe it. Ephedrine, used in China
more than 2000 years ago, has the longest history of use of any
antiasthmatic. It has a longer duration of action, lower potency,
and greater oral activity than epinephrine. However, it has
marked adverse effects, particularly in the CNS, and is rarely
administered. Isoproterenol is characterized by a rapid onset of
action, with peak bronchodilation occurring within 15 minutes
of injection.

Catecholamine Action on α and β Receptors of Heart and Bronchial Tree

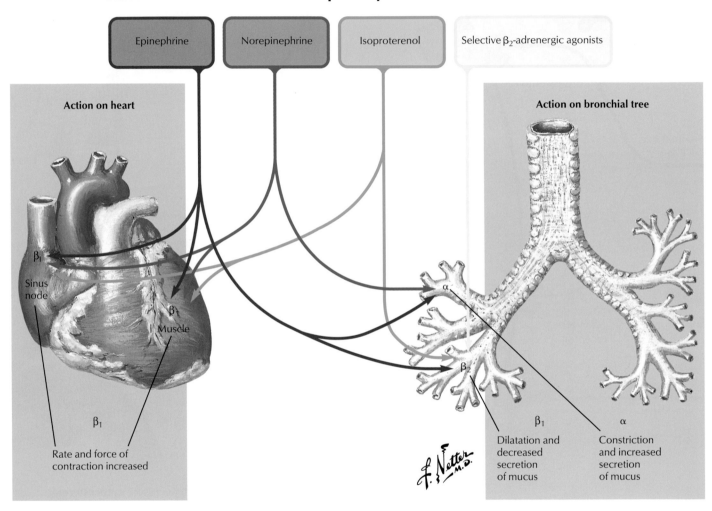

FIGURE 7-16 SELECTIVE β₂-ADRENERGIC AGONISTS

Selective β₂-adrenoceptor activators are the most widely prescribed sympathomimetic drugs because of their β₂ selectivity, oral activity, and rapid onset and long duration of action (4 hours). The major drugs—metaproterenol, terbutaline, albuterol, salmeterol, and formoterol—have minimal β₁-mediated effects on the nervous and cardiac systems. The inhalation route allows the greatest local effects with the fewest adverse effects. Inhaled agents cause bronchodilation that equals that of isoproterenol and persists for 4 hours. Terbutaline, metaproterenol, and albuterol can be given orally as tablets. Terbutaline, the only drug that can be used subcutaneously, is given for severe asthma attacks or if insensitivity to inhaled agents exists. Two new drugs, salmeterol and formoterol, have a long duration of action and high lipid solubility. Both drugs at high concentrations move slowly into airway smooth muscle, so effects can last up to 12 hours. Both also enhance antiasthmatic actions of corticosteroids.

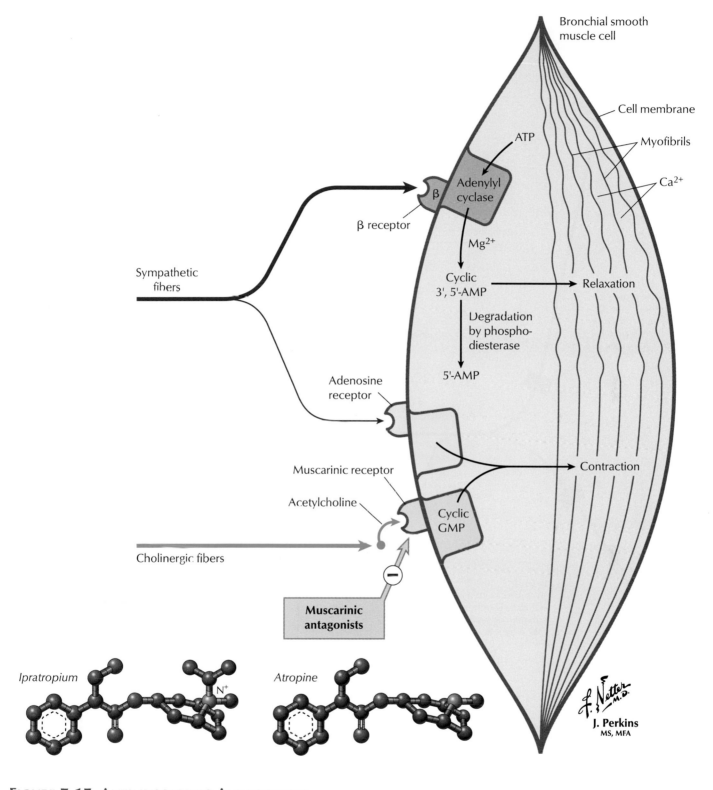

Bronchial smooth
muscle cell

Cell membrane

Myofibrils

Ca^{2+}

ATP

Adenylyl
cyclase

β

β receptor

Mg^{2+}

Cyclic
3', 5'-AMP

Relaxation

Sympathetic
fibers

Degradation
by phospho-
diesterase

5'-AMP

Adenosine
receptor

Muscarinic receptor

Contraction

Acetylcholine

Cyclic
GMP

Cholinergic fibers

−

**Muscarinic
antagonists**

Ipratropium

N^+

Atropine

J. Perkins
MS, MFA

FIGURE 7-17 ANTIMUSCARINIC ANTAGONISTS

Acetylcholine mediates its physiologic effects via 2 types of receptors: muscarinic and cholinergic. Muscarinic receptors are GPCRs that are densely expressed in the airways. When stimulated, muscarinic receptors cause muscle contraction, which leads to narrowing of the airways and bronchoconstriction. Muscarinic antagonists, or anticholinergics, prevent acetylcholine from producing smooth muscle contractions and excess mucus in the bronchi. Ipratropium bromide and atropine are most commonly used. Anticholinergics are less effective than β_2-adrenergic activators. However, these drugs enhance bronchodilation induced by β_2-adrenoceptor agonists, so patients often take both anticholinergics and β_2 agonists. Dry mouth, bitter taste, scratchy throat, and headache are the major adverse effects.

Corticosteroid Actions in Bronchial Asthma

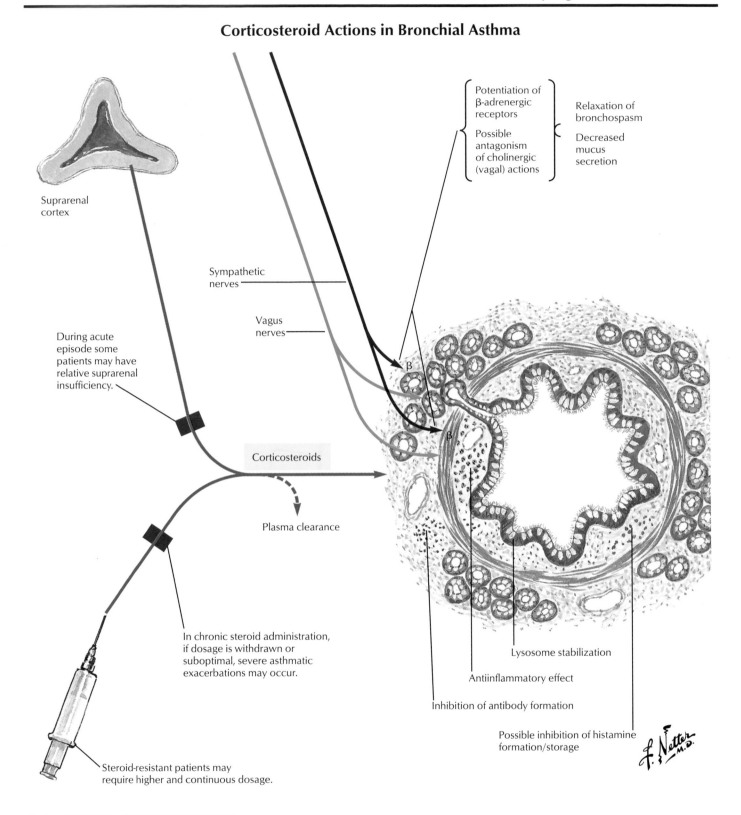

Potentiation of β-adrenergic receptors

Possible antagonism of cholinergic (vagal) actions

Relaxation of bronchospasm

Decreased mucus secretion

Suprarenal cortex

Sympathetic nerves

Vagus nerves

During acute episode some patients may have relative suprarenal insufficiency.

Corticosteroids

Plasma clearance

In chronic steroid administration, if dosage is withdrawn or suboptimal, severe asthmatic exacerbations may occur.

Steroid-resistant patients may require higher and continuous dosage.

Lysosome stabilization

Antiinflammatory effect

Inhibition of antibody formation

Possible inhibition of histamine formation/storage

FIGURE 7-18 CORTICOSTEROIDS

Corticosteroids are antiinflammatory drugs similar to natural corticosteroid hormones produced by the adrenal cortex. Treatment with these agents improves symptoms of asthma, allergic rhinitis, eczema, and rheumatoid arthritis. Corticosteroids inhibit late phase allergic reactions (including late asthmatic response to antigen challenge) by various mechanisms, eg, reduced (1) number of mast cells lining the surfaces of airway mucosal cells; (2) chemotaxis and activation of eosinophils; and (3) cytokine production by eosinophils, monocytes, mast cells, and lymphocytes. Corticosteroids taken regularly reduce bronchial reactivity, enhance airway quality, and decrease the severity and frequency of asthma attacks. However, corticosteroids do not directly relax smooth muscle. These drugs would be the only ones needed to treat asthma if their adverse effects were not so pronounced. Commonly used agents are prednisone, methylprednisone, beclomethasone, flunisolide, budesonide, and mometasone.

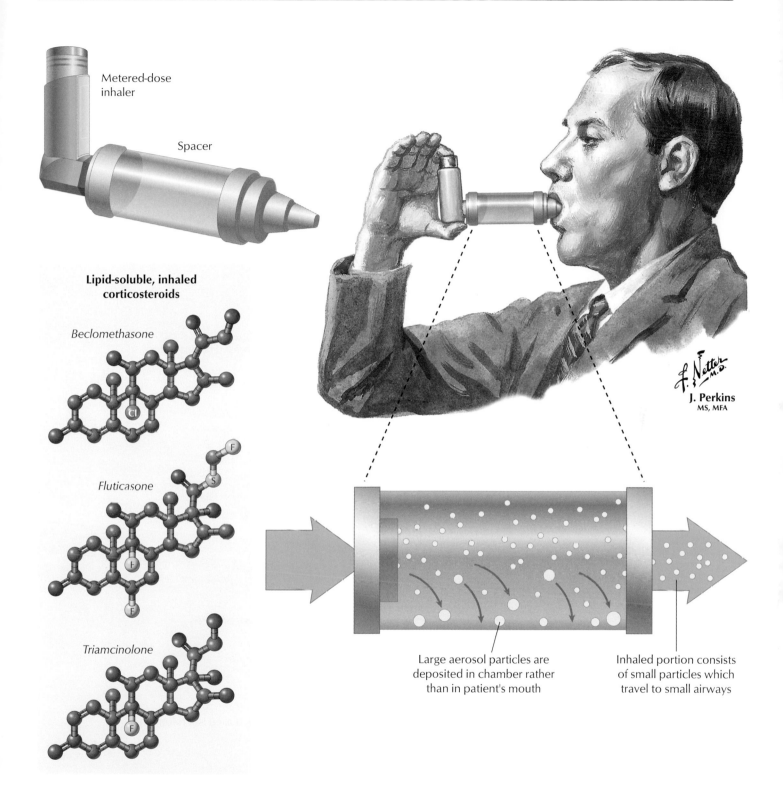

Metered-dose inhaler

Spacer

Lipid-soluble, inhaled corticosteroids

Beclomethasone

Fluticasone

Triamcinolone

J. Perkins
MS, MFA

Large aerosol particles are deposited in chamber rather than in patient's mouth

Inhaled portion consists of small particles which travel to small airways

FIGURE 7-19 CORTICOSTEROIDS: CLINICAL USES

Corticosteroids have marked adverse effects on nonrespiratory systems, so inhalation (maintenance therapy in asthma, via inhaler) or the intranasal (in allergy, as nasal spray) route is preferred. Intranasal corticosteroids relieve stuffy nose, nasal irritation, and other discomforts. Corticosteroids inhaled by mouth effectively prevent asthma attacks. Spacers (chambers) can be attached to metered-dose inhalers to reduce the velocity and particle size of the drug; the amount of drug reaching the lungs is maximized, and the quantity of drug deposited in the mouth is minimized. Spacers are crucial for therapy with corticosteroids, which have many adverse effects. Regular doses of aerosol agents are smaller than doses used in pill form. The smaller, regular doses reduce side effect risk and may eliminate a need for aerosol steroids. Oral prednisone or IV methylprednisone is used only when patients are insensitive to the inhaled drugs or need urgent treatment for severe asthma attacks.

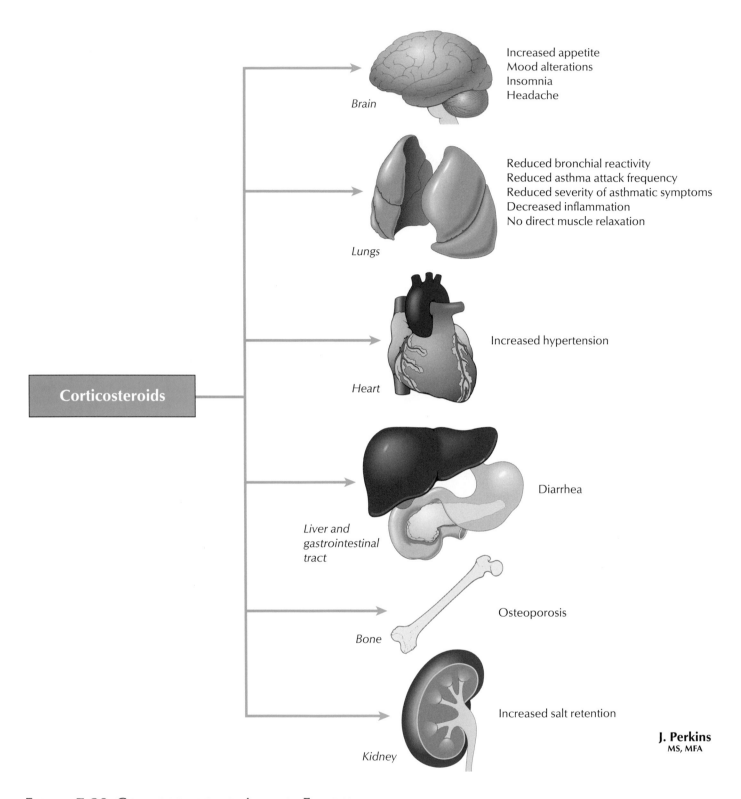

Brain
Increased appetite
Mood alterations
Insomnia
Headache

Lungs
Reduced bronchial reactivity
Reduced asthma attack frequency
Reduced severity of asthmatic symptoms
Decreased inflammation
No direct muscle relaxation

Corticosteroids

Heart
Increased hypertension

Liver and
gastrointestinal
tract
Diarrhea

Bone
Osteoporosis

Kidney
Increased salt retention

J. Perkins
MS, MFA

FIGURE 7-20 CORTICOSTEROIDS: ADVERSE EFFECTS

Taking corticosteroids orally (prednisone) and intravenously (methylprednisone) can cause unwanted side effects. Short-term use (days) of prednisone can lead to increased appetite, weight gain, diarrhea, headache, mood changes, and insomnia, and possibly hyperglycemia and hypertension. Cessation of short-term corticosteroid use or taking smaller doses of these agents usually minimizes or eliminates the effects. Adverse effects that accompany long-term (months to years) oral and IV therapy are suppressed immune system, increased cholesterol levels, and rapid weight gain. Long-term use may also promote osteoporosis, cataracts, and thinning of the skin. Efforts to develop safer corticosteroids with antiinflammatory properties but lacking adverse effects are ongoing. Lipophilic steroids, such as beclomethasone, flunisolide, budesonide, and mometasone, have a strong safety profile and are almost devoid of the orally precipitated systemic effects.

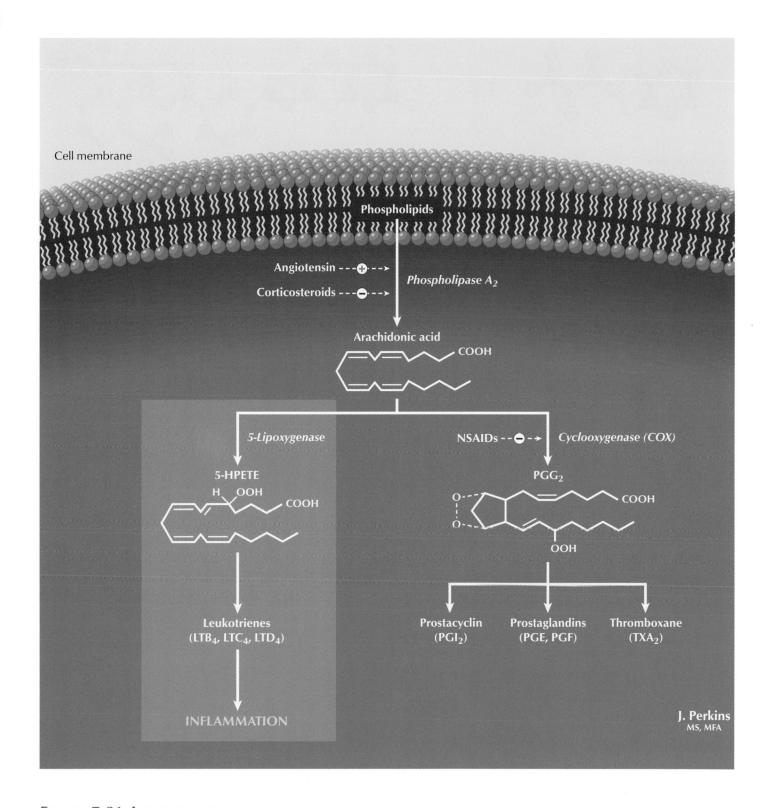

FIGURE 7-21 LEUKOTRIENES

Leukotrienes are arachidonic acid derivatives that are involved in inflammatory processes including asthma and anaphylaxis. The enzyme 5-lipoxygenase catalyzes synthesis of arachidonic acid into unstable intermediates, which are converted into leukotrienes. A number of airway cells (including mast cells, macrophages, eosinophils, and basophils) synthesize, store, and secrete several subtypes of proinflammatory leukotrienes. Leukotriene B_4 (LTB_4) attracts additional leukocytes, and LTC_4 and LTD_4 increase bronchial reactivity, bronchoconstriction, and secretion of mucus. Evidence that inhaled leukotrienes increase bronchial reactivity and that antigen challenge in sensitized airways augments leukotriene synthesis supports a role for these mediators in asthma and a rationale for development of drugs that block leukotriene or 5-lipoxygenase action.

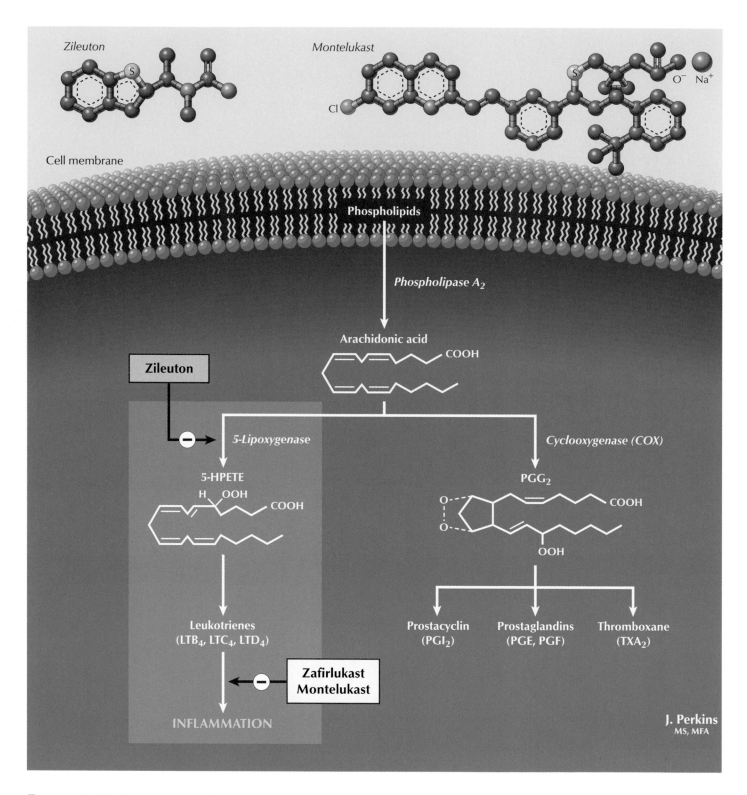

FIGURE 7-22 LEUKOTRIENE ANTAGONISTS

Efforts to develop drugs that disrupt proinflammatory actions of leukotrienes produced 2 types of drugs: 5-lipoxygenase inhibitors and leukotriene antagonists. Zileuton reduces the leukotriene synthesis rate by blocking 5-lipoxygenase. Zafirlukast and montelukast, LTD_4 antagonists, block leukotriene receptors and prevent these mediators from causing an asthmatic response. When taken regularly, these drugs work as well as inhaled corticosteroids in reducing the frequency of asthma attacks. However, leukotriene antagonists are less successful for relieving symptoms, reducing bronchial reactivity, and improving airway quality. These drugs are effective and safe when taken orally, an advantage compared with inhaled corticosteroids. The strong safety profile and excellent oral activity account for the popularity of leukotriene antagonists for children. Leukotriene antagonists also reduce responses in aspirin-induced asthma, a disorder affecting nearly 10% of patients with asthma.

Causes of Chronic Cough

Etiology of Chronic Cough With a Normal Chest Radiograph

Cause	Prevalence
Postnasal drip	28-41%
Asthma	24-33%
GERD	10-21%
Chronic bronchitis Postinfectious (often, viral URI) bronchial hyperresponsiveness	5-10% 10%
Bronchiectasis	4%
ACE inhibitors, tracheomalacia, eosinophilic bronchitis, psychogenic, etc	5%

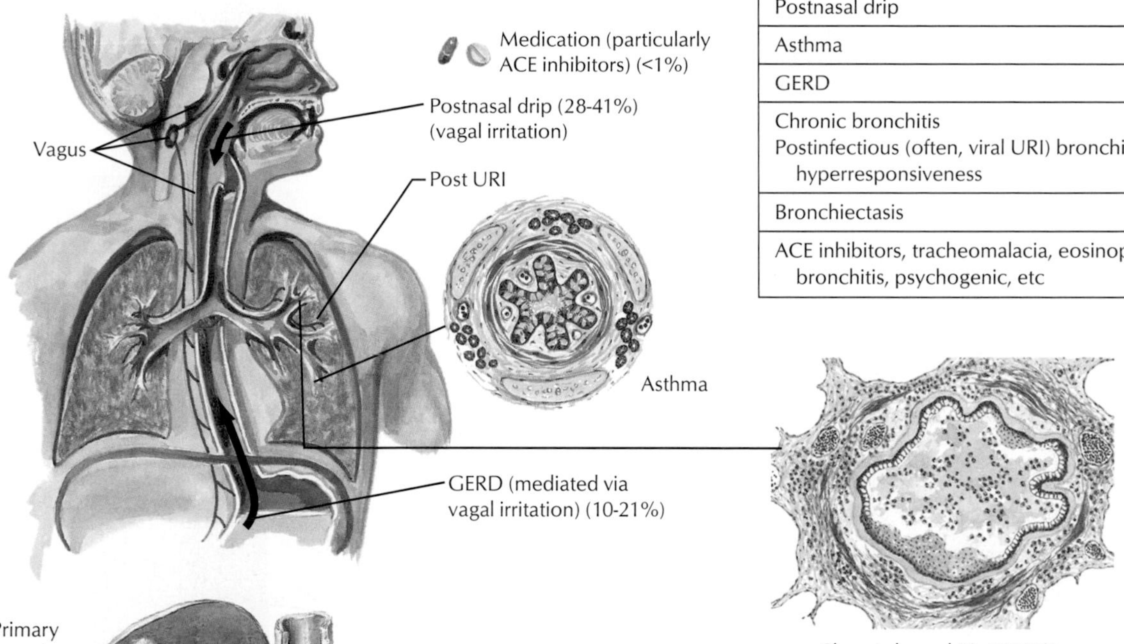

Medication (particularly ACE inhibitors) (<1%)

Postnasal drip (28-41%) (vagal irritation)

Post URI

Vagus

Asthma

GERD (mediated via vagal irritation) (10-21%)

Chronic bronchitis (5-10%)

Causes of Chronic Cough With Abnormal Chest Radiograph

Primary complex

Involved nodes

Pulmonary tuberculosis

Fctatic mucus-filled spaces

Cystic fibrosis and bronchietasis

Dilated air sacks

Carcinoma of lung

L. ventricular hypertrophy and dilation

Left-sided congestive heart failure and pulmonary hypertension

COPD (pulmonary emphysema)

JOHN A. CRAIG—AD
D. Mascaro

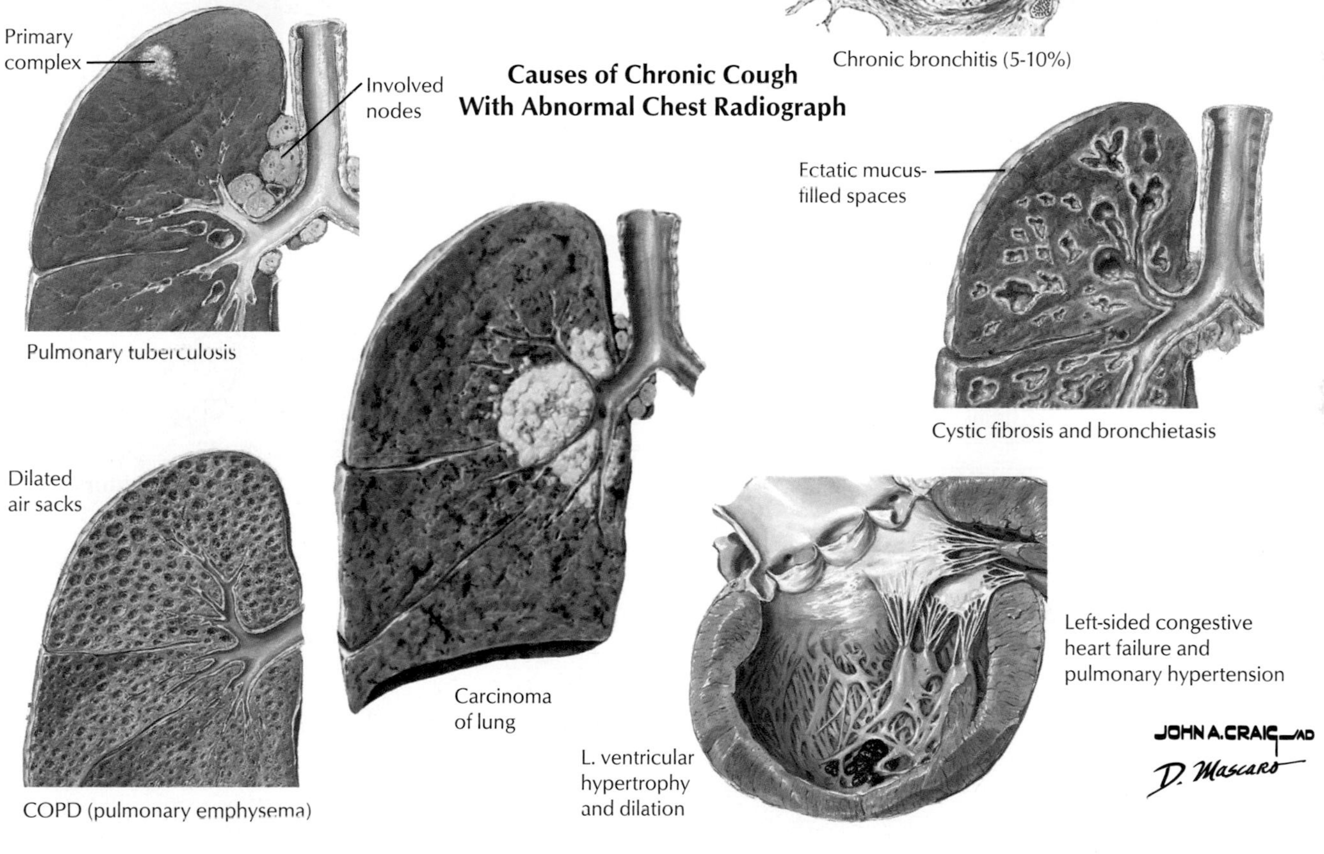

FIGURE 7-23 COUGH

Cough—forceful release of air from lungs—is a sudden, often involuntary reflex and a major defense mechanism. Airway irritation activates the reflex, which forcefully removes irritants, by stimulating the airways, which then activates afferent nerves going from respiratory passages through the vagus nerve to the medulla. Activated cough receptors in the medulla drive a reflex that initiates inspiration (2.5 L of air); increases contraction of diaphragmatic, abdominal, and intercostal (rib) muscles; increases lung pressure; and emits air and irritants (at 100 mph). Coughs triggered by drainage of mucus from nasal passages into airways are treated with cough suppressants (antitussives). Infection-related coughs (eg, in bronchitis) last for approximately 2 weeks. Persistent, chronic coughs (eg, in smokers) must be evaluated. Coughs occurring with blood, chest pain, shortness of breath, weight loss, or dyspnea may indicate serious disease. Coughs in infants may indicate a serious lung disorder.

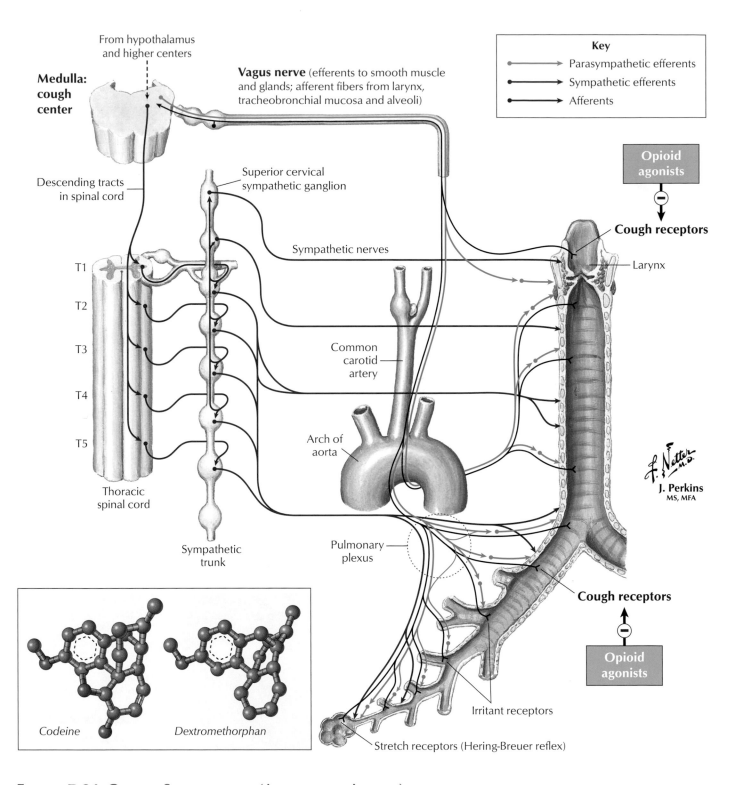

Key
- Parasympathetic efferents
- Sympathetic efferents
- Afferents

From hypothalamus and higher centers

Medulla: cough center

Vagus nerve (efferents to smooth muscle and glands; afferent fibers from larynx, tracheobronchial mucosa and alveoli)

Descending tracts in spinal cord

Superior cervical sympathetic ganglion

Opioid agonists

⊖

Cough receptors

Sympathetic nerves

Larynx

T1

T2

T3

T4

T5

Common carotid artery

Thoracic spinal cord

Arch of aorta

Sympathetic trunk

Pulmonary plexus

Cough receptors

⊖

Opioid agonists

Irritant receptors

Codeine   *Dextromethorphan*

Stretch receptors (Hering-Breuer reflex)

J. Perkins
MS, MFA

FIGURE 7-24 COUGH SUPPRESSANTS (ANTITUSSIVE AGENTS)

Cough suppressants are opioids that reduce the sensitivity of central cough receptors to peripherally activated afferents. Receptor desensitization disrupts the reflex and minimizes coughing. Opioids include opiates (morphine and drugs derived from the opium poppy plant, such as hydromorphone, hydrocodone, and codeine) and synthetic drugs that mimic effects of morphine. Opioids desensitize central cough receptors, reduce airway mucous secretion, and alter mucous composition. These drugs also produce many adverse effects, including analgesia,

addiction, sedation, euphoria, respiratory depression, nausea, vomiting, and constipation. The doses of opioids needed to suppress cough are lower than doses that evoke most of the undesirable effects, particularly analgesia and addiction. Dextromethorphan, a morphine derivative and glutamate antagonist, suppresses the cough center and has fewer adverse effects than other opioids, which accounts for its popularity in over-the-counter preparations.

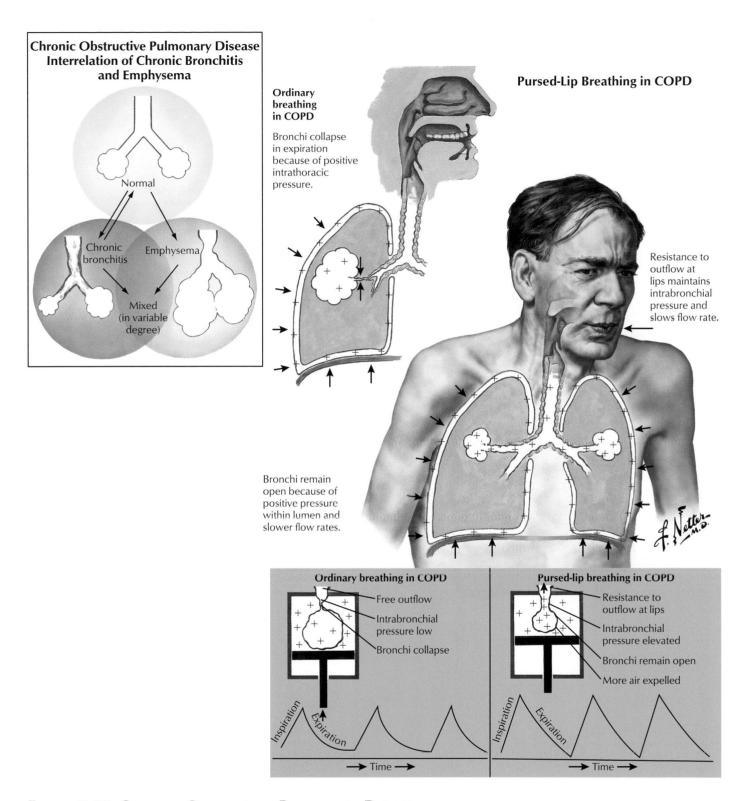

Chronic Obstructive Pulmonary Disease Interrelation of Chronic Bronchitis and Emphysema

Normal

Chronic bronchitis

Emphysema

Mixed (in variable degree)

Ordinary breathing in COPD

Bronchi collapse in expiration because of positive intrathoracic pressure.

Pursed-Lip Breathing in COPD

Resistance to outflow at lips maintains intrabronchial pressure and slows flow rate.

Bronchi remain open because of positive pressure within lumen and slower flow rates.

Ordinary breathing in COPD

Free outflow
Intrabronchial pressure low
Bronchi collapse

Inspiration
Expiration
→ Time →

Pursed-lip breathing in COPD

Resistance to outflow at lips
Intrabronchial pressure elevated
Bronchi remain open
More air expelled

Inspiration
Expiration
→ Time →

FIGURE 7-25 CHRONIC OBSTRUCTIVE PULMONARY DISEASE

Chronic obstructive pulmonary disease, the term used to describe airflow obstruction, encompasses emphysema and chronic bronchitis. Long-term smoking is the most frequent cause of COPD and accounts for approximately 90% of all cases. Heredity, secondhand smoke, exposure to air pollution, and history of childhood respiratory infections are also major risk factors. COPD symptoms are chronic cough, chest tightness, shortness of breath, and increased production of mucus. Emphysema causes irreversible lung damage by weakening and destroying air sacs within the lungs, which reduces lung elasticity and causes airway collapse and obstruction. *Chronic bronchitis* is an inflammatory disease that begins in smaller lung airways and advances gradually to larger airways. Increased mucus in the airways and more frequent bacterial infections in the bronchia result, which, in turn, impedes airflow. Ipratropium, theophylline, and albuterol are among drugs used for treatment.

231

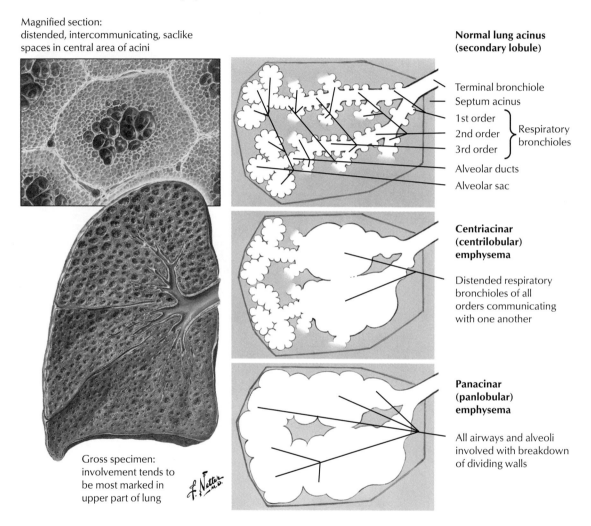

Centriacinar (centrilobular) emphysema

Magnified section:
distended, intercommunicating, saclike
spaces in central area of acini

**Normal lung acinus
(secondary lobule)**

Terminal bronchiole
Septum acinus
1st order
2nd order } Respiratory bronchioles
3rd order
Alveolar ducts
Alveolar sac

**Centriacinar
(centrilobular)
emphysema**

Distended respiratory
bronchioles of all
orders communicating
with one another

**Panacinar
(panlobular)
emphysema**

All airways and alveoli
involved with breakdown
of dividing walls

Gross specimen:
involvement tends to
be most marked in
upper part of lung

FIGURE 7-26 EMPHYSEMA

Emphysema is a condition in which structures in alveoli are overinflated. The lungs loose elasticity and cannot fully expand and contract. Patients can inhale, but exhalation is difficult and inefficient. Emphysema in children is usually caused by congenital abnormalities of the lung and α_1-antitrypsin deficiency. Although emphysema ranks ninth among chronic conditions that reduce activity, the seriousness of the disease varies. Some persons never reach a stage of incapacity and live with relatively little inconvenience. In others, the disease worsens until breathing becomes impossible. Shortness of breath, chronic cough, cyanosis (bluish coloration of skin caused by lack of oxygen), and exertion-induced wheezing are the most common symptoms. Dizziness, anxiety, stress, impotence, fatigue, impaired ability to concentrate, excessive daytime sleepiness, and insomnia may also occur.

Effect of Emphysema on Compliance and Diffusing Capacity (DL_{CO})

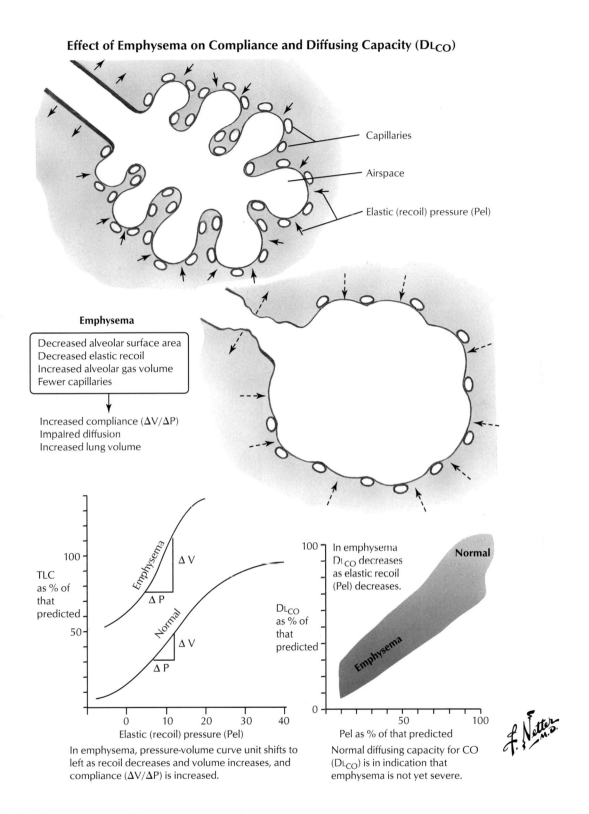

Capillaries

Airspace

Elastic (recoil) pressure (Pel)

Emphysema

Decreased alveolar surface area
Decreased elastic recoil
Increased alveolar gas volume
Fewer capillaries

Increased compliance (ΔV/ΔP)
Impaired diffusion
Increased lung volume

TLC as % of that predicted

Emphysema

ΔV

ΔP

Normal

ΔV

ΔP

100

50

0   10   20   30   40
Elastic (recoil) pressure (Pel)

In emphysema, pressure-volume curve unit shifts to left as recoil decreases and volume increases, and compliance (ΔV/ΔP) is increased.

In emphysema Dl_{CO} decreases as elastic recoil (Pel) decreases.

100

DL_{CO} as % of that predicted

Normal

Emphysema

0
50   100
Pel as % of that predicted

Normal diffusing capacity for CO (DL_{CO}) is in indication that emphysema is not yet severe.

F. Netter M.D.

FIGURE 7-27 EMPHYSEMA: CAUSES

The primary cause of emphysema is cigarette smoking. Tobacco smoke and other pollutants promote release of chemicals within alveoli that damage the walls of air sacs. The alveoli play a critical role in respiration because they facilitate exchange of oxygen from the air for carbon dioxide in the blood. Gases diffuse easily through the thin and fragile alveolar walls. Damage to air sac walls is irreversible and results in permanent holes in tissues of the lower lungs. The lungs can thus transfer less oxygen to the bloodstream, which causes shortness of breath. Lungs also lose elasticity, and the patient exhales with great difficulty. Emphysema does not develop suddenly; it occurs after years of exposure to cigarette smoke, air pollution, and irritating fumes.

Hypothesis of the Role of α_1 Antitrypsin

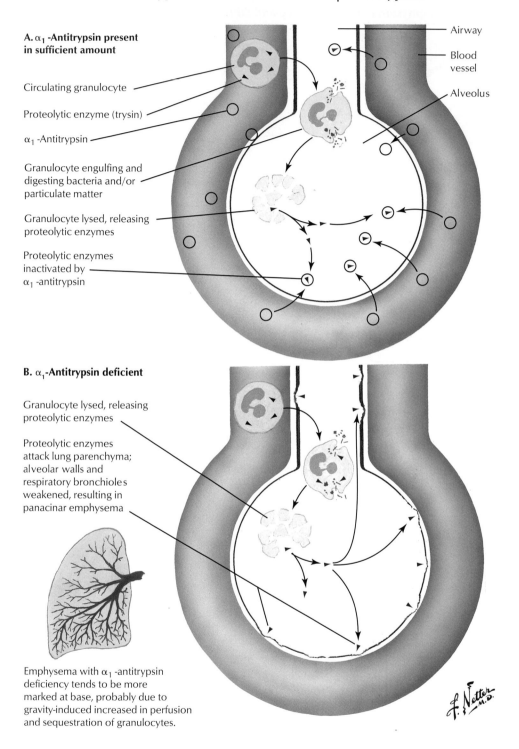

A. α_1-Antitrypsin present in sufficient amount

Circulating granulocyte

Proteolytic enzyme (trysin)

α_1-Antitrypsin

Granulocyte engulfing and digesting bacteria and/or particulate matter

Granulocyte lysed, releasing proteolytic enzymes

Proteolytic enzymes inactivated by α_1-antitrypsin

Airway

Blood vessel

Alveolus

B. α_1-Antitrypsin deficient

Granulocyte lysed, releasing proteolytic enzymes

Proteolytic enzymes attack lung parenchyma; alveolar walls and respiratory bronchioles weakened, resulting in panacinar emphysema

Emphysema with α_1-antitrypsin deficiency tends to be more marked at base, probably due to gravity-induced increased in perfusion and sequestration of granulocytes.

FIGURE 7-28 INHERITED EMPHYSEMA

Inherited emphysema involves deficiency of α_1-antitrypsin, a major blood protein of many genetic variations, only a few of which cause lung disease. This protein is produced by hepatic cells and protects lungs by blocking effects of enzymes called *elastases*. Elastases, carried in leukocytes, protect lungs by killing inhaled bacteria and removing tiny particles. α_1-Antitrypsin blocks elastase action after protective enzymatic work ends. Elastases destroy air sacs of lungs in people who lack α_1-antitrypsin.

Intravenous α_1-proteinase inhibitor, a novel therapy for this deficiency, replaces α_1-antitrypsin in the blood. Symptoms of inherited emphysema are also managed by exercise, avoiding infection, oxygen therapy, and pulmonary rehabilitation. Smoking accelerates progression of the disease and shortens lifespan, so avoiding cigarettes and secondhand smoke is critical. Lung transplantation and lung reduction surgery are options for patients with serious effects of α_1-antitrypsin deficiency.

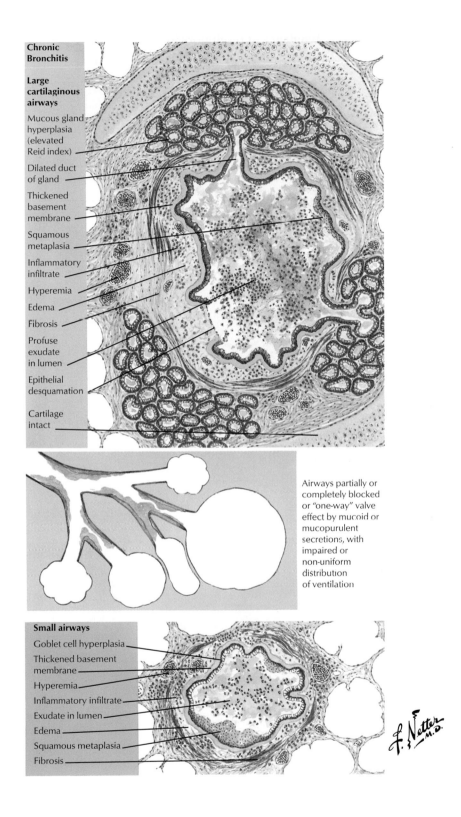

Chronic Bronchitis

Large cartilaginous airways

- Mucous gland hyperplasia (elevated Reid index)
- Dilated duct of gland
- Thickened basement membrane
- Squamous metaplasia
- Inflammatory infiltrate
- Hyperemia
- Edema
- Fibrosis
- Profuse exudate in lumen
- Epithelial desquamation
- Cartilage intact

Airways partially or completely blocked or "one-way" valve effect by mucoid or mucopurulent secretions, with impaired or non-uniform distribution of ventilation

Small airways
- Goblet cell hyperplasia
- Thickened basement membrane
- Hyperemia
- Inflammatory infiltrate
- Exudate in lumen
- Edema
- Squamous metaplasia
- Fibrosis

FIGURE 7-29 CHRONIC BRONCHITIS

Bronchi are air passages that connect the trachea, or windpipe, with alveoli. *Bronchitis* is inflammation of the bronchi causing excessive production of mucus and swelling of bronchial walls. Many people with a severe cold experience a brief attack of acute bronchitis, which is usually accompanied by fever, cough, wheezing, and spitting. The term *chronic bronchitis* is applied when these symptoms persist for months. Also, in chronic bronchitis, the episodes recur and generally last longer each time. Obstruction to airflow in air passages caused by swelling of the bronchial wall and the presence of mucus that cannot be cleared eventually produces shortness of breath after mild exertion. Chest infections are more prevalent in patients with chronic bronchitis.

A. Avoidance of respiratory irritants

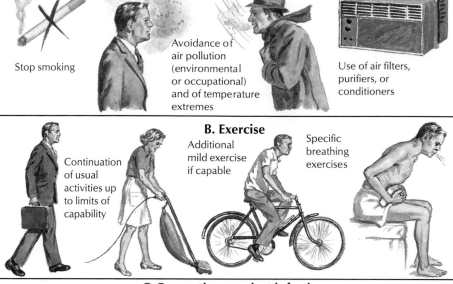

Stop smoking

Avoidance of air pollution (environmental or occupational) and of temperature extremes

Use of air filters, purifiers, or conditioners

B. Exercise

Continuation of usual activities up to limits of capability

Additional mild exercise if capable

Specific breathing exercises

C. Precautions against infection

Avoidance of crowds and persons with respiratory infections; use of influenza and pneumococcal vaccine important

Prompt treatment of respiratory infections with antibiotics, bed rest, and other indicated measures

D. Adequate hydration
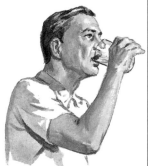

At least 3 L/24 h

E. Adequate nutrition
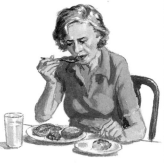

Frequent small meals, bedtime snacks, etc

F. Practice of pursed-lip breathing
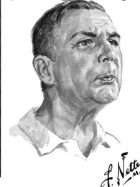

FIGURE 7-30 COPD: GENERAL TREATMENT MEASURES

Various treatments are available for people with severe COPD (ie, chronic bronchitis and emphysema). Traditional management has involved medicines, inhalers, cessation of smoking, regular exercise, and oxygen therapy. Exercise is particularly crucial and should be continued to the point of exertion and shortness of breath. Breathing exercises, along with regular physical activity, are also used to strengthen respiratory muscles. Medicines may provide some relief but rarely have a major impact on physical limitations brought on by COPD. Such drugs include antibiotics for bacterial infections, oral medications, bronchodilators, and other inhaled medications. Oxygen supplementation from portable containers, lung reduction surgery to remove damaged lung tissue, and lung transplantation are used in extreme cases of COPD.

Specific Measures in Management of Chronic Obstructive Pulmonary Disease

A. Bronchodilator therapy

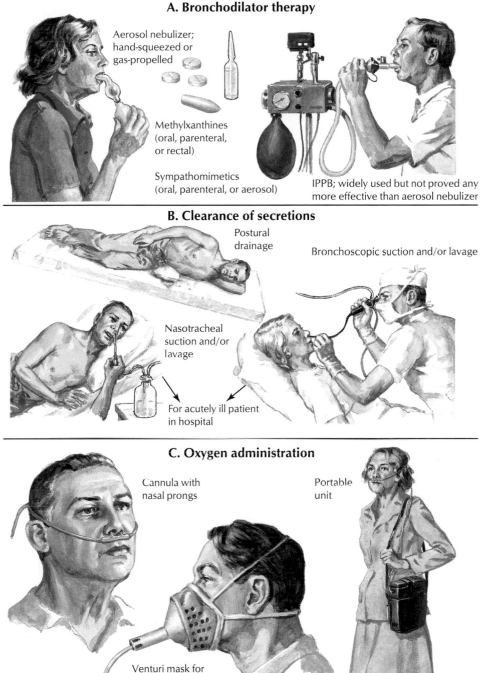

Aerosol nebulizer; hand-squeezed or gas-propelled

Methylxanthines (oral, parenteral, or rectal)

Sympathomimetics (oral, parenteral, or aerosol)

IPPB; widely used but not proved any more effective than aerosol nebulizer

B. Clearance of secretions

Postural drainage

Bronchoscopic suction and/or lavage

Nasotracheal suction and/or lavage

For acutely ill patient in hospital

C. Oxygen administration

Cannula with nasal prongs

Portable unit

Venturi mask for acutely ill patient in hospital

FIGURE 7-31 COPD: SPECIFIC DRUG TREATMENTS

Specific medications prescribed for people with COPD are short-acting β_2 agonists (eg, albuterol), anticholinergic bronchodilators (eg, ipratropium), and long-acting bronchodilators (eg, salmeterol), which all help to open narrowed airways. Corticosteroids that are inhaled or taken orally minimize inflammation. The role of the antiinflammatory medications is not well defined, and, although clinical trials are ongoing, these agents are not approved in the United States for treatment of COPD. Oxygen is given in cases of acute COPD (severe hypoxemia). Antibiotics are often given at the first sign of respiratory infection to prevent further damage of diseased lungs. Finally, expectorants, which help to loosen and expel mucus from the airways, can facilitate respiration. Adverse effects of bronchodilators and corticosteroids can include arrhythmias, cough, steroid myopathy, osteopenia, and cataracts.

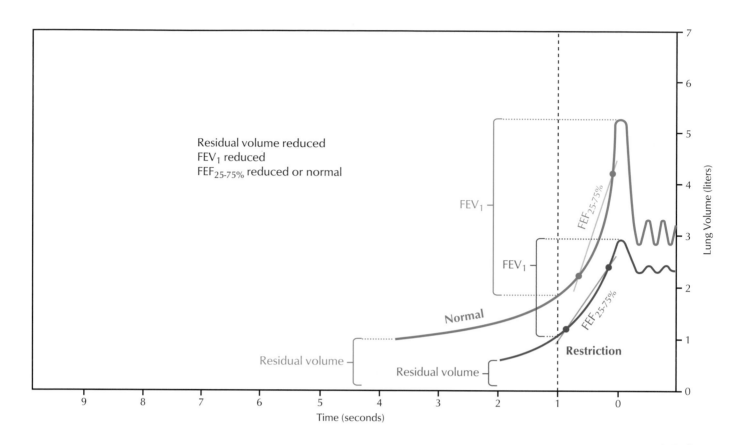

Residual volume reduced
FEV$_1$ reduced
FEF$_{25-75\%}$ reduced or normal

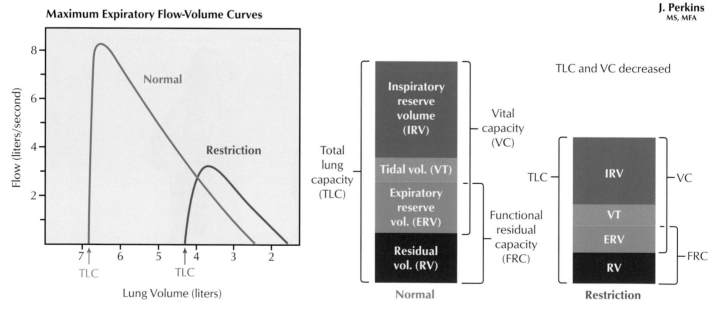

FIGURE 7-32 RESTRICTIVE PULMONARY DISEASE

Restrictive lung disease reduces the amount of inhaled air because of decreased elasticity or amount of lung tissue. Reduced lung volume results from altered lung parenchyma or disease of the pleura, chest wall, or neuromuscular apparatus. Lower total lung capacity, vital capacity, or resting lung volume often occurs. These disorders are classified on the basis of anatomical structure: (1) Intrinsic lung diseases, or diseases of lung parenchyma, cause inflammation or scarring of lung tissue or result in filling of airspaces with debris (pneumonitis). These diseases are idiopathic fibrotic, connective tissue, drug-induced lung, and primary lung diseases (eg, sarcoidosis). (2) Extrinsic, or extraparenchymal, diseases affect chest wall, pleura, and respiratory muscles (respiratory pump components), with resultant lung restriction, impaired ventilatory function, and respiratory failure. Corticosteroids, immunosuppressants, and cytotoxic agents are major drugs for restrictive lung disease.

Pneumococcal Pneumonia

A. Lobar pneumonia; r. upper lobe. Mixed red and gray hepatization (transition stage); pleural fibrinous exudate

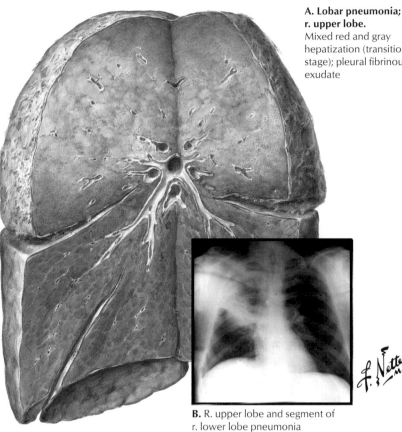

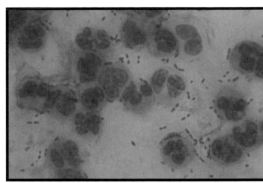

C. Purulent sputum with pneumococci (Gram stain)

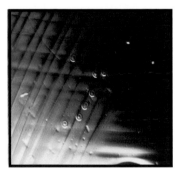

D. Colonies of pneumococci growing on agar plate

B. R. upper lobe and segment of r. lower lobe pneumonia

E. Pathologic changes in zones of the pneumonic lesion

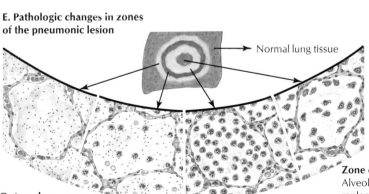

Normal lung tissue

Zone of resolution
Alveolar macrophages replace leukocytes

Outer edema zone
Alveoli filled with edema fluid containing pneumococci

Zone of early consolidation
Polymorphonuclear and some red cell exudation

Zone of advanced consolidation
Intense polymorphonuclear outpouring; pneumococci phagocytized and destroyed

Septic arthritis

Intravascular coagulopathy (in asplenic patient)

Purulent pericarditis

Endocarditis

Empyema

Sterile pleural effusion

F. Complications of pneumococcal pneumonia

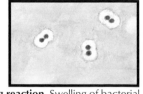

G. Quellung reaction. Swelling of bacterial capsule when exposed to antibody

FIGURE 7-33 PNEUMONIA

Pneumonia is inflammation of the lung, with consolidation of the diseased part and alveolar air spaces filled with exudate, inflammatory cells, and fibrin. Most cases result from infection caused by various microorganisms, including viruses, bacteria (eg, *Streptococcus pneumoniae*), and parasites. Pneumonia often begins after an upper respiratory tract infection, with infections of the nose and throat being the most common culprits. Symptoms vary and depend on the patient's age and the cause of the

Infectious Agents Causing Pneumonia

Class	Etiologic Agent	Type of Pneumonia
Bacteria	*Streptococcus pneumoniae* *Streptococcus pyogenes* *Staphylococcus aureus* *Klebsiella pneumoniae* *Pseudomonas aeruginosa* *Escherichia coli* *Yersinia pestis* *Legionnaires bacillus* *Peptostreptococcus, Peptococcus* *Bacteroides* *Fusobacterium* *Veillonella*	Bacterial pneumonias Legionnaires disease Aspiration (anaerobic) pneumonia
Actinomycetes	*Actinomyces israelii* *Nocardia asteroides*	Pulmonary actinomycosis Pulmonary nocardiosis
Fungi	*Coccidioides immitis* *Histoplasma capsulatum* *Blastomyces dermatitidis* *Aspergillus* *Phycomycetes*	Coccidioidomycosis Histoplasmosis Blastomycosis Aspergillosis Mucormycosis
Rickettsia	*Coxiella burnetii*	Q fever
Chlamydia	*Chlamydia psittaci*	Psittacosis Ornithosis
Mycoplasma	*Mycoplasma pneumoniae*	Mycoplasmal pneumonia
Viruses	Influenza virus, adenovirus, respiratory syncytial virus, etc	Viral pneumonia
Protozoa	*Pneumocystis carinii*	*Pneumocystis* pneumonia (plasma cell pneumonia)

FIGURE 7-33 PNEUMONIA (continued) ─────────────────────

infection. The symptoms, which begin after 2 or 3 days of a cold or sore throat, include fever, chills, cough, rapid ventilation, wheezing, emesis, chest pain, abdominal pain, decreased activity, and loss of appetite. In extreme cases, lips and fingernails may appear bluish or gray, particularly in children. Treatment aims to cure a bacterial infection with antibiotics, which do not attack viruses. It may be hard to distinguish between viral and bacterial pneumonia, so antibiotics may be given.

Influenza Virus and Its Epidemiology

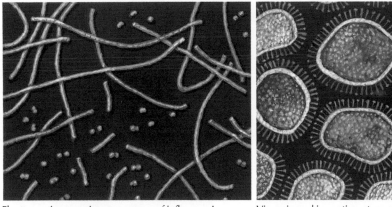

Electron microscopic appearance of influenza A₂ virus; filaments and spherical forms (×10,000)

Virus viewed in section at much higher magnification (×300,000)

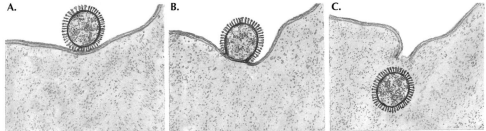

A. **B.** **C.**

Influenza virus invasion of chorioallantoic membrane cell of chick embryo. **A.** Attachment to cell membrane. **B.** Fusion of viral envelope with cell membrane. **C.** Penetration into cell cytoplasm.

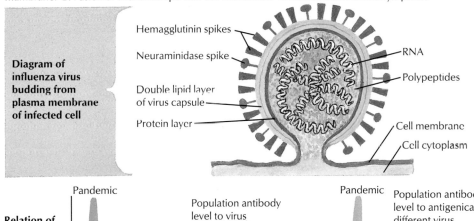

Diagram of influenza virus budding from plasma membrane of infected cell

- Hemagglutinin spikes
- Neuraminidase spike
- Double lipid layer of virus capsule
- Protein layer
- RNA
- Polypeptides
- Cell membrane
- Cell cytoplasm

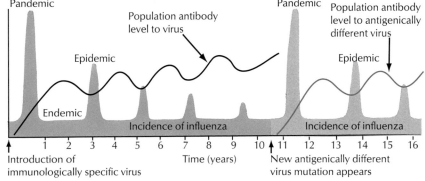

Relation of influenza incidence to population antibody levels*

*Modified after Kilbourne

Pandemic
Population antibody level to virus
Pandemic
Population antibody level to antigenically different virus
Epidemic
Epidemic
Endemic
Incidence of influenza
Incidence of influenza

Introduction of immunologically specific virus
Time (years)
New antigenically different virus mutation appears

Figure 7-34 Viral Pneumonia

Viral pneumonia is an inflammation of the lungs caused by infection with a virus such as influenza or parainfluenza virus, adenovirus, rhinovirus, herpes simplex virus, respiratory syncytial virus, Hantavirus, or cytomegalovirus. Vaccines against influenza virus and respiratory syncytial virus are available for high-risk patients. Antibiotics are ineffective for treating viral pneumonia, but some more serious forms can be treated with antiviral medications (eg, ribavirin). Other supportive care for viral pneumonia

Influenzal Pneumonia

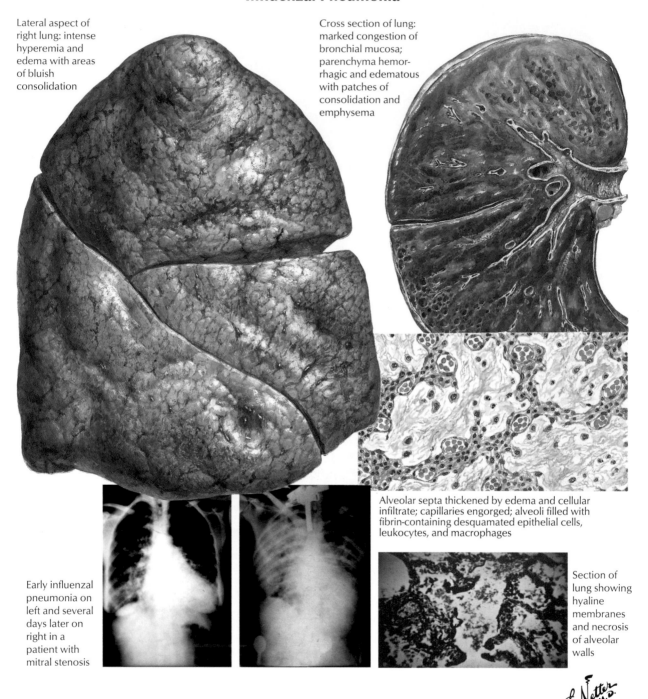

Lateral aspect of right lung: intense hyperemia and edema with areas of bluish consolidation

Cross section of lung: marked congestion of bronchial mucosa; parenchyma hemorrhagic and edematous with patches of consolidation and emphysema

Alveolar septa thickened by edema and cellular infiltrate; capillaries engorged; alveoli filled with fibrin-containing desquamated epithelial cells, leukocytes, and macrophages

Early influenzal pneumonia on left and several days later on right in a patient with mitral stenosis

Section of lung showing hyaline membranes and necrosis of alveolar walls

FIGURE 7-34 VIRAL PNEUMONIA (continued)

includes use of humidified air, increased fluids, and oxygen. Most episodes of viral pneumonia improve without treatment within 1 to 3 weeks, but some last longer and cause more serious symptoms that require hospital stays. Serious infections can cause respiratory failure, liver failure, and heart failure.

Staphylococcal Pneumonia

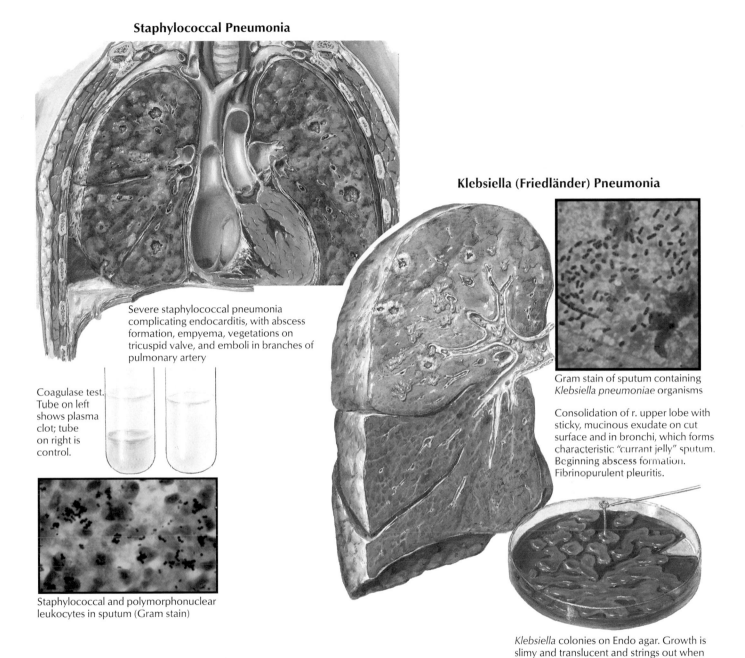

Severe staphylococcal pneumonia complicating endocarditis, with abscess formation, empyema, vegetations on tricuspid valve, and emboli in branches of pulmonary artery

Coagulase test. Tube on left shows plasma clot; tube on right is control.

Staphylococcal and polymorphonuclear leukocytes in sputum (Gram stain)

Klebsiella (Friedländer) Pneumonia

Gram stain of sputum containing *Klebsiella pneumoniae* organisms

Consolidation of r. upper lobe with sticky, mucinous exudate on cut surface and in bronchi, which forms characteristic "currant jelly" sputum. Beginning abscess formation. Fibrinopurulent pleuritis.

Klebsiella colonies on Endo agar. Growth is slimy and translucent and strings out when drawn up on a loop.

FIGURE 7-35 BACTERIAL PNEUMONIA

Bacterial pneumonia, an infection that causes lung irritation, swelling, and congestion, occurs most often in winter. It usually follows a cold and starts suddenly with fever and chills. Painful breathing and a cough with bloody or yellow sputum are common; other signs are rapid breathing, tiredness, abdominal pain, and blue lips. Antibiotics and a humidifier (to loosen sputum and facilitate expectoration) are common remedies. Most cases of infectious pneumonia are caused by bacteria, and nearly 70%

these cases are due to *S pneumoniae*. These bacteria cause disease when they move to the lower respiratory tract in susceptible individuals. Pneumococci are spread by droplets or direct contact with an infected person. The incubation period is 1 to 3 days. Therapy with penicillin or erythromycin makes the patient noninfective and usually leads to rapid recovery. Vaccines for pneumococcal pneumonia are available for patients at highest risk of fatal infection (eg, those older than 65 years).

CHAPTER 8

DRUGS USED IN DISORDERS OF THE REPRODUCTIVE SYSTEM

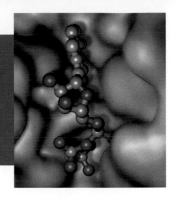

OVERVIEW

Sex hormones include androgens, progestins, and estrogens. They are produced by the gonads and the adrenal glands and are necessary for conception, embryonic maturation, and development of primary and secondary sexual characteristics during puberty. These hormones are used therapeutically as contraceptives, as therapy for postmenopausal complications and breast cancer, and as replacement therapy in hypogonadism.

Combination oral contraceptives (COCs) are effective in blocking ovulation in approximately 98% of patients and come in many different formulations. Ethinyl estradiol and mestranol are the commonly used estrogens; desogestrel and norgestimate are commonly used progestins. Also used for contraception are progestin-only formulations to inhibit or delay ovulation and emergency preparations such as mifepristone (RU-486), given along with misoprostol, for medical termination of intrauterine pregnancy. Although COCs do have adverse effects, they are associated with benefits unrelated to contraception, such as a reduced risk of ovarian cysts, and can also ameliorate other menstrual and reproductive system abnormalities, acne, and hirsutism. Their ability to induce neoplasms is controversial.

The doses of estrogen used in hormone replacement therapy (HRT) for treatment of postmenopausal symptoms including vasomotor manifestations, genitourinary atrophy, and osteoporosis are substantially less than those used in oral contraceptives (OCs). The risks and benefits of estrogen in postmenopausal women with regard to cardioprotection, neuroprotection, and carcinogenicity have been a subject of much debate and are the focus of considerable research efforts.

Certain hormonelike drugs whose estrogenic activities are tissue selective (the selective estrogen receptor modulators, or SERMs) have different therapeutic uses, including prevention and treatment of breast cancer (tamoxifen) and osteoporosis (raloxifene).

Infertility associated with anovulatory menstrual cycles can be treated by use of antiestrogens such as clomiphene.

In female patients with failure of ovarian development, therapy with estrogen, usually in combination with progestin, replicates most of the events of puberty. Testosterone replacement therapy is used for male patients with hypogonadism.

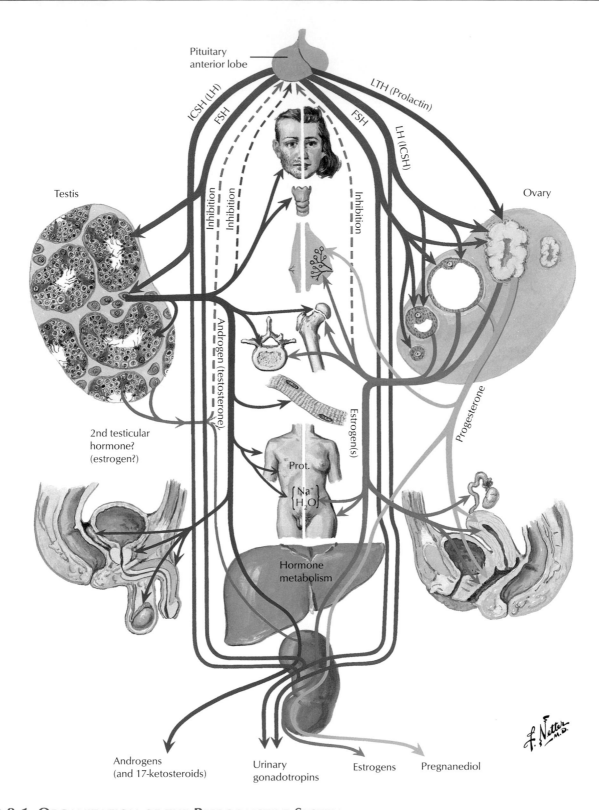

FIGURE 8-1 ORGANIZATION OF THE REPRODUCTIVE SYSTEM

Sex hormones include progestins, estrogens, and androgens. They are produced by the gonads and adrenal glands and are necessary for conception, embryonic maturation, and development of primary and secondary sexual characteristics. As one example of these functional gonadal relations, the menstrual cycle is controlled by a neuroendocrine cascade involving the hypothalamus, pituitary, and ovaries. For control of this cycle, the hypothalamus releases gonadotropin-releasing hormone (GnRH), which triggers the anterior pituitary to release the gonadotropins luteinizing hormone (LH) and follicle-stimulating hormone (FSH), with effects on the ovaries. Androgens are steroids with anabolic and masculinizing effects in both males and females. Testosterone, the main androgen in humans, is synthesized and secreted primarily by testicular Leydig cells, as well as by ovaries in women and by adrenal glands. Testosterone secretion is also controlled by the hypothalamus-pituitary cascade.

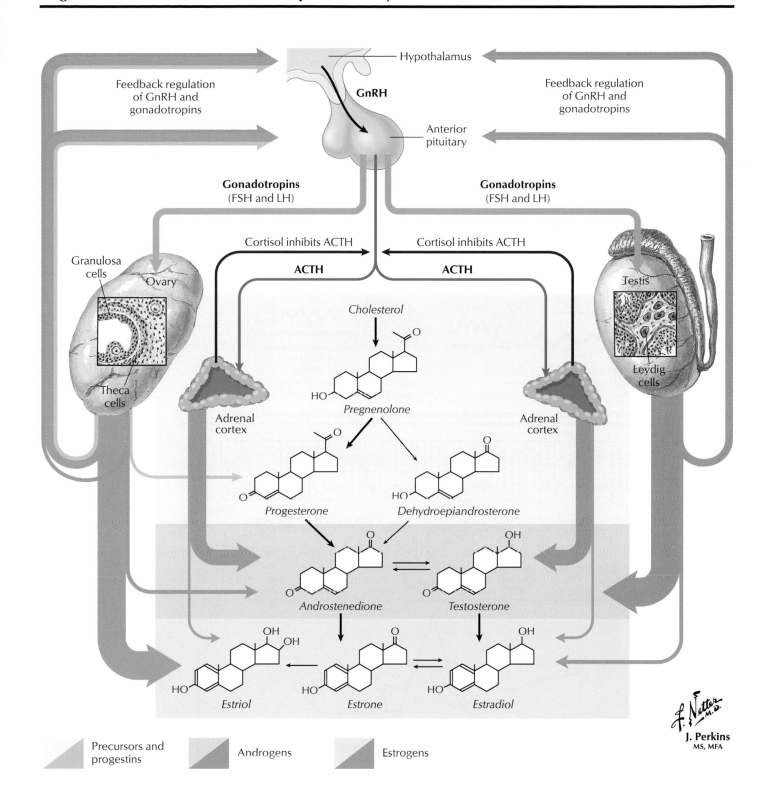

FIGURE 8-2 REGULATION OF ESTROGEN AND TESTOSTERONE

Estrogen is synthesized in several forms, estradiol being the most potent and estrone and estriol having one tenth its potency. Many organs and processes in women are under the influence of estrogen, but the menstrual cycle shows its greatest effects. For control of this cycle, the hypothalamus periodically releases GnRH, which triggers the anterior pituitary to release the gonadotropins LH and FSH. LH and FSH, which are responsible for growth and maturation of ovarian follicles, also control ovarian production of estrogen and progesterone, which exert feedback regulation on the pituitary and hypothalamus and signal them when to start and stop releasing GnRH, FSH, and LH. In males, the hypothalamus and anterior pituitary also effect release of FSH (starts spermatogenesis) and LH (triggers steroidogenesis in Leydig cells). The testosterone resulting from steroidogenesis inhibits hormone production via negative feedback on the pituitary and hypothalamus, and release of GnRH, FSH, and LH ends.

Neuroendocrine Regulation of Menstrual Cycle

Hypothalamic regulation of pituitary gonadotrophin production and release

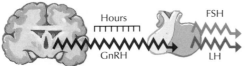

Pulsed release of GnRH by hypothalamus (1 pulse/1-2 hr) permits anterior pituitary production and release of FSH and LH (normal).

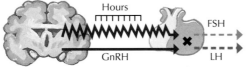

Continuous, excessive, absent, or more frequent GnRH release inhibits FSH and LH production and release (downloading).

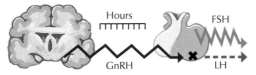

Decreased pulsed release of GnRH decreases LH secretion but increases FSH secretion (slow-pulsing model).

Ovarian feedback modulation of pituitary gonadotropin production and release

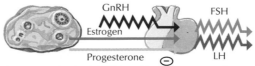

Presence of pulsed GnRH and low estrogen and progesterone levels result in increased levels of pulsed LH and FSH (negative feedback).

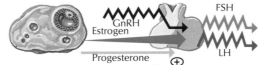

Presence of pulsed GnRH, rapidly increasing levels of estrogen, and small amounts of progesterone result in high pulsed LH and moderately increased pulsed FSH levels (positive feedback).

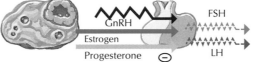

Presence of pulsed GnRH and high levels of estrogen and progesterone result in decreased LH and FSH levels (negative feedback).

Correlation of serum gonadotrophic and ovarian hormone levels and feedback mechanisms

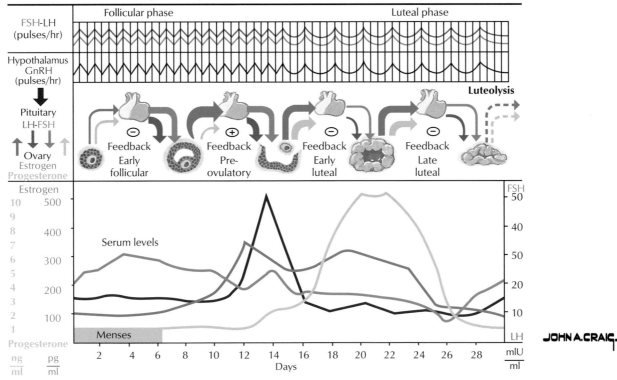

FIGURE 8-3 EVENTS OF THE NORMAL MENSTRUAL CYCLE

In the early (follicular) phase, the hypothalamus releases GnRH, which triggers the anterior pituitary to release LH and FSH. These gonadotropins cause the graafian follicle to mature and secrete estrogen. Estrogen inhibits the pituitary; it reduces the gland's release of LH and FSH (negative feedback loop). In midcycle, however, estrogen triggers a surge in gonadotropin release from the pituitary (a brief positive feedback effect), which stimulates follicular rupture and ovulation. The ruptured follicle becomes the corpus luteum, which produces progesterone and estrogen under the influence of LH during the second half of the cycle (luteal phase). Progesterone promotes development of a secretory endometrium that can accommodate embryo implantation. Conception causes progesterone secretion to continue, with the endometrium maintained as suitable for pregnancy. Without conception, the corpus luteum stops progesterone release and ceases to function, hormone levels decrease, and menstruation begins.

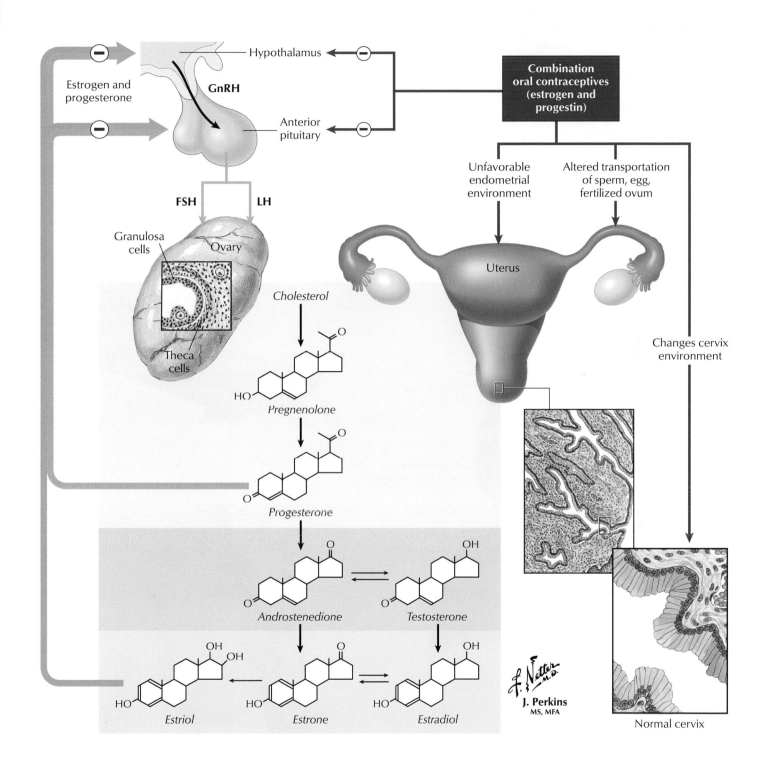

FIGURE 8-4 COMBINATION ORAL CONTRACEPTIVES

Combination oral contraceptives contain both estrogen and progestin and prevent pregnancy through several mechanisms. They inhibit ovulation via a negative feedback mechanism on the hypothalamus, which alters the normal pattern of FSH and LH secretion by the anterior pituitary. Estrogen suppresses FSH release from the pituitary during the follicular phase of the menstrual cycle and inhibits the midcycle surge of gonadotropins.

Progestin inhibits the estrogen-induced LH surge. COCs also produce alterations in the genital tract. Progestin is likely responsible for changing the cervical mucus and rendering it unfavorable for sperm penetration even if ovulation occurs. COCs induce an environment in the endometrium that is unfavorable for implantation. COCs may also alter the tubal transport of the sperm, egg, and fertilized ovum through the fallopian tubes.

Migraine Attack

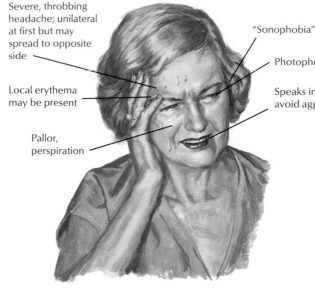

Severe, throbbing headache; unilateral at first but may spread to opposite side

"Sonophobia"

Photophobia

Speaks in low voice to avoid aggravating pain

Local erythema may be present

Pallor, perspiration

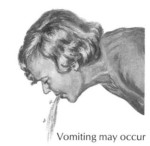

Vomiting may occur

Cluster Headache

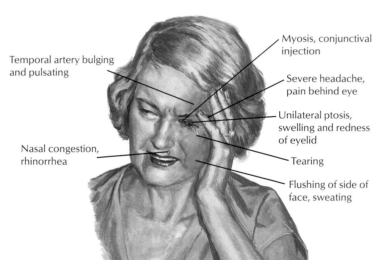

Temporal artery bulging and pulsating

Myosis, conjunctival injection

Severe headache, pain behind eye

Unilateral ptosis, swelling and redness of eyelid

Nasal congestion, rhinorrhea

Tearing

Flushing of side of face, sweating

Pitting edema

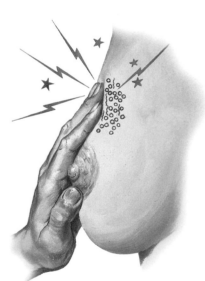

Schema of clinical syndrome: tender, granular swelling

FIGURE 8-5 MAJOR ADVERSE EFFECTS OF COMBINATION ORAL CONTRACEPTIVES

Major effects, related to excess or lack of estrogen or progestin, include breast fullness, depression, dizziness, edema, migraine, and vomiting. Serum lipoprotein profiles can change: estrogen increases HDL levels and decreases LDL levels; progestins (especially norgestrel) cause the unwanted opposite effect. COCs are associated with gallbladder disease, cholestasis, and abnormal glucose tolerance and are not used if cerebrovascular and thromboembolic disease, estrogen-dependent neoplasms, abnormal genital bleeding, chronic diabetes, or liver disease exists. Benefits include reduced risk of ovarian cysts, benign breast disease, and ectopic pregnancy and improved premenstrual symptoms, dysmenorrhea, endometriosis, acne, and hirsutism. COCs reduce endometrial and ovarian tumor incidence; their cause of other neoplasms is controversial. Other drugs—antibiotics (eg, tetracycline), rifampin, rifabutin, anticonvulsants—may decrease the efficacy of COCs.

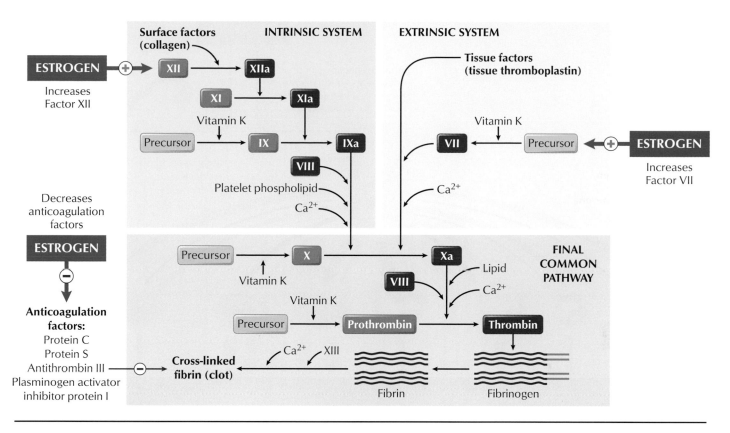

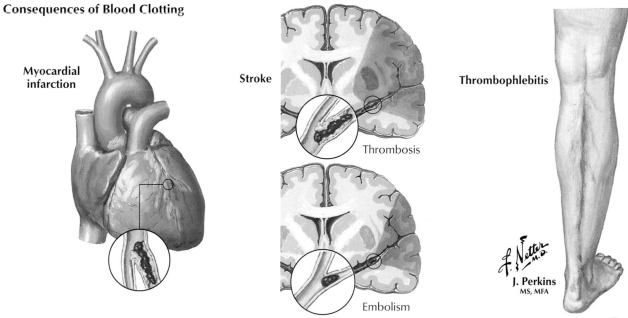

Consequences of Blood Clotting

Myocardial infarction

Stroke

Thrombophlebitis

Thrombosis

Embolism

J. Perkins
MS, MFA

FIGURE 8-6 ESTROGEN AND COAGULATION

Estrogens may affect fibrinolytic pathways and cause a small increase in coagulation factors VII and XII and a decrease in anticoagulation factors protein C, protein S, plasminogen-activator inhibitor protein I, and antithrombin III. By causing this imbalance between coagulation and anticoagulation, estrogens may produce serious associated complications, including thromboembolism, thrombophlebitis, myocardial infarction, and cerebral and coronary thrombosis. These complications are more likely to occur in women who smoke and are older than 35 years.

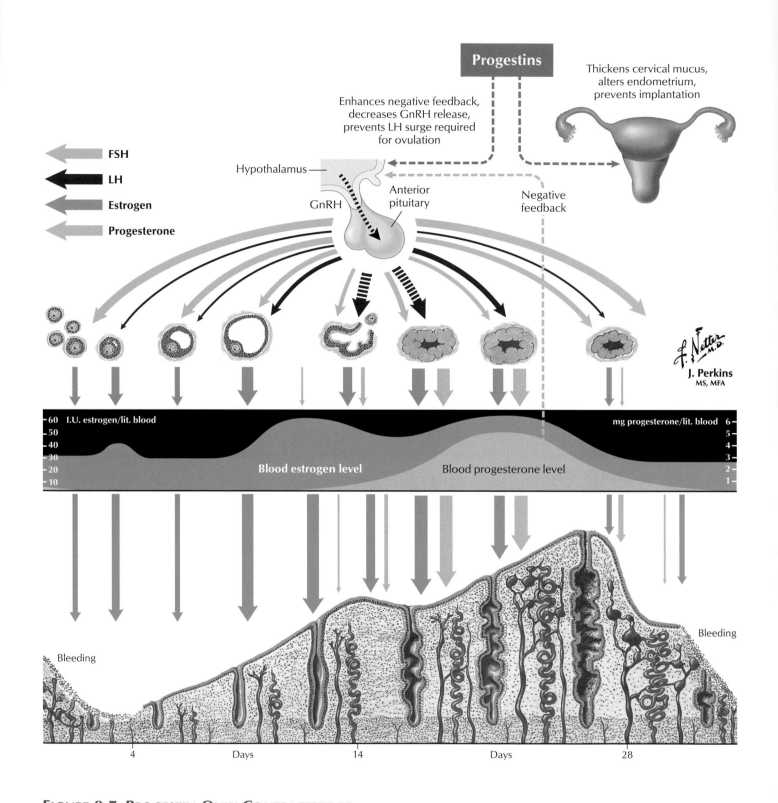

FIGURE 8-7 PROGESTIN-ONLY CONTRACEPTIVES

Progestin thickens cervical mucus, which decreases sperm penetration and alters the endometrium, thus preventing implantation. Progestin-only formulations are available as pills ("minipills"), depot injections, and implants. Pills contain norethindrone or norgestrel, taken daily on a continuous schedule; they are less effective than COCs because they block ovulation in only 60% to 80% of cycles. Depot injections of medroxyprogesterone acetate (MPA) impair implantation and produce plasma drug levels that are high enough to prevent ovulation in virtually all patients by slowing GnRH release, which thus prevents the LH surge required for ovulation. Progestin implants (subdermal capsules containing levonorgestrel) offer contraception for approximately 5 years. They are nearly as effective as sterilization, with completely reversible effects if the implants are surgically removed. Drug-related effects are weight gain, breast tenderness, headaches, and frequent occurrence of irregular menstrual bleeding.

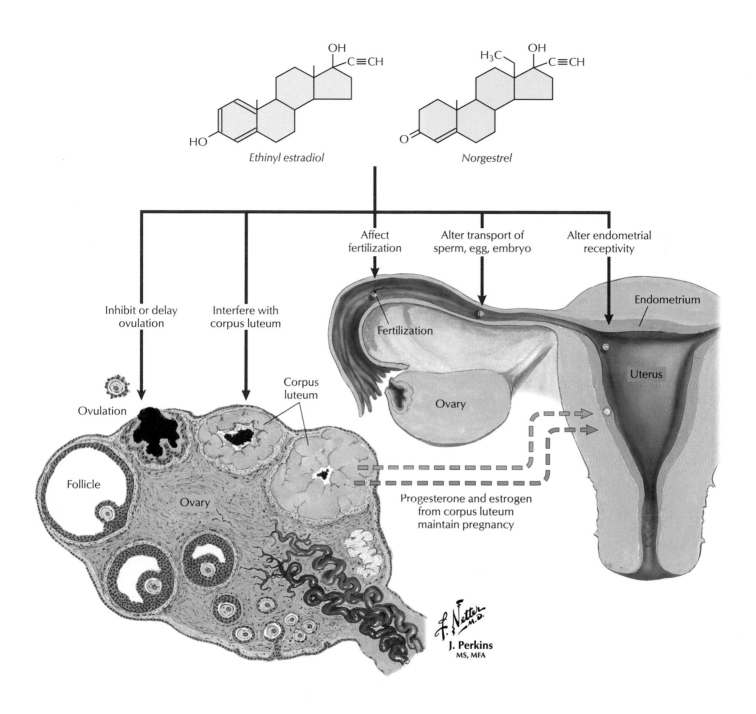

Ethinyl estradiol

Norgestrel

Affect fertilization

Alter transport of sperm, egg, embryo

Alter endometrial receptivity

Inhibit or delay ovulation

Interfere with corpus luteum

Fertilization

Endometrium

Corpus luteum

Ovulation

Uterus

Follicle

Ovary

Ovary

Progesterone and estrogen from corpus luteum maintain pregnancy

J. Perkins
MS, MFA

FIGURE 8-8 THE MORNING-AFTER PILL

Postcoital, or emergency, contraceptives consist of high-dose estrogen (ethinyl estradiol), administered within 72 hours of coitus and continued twice daily for 5 days. Alternatively, 2 doses of ethinyl estradiol plus norgestrel can be used within 72 hours of coitus, followed by another 2 doses 12 hours later. The hormones may inhibit or delay ovulation if taken during the first half of the cycle. They may also alter endometrial receptivity for implantation, interfere with the functions of the corpus luteum that maintains pregnancy, decrease sperm penetration, affect fertilization, and alter the transport of sperm, egg, or embryo. Emergency contraception does not interrupt an established pregnancy, which officially begins with implantation. Emergency contraceptives are associated with a high incidence of nausea and vomiting because of the high doses of hormones used.

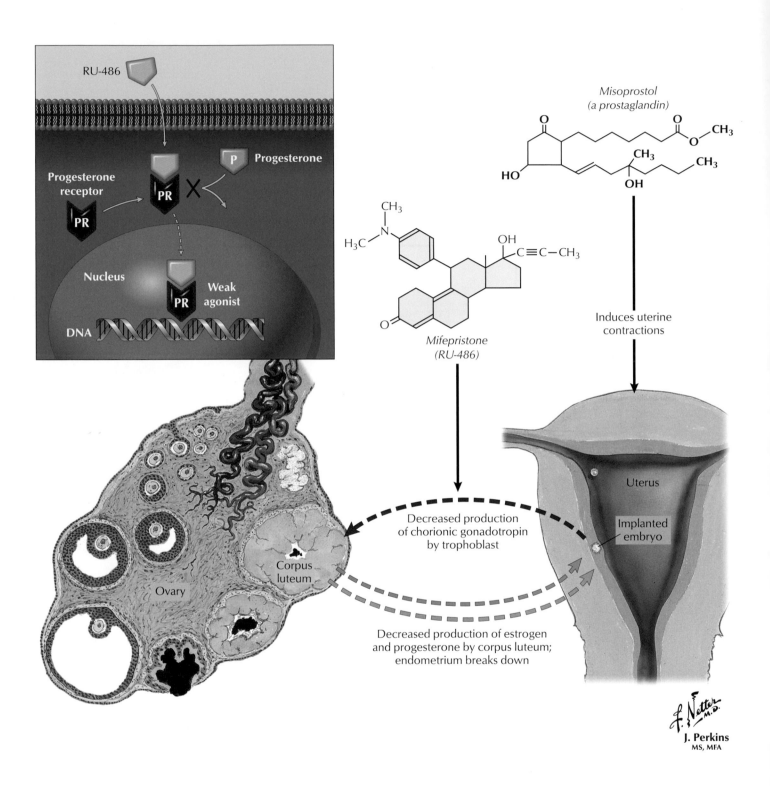

FIGURE 8-9 THE ABORTION PILL

A progestin antagonist with partial agonist activity, mifepristone (RU-486) is used for medical termination of intrauterine pregnancy through 49 days of pregnancy. Taken early in pregnancy, mifepristone interferes with progesterone, causing a decline in human chorionic gonadotropin and subsequent abortion of the fetus. Mifepristone is also known to sensitize the endometrium to prostaglandins, which terminate gestation by inducing uterine contractions. Therefore, it is rational to use mifepristone with the prostaglandin misoprostol, especially because mifepristone alone is more likely to cause an incomplete abortion. The regimen consists of a single dose of mifepristone, followed by a single dose of misoprostol 2 days later. Expected major adverse effects are cramping and bleeding, which are similar to symptoms of a spontaneous abortion. Incomplete abortion is also possible.

Pelvis: Sites of Implantation

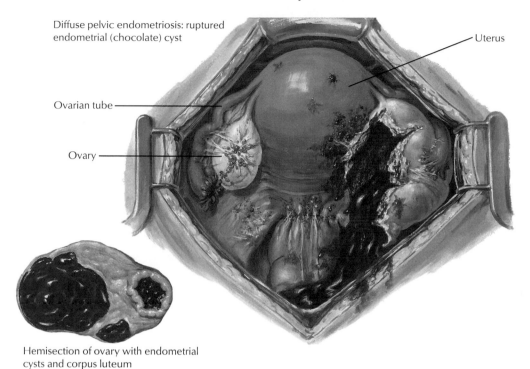

Diffuse pelvic endometriosis: ruptured endometrial (chocolate) cyst

Uterus

Ovarian tube

Ovary

Hemisection of ovary with endometrial cysts and corpus luteum

Laparoscopic Views

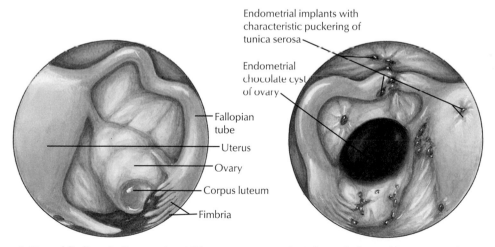

Endometrial implants with characteristic puckering of tunica serosa

Endometrial chocolate cyst of ovary

Fallopian tube

Uterus

Ovary

Corpus luteum

Fimbria

A. Normal findings (indigo carmine visible at end of tube)

B. Endometriosis (involving ovary and distorting fallopian tube)

FIGURE 8-10 ENDOMETRIOSIS

Endometriosis is characterized by the presence of endometrial tissue on ovaries, fallopian tubes, and peritoneum or on more remote extrauterine sites such as the bowel, rectum, kidneys, and lungs. The most frequent symptoms of genital tract endometriosis include dyspareunia, dysmenorrhea, low back pain, menstrual irregularities, and infertility. The pathogenesis of endometriosis is multifactorial, but essentially it involves retrograde menstruation, in which endometrial cells implant in the pelvis and create "endometrial islands" that bleed and cause local inflammation in response to cyclic hormonal stimulation. Endometriosis is likely to remain problematic as long as menstruation continues. Therefore, the mainstay of medical therapy involves interrupting or decreasing menstruation.

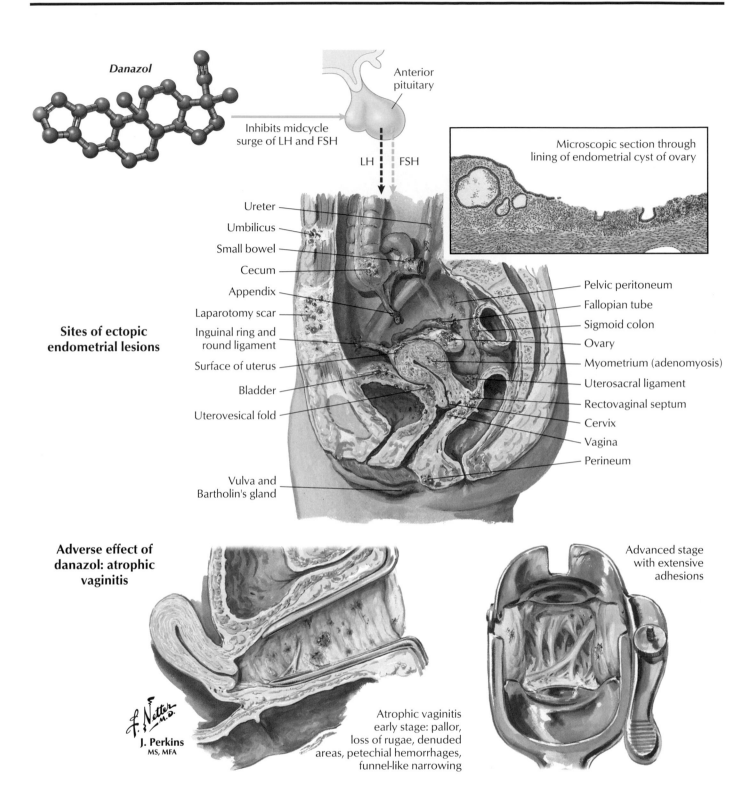

Danazol

Inhibits midcycle surge of LH and FSH

Anterior pituitary

LH   FSH

Microscopic section through lining of endometrial cyst of ovary

Sites of ectopic endometrial lesions

Ureter
Umbilicus
Small bowel
Cecum
Appendix
Laparotomy scar
Inguinal ring and round ligament
Surface of uterus
Bladder
Uterovesical fold
Vulva and Bartholin's gland

Pelvic peritoneum
Fallopian tube
Sigmoid colon
Ovary
Myometrium (adenomyosis)
Uterosacral ligament
Rectovaginal septum
Cervix
Vagina
Perineum

Adverse effect of danazol: atrophic vaginitis

Advanced stage with extensive adhesions

Atrophic vaginitis early stage: pallor, loss of rugae, denuded areas, petechial hemorrhages, funnel-like narrowing

J. Netter M.D.
J. Perkins
MS, MFA

FIGURE 8-11 DANAZOL

Danazol is a synthetic androgen that suppresses ovarian estrogen production by inhibiting the midcycle surge of LH and FSH from the pituitary. The resultant relatively hypoestrogenic state leads to atrophy of ectopic endometrial lesions and pain relief. Danazol is started when the patient is menstruating and is continued for 6 to 9 months, depending on disease severity. During therapy, the patient is usually amenorrheic, but ovulation may still occur. Patients should use nonhormonal contraception, because use of danazol during pregnancy should be avoided. Regular ovulatory cycles are resumed within 4 weeks after ending danazol therapy. Adverse effects are characteristic of estrogen deficiency and include headache, flushing, sweating, and atrophic vaginitis. Androgenic side effects include acne, edema, hirsutism, deepening of the voice, and weight gain. Although danazol has been highly effective in relieving the symptoms of endometriosis, newer, better-tolerated treatments have reduced its use.

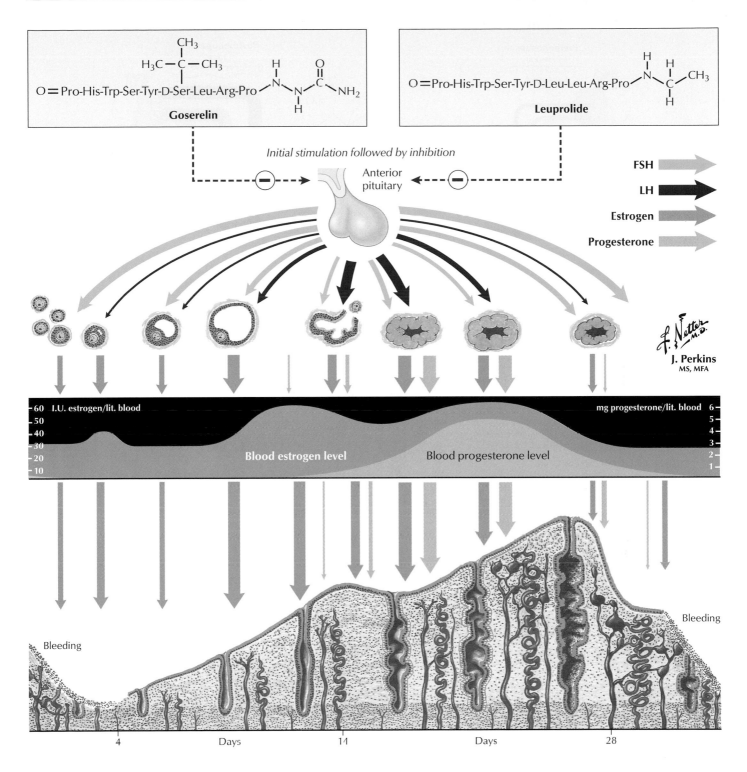

FIGURE 8-12 GONADOTROPIN-RELEASING HORMONE AGONISTS, COMBINATION ORAL CONTRACEPTIVES, AND PROGESTIN

Gonadotropin-releasing hormone agonists (eg, leuprolide, goserelin) create a temporary medical oophorectomy by causing paradoxical effects on the pituitary: initial stimulation of LH and FSH release, and then inhibition of hormone release. These effects result in reduced sex hormone levels and regression of endometriosis-related lesions. Long-acting formulations are usually given every 28 days for approximately 6 months. GnRH agonists are contraindicated in pregnancy and have hypoestrogenic side effects, eg, mild bone loss (which reverses after the drug is stopped). Because of concerns about osteopenia, add-back low-dose estrogen therapy has been used. COCs and progestins also suppress LH and FSH, so they render endometrial tissue thin and compact, thus alleviating endometriosis. COCs can be taken continuously or cyclically. Therapy can be stopped after 6 to 12 months or continued indefinitely. Progestins may have greater adverse effects than COCs; a depot form may delay return to fertility.

Pituitary and Ovarian Hormone Changes in Menopause

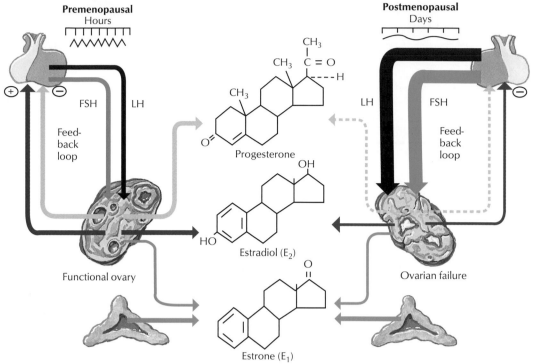

Hormone levels increase and decrease cyclically during menstrual cycle. Modulation occurs by pulsatile release of gonadotropins and positive and negative feedback loops.

In postmenopausal period, gonadotropin levels increase and ovarian hormone levels decrease secondary to ovarian failure. Endogenous estrogen is primarily of adrenal origin, and E_1 to E_2 ratio is reversed.

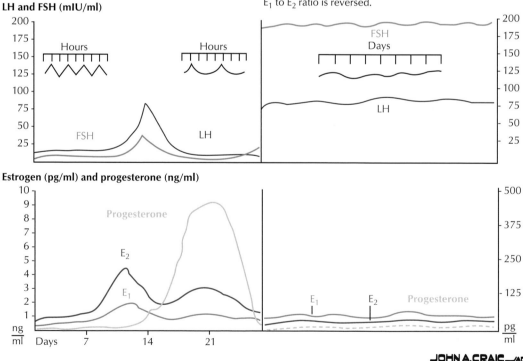

Figure 8-13 Estrogen Decline

In the premenopausal period, ovarian secretion of estradiol, the most potent form of estrogen, is the major source of estrogen production. In menopause, production of estradiol diminishes as the ovaries cease to function. In the postmenopausal period (1 year after amenorrhea), gonadotropin levels increase and ovarian hormone levels decrease secondary to ovarian failure. Peripheral conversion of adrenal androstenedione to estrone (one tenth the potency of estradiol) becomes the principal source of estrogen. Consequences of this estrogen deficiency include vasomotor symptoms, genitourinary atrophy, and osteoporosis.

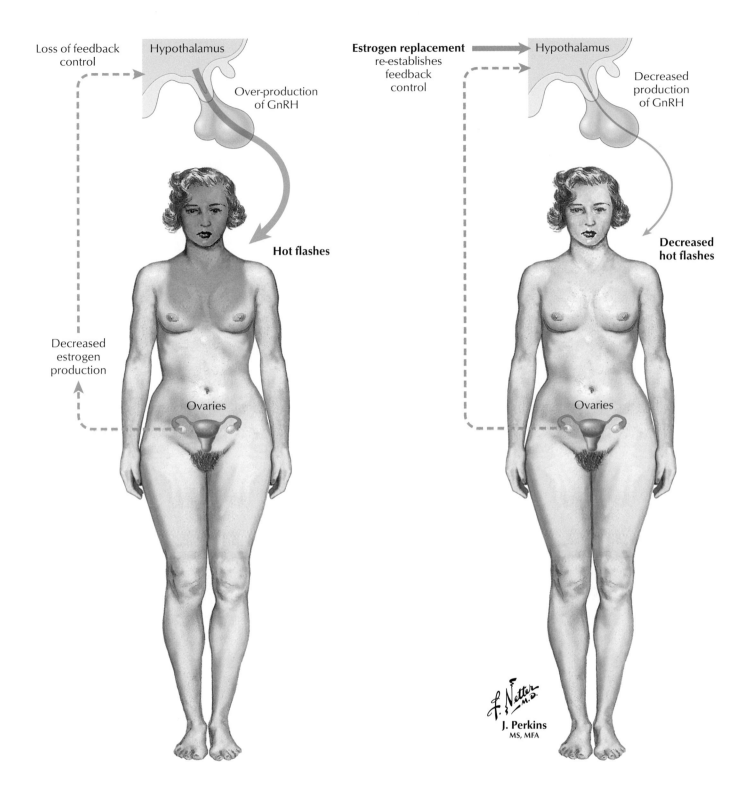

FIGURE 8-14 VASOMOTOR SYMPTOMS

The chief vasomotor symptoms reported by women are described as hot flashes, which occur over the anterior part of the body, especially the face, neck, and chest. Usually lasting a few minutes but varying in frequency and severity, these symptoms are caused by a decrease in the tone of arterioles. This compromised state results in increased blood flow to the skin and a subsequent increase in skin temperature.

Hot flashes seem to be synchronous with the increased hypothalamic release of GnRH that occurs in response to estrogen deficiency. GnRH neurons are coincidentally close to the hypothalamic centers that regulate temperature. Estrogen replacement therapy reestablishes feedback control of hypothalamic secretion of GnRH, leading to a decreased incidence of hot flashes.

Aging Ovary

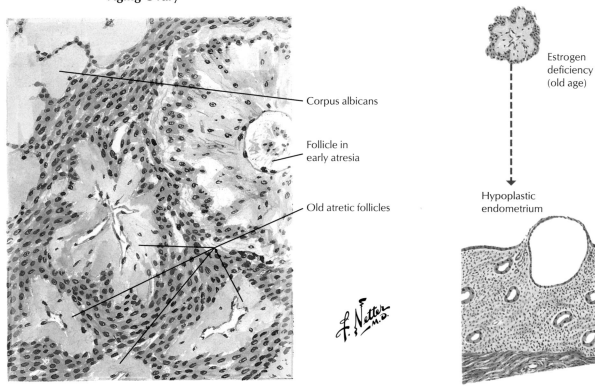

Corpus albicans

Follicle in early atresia

Old atretic follicles

Estrogen deficiency (old age)

Hypoplastic endometrium

FIGURE 8-15 GENITOURINARY ATROPHY

Postmenopausal estrogen deficiency leads to several changes in the vagina, including thinning of the epithelium, a decreased blood supply, dryness, and a change from acidic to a neutral or alkaline pH that predisposes to infection. Chief symptoms include vaginal discharge secondary to infection and painful intercourse from dryness, as well as dysuria and urinary incontinence from bladder atrophy. Estrogen increases the vascularity and epithelial proliferation of the vagina, which allows greater lubrication, increased protection from vaginitis, and reduced vaginal trauma from intercourse. Estrogen also reverses atrophy of the bladder.

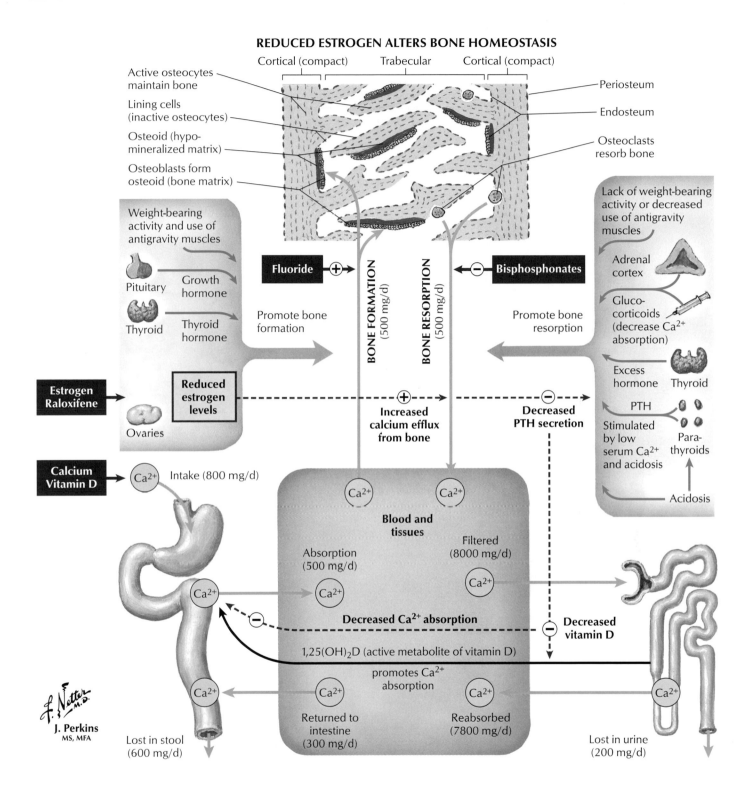

FIGURE 8-16 OSTEOPOROSIS AND ESTROGEN

Lower estrogen levels enhance calcium efflux from bone mineral stores and increases serum Ca^{2+} levels. These effects suppress parathyroid hormone secretion, which reduces vitamin D3 synthesis, thus decreasing intestinal calcium absorption. Estrogen deficiency and advanced age also reduce secretion of the hormone calcitonin, which inhibits bone resorption. Bones thin and weaken, with increased risk of fractures, especially compression fractures of vertebrae (and thus height loss) and minimal-trauma hip and wrist fractures. Preventive and therapeutic measures include use of estrogen, calcium, vitamin D, calcitonin, fluoride, bisphosphonates, and drugs such as raloxifene. Therapeutic estrogen primarily decreases bone resorption, which reduces bone loss (does not restore bone mass); decreases calcium excretion, producing a premenopausal calcium balance; increases vitamin D3 synthesis; increases serum calcitonin levels; and (given with calcium) decreases hip fracture occurrence.

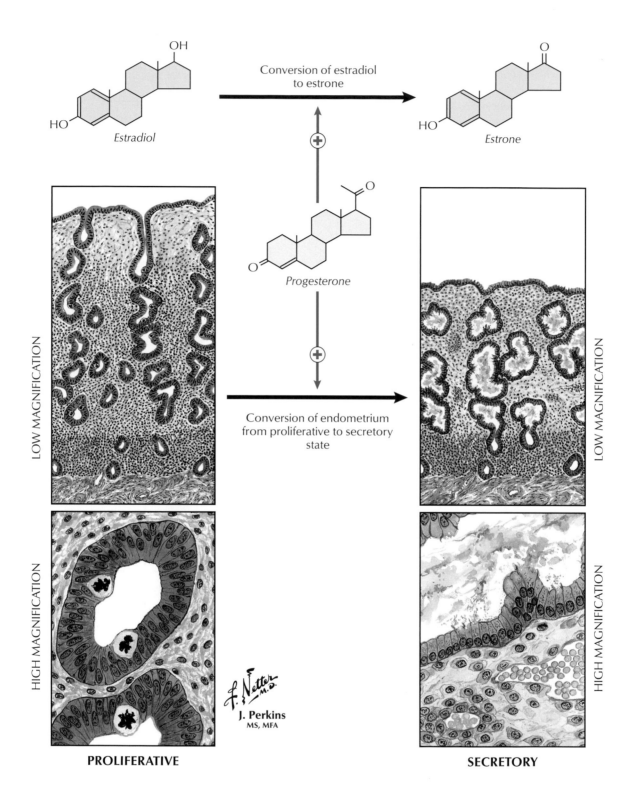

FIGURE 8-17 ROLE OF PROGESTINS IN HORMONE REPLACEMENT THERAPY

Unopposed estrogen is associated with a large increase in the incidence of endometrial carcinoma, which is thought to be due to the hormone's continuous stimulation of endometrial hyperplasia. In patients with an intact uterus, progestin is added to estrogen therapy because it reduces endometrial hyperplasia by increasing local conversion of estradiol to the less potent estrone, converting the endometrium from a proliferative to a secretory state, or both. Progestin also reduces the risk of estrogen-induced irregular bleeding. Patients who have undergone a hysterectomy can use unopposed estrogen therapy; progestin is unnecessary, especially because it may unfavorably alter the HDL/LDL ratio.

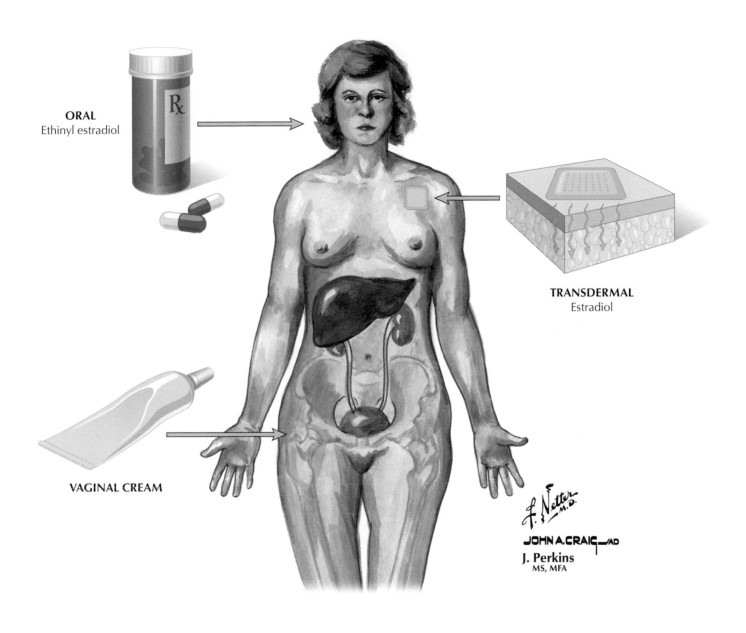

ORAL
Ethinyl estradiol

TRANSDERMAL
Estradiol

VAGINAL CREAM

FIGURE 8-18 ROUTE OF HORMONE ADMINISTRATION

A major pharmacologic consideration in HRT is the route of administration. Oral dosage forms of estrogen go through portal circulation and thus expose the liver to high hormone concentrations. Also, oral administration is associated with a more rapid conversion of estradiol to estrone. Transdermal estradiol overcomes these problems and still relieves vasomotor and genitourinary symptoms and protects against bone loss. Vaginally applied estrogen cream can be used to treat genitourinary symptoms, but the response may be lost after 14 days because of tissue cornification or down-regulation of estrogen receptors. Stopping treatment for 7 to 14 days and then restarting can overcome this effect. Conjugated estrogen vaginal cream and its equivalents have 4 times the activity of oral estrogens on local tissues. Because estrogen in the cream may enter the systemic circulation, warnings related to its use are essentially the same as those for systemic preparations.

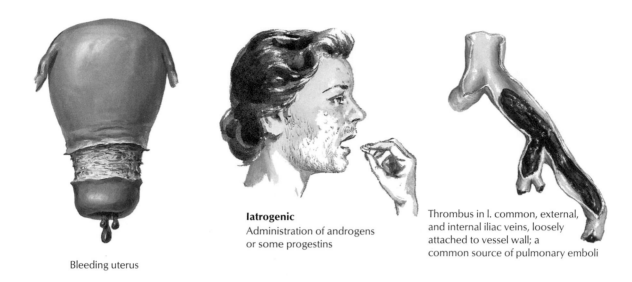

Bleeding uterus

Iatrogenic
Administration of androgens
or some progestins

Thrombus in l. common, external,
and internal iliac veins, loosely
attached to vessel wall; a
common source of pulmonary emboli

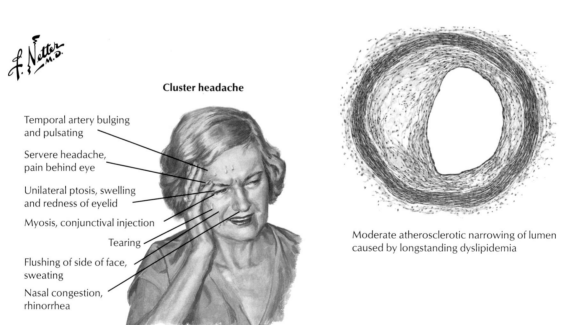

Cluster headache

Temporal artery bulging
and pulsating

Servere headache,
pain behind eye

Unilateral ptosis, swelling
and redness of eyelid

Myosis, conjunctival injection

Tearing

Flushing of side of face,
sweating

Nasal congestion,
rhinorrhea

Moderate atherosclerotic narrowing of lumen
caused by longstanding dyslipidemia

Figure 8-19 General Adverse Effects

The doses of estrogen used in HRT are substantially less than those used in OCs, so adverse effects of HRT tend to be less severe than those of OCs. Estrogen may cause nausea, vomiting, edema, headache, hypertension, and breast tenderness. Estrogen is also a major cause of postmenopausal uterine bleeding, which is more likely to occur during the withdrawal period if estrogen is given cyclically with progestin. Progestin is likely responsible for edema and depression. Androgen-like progestins can increase the LDL/HDL ratio and cause thrombophlebitis, hirsutism, weight gain, and acne.

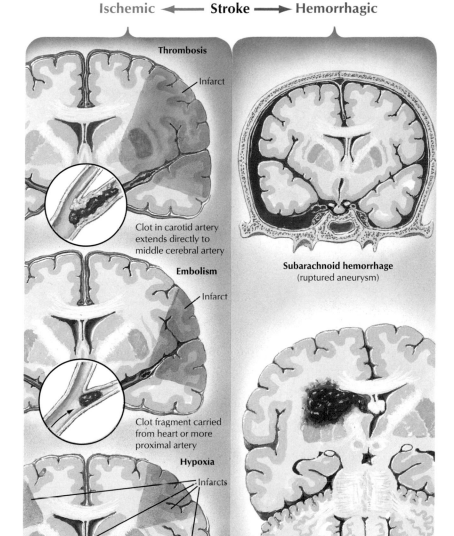

Diagnosis of Stroke

Ischemic ◄──── **Stroke** ────► Hemorrhagic

Thrombosis

Infarct

Clot in carotid artery extends directly to middle cerebral artery

Embolism

Infarct

Clot fragment carried from heart or more proximal artery

Hypoxia

Infarcts

Hypotension and poor cerebral perfusion: border zone infarcts, no vascular occlusion

Subarachnoid hemorrhage
(ruptured aneurysm)

Intracerebral hemorrhage
(hypertensive)

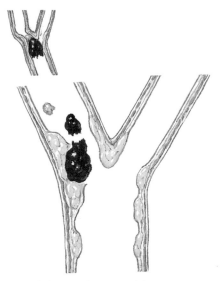

Embolization of contents of plaque (cholesterol) and/or platelet-fibrin; occlusion of blood vessels distally in arterial tree

FIGURE 8-20 CARDIOVASCULAR AND NEUROLOGIC RISKS

Risks and benefits of estrogen with regard to cardioprotection, neuroprotection, and carcinogenicity in postmenopausal women have been a subject of much debate. Estrogen had been believed to be cardioprotective, possibly through favorable changes in lipid metabolism and direct vasodilatory effects. However, a landmark trial (Women's Health Initiative) found estrogen-progestin HRT to be associated with an increased risk of stroke, venous thromboembolism, coronary heart disease, nonfatal myocardial infarction, and death from heart disease. Also, estrogen alone or with progestin did not affect the progression of atherosclerotic lesions in older postmenopausal women with at least 1 coronary artery lesion. Estrogen increased the risk of Alzheimer disease, a finding that contradicts earlier data indicating a possible association between estrogen and neuroprotection.

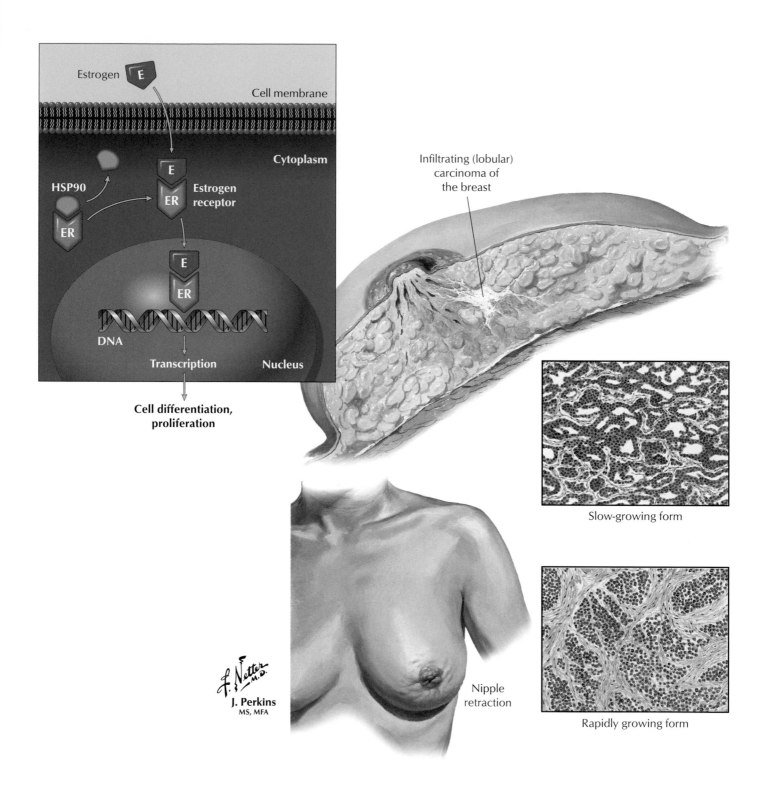

Estrogen

E

Cell membrane

Cytoplasm

HSP90

E

ER Estrogen receptor

ER

E

ER

DNA

Transcription

Nucleus

Cell differentiation, proliferation

Infiltrating (lobular) carcinoma of the breast

Slow-growing form

J. Perkins
MS, MFA

Nipple retraction

Rapidly growing form

FIGURE 8-21 CANCER RISKS

Estrogen was shown in the Women's Health Initiative trial and another large study to increase the risk of breast cancer. The latter trial evaluated HRT in more than 1 million British women and found that those who received HRT (especially both estrogen and progestin) had an increased risk of development of and death resulting from breast cancer. The risk of development of cancer increased with duration of HRT use, but it also declined after discontinuation of HRT. The trial indicated that estrogen-progestin reduced the risk of colorectal cancer and confirmed beneficial effects on reduction of hip and vertebral fractures. However, these benefits do not seem to outweigh the risks. As a result, in 2003, the US FDA urged clinicians to limit the use of HRT to a few months for temporary relief of postmenopausal symptoms.

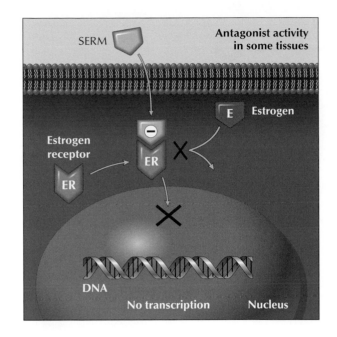

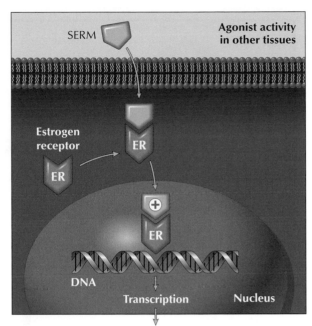

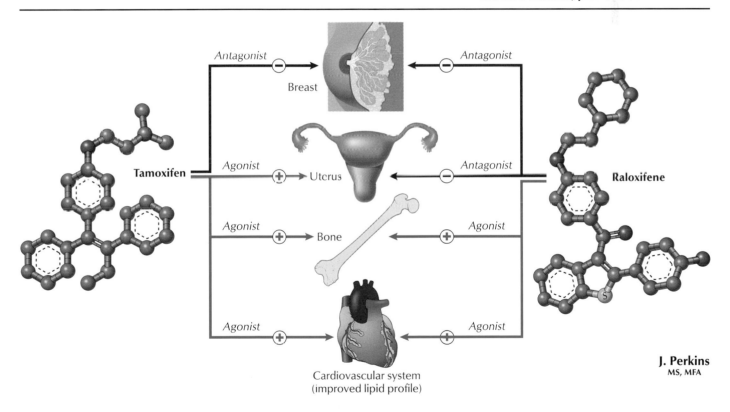

FIGURE 8-22 SELECTIVE ESTROGEN RECEPTOR MODULATORS

Selective estrogen receptor modulators (SERMs), hormonelike drugs with tissue-selective estrogenic activities, act as competitive antagonists or weak agonists: estrogenic in bone but no effect or antagonistic in breast and endometrium. Tamoxifen, first classed as antiestrogenic, is used to prevent and treat hormone-responsive breast cancer (inhibits cell proliferation and reduces tumors, as a result of estrogen receptor antagonism). It has estrogenic actions in the uterus (stimulates endometrial proliferation and thickening, which increases carcinoma risk) and in the skeletal and cardiovascular systems (reduces bone loss; improves lipid profiles). Hot flashes, menstrual abnormalities, thrombosis, and pulmonary embolism are adverse effects. Raloxifene is used to prevent and treat osteoporosis: it has estrogen agonist action in bone and on lipid metabolism and antagonist action in breast and uterus; it is antiproliferative for estrogen-positive breast cancer cells. Adverse effects are hot flashes, leg cramps, and venous thromboembolism.

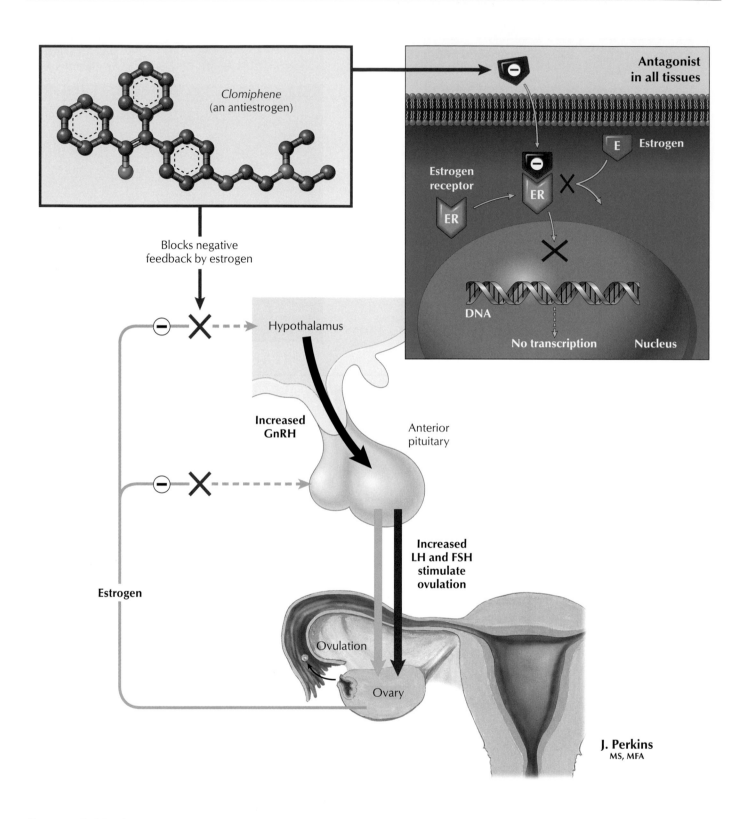

FIGURE 8-23 ANTIESTROGENS

Antiestrogens are distinguished from SERMs in that they act as pure antagonists in all tissues. The antiestrogen clomiphene binds competitively to estrogen receptors and decreases the sites available to endogenous estrogen, including hypothalamic and pituitary estrogen receptors. This inhibition leads to a disruption in the negative feedback of estrogens on the hypothalamus and pituitary, a subsequent increase in secretion of GnRH and gonadotropins, and ultimately stimulation of ovulation. The agent is used to treat infertility associated with anovulatory menstrual cycles, but it is effective only in women with a functional hypothalamus and adequate endogenous estrogen production. Adverse effects are dose related and include ovarian enlargement, vasomotor symptoms, and visual disturbances.

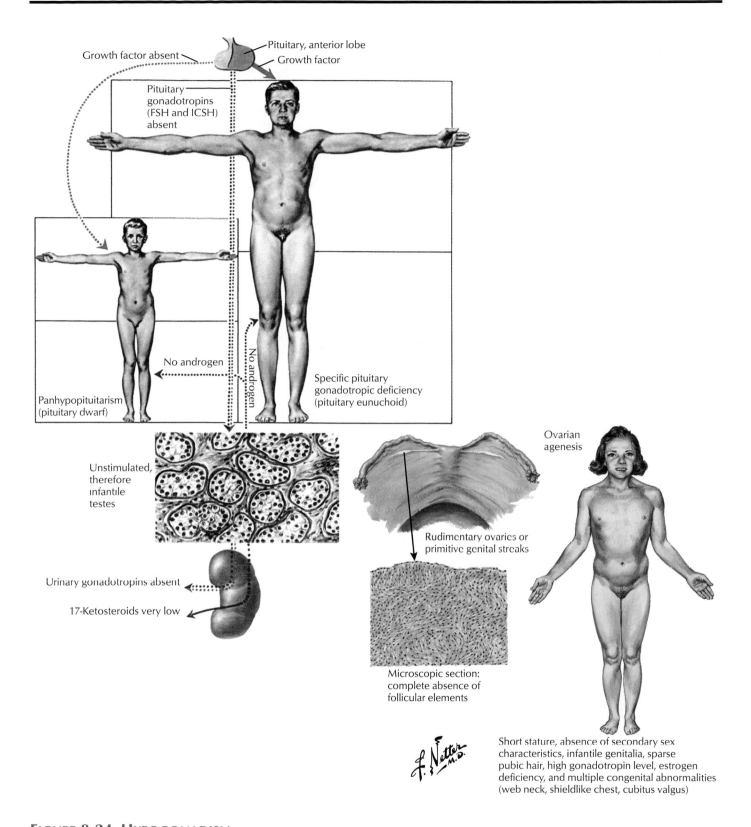

Growth factor absent
Pituitary, anterior lobe
Growth factor

Pituitary gonadotropins (FSH and ICSH) absent

No androgen

No androgen

Panhypopituitarism (pituitary dwarf)

Specific pituitary gonadotropic deficiency (pituitary eunuchoid)

Unstimulated, therefore infantile testes

Urinary gonadotropins absent

17-Ketosteroids very low

Rudimentary ovaries or primitive genital streaks

Microscopic section: complete absence of follicular elements

Ovarian agenesis

Short stature, absence of secondary sex characteristics, infantile genitalia, sparse pubic hair, high gonadotropin level, estrogen deficiency, and multiple congenital abnormalities (web neck, shieldlike chest, cubitus valgus)

FIGURE 8-24 HYPOGONADISM

In several conditions in females, such as Turner syndrome (ovarian dysgenesis and dwarfism), the ovaries do not develop (or have no primordial follicles and may be represented only by a fibrous streak), and puberty does not occur. Other characteristics include short stature, primary amenorrhea, sexual infantilism, high gonadotropin levels, and multiple congenital abnormalities. Conception is impossible. In males, dysfunction of Leydig cells or failure of the hypothalamic-pituitary system can lead to inadequate secretion of androgens, for which testosterone replacement therapy is used. If testosterone deficiency occurs before puberty, it results in failure to complete puberty. After completion of puberty, testosterone deficiency can lead to loss of libido and energy, decreased muscle mass and strength, decreased hematocrit and hemoglobin, and decreased bone mineral density.

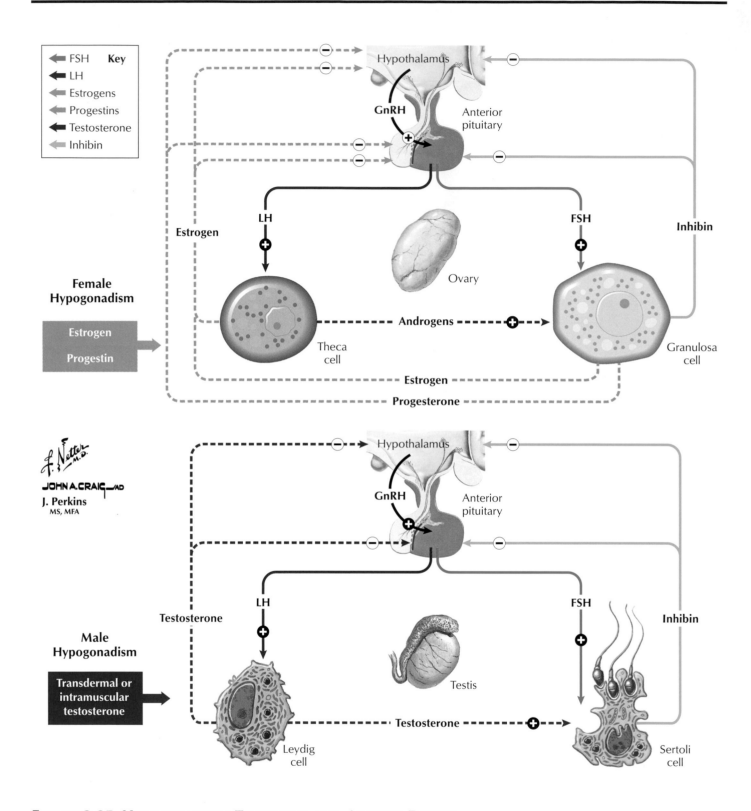

Key
- FSH
- LH
- Estrogens
- Progestins
- Testosterone
- Inhibin

Female Hypogonadism

Estrogen
Progestin

Hypothalamus

GnRH

Anterior pituitary

LH

Estrogen

FSH

Inhibin

Ovary

Theca cell

Androgens

Granulosa cell

Estrogen

Progesterone

Male Hypogonadism

Transdermal or intramuscular testosterone

Hypothalamus

GnRH

Anterior pituitary

LH

Testosterone

FSH

Inhibin

Testis

Leydig cell

Testosterone

Sertoli cell

FIGURE 8-25 HYPOGONADISM TREATMENT AND ADVERSE EFFECTS

For females, appropriate therapy with estrogen, usually with pro-gestin, replicates most events of puberty. Genital structures grow to normal size, breasts develop, axillary and pubic hair grows, and the body achieves a normal feminine contour. Estrogen may increase growth, but if used too soon, it can accelerate epiphyseal fusion and cause a short final height (treated with androgens and growth hormone). For male testosterone deficiency, an oral drug is ineffective because of liver metabolism. Intramuscular (cypionate or enanthate) or transdermal testosterone overcomes first-pass metabolism to reach normal serum concentrations. In prepubertal children, testosterone causes acne, hirsutism, gynecomastia, and sexual aggression as well as growth disturbances. Excess androgen in men can cause priapism, impotence, reduced spermatogenesis, and gynecomastia. Androgens can also cause edema and an increased LDL/HDL ratio, which may be harmful to those with hyperlipidemia or CHF.

CHAPTER 9

DRUGS USED TO AFFECT RENAL FUNCTION

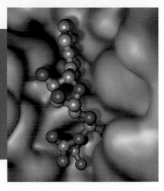

OVERVIEW

For many drugs, the kidney is the major organ of elimination. In the healthy human, the kidney receives between 20% and 25% of the blood pumped by each beat of the heart. The kidney's primary function is 2-fold: to eliminate unwanted substances (eg, toxic substances, drugs, and their metabolites) and to retain (reabsorb, recycle) wanted materials (eg, water and electrolytes). The amount of drug and metabolites eliminated (cleared) from the body depends on several factors, including the glomerular filtration rate (GFR), the urine flow rate, and the pH. The rate of renal elimination is the net result of glomerular filtration, secretion, and reabsorption.

The functional microscopic unit of the kidney is the nephron, a tube that is open at one end and closed at the other end by a semipermeable membrane. The nephron has 5 distinct anatomical and functional units: glomerulus, proximal convoluted tubule, loop of Henle, distal convoluted tubule, and collecting duct. Large drug molecules (>5-6 kd) and drug molecules that are bound to plasma proteins do not pass into the nephron of a healthy kidney. Most of the water and other substances that enter the nephron are reabsorbed into the surrounding tissue and blood supply. The small residual amount is excreted as the urine.

The flow and contents of the urine are determined by 3 processes, most of which are coupled: filtration through the glomerulus, reabsorption of water and other substances from the tubule, and secretion of substances into the tubule. Many processes involve active transport, passive transport, or osmotic gradients. Most of the water and solutes (eg, sodium, glucose, bicarbonate, amino acids) are reabsorbed during passage through the proximal convoluted tubule, and further concentration occurs in the countercurrent system of the loop of Henle. The thick ascending limb and the distal convoluted tubule are involved in Na^+-K^+ and H^+ exchange under tight homeostatic control and hormonal influence, including adrenal steroid hormones such as aldosterone. The collecting duct is the primary site of action of antidiuretic hormone (ADH).

Drugs that target the renal system, primarily diuretic agents, have been a major advance in treatment of hypertension, heart failure, and other disorders. Each class of diuretics affects different processes located at different sites along nephrons. Therefore, each class has its own set of associated therapeutic advantages or drawbacks. Each also has characteristic effects on electrolyte balance, which is an important consideration for long-term use. Many effects can be anticipated on the basis of a drug's mechanism of diuretic action and can be ameliorated by dietary or drug regimens. Combinations of diuretics may offer a remedy for resistance to a single agent.

A decline in renal function, whether caused by advanced age or disease, has a significant effect on clearance of drugs that are eliminated predominantly via the kidney. Dosages must be adjusted in these situations.

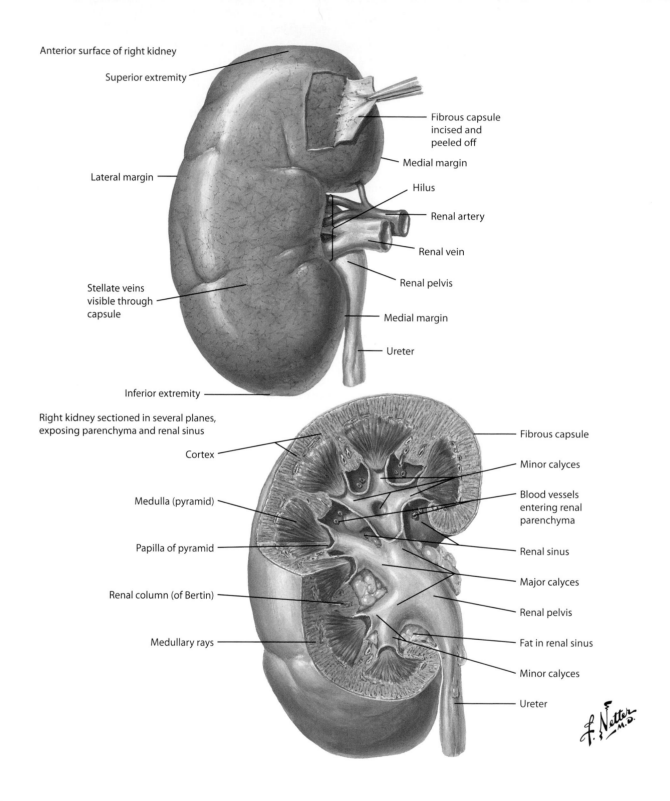

Anterior surface of right kidney

Superior extremity

Fibrous capsule incised and peeled off

Medial margin

Lateral margin

Hilus

Renal artery

Renal vein

Renal pelvis

Stellate veins visible through capsule

Medial margin

Ureter

Inferior extremity

Right kidney sectioned in several planes, exposing parenchyma and renal sinus

Cortex

Fibrous capsule

Minor calyces

Blood vessels entering renal parenchyma

Medulla (pyramid)

Papilla of pyramid

Renal sinus

Renal column (of Bertin)

Major calyces

Renal pelvis

Medullary rays

Fat in renal sinus

Minor calyces

Ureter

FIGURE 9-1 MACROSCOPIC ANATOMY

The *kidneys* are a pair of specialized, retroperitoneal organs located at the level between the lower thoracic and upper lumbar vertebrae. Each kidney is reddish brown and has a characteristic shape: a convex lateral edge and concave medial border with a marked depression or notch termed the *hilus*. Each adult kidney is approximately 11 cm long, 2.5 cm thick, and 5 cm wide and weighs 120 to 170 g. Kidneys contribute to several important processes, including regulation of fluid volume;

regulation of electrolyte balance; excretion of metabolic wastes; and elimination of toxic compounds, drugs, and their metabolites. It also acts as an endocrine organ. Each kidney is divided into a cortex and a medulla, both parts containing nephrons (approximately 1.25 million per kidney). The fluid that exits a nephron flows out the papilla of a pyramid (8-15 per medulla), enters a minor calyx, joins effluent of other minor calyces in the major calyx, and is eliminated as urine through the ureter.

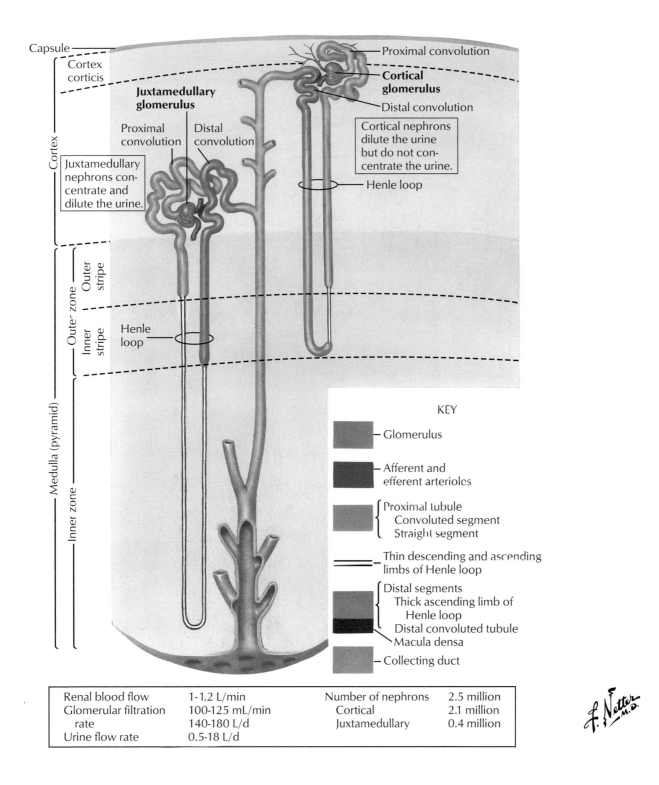

KEY

- Glomerulus
- Afferent and efferent arterioles
- { Proximal tubule
  Convoluted segment
  Straight segment
- Thin descending and ascending limbs of Henle loop
- { Distal segments
  Thick ascending limb of Henle loop
  Distal convoluted tubule
  Macula densa
- Collecting duct

Renal blood flow	1-1.2 L/min	Number of nephrons	2.5 million
Glomerular filtration rate	100-125 mL/min	Cortical	2.1 million
	140-180 L/d	Juxtamedullary	0.4 million
Urine flow rate	0.5-18 L/d		

FIGURE 9-2 THE NEPHRON

Each kidney contains approximately 1 to 3 million tubular nephrons (Greek *nephros*, meaning kidney). A nephron originates in the glomerular apparatus. The part adjoining this corpuscle is termed the *proximal convoluted tubule* because of its tortuous course that remains close to its point of origin. The tubule then straightens in the direction of the center of the kidney and forms the Henle loop, by making a hairpin turn and returning to the vascular pole of its parent renal corpuscle. The loop extends to the distal convoluted tubule and then to the collecting tubule. Collecting tubules unite to form larger collecting ducts. Most nephrons originate in the kidney cortex, are short, and extend only to the outer medullary zone. Other nephrons originate close to the medullary level (juxtamedullary glomeruli) and extend deep into the medulla, almost as far as the papilla. Each part of the nephron acts in physiologic processes that affect or are affected by metabolism of drug molecules (or their metabolites).

Pattern of Blood Vessels in Parenchyma of Kidney: Schema

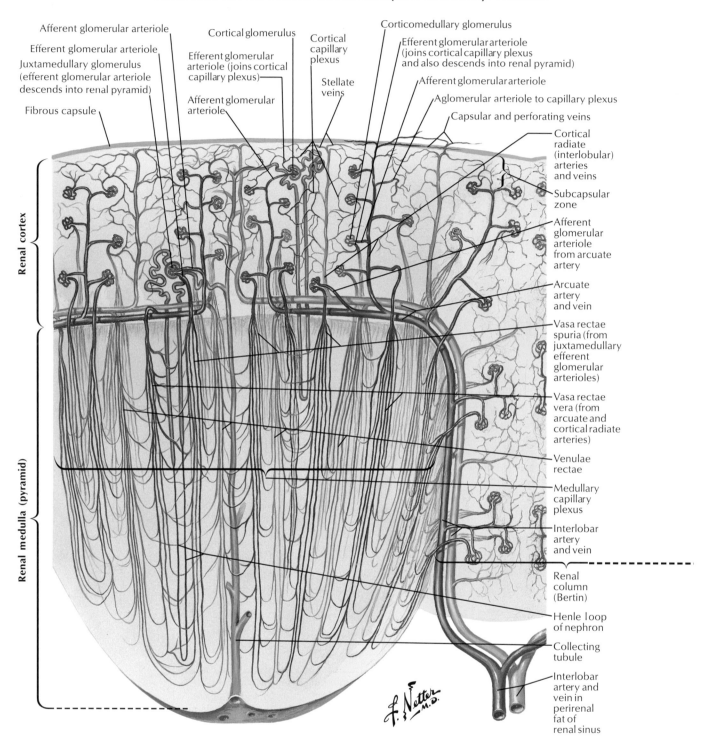

FIGURE 9-3 BLOOD VESSELS SURROUNDING NEPHRONS

Critical to multiple kidney functions is close association of nephrons with blood vessels, in that water and other substances pass from nephron to blood and vice versa. Kidneys have a great influence on volume and composition of plasma and urine, so the architecture of renal vasculature reflects functions other than tissue oxygenation. In the outer renal cortex, each afferent arteriole enters a glomerulus, divides, forms a capillary network, becomes an efferent arteriole, and exits the glomerulus.

Neurotransmitters, drugs, and environmental factors that relax the afferent arteriole or constrict the efferent arteriole increase the GFR; those that constrict the afferent arteriole or relax the efferent arteriole reduce the GFR. Blood vessels surround and outnumber tubular segments of each nephron and form a peritubular network of capillaries that allows exchange of water, electrolytes, and other substances. This exchange is the target for actions of many drugs, especially diuretics.

Histology of Renal Corpuscle

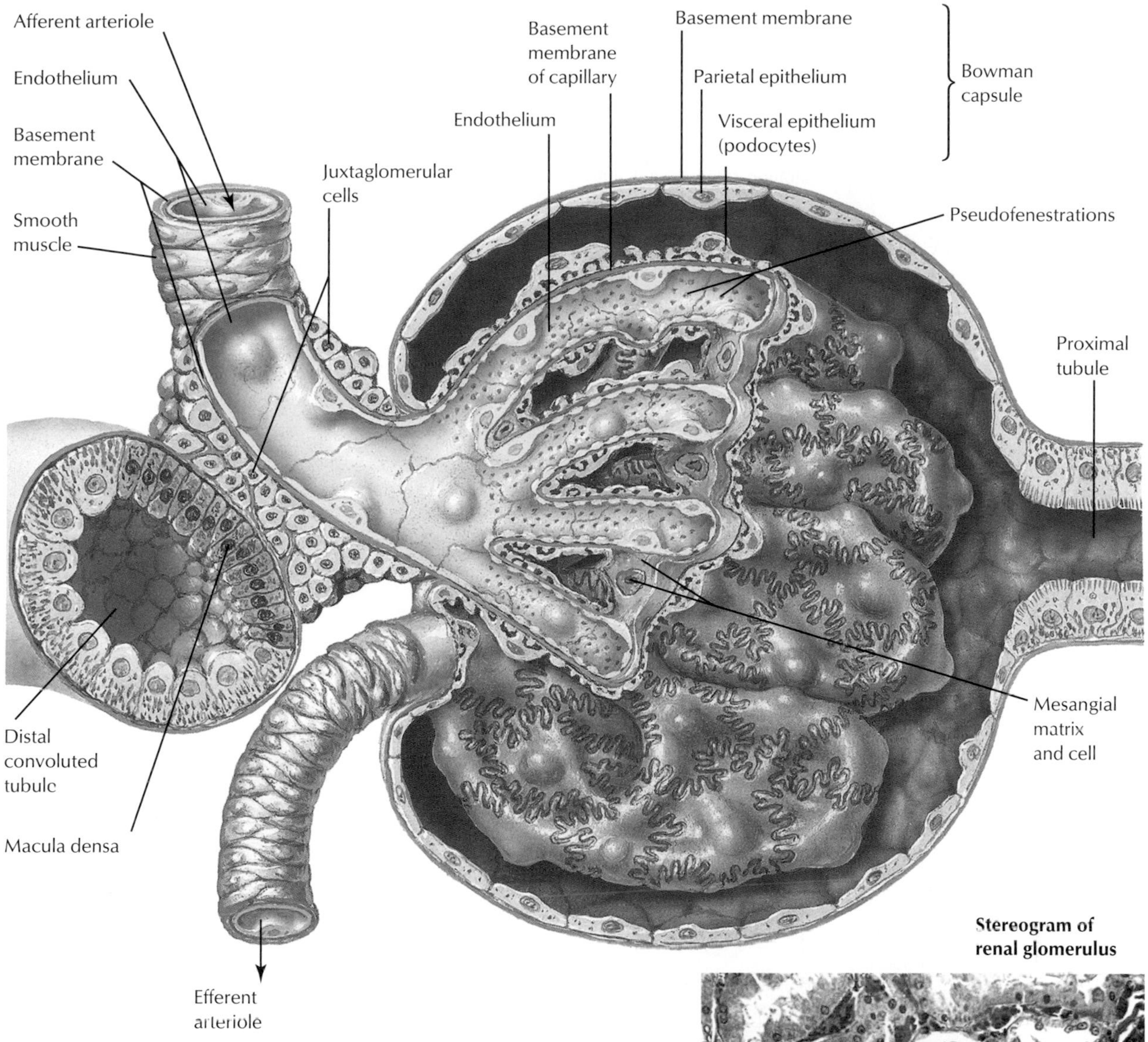

Afferent arteriole

Endothelium

Basement membrane

Smooth muscle

Juxtaglomerular cells

Basement membrane of capillary

Endothelium

Basement membrane

Parietal epithelium

Visceral epithelium (podocytes)

Bowman capsule

Pseudofenestrations

Proximal tubule

Distal convoluted tubule

Macula densa

Efferent arteriole

Mesangial matrix and cell

Stereogram of renal glomerulus

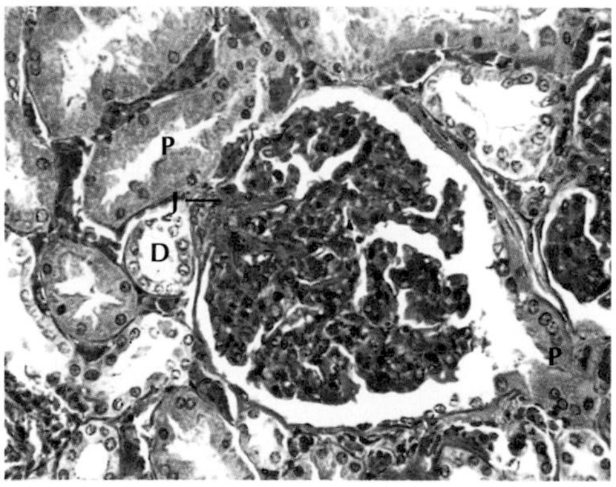

Glomerulus (human); H and E stain, 3350
P = Proximal tubule
D = Distal tubule
P = Juxtaglomerular cells

FIGURE 9-4 THE GLOMERULUS

The glomerulus is an important interface between afferent arteriolar blood flow and the nephron. The glomerulus filters plasma, and the fluid, minus cells, enters the nephron as an ultrafiltrate. The glomerulus is also a barrier to molecules larger than approximately 5 kd (eg, plasma proteins). Thus, plasma proteins and drug molecules bound to them do not pass into nephrons of a healthy kidney; only smaller free drug or metabolite molecules do so. However, damaged glomeruli allow passage of plasma proteins, and the presence of these proteins in the urine indicates a renal disorder. In renal disease, drugs enter the nephron and are excreted at a rate greater than normal, which is noted as a shorter plasma half-life of drugs (or metabolites). Hormones and hormone-mimetic drugs that alter the GFR include angiotensin II (constricts afferent arterioles and thereby reduces the GFR) and atrial natriuretic peptide and prostaglandin E_2 (dilate afferent arterioles and thus increase it).

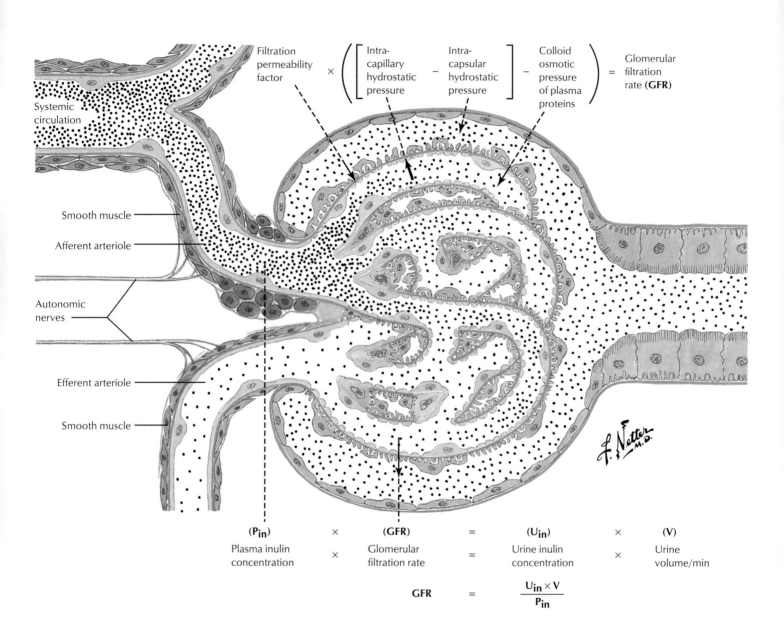

Filtration permeability factor $\times \left(\left[\begin{array}{c} \text{Intra-capillary hydrostatic pressure} \end{array} - \begin{array}{c} \text{Intra-capsular hydrostatic pressure} \end{array} \right] - \begin{array}{c} \text{Colloid osmotic pressure of plasma proteins} \end{array} \right) = \begin{array}{c} \text{Glomerular filtration rate (GFR)} \end{array}$

Systemic circulation

Smooth muscle

Afferent arteriole

Autonomic nerves

Efferent arteriole

Smooth muscle

(P_{in})	$\times$	(GFR)	$=$	(U_{in})	$\times$	(V)
Plasma inulin concentration	$\times$	Glomerular filtration rate	$=$	Urine inulin concentration	$\times$	Urine volume/min

$$GFR = \frac{U_{in} \times V}{P_{in}}$$

FIGURE 9-5 PRACTICAL APPLICATION: MEASURING THE GLOMERULAR FILTRATION RATE

The GFR is an important characteristic of kidney functioning and an important variable in elimination of drugs and their metabolites. In general, the greater the GFR is, the greater the rate of elimination is. The GFR can be measured noninvasively by determining the rate at which a substance is removed from plasma (or appears in urine), which requires the use of a substance that is freely filtered by the glomerulus and is neither reabsorbed nor secreted within the nephron. These criteria are fulfilled by the 5-kd fructose polysaccharide inulin. For the assay, after a uniform blood level of inulin is established, measurement of the concentration of inulin in plasma (P_{in}), the concentration of inulin in urine (U_{in}), and urine flow rate (V) yields the GFR from the equation: GFR = (V × U_{in})/P_{in}. The GFR of a healthy adult kidney is approximately 120 mL/min. Decreased clearance, which is common in the elderly, usually results in slower drug elimination and requires an appropriate dosage adjustment.

Stereogram of Proximal Segment of Renal Tubule

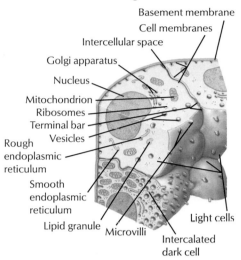

Labels: Basement membrane; Microvilli (brush border); Cell margins interdigitating; Rough endoplasmic reticulum; Invagination; Vacuole; Mitochondria; Basal infoldings; Basal process; Lateral process full height of cell; Ribosomes; Nucleus; Golgi apparatus; Terminal bar; Intercellular space; Cell borders; Basal infolding and process from adjacent cell; Lysosome (or protein granule)

Stereogram of Cells of Collecting Tubule

Labels: Basement membrane; Cell membranes; Intercellular space; Golgi apparatus; Nucleus; Mitochondrion; Ribosomes; Terminal bar; Vesicles; Rough endoplasmic reticulum; Smooth endoplasmic reticulum; Lipid granule; Microvilli; Light cells; Intercalated dark cell

Stereogram of Thin Segment of Renal Tubule

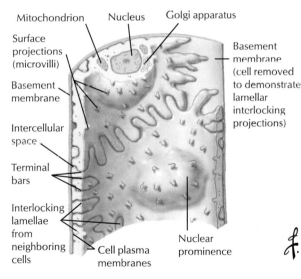

Labels: Mitochondrion; Nucleus; Golgi apparatus; Surface projections (microvilli); Basement membrane; Intercellular space; Terminal bars; Interlocking lamellae from neighboring cells; Cell plasma membranes; Nuclear prominence; Basement membrane (cell removed to demonstrate lamellar interlocking projections)

Stereogram of Distal Segment Cells of Renal Tubule

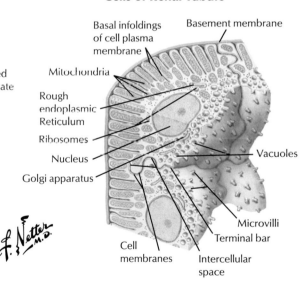

Labels: Basal infoldings of cell plasma membrane; Basement membrane; Mitochondria; Rough endoplasmic Reticulum; Ribosomes; Nucleus; Golgi apparatus; Cell membranes; Intercellular space; Terminal bar; Microvilli; Vacuoles

F. Netter M.D.

FIGURE 9-6 TUBULAR SEGMENTS

The structure and function of tubular segments are important for understanding drug effects on the kidney. The proximal portion and thick segment of the descending limb have a similar structure (slight variation in cell size and shape). Tight junctions between cells prevent escape of material in the tubular lumen. Proximal segment cells act to reabsorb water and other substances. The proximal segment's brush border is replaced in the thin tubular segment by fewer short microvilli. Permeability to water and position of descending and ascending limbs of the Henle loop create a countercurrent multiplier for urine concentration. The distal segment of the nephron consists of the thick ascending limb of the Henle loop and the distal convoluted tubule. The ultrastructure and large surface area of the distal segment serve the energy requirements of active Na^+ transport from luminal fluid, formation of ammonia, and urine acidification. Drug action in each segment alters kidney function in specific ways.

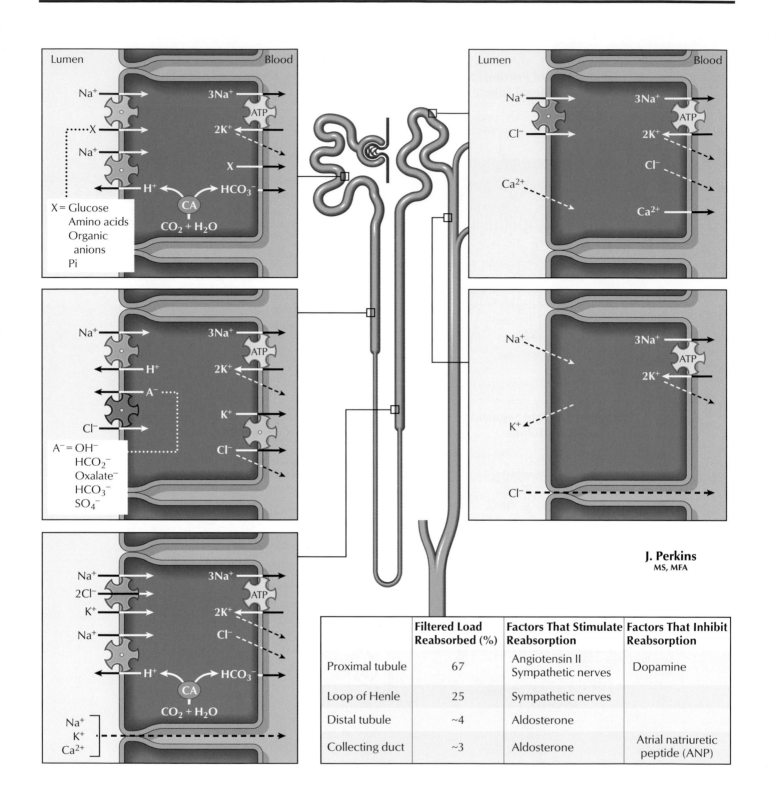

	Filtered Load Reabsorbed (%)	Factors That Stimulate Reabsorption	Factors That Inhibit Reabsorption
Proximal tubule	67	Angiotensin II Sympathetic nerves	Dopamine
Loop of Henle	25	Sympathetic nerves	
Distal tubule	~4	Aldosterone	
Collecting duct	~3	Aldosterone	Atrial natriuretic peptide (ANP)

J. Perkins
MS, MFA

FIGURE 9-7 ION AND WATER REABSORPTION

More than 99% of glomerular ultrafiltrate is reabsorbed from the tubular lumen. The kidney is thus more an organ of retention than of elimination. The driving factor for water and Na^+ reabsorption in the nephron is active Na^+ transport. Drugs affecting Na^+ transport can alter urine flow and composition. Na^+ reabsorption occurs against concentration and electrical potential gradients (the lumen is electrically negative compared with peritubular fluid) and is an active process requiring energy (supplied by ATP). The active uptake mechanism (pump) for Na^+ involves a cotransporter that exchanges Na^+ for K^+, an important factor for drugs that affect Na^+ transport. Cl^- and other ions move by cotransport with Na^+ or other ions or by passive diffusion. The osmotic gradient (established by ion transport) drives water out of the lumen. Hormones and drugs that decrease ion transport or the osmotic gradient reduce ion and water reabsorption and thus increase urine flow (diuresis) and ion content.

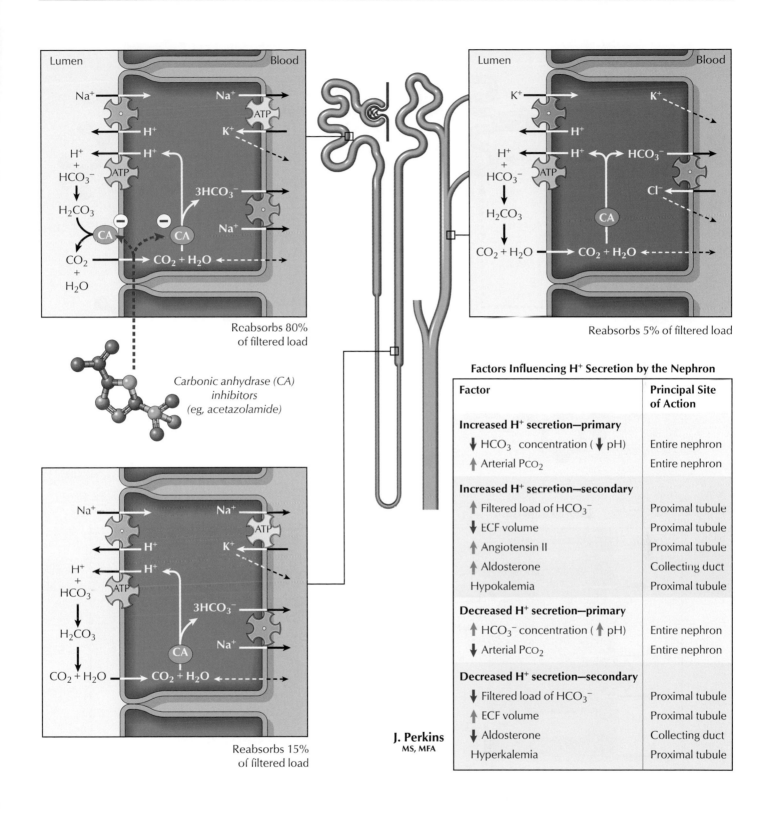

Reabsorbs 80%
of filtered load

*Carbonic anhydrase (CA)
inhibitors
(eg, acetazolamide)*

Reabsorbs 5% of filtered load

Reabsorbs 15%
of filtered load

J. Perkins
MS, MFA

Factors Influencing H⁺ Secretion by the Nephron

Factor	Principal Site of Action
Increased H⁺ secretion—primary	
↓ HCO₃ concentration (↓ pH)	Entire nephron
↑ Arterial P_{CO_2}	Entire nephron
Increased H⁺ secretion—secondary	
↑ Filtered load of HCO_3^-	Proximal tubule
↓ ECF volume	Proximal tubule
↑ Angiotensin II	Proximal tubule
↑ Aldosterone	Collecting duct
Hypokalemia	Proximal tubule
Decreased H⁺ secretion—primary	
↑ HCO_3^- concentration (↑ pH)	Entire nephron
↓ Arterial P_{CO_2}	Entire nephron
Decreased H⁺ secretion—secondary	
↓ Filtered load of HCO_3^-	Proximal tubule
↑ ECF volume	Proximal tubule
↓ Aldosterone	Collecting duct
Hyperkalemia	Proximal tubule

FIGURE 9-8 BICARBONATE REABSORPTION

A notable ion with regard to drug metabolism is bicarbonate, or HCO_3^-. HCO_3^- and Cl^- are the most relevant ions for the class of diuretic drugs known as carbonic anhydrase inhibitors. HCO_3^- is freely filtered through the glomerulus and enters the nephron. Almost all of it is reabsorbed along the tubule—most of it (80%–85%) in the proximal convoluted tubule—in a process that involves H⁺ secretion, and thus reabsorption of HCO_3^- is inhibited by carbonic anhydrase inhibitors. Although usually all the filtered HCO_3^- is reabsorbed and none is excreted in the urine, a number of factors influence H⁺ secretion by the nephron, and a small amount of HCO_3^- can be lost in the urine. The kidneys generate new HCO_3^- to replenish this loss. Acetazolamide is a diuretic that affects HCO_3^- exchange, predominantly at the proximal convoluted tubule (see Figure 9-14).

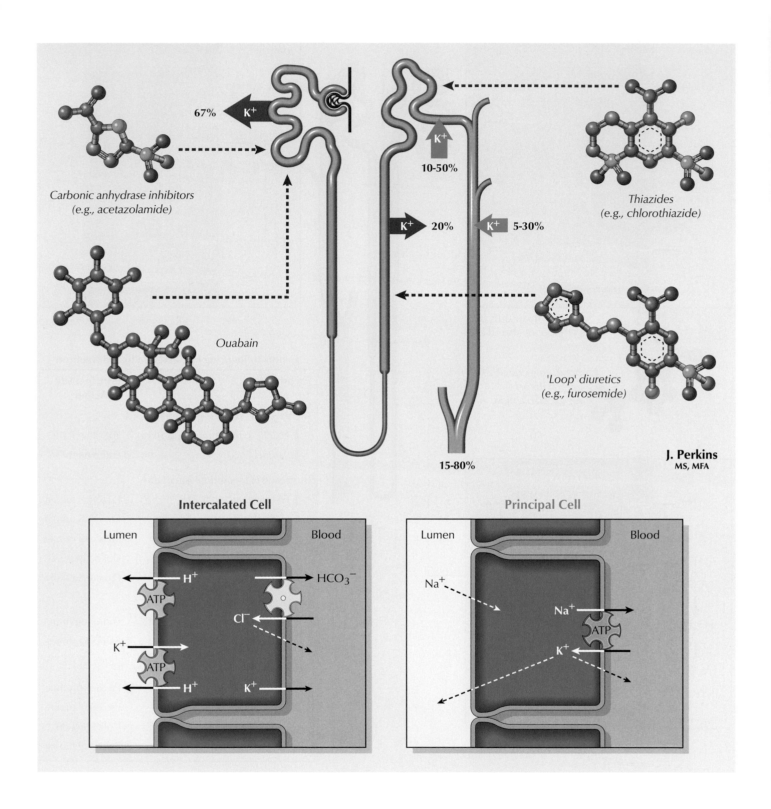

FIGURE 9-9 POTASSIUM EXCRETION

The kidneys are the primary route of excretion of K⁺ from the body. Although a large fraction of the filtered K⁺ is reabsorbed along the proximal convoluted tubule and the loop of Henle, the amount of K⁺ excretion in the urine is determined mainly by the highly variable secretory activity of the distal convoluted tubule. Several diuretics and other drugs cause excess urinary K⁺ loss as a side effect by increasing the distal tubular flow rate and Na⁺ delivery (eg, ethacrynic acid and furosemide), by alkalinizing the distal tubular fluid (eg, carbonic anhydrase inhibitors such as acetazolamide), or by blocking tubular K⁺ reabsorption (eg, oua-bain). Some diuretics, known as *potassium-sparing diuretics*, do not cause K⁺ loss (see Figure 9-16).

ADH is produced in supraoptic and paraventricular nuclei of hypothalamus and descends along nerve fibers to neurohypophysis, where it is stored for subsequent release.

Blood osmolality and volume are modified by fluid intake (oral or parenteral); water and electrolyte exchange with tissues, normal or pathologic (edema); loss via gut (vomiting, diarrhea); loss into body cavities (ascites, effusion); or loss externally (hemorrhage, sweat).

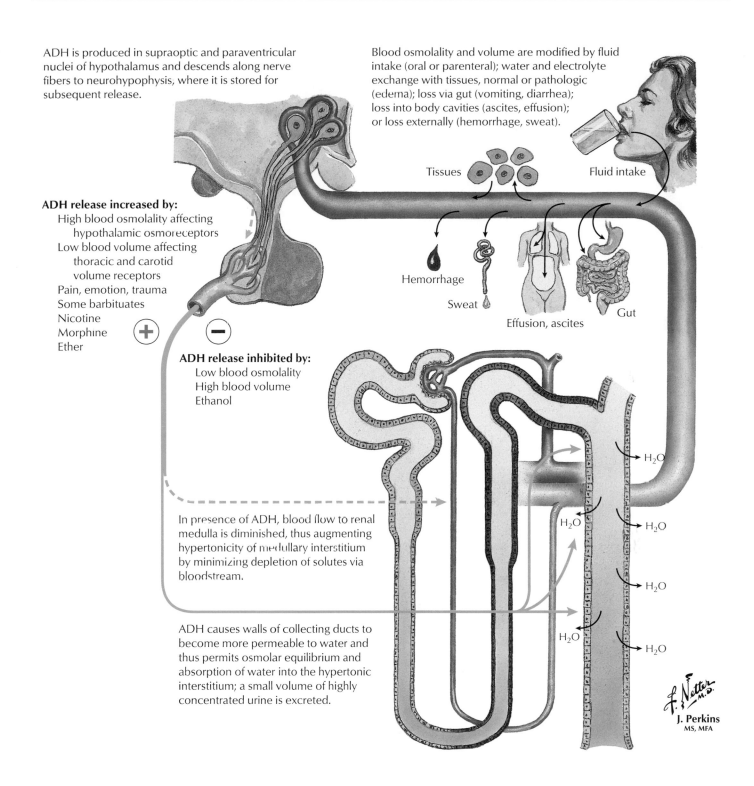

ADH release increased by:
High blood osmolality affecting
hypothalamic osmoreceptors
Low blood volume affecting
thoracic and carotid
volume receptors
Pain, emotion, trauma
Some barbituates
Nicotine
Morphine
Ether

ADH release inhibited by:
Low blood osmolality
High blood volume
Ethanol

In presence of ADH, blood flow to renal medulla is diminished, thus augmenting hypertonicity of medullary interstitium by minimizing depletion of solutes via bloodstream.

ADH causes walls of collecting ducts to become more permeable to water and thus permits osmolar equilibrium and absorption of water into the hypertonic interstitium; a small volume of highly concentrated urine is excreted.

J. Perkins
MS, MFA

FIGURE 9-10 ANTIDIURETIC HORMONE

Antidiuretic hormone, also known as *arginine vasopressin* in humans, is a 1-kd nonapeptide that is synthesized in the hypothalamus and released into the blood from the posterior pituitary gland. It is structurally similar to oxytocin but is a more potent (>100 times) antidiuretic. ADH alters the morphology of cells of the collecting duct and increases their permeability. Water passes from the collecting duct lumen into the renal interstitium, so an osmotic equilibrium between interstitium and fluid in the duct occurs. In the presence of ADH, the amount of water that can be reabsorbed from collecting ducts is limited only by the amount flowing through them. Various stimuli induce ADH release (and thus production of a small volume of concentrated urine): plasma osmolality, pain, emotion, trauma, and drugs (eg, nicotine, morphine, ether, some barbiturates). ADH is inhibited by ethanol.

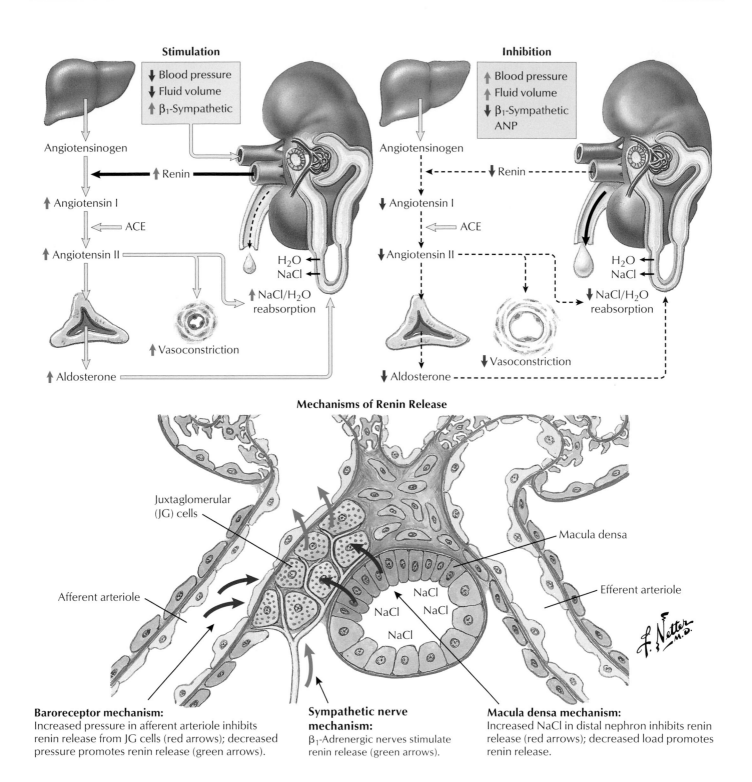

Mechanisms of Renin Release

Juxtaglomerular (JG) cells

Macula densa

Afferent arteriole

Efferent arteriole

NaCl
NaCl   NaCl
NaCl

Baroreceptor mechanism:
Increased pressure in afferent arteriole inhibits renin release from JG cells (red arrows); decreased pressure promotes renin release (green arrows).

Sympathetic nerve mechanism:
β₁-Adrenergic nerves stimulate renin release (green arrows).

Macula densa mechanism:
Increased NaCl in distal nephron inhibits renin release (red arrows); decreased load promotes renin release.

Stimulation
- ↓ Blood pressure
- ↓ Fluid volume
- ↑ β₁-Sympathetic

Angiotensinogen
↑ Angiotensin I
← ACE
↑ Angiotensin II
↑ Aldosterone
↑ Renin
↑ NaCl/H₂O reabsorption
↑ Vasoconstriction
H₂O
NaCl

Inhibition
- ↑ Blood pressure
- ↑ Fluid volume
- ↓ β₁-Sympathetic
  ANP

Angiotensinogen
↓ Angiotensin I
← ACE
↓ Angiotensin II
↓ Aldosterone
↓ Renin
↓ NaCl/H₂O reabsorption
↓ Vasoconstriction
H₂O
NaCl

FIGURE 9-11 RENIN-ANGIOTENSIN-ALDOSTERONE SYSTEM

In addition to ADH, a second volume-regulating system—the renin-angiotensin-aldosterone system—involves the kidney. The kidneys synthesize and secrete renin, a proteolytic enzyme of approximately 40 kd, in response to decreased blood pressure, fluid volume, and Na^+ and increased H^+. Renin secretion results in conversion of angiotensinogen (a blood-borne α globulin produced by the liver) to the decapeptide angiotensin I. Angiotensin I is converted (primarily in lungs) to angiotensin II, which is a potent vasoconstrictor and a stimulator of aldosterone release from the adrenal gland. Angiotensin II and aldosterone stimulate NaCl and water reabsorption by the proximal convoluted tubule and the collecting duct, respectively. The enzyme that catalyzes conversion of angiotensin I to angiotensin II, termed *angiotensin-converting enzyme* (ACE), is the target of the ACE inhibitor class of antihypertensive drugs.

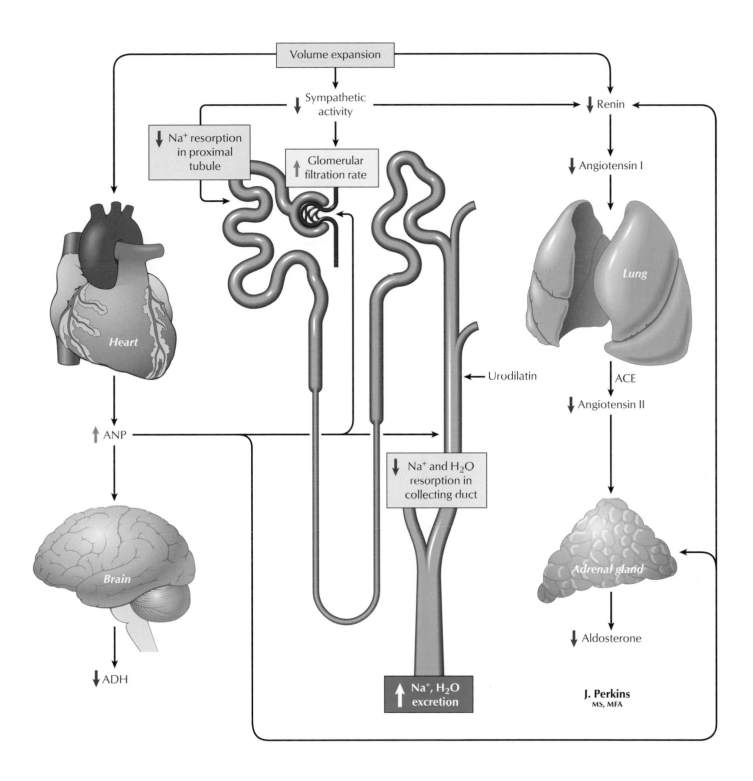

FIGURE 9-12   GENERAL CONSIDERATIONS: VOLUME HOMEOSTASIS

The kidneys are part of an integrated homeostatic mechanism for maintaining the volume of the extracellular fluid. Other organs involved in this mechanism include the heart (eg, cardiac output and heart rate), the CNS (eg, sympathetic tone and ADH release), the lungs (eg, conversion of angiotensin I to angiotensin II), and the adrenal gland (eg, release of aldosterone). Several feedback control mechanisms operate among the components of this control mechanism, which ensure responses to volume expansion

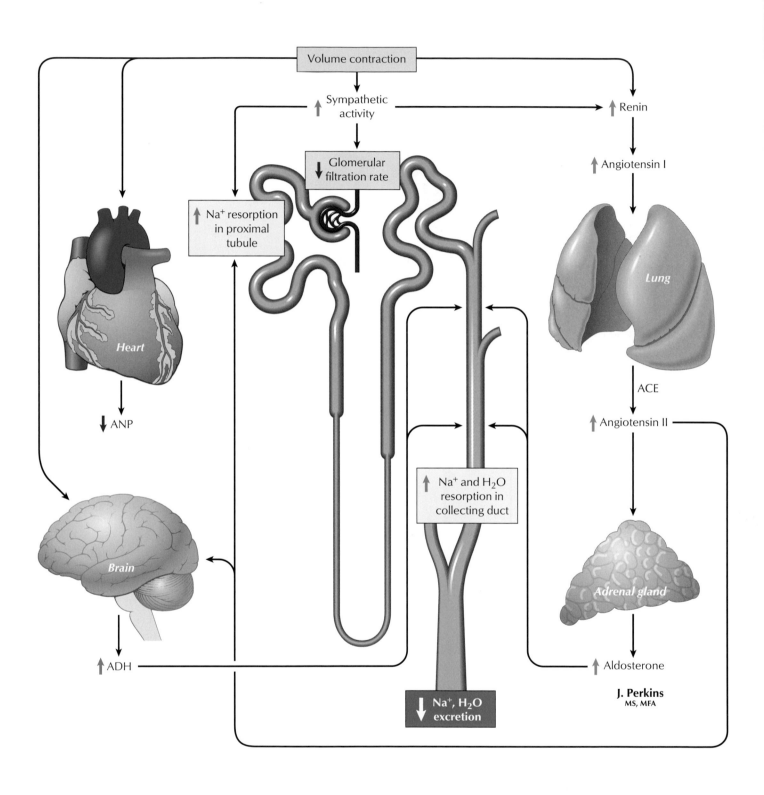

FIGURE 9-12 GENERAL CONSIDERATIONS: VOLUME HOMEOSTASIS (continued)

(increased extracellular fluid) and volume contraction (decreased extracellular fluid). The design of drugs that selectively target the components of this system has led to major advances in therapy for cardiovascular diseases such as hypertension and heart failure (discussed in chapter 4).

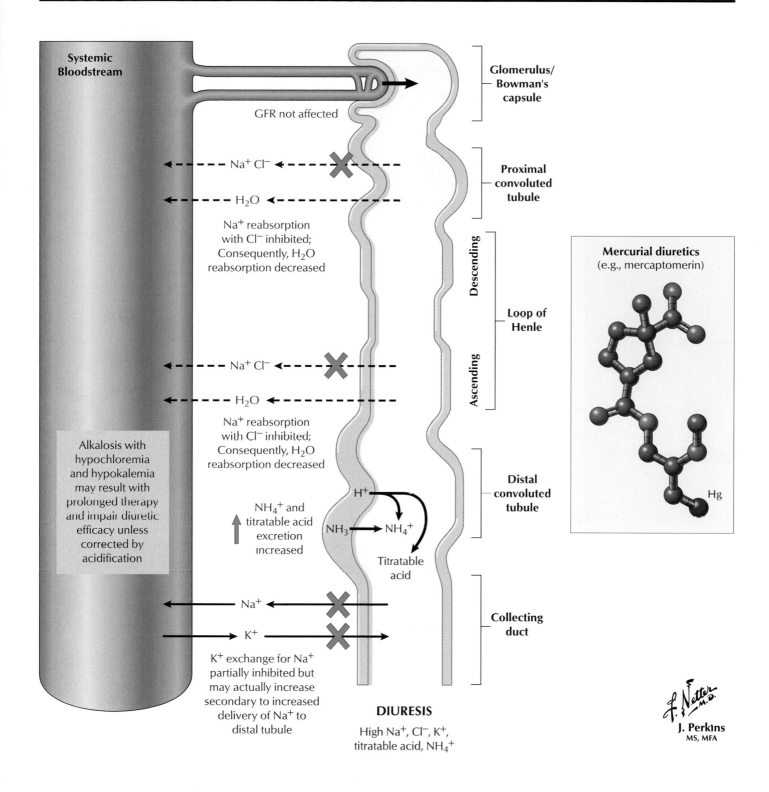

Systemic Bloodstream

Glomerulus/ Bowman's capsule

GFR not affected

$Na^+ Cl^-$

H_2O

Proximal convoluted tubule

Na^+ reabsorption with Cl^- inhibited; Consequently, H_2O reabsorption decreased

Descending

Loop of Henle

Mercurial diuretics (e.g., mercaptomerin)

$Na^+ Cl^-$

H_2O

Ascending

Na^+ reabsorption with Cl^- inhibited; Consequently, H_2O reabsorption decreased

Alkalosis with hypochloremia and hypokalemia may result with prolonged therapy and impair diuretic efficacy unless corrected by acidification

H^+

NH_4^+ and titratable acid excretion increased

$NH_3 \rightarrow NH_4^+$

Titratable acid

Distal convoluted tubule

Na^+

K^+

Collecting duct

K^+ exchange for Na^+ partially inhibited but may actually increase secondary to increased delivery of Na^+ to distal tubule

DIURESIS

High Na^+, Cl^-, K^+, titratable acid, NH_4^+

J. Netter M.D.

J. Perkins
MS, MFA

FIGURE 9-13 MERCURIAL DIURETICS

Organomercurial agents inhibit active Cl^- transport, especially in the ascending limb of the Henle loop. In acidic conditions, Hg^{2+} dissociates, binds to, and inhibits sulfhydryl enzymes. Na^+ reabsorption is thus decreased; more Na^+ and Cl^- are excreted. Because more Na^+ is delivered to the distal nephron during diuresis, K^+ and H^+ excretion (sum of urinary NH_4^+ + titratable acid − urinary HCO_3^-) may increase. In alkaline conditions, Hg^{2+} does not dissociate, and patients become refractory to mercurials. Acidifying agents (eg, NH_4Cl) can be used to counteract this effect. Mercurial diuretics (eg, mercaptomerin) are poorly absorbed when taken orally, so an intramuscular route is required. Because of this difficulty and their toxicity (eg, systemic poisoning, cardiac toxicity, hypersensitivity, worsening of renal insufficiency), mercurials are largely obsolete. They are sometimes used for CHF, cirrhosis, and portal obstruction because they do not deplete K^+.

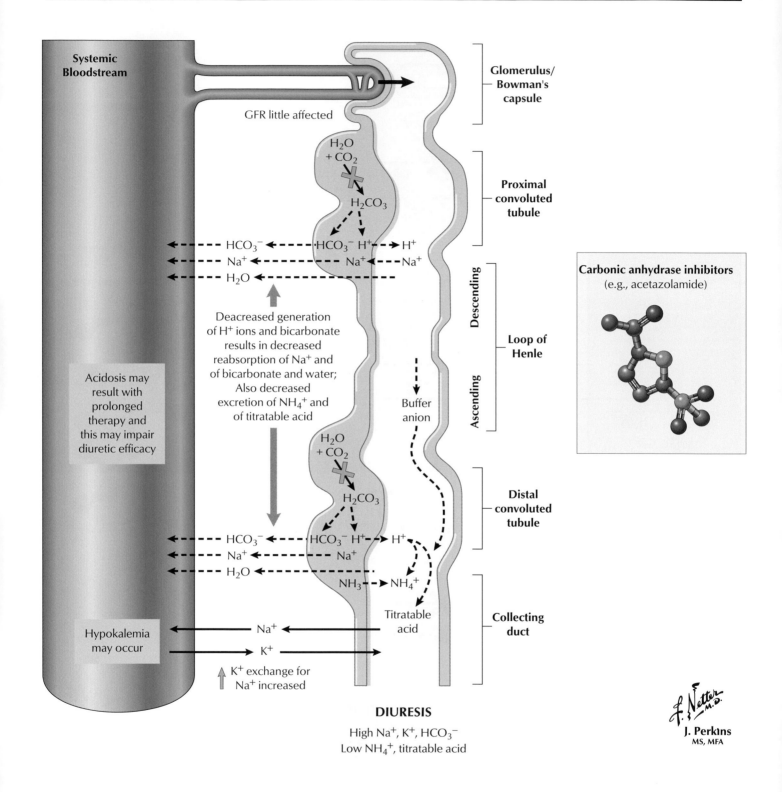

Systemic Bloodstream

GFR little affected

Glomerulus/ Bowman's capsule

$H_2O + CO_2$

H_2CO_3

Proximal convoluted tubule

HCO_3^- HCO_3^- H^+ H^+

Na^+ Na^+ Na^+

H_2O

Descending

Loop of Henle

Deacreased generation of H^+ ions and bicarbonate results in decreased reabsorption of Na^+ and of bicarbonate and water; Also decreased excretion of NH_4^+ and of titratable acid

Ascending

Buffer anion

Acidosis may result with prolonged therapy and this may impair diuretic efficacy

$H_2O + CO_2$

H_2CO_3

Distal convoluted tubule

HCO_3^- HCO_3^- H^+ H^+

Na^+ Na^+

H_2O

NH_3 NH_4^+

Titratable acid

Collecting duct

Hypokalemia may occur

Na^+ Na^+

K^+ K^+

↑ K^+ exchange for Na^+ increased

Carbonic anhydrase inhibitors
(e.g., acetazolamide)

DIURESIS
High Na^+, K^+, HCO_3^-
Low NH_4^+, titratable acid

J. Perkins
MS, MFA

FIGURE 9-14 CARBONIC ANHYDRASE INHIBITORS

Diuretic drugs such as acetazolamide, brinzolamide, dichlorphenamide, and dorzolamide inhibit carbonic anhydrase, particularly at the proximal convoluted tubule. Carbonic anhydrase catalyzes dehydration of carbonic acid (H_2CO_3). As a result, H^+ needed for Na^+-H^+ exchange is reduced, HCO_3^- and Na^+ reabsorption in proximal tubules is suppressed, and diuresis is promoted. Because of the decreased reabsorption of Na^+, Na^+-K^+ exchange increases in the distal convoluted tubules. Increased amounts of Na^+, K^+, and HCO_3^- are excreted in the urine, and Cl^- is retained. Acidosis that may result eventually leads to a refractory response to the diuretic. Carbonic anhydrase inhibitors are relatively weak diuretics. They are also used for glaucoma (to reduce formation of aqueous humor), petit mal epilepsy (mechanism unclear), and salicylate or HCO_3^- poisoning (to alkalinize urine). These agents can cause CNS effects, hypokalemia, and hyperglycemia.

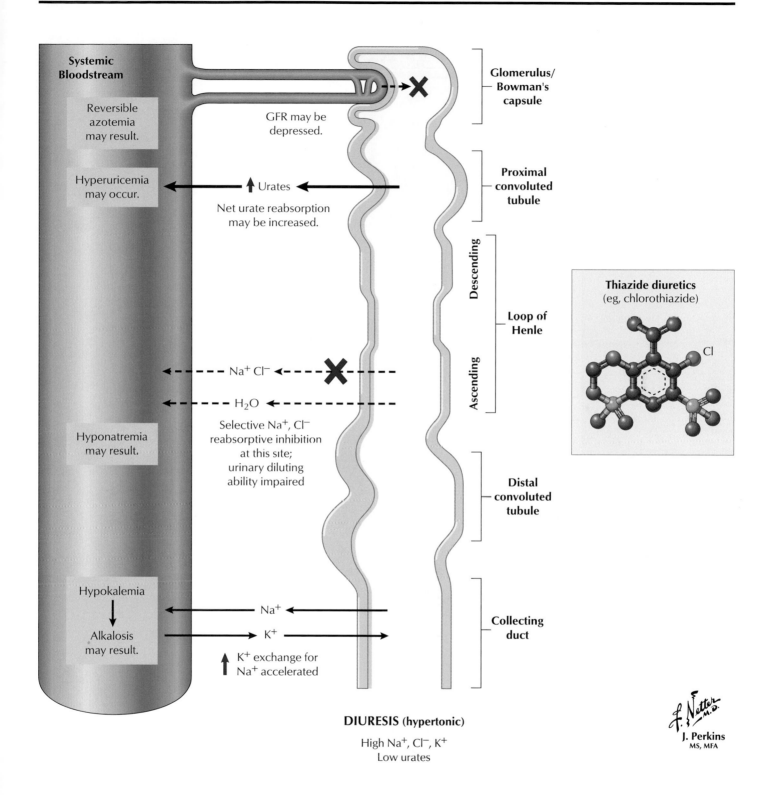

Systemic Bloodstream

Reversible azotemia may result.

Hyperuricemia may occur.

Hyponatremia may result.

Hypokalemia
↓
Alkalosis may result.

Glomerulus/ Bowman's capsule

GFR may be depressed.

↑ Urates

Net urate reabsorption may be increased.

Proximal convoluted tubule

Descending

Loop of Henle

Ascending

Na⁺ Cl⁻

H₂O

Selective Na⁺, Cl⁻ reabsorptive inhibition at this site; urinary diluting ability impaired

Distal convoluted tubule

Na⁺

K⁺

↑ K⁺ exchange for Na⁺ accelerated

Collecting duct

Thiazide diuretics
(eg, chlorothiazide)

Cl

DIURESIS (hypertonic)

High Na⁺, Cl⁻, K⁺
Low urates

J. Perkins
MS, MFA

FIGURE 9-15 THIAZIDE DIURETICS

Thiazide (benzothiadiazide) diuretics—bendroflumethiazide, chlorothiazide, hydrochlorothiazide, hydroflumethiazide, methyclothiazide, polythiazide, trichlormethiazide—inhibit Cl⁻ reabsorption, especially in the distal portion of the ascending limb of the Henle loop and the proximal portion of the distal convoluted tubule. Excretion of Na⁺, K⁺, Cl⁻, and HCO₃⁻ is increased; refractoriness does not develop to the diuretic effect. Thiazide diuretics are often used to treat chronic edema and essential hypertension and, less often, nephrosis, some forms of diabetes insipidus, and hypercalciuria. Common adverse effects are hypokalemia (K⁺ supplements are recommended), which may lead to alkalosis, and hyperglycemia. Extra caution is needed when these agents are used with digitalis for CHF because of greater digitalis toxicity in conditions of low K⁺. Because thiazides are excreted via glomerular filtration and tubular secretion, they compete with uric acid for tubular secretion.

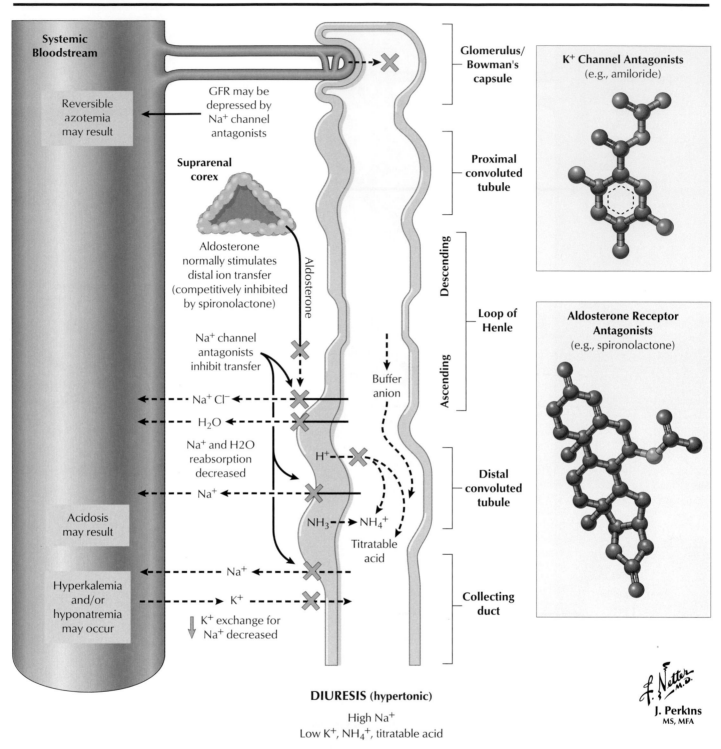

FIGURE 9-16 POTASSIUM-SPARING AGENTS

Two major categories of K+-sparing diuretic drugs are Na+ channel antagonists (eg, amiloride, triamterene) and aldosterone receptor antagonists (eg, spironolactone). The former inhibit active Na+ reuptake. Enhanced Na+ and Cl− excretion disrupts Na+ transport and reduces K+ secretion. These drugs moderately increase Na+, Cl−, and HCO3− excretion; when they are used with other diuretics, Na+ excretion increases and K+ is retained. Reversible azotemia can occur. Triamterene can increase serum uric acid levels, so caution is needed for its use in patients with gout. Spironolactone reduces aldosterone-mediated Na+-K+ exchange at the distal convoluted tubule, which increases Na+ loss while reducing K+ excretion. Adverse effects of both types of drugs include hyperkalemia (especially when impaired renal function exists). Combination therapy with K+-sparing drugs is not usually advised, but they are often used with diuretics (eg, thiazides) that increase K+ excretion.

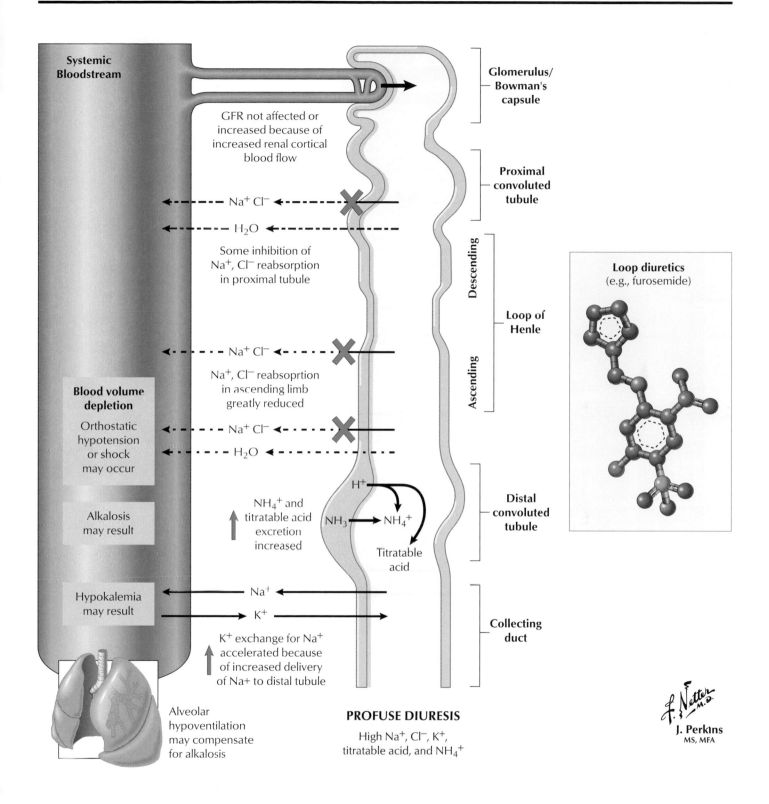

Systemic Bloodstream

GFR not affected or increased because of increased renal cortical blood flow

$Na^+ Cl^-$

H_2O

Some inhibition of Na^+, Cl^- reabsorption in proximal tubule

$Na^+ Cl^-$

Na^+, Cl^- reabsorption in ascending limb greatly reduced

Blood volume depletion

Orthostatic hypotension or shock may occur

$Na^+ Cl^-$

H_2O

Alkalosis may result

NH_4^+ and titratable acid excretion increased

Hypokalemia may result

Na^+

K^+

K^+ exchange for Na^+ accelerated because of increased delivery of Na^+ to distal tubule

Alveolar hypoventilation may compensate for alkalosis

Loop diuretics (e.g., furosemide)

Glomerulus/ Bowman's capsule

Proximal convoluted tubule

Descending

Loop of Henle

Ascending

H^+

$NH_3 \rightarrow NH_4^+$

Titratable acid

Distal convoluted tubule

Collecting duct

PROFUSE DIURESIS

High Na^+, Cl^-, K^+, titratable acid, and NH_4^+

J. Perkins
MS, MFA

FIGURE 9-17 LOOP (HIGH-CEILING) DIURETICS

This class of diuretic drugs (eg, bumetanide, ethacrynic acid, furosemide, torsemide) acts mainly on the thick ascending limb of the Henle loop. Because they elicit the greatest diuresis possible, they are also termed *high-ceiling diuretics*. They act at the luminal nephron surface and inhibit electrolyte reabsorption, with resultant greater Na^+, Cl^-, K^+, Mg^{2+}, and Ca^{2+} excretion. Inhibition of NaCl reabsorption in the Henle loop decreases the strength of the countercurrent concentrating mechanism and

causes greatly increased urine output. Bumetanide, furosemide, and torsemide are weak inhibitors of carbonic anhydrase; ethacrynic acid, which is not a sulfonamide, does not inhibit this enzyme. The drugs increase Cl^- more than Na^+ excretion, which can lead to hypochloremic alkalosis. Refractoriness does not occur. Loop diuretics are used for acute pulmonary edema, edema associated with CHF, cirrhosis, and renal disease. Fluid and electrolyte imbalances are the most common adverse effects.

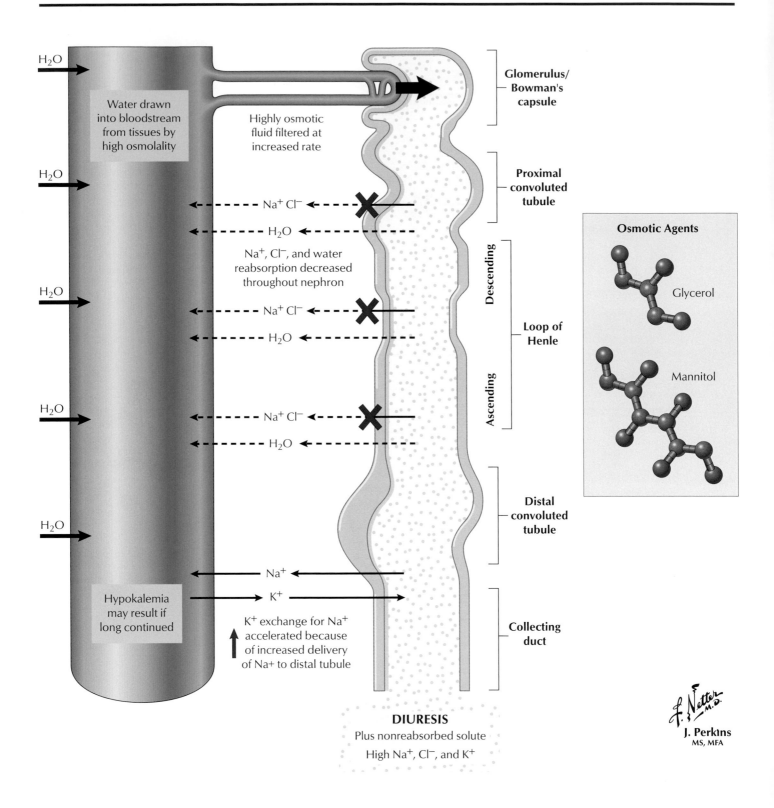

Osmotic Agents

Glycerol

Mannitol

H$_2$O

Water drawn into bloodstream from tissues by high osmolality

H$_2$O

Highly osmotic fluid filtered at increased rate

Glomerulus/ Bowman's capsule

Proximal convoluted tubule

Na$^+$ Cl$^-$

H$_2$O

Na$^+$, Cl$^-$, and water reabsorption decreased throughout nephron

H$_2$O

Na$^+$ Cl$^-$

H$_2$O

Descending

Ascending

Loop of Henle

H$_2$O

Na$^+$ Cl$^-$

H$_2$O

Distal convoluted tubule

H$_2$O

Na$^+$

K$^+$

Hypokalemia may result if long continued

K$^+$ exchange for Na$^+$ accelerated because of increased delivery of Na+ to distal tubule

Collecting duct

DIURESIS
Plus nonreabsorbed solute
High Na$^+$, Cl$^-$, and K$^+$

J. Perkins
MS, MFA

FIGURE 9-18 OSMOTIC AGENTS

Osmotic diuretics (eg, mannitol, glycerol) enter the nephron through the glomerulus but are poorly reabsorbed along the nephron because of their relatively large molecular size. The presence of unabsorbed molecules in the tubule lumen creates a concentration (osmotic) gradient across the tubular membrane. In the proximal convoluted tubule, reabsorption of Na$^+$ and water decreases, which produces diuresis without marked changes in Na$^+$ or Cl$^-$ excretion. Mannitol, the agent used most

often, is a hexacarbon sugar alcohol that is given intravenously; it is not metabolized. Osmotic diuretics are used to treat cerebral edema and glaucoma (by reducing cerebrospinal or intraocular fluid pressure), oliguria and anuria, and certain phases of acute renal failure (as prophylaxis). Because osmotic diuretics increase blood volume, adverse effects include decompensation in patients with CHF. Hyperosmolarity or hyponatremia can occur during therapy of renal failure or cirrhosis.

DRUG	ROUTE OF ADMIN.	MAJOR SITES OF ACTION	MAJOR EFFECT ON Na$^+$ REABSORPTION
Mercurial diuretics (e.g., meralluride, chlormerodrin)	Intra-muscular	Proximal and/or distal tubules and loop of Henle	Block isosmotic Na$^+$, Cl$^-$, reabsorption
Carbonic anhydrase inhibitors (e.g., acetazolamide, dichlorphenamide)	Oral	Proximal tubules	Reduce secretion of H$^+$ and net Na$^+$, HCO$_3^-$ reabsorption by inhibition of carbonic anhydrase
Thiazides (e.g., chlorothiazide)	Oral	Loop of Henle and distal tubule within renal cortex	Inhibit selective Na$^+$, Cl$^-$ reabsorption at distal diluting segment (urinary dilution impaired)
Potassium-sparing diuretics (e.g., amiloride, triamterene, spironolactone)	Oral	Distal tubules, collecting ducts	Amiloride/Triamterene: Directly inhibit distal Na$^+$, Cl$^-$ reabsorption and distal Na$^+$ exchange for H$^+$, K$^+$ Spironolactone: Competitive antagonist of aldosterone-stimulated reabsorption of Na$^+$ with Cl$^-$ and of Na$^+$ reabsorption in exchange for H$^+$ and K$^+$
Loop diuretics (e.g., furosemide, ethacrynic acid)	Oral or parenteral	Ascending limb of Henle's loop	Block selective Cl$^-$ and Na$^+$ reabsorption, inhibiting ability of kidney to dilute or concentrate urine
Osmotic agents (e.g., glycerol, mannitol)	Intravenous	Proximal tubules, ascending limb of Henle's loop	Presence of osmotic particles within nephron retards H$_2$O reabsorption and reduces net Na$^+$, Cl$^-$ transport

FIGURE 9-19 SUMMARY OF THERAPEUTICS

Each class of diuretic drug affects various transport processes that are located along different segments of the tubular nephron. Because the drugs tend to have relatively selective actions on specific transport processes and predominant actions on specific segments, they produce characteristic effects on electrolyte and acid-base balances in patients. It is therefore possible to provide

Relative Potency	Effect on K⁺	Effect on Acid Secretion	Effect on Renal Hemodynamics	Particularly Useful for:	Side Effects of Diuresis
+ + + +	Partial inhibition of distal K⁺ secretion but hypokalemia may occur	H⁺ secretion increased	No effect on RPF or GFR	Patients with dilutional hyponatremia; moderate to extensive edema	Hypokalemia and hypochloremic alkalosis; nephrotoxicity in patients with renal disease; hypersensitivity reactions
+ +	K⁺ secretion increased	H⁺ excretion diminished (bicarbonate diuresis)	Little effect on RPF or GFR	Patients with metabolic alkalosis; cor pulmonale	Hyperchloremic acidosis; hypokalemia
+ + +	K⁺ secretion increased	Little effect on net acid-base	May depress RPF or GFR	Mild to moderate edema	Hypokalemia; hypochloremia and metabolic alkalosis; dilutional hyponatremia, prerenal azotemia; hyperuricemia
+	Amiloride/ Triamterene: Depress K⁺ excretion Spironolactone: Retards K⁺ secretion stimulated by aldosterone	Amiloride/ Triamterene: Inhibit distal H⁺ excretion Spironolactone: Retards aldosterone-stimulated H⁺ excretion	Amiloride/ Triamterene: May depress GFR Spironolactone: No effect on RPF	Patients with hyperaldoster-onism (cirrhosis with ascites, nephrosis, severe cardiac failure)	Hyperkalemia; metabolic acidosis; azotemia
+ + + + +	K⁺ secretion increased	H⁺ excretion accelerated	Little effect at low doses; large doses may increase RPF and GFR	Patients with pulmonary edema; edema complicated by azotemia, electrolyte or acid-base disorders	Hypokalemia, hypochloremia; metabolic alkalosis; may lead to extracellular fluid depletion; ototoxicity in patients with renal disease; hyperuricemia
Variable; related to dose	K⁺ secretion slightly increased	H⁺ excretion little affected (some increase in HCO₃⁻ excretion)	RPF and GFR increased	Prerenal azotemia; cerebral edema; poisonings	May produce pulmonary edema in cardiac patients; cellular dehydration; extracellular fluid depletion; hyponatremia if urinary losses are insufficiently replaced

FIGURE 9-19 SUMMARY OF THERAPEUTICS (continued) ————————————

the general mechanistic and adverse effect characteristics of each class of drug. Consideration of the characteristics of each class may facilitate the choice of diuretic or combination of diuretics.

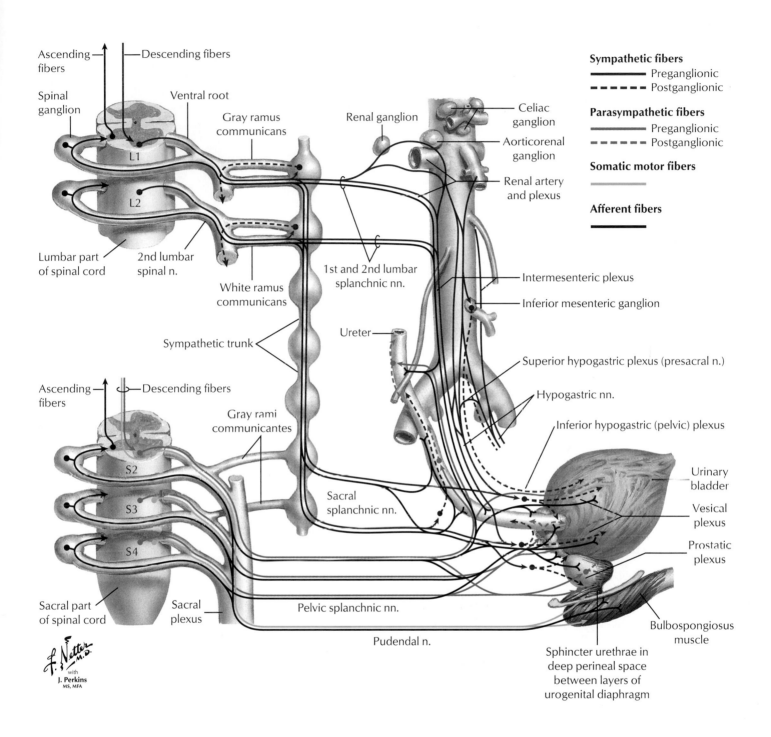

Sympathetic fibers
——— Preganglionic
- - - - Postganglionic

Parasympathetic fibers
——— Preganglionic
- - - - Postganglionic

Somatic motor fibers

Afferent fibers

Ascending fibers — Descending fibers

Spinal ganglion

Ventral root

Gray ramus communicans

Renal ganglion

Celiac ganglion

Aorticorenal ganglion

Renal artery and plexus

L1

L2

Lumbar part of spinal cord

2nd lumbar spinal n.

White ramus communicans

Sympathetic trunk

1st and 2nd lumbar splanchnic nn.

Intermesenteric plexus

Inferior mesenteric ganglion

Ureter

Ascending fibers — Descending fibers

Gray rami communicantes

S2

S3

S4

Superior hypogastric plexus (presacral n.)

Hypogastric nn.

Inferior hypogastric (pelvic) plexus

Urinary bladder

Vesical plexus

Prostatic plexus

Sacral splanchnic nn.

Sacral part of spinal cord

Sacral plexus

Pelvic splanchnic nn.

Pudendal n.

Sphincter urethrae in deep perineal space between layers of urogenital diaphragm

Bulbospongiosus muscle

J. Netter M.D.
with
J. Perkins
MS, MFA

FIGURE 9-20 URINARY INCONTINENCE

Urinary retention is normally under autonomic or voluntary control. Incontinence (an increased stimulus to void, a decreased ability to prevent voiding, or both) results when these pathways are interrupted or are overactivated or underactivated, or when smooth muscle of the bladder contracts weakly, incoordinately, or inappropriately. Although incontinence is not life threatening, it has significant medical and social consequences. It is often cited as a primary reason for inability of families to care for elders at home. Drugs for treatment are far from ideal but include those that reduce bladder contraction, such as cholinergic antagonists (eg, oxybutynin, prophantheline, tolterodine); those that increase bladder outlet function, such as α-adrenoceptor agonists (eg, phenylpropanolamine, pseudoephedrine); and those for which the mechanism is not fully understood, such as tricyclic antidepressants (possibly related to anticholinergic actions) and estrogens (in postmenopausal women).

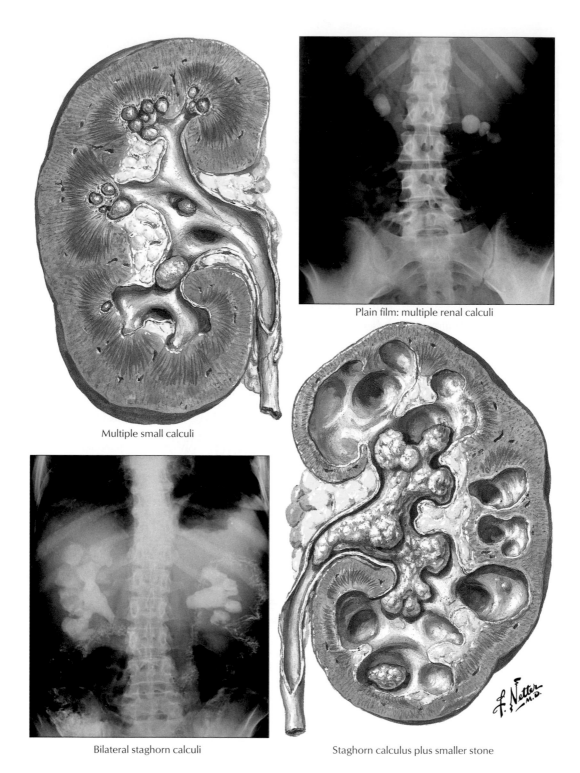

Multiple small calculi

Plain film: multiple renal calculi

Bilateral staghorn calculi

Staghorn calculus plus smaller stone

FIGURE 9-21 URINARY TRACT CALCULI (KIDNEY STONES)

Urinary calculi are hardened crystals composed of a nucleus (often urate) and surrounding layers of precipitated minerals, such as calcium and magnesium salts, and other components of the urine (including metabolites of drugs excreted in the urine). These stones are usually found in the kidney, but they also occur in the ureter and the bladder (in the latter, the stones are usually passed from the kidney). They occur in all age groups but primarily in persons aged between 20 and 55 years. Treatment (surgical or pharmacologic) depends on the cause, size, and location of the stone. Two common types for which drugs are used are due to hypercalciuria and hyperuricuria. Drugs for hypercalciuria include sodium cellulose phosphate (inhibits calcium reabsorption) and thiazides (mild diuresis stimulates convoluted tubule reabsorption of calcium). Drugs for hyperuricuria include allopurinol (decreases urate formation) and alkali (increases urinary citrate, which inhibits stone formation).

NORMAL

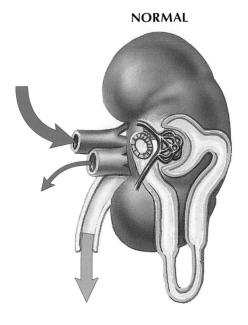

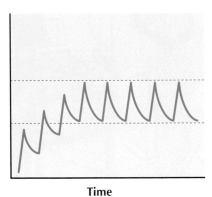

Circulating drug concentration

Time

INSUFFICIENCY

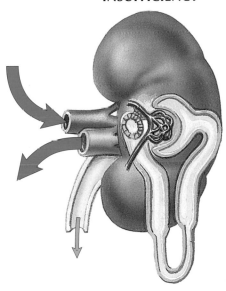

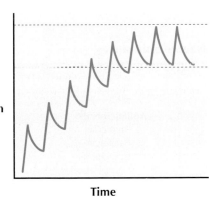

Circulating drug concentration

Time

J. Perkins
MS, MFA

FIGURE 9-22 EFFECT OF RENAL INSUFFICIENCY ON DRUG ACTION

Many drugs and drug metabolites are excreted via the kidneys, so changes (eg, advanced age, disease) that alter renal function affect the elimination (half-life) of many agents. Blood levels of a drug or its metabolites are greater when decreased renal clearance exists than during normal renal clearance. This change is clinically relevant for drugs eliminated primarily by kidneys and becomes more critical for drugs with a small therapeutic index. Sometimes the effect of renal insufficiency on a drug metabolite (eg, normeperidine) is more important than that on the drug itself (ie, meperidine). Renal function usually declines with age, so elderly patients are often given reduced doses of drugs eliminated mainly via the kidneys. Examples of altered drug action in renal insufficiency are enhanced hyperkalemia with K$^+$-sparing diuretics or NSAIDs; delayed or decreased diuretic effectiveness; and greater risk of NSAID-induced GI bleeding.

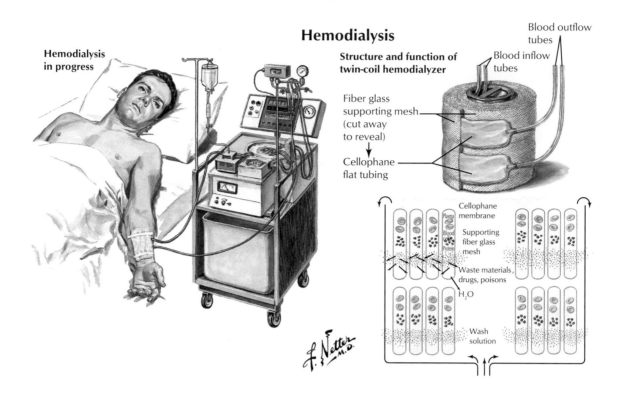

Hemodialysis

Hemodialysis in progress

Structure and function of twin-coil hemodialyzer

Blood outflow tubes

Blood inflow tubes

Fiber glass supporting mesh (cut away to reveal)

Cellophane flat tubing

Cellophane membrane

Supporting fiber glass mesh

Waste materials, drugs, poisons

H_2O

Wash solution

Currently Known Dialyzable Substances

Analgesics	Tricyclic secondary amines	Polymyxin	**Depressants, Sedatives, and**
Acetophenetidin	Tricyclic tertiary amines	Quinine	**Tranquilizers**
Acetylsalicylic acid*		Streptomycin	Chloral hydrate
Dextropropoxyphene	**Antimicrobials**	Sulfonamides	Diphenhydramine
Methylsalicylate*	Ampicillin	Tetracycline	Diphenylhydantoin
Paracetamol	Bacitracin	Vancomycin	Ethchlorvynol*
	Carbenicillin		Ethinamate
Antidepressants	Cephalosporins	**Barbiturates***	Gallamine triethiodide
Amphetamine	Chloramphenicol	Amobarbital	Glutethimide*
Isocarboxazid	Cycloserine	Barbital	Heroin
Methamphetamine	Isoniazid	Butabarbital	Meprobamate
Monoamine oxidase inhibitors	Kanamycin	Butalbital	Methaqualone
Pargyline	Neomycin	Cyclobarbital	Methyprylon
Phenelzine	Nitrofurantoin	Pentobarbital	Paraldehyde
Tranylcypromine	Penicillin	Phenobarbital	Primidone
		Secobarbital	

*Kinetics of dialysis thoroughly studied and/or clinical experience extensive.
Based on Schreiner GE, Teehan BP: Dialysis of poisons and drugs: annual review. *Trans Amer Soc Artif Intern Organs*. 1973;17:513.
For complete details and supporting data, the reader is advised to consult the original reference.

FIGURE 9-23 EFFECT OF HEMODIALYSIS ON DRUG ACTION

Hemodialysis is used as maintenance therapy for patients with renal failure and to clear toxic substances from the blood of patients who ingested poisons or overdoses of drugs. The fundamental physiologic principle in dialysis is that of a solute moving across a semipermeable membrane in a direction and at a rate consistent with concentration and osmotic gradients. This principle is the basis for operation of artificial or mechanical kidneys. If a patient receives therapy with a drug that can be dialyzed (ie, pass through the membrane), the amount lost during dialysis must be considered, and supplementary doses may be needed to replace the lost drug.

CHAPTER 10

DRUGS USED IN INFECTIOUS DISEASE

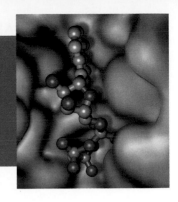

OVERVIEW

The goal of the drugs discussed in this chapter is total destruction of a disease-causing organism (bacteria, fungus, or virus). Because antimicrobials are by design cytotoxic, the distinguishing feature of each agent is relative selectivity for particular pathogens rather than the host. The greater the selectivity for the pathogen is, the fewer the adverse effects of the drug are. A major concern for this therapeutic class is the emergence of resistance of pathogens to drugs.

Antimicrobials selectively kill or inhibit replication of a pathogen by interfering with a phase of cell physiology that is required by the pathogen. Antibiotics are typically classified and subclassified according to mechanism of action, chemical structure, and spectrum of activity against particular organisms. Narrow-spectrum antibiotics act on a single group or a limited number of groups of organisms, whereas broad-spectrum agents are effective against a wide variety of microbes. Tetracyclines have the broadest antibacterial spectrum of any class of antibiotics. They bind reversibly to the 30S and 50S subunits of the bacterial ribosome, thereby inhibiting protein synthesis. Aminoglycosides and macrolides inhibit bacterial protein synthesis by binding directly and irreversibly to 30S and 50S subunits, respectively, of the bacterial ribosome. β-Lactam antibiotics (penicillins, cephalosporins, carbapenems, monobactams, and vancomycin) act by interfering with bacterial wall synthesis, which causes rapid cell lysis. However, β-lactam antibiotics are subject to inactivation by β lactamase–producing organ-

isms, so many of these agents are used in combination with β-lactamase inhibitors. Carbapenems are the broadest spectrum β-lactam antibiotics. Quinolones are broad-spectrum bacteriocidal antibiotics that inhibit intracellular DNA topoisomerase II (DNA gyrase) or topoisomerase IV, which are essential for duplication, transcription, and repair of bacterial DNA.

Fungi have more rigid cell walls than bacteria and are resistant to antibiotics. Drugs used to treat systemic fungal infections include amphotericin B, the azole antifungals, caspofungin, and voriconazole. All of these drugs interfere with critical components of the normal physiology of fungi.

Human immunodeficiency virus infection is a particularly difficult viral infection to treat because of the ability of the virus to rapidly mutate to drug-resistant forms. HIV attacks and binds to the CD4 receptor on specific cells of the immune system. Over time, HIV causes host cell lysis and prevents production of new $CD4^+$ cells. Nucleoside reverse transcriptase inhibitors (NRTIs) suppress viral replication by inhibiting the enzyme responsible for conversion of viral RNA into DNA. Protease inhibitors (PIs) inhibit the enzyme required for the proteolysis of viral polyprotein precursors into individual functional proteins—a conversion essential for HIV to be infectious. Nonnucleoside reverse transcriptase inhibitors (NNRTIs) prevent viral replication through noncompetitive inhibition of the reverse transcriptase enzyme. These and other drugs are often used in multidrug cocktails to enhance their effectiveness and minimize resistance.

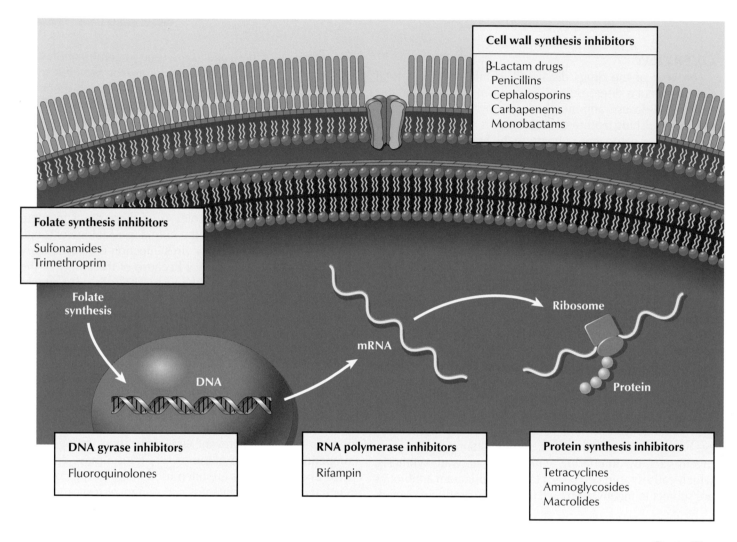

Cell wall synthesis inhibitors

β-Lactam drugs
  Penicillins
  Cephalosporins
  Carbapenems
  Monobactams

Folate synthesis inhibitors

Sulfonamides
Trimethroprim

Folate
synthesis

DNA

mRNA

Ribosome

Protein

DNA gyrase inhibitors

Fluoroquinolones

RNA polymerase inhibitors

Rifampin

Protein synthesis inhibitors

Tetracyclines
Aminoglycosides
Macrolides

FIGURE 10-1 CLASSIFICATION OF ANTIBIOTICS

The clinical utility of antimicrobials is based on their ability to selectively kill or inhibit replication of invading organisms without causing significant harm to host cells. Designed to interfere with a phase of cell physiology that is unique to the pathogen, antimicrobials essentially make use of inherent structural differences among human, bacterial, viral, and fungal cells. Antibiotics are typically classified according to mechanism of action, chemical structure, and spectrum of activity against particular organisms. Drug classes include cell wall synthesis inhibitors (β-lactam drugs such as penicillins, cephalosporins, carbapenems, monobactams); protein synthesis inhibitors (eg, tetracyclines, aminoglycosides, macrolides); DNA gyrase inhibitors (fluoroquinolones); RNA polymerase inhibitor (rifampin); and folate synthesis inhibitors (eg, sulfonamides).

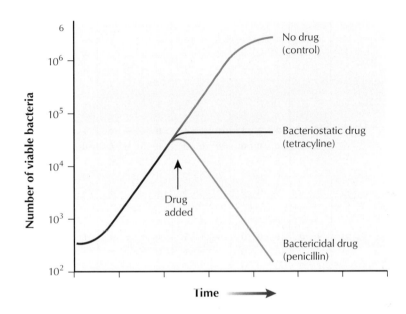

FIGURE 10-2 DEFINITIONS: BACTERIOSTATIC VERSUS BACTERICIDAL

When characterizing the mechanism of action of an antibiotic, it is important to establish whether the agent is bacteriostatic or bactericidal. Bacteriostatic antibiotics arrest microbial growth and replication, which limits the spread of infection while the host's immune system naturally eliminates the pathogens. If therapy ends before the immune system completely eliminates the organisms, a second cycle of infection may begin. Bactericidal agents kill bacteria, which leads directly to a reduced total number of viable pathogens in the host. Bactericidal agents are preferred for patients with neutropenia because these individuals have compromised immune systems and may not be able to eliminate remaining pathogens. Life-threatening infections such as endocarditis and meningitis should also be treated with bactericidal agents.

Comparison of Antimicrobial Spectra

Columns are grouped under **Penicillins, Carbapenems, Aztreonam, Fluoroquinolones**: Anti-staphylococcal Penicillins (Methicillin; Nafcillin/Oxacillin; Cloxacillin/Dicloxacillin); Aminopenicillins (Amp/Amox; Amox/Clav; Amp/Sulb); Anti-pseudomonal Penicillins (Ticarcillin; Ticar/Clav; Pip/Tazo; Piperacillin); Carbapenems/Aztreonam (Ertapenem; Imipenem; Meropenem; Aztreonam); Fluoroquinolones (Ciprofloxacin; Ofloxacin; Lomefloxacin; Perfloxacin; Levofloxacin; Moxifloxacin; Gemifloxacin; Gatifloxacin).

Organisms	Pen G	Pen V	Methicillin	Nafcillin/Oxacillin	Cloxacillin/Dicloxacillin	Amp/Amox	Amox/Clav	Amp/Sulb	Ticarcillin	Ticar/Clav	Pip/Tazo	Piperacillin	Ertapenem	Imipenem	Meropenem	Aztreonam	Ciprofloxacin	Ofloxacin	Lomefloxacin	Perfloxacin	Levofloxacin	Moxifloxacin	Gemifloxacin	Gatifloxacin
Gram positive																								
Strep group A, B, C, G	+	+	+	+	+	+	+	+	+	+	+	+	+	+	+	0	±	±	0	0	+	+	+	+
Strep pneumoniae	+	+	+	+	+	+	+	+	+	+	+	+	+	+	+	0	±	±	0	0	+	+	+	+
Viridans strep	±	±	±	±	±	±	±	±	±	±	±	±	+	+	+	0	0	0			+	+	+	+
Strep milleri	+	+	+	+	+	+	+	+	+	+	+	+	+	+	+	0	0	0			+	+	+	+
Enterococcus faecalis	+	+	0	0	0	+	+	+	±	±	+	+	±	+	±	0	*	*		0	+	+		+
Enterococcus faecium	±	±	0	0	0	+	+	+	±	±	±	±	0	±	0	0	0	0			0	0	±	±
Staph aureus (MSSA)	0	0	+	+	+	0	+	+	0	+	+	0	+	+	+	0	+	+	+	+	+	+	+	+
Staph aureus (MSSA)	0	0	0	0	0	0	0	0	0	0	0	0	0	0	0	0	0	0	0	0	0	±		±
Staph epidermidis	0	0	±	±	±	±	+	+	±	±	+	0	+	+	+	0	+	+	+	+	+	+		+
C jeikeium	0	0	0	0	0	0	0	0	0	0		0	0	0		0	0	0						
L monocytogenes	+	0	0	0	0	+		+	+			+	±	+	+	0	+							
Gram negative																								
N gonorrhoeae	0	0	0	0	0	0	+	+	+	+	+	+	+	+	+	+	+	+	+	+	+	+		+
N meningitidis	+	0	0	0	0	+	+	+	+	+	+	+	+	+	+	+	+	+			+	+	+	+
M catarrhalis	0	0	0	0	0	0	+	+	0	+	+	±	+	+	+	+	+	+	+	+	+	+		+
H influenzae	0	0	0	0	0	±	+	+	±	+	±	±	+	+	+	+	+	+	+	+	+	+		+
E coli	0	0	0	0	0	±	+	+	±	+	+	+	+	+	+	+	+	+	+	+	+	+		+
Klebsiella species	0	0	0	0	0	0	+	+	0	+	+	+	+	+	+	+	+	+	+	+	+	+		+
Enterobacter species	0	0	0	0	0	0	0	0	+	+	+	+	+	+	+	+	+	+	+	+	+	+		+
Serratia species	0	0	0	0	0	0	0	0	+	+	+	0	+	+	+	+	+	+	+	+	+	+		+
Salmonella species	0	0	0	0	0	±	+	+	+	+	+		+	+	+		+	+			+	+	+	+
Shigella species	0	0	0	0	0	±	+	+	+			+	+	+	+	+	+	+			+	+	+	+
Proteus mirabilis	0	0	0	0	0	+	+	+	+	+	+	+	+	+	+	+	+	+			+	+	+	+
Proteus vulgaris	0	0	0	0	0	0	+	+	+	+	+	+	+	+	+	+	+	+			+	+	+	+
Providencia species	0	0	0	0	0	0	+	+	+	+	+	+	+	+	+	+	+	+			+	+	+	+
Morganella species	0	0	0	0	0	0	±	+	+	+	+	+	+	+	+	+	+	+			+	+	+	+
Citrobacter species	0	0	0	0	0	0	0	0	+	+	+	+	+	+	+	+	+	+			+	+	+	+
Aeromonas species	0	0	0	0	0	0	+	+	+	+	+	+	+	+	+	+	+	+			+	+	+	+
Acinetobacter species	0	0	0	0	0	0	0	+	0	±	+	0	±	+	+	0	±	±			±	±		±
Ps aeruginosa	0	0	0	0	0	0	0	0	+	+	+	+	±	+	+	+	+	+	±		±	±		±
B (Ps) cepacia	0	0	0	0	0	0	0	0	0				0	0	+	0	0	0	0			0		0
S (X) maltophilia	0	0	0	0	0	0	0	0		±	±	±	0	0	0	0	0	0	0	0	0	±	+	
Y enterocolitica	0	0	0	0	0	0	±	±	±	+		+		+		+	+	+	+	+	+	+		+
Legionella species	0	0	0	0	0	0	0	0	0	0	0	0	0	0	0	0	+	+			+	+		+
P multocida	+	+	0	0	0	+	+	+	+	+		+	+	+		+	+	+			+	+		+
H ducreyi	+					0	+	+																

*Most strains ±, can be used in UTI, not in systemic infection. With permission from Gilbert DN et al, eds. *The Sanford Guide to Antimicrobial Therapy.* 32nd ed. Hyde Park, Vt: Antimicrobial Therapy, Inc; 2002.

FIGURE 10-3 SPECTRUM OF ACTIVITY

An antibiotic's *spectrum of activity* refers to the range of pathogenic organisms affected by that drug. Antibiotics with a narrow spectrum of activity act on a single organism or a few groups of organisms; broad-spectrum agents such as fluoroquinolones are effective against a wide variety of microbes. Extended-spectrum antibiotics such as ampicillin-sulfbactam have an intermediate range of activity and target gram-positive organisms and some gram-negative species. Because broad- and extended-spectrum antibiotics eliminate a wide variety of microbial species, these agents can alter the non-pathogenic bacterial flora that normally colonizes the host and result in superinfection by organisms (eg, *Candida*, *Clostridium difficile*) whose growth would otherwise be suppressed.

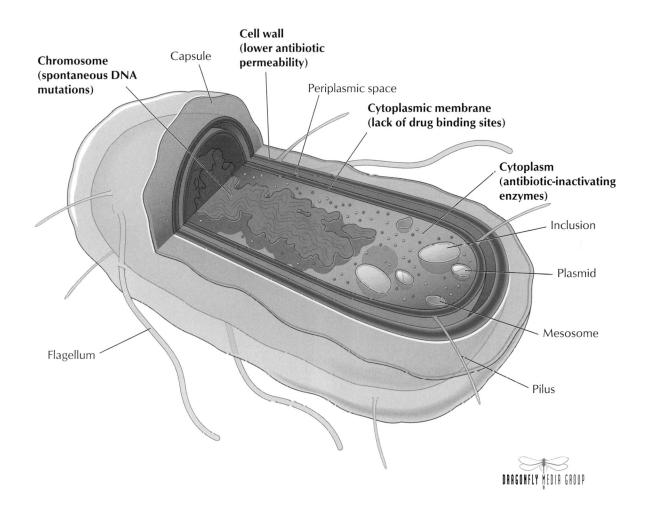

Chromosome
(spontaneous DNA
mutations)

Capsule

Cell wall
(lower antibiotic
permeability)

Periplasmic space

Cytoplasmic membrane
(lack of drug binding sites)

Cytoplasm
(antibiotic-inactivating
enzymes)

Inclusion

Plasmid

Mesosome

Pilus

Flagellum

DRAGONFLY MEDIA GROUP

FIGURE 10-4 MECHANISMS OF RESISTANCE

Bacteria such as *Staphylococcus* strains are resistant if their growth is not halted by the maximal level of an antibiotic that is tolerated by the host. Organisms develop into more virulent strains through mechanisms such as spontaneous DNA mutations. Main mechanisms of resistance are lower permeability of the antibiotic through the cell wall (eg, ampicillin), presence of antibiotic-inactivating enzymes (eg, β lactamases), and lack of drug-binding sites (eg, penicillin). Various factors contribute to the emergence of resistant strains, one of which is overprescribing of antibiotics in the community setting. Diagnostic uncertainty may be responsible: rapid diagnostic testing is available for only a few infections, so community physicians often distinguish between viral and bacterial infections on the basis of symptoms alone. For an uncertain diagnosis, physicians tend to use antibiotics. Other factors include inappropriate or indiscriminate drug use and patients' not completing courses of treatment.

Tuberculosis: Sputum Examination
(Stained Smear)

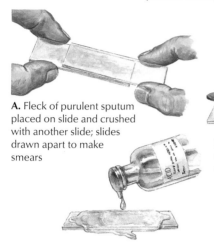

A. Fleck of purulent sputum placed on slide and crushed with another slide; slides drawn apart to make smears

B. Slide flooded with carbolfuchsin and then heated

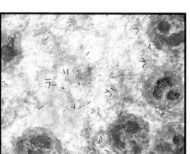

C. Slide rinsed with water, decolorized with acid alcohol, and rinsed again

D. Counterstained with methylene blue or malachite green for 30 seconds, rinsed again, and dried

E. Slide of sputum stained with carbolfuchsin (Ziehl-Neelsen method as above), viewed under oil immersion, showing acid-fast bacilli (*M tuberculosis*) as bright red rods

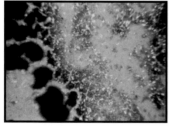

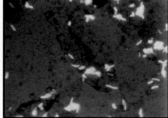

F. *M tuberculosis* stained with auramine O, which causes acid-fast bacilli to fluoresce ((×200)

G. Auramine O stain of *M kansasii* (acid-fast "atypical" mycobacteria), which are much larger than *M tuberculosis* (×200)

Pneumococcal Pneumonia

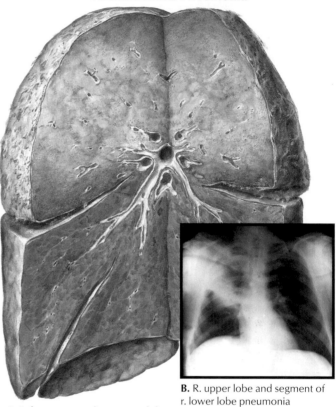

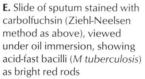

A. Lobar pneumonia; r. upper lobe. Mixed red and gray hepatization (transition stage); pleural fibrinous exudate

B. R. upper lobe and segment of r. lower lobe pneumonia

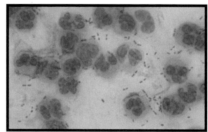

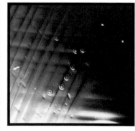

C. Purulent sputum with pneumococci (Gram stain)

D. Colonies of pneumococci growing on agar plate

FIGURE 10-5 EXAMPLES OF RESISTANCE

Increasing bacterial resistance to antibiotics in the outpatient setting now seems to affect hospitals. Second- or third-generation cephalosporins, with or without a macrolide, are often given to patients who stay in the hospital for multidrug-resistant pneumococcal infections. However, overprescribing of these cephalosporins in communities has left hospitals with few options for patients who are already using these agents and present with such resistant infections. Penicillin-resistant *Streptococcus pneu-* *moniae* strains are increasingly found (now in 20% of all pneumococcal infections), with growing numbers of strains resistant to multiple drug classes, including macrolides and β-lactam antibiotics. Vancomycin is the fallback for therapy in such cases, but the utility of this drug may be limited because other bacteria such as *Enterococcus* and *Staphylococcus aureus* now have resistant strains. *Mycobacterium tuberculosis* strains can now evade many drugs, so this disease has become difficult to treat.

Superficial Syphilitic Lesions

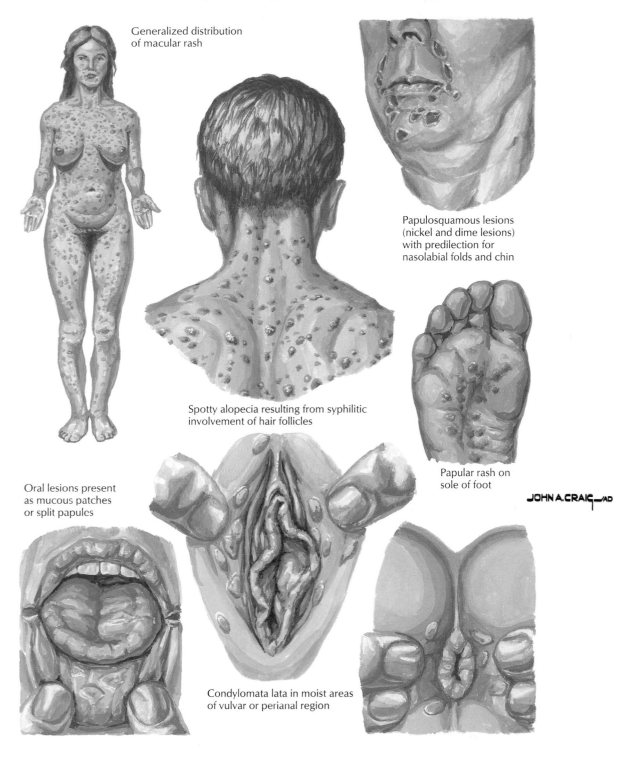

Generalized distribution of macular rash

Papulosquamous lesions (nickel and dime lesions) with predilection for nasolabial folds and chin

Spotty alopecia resulting from syphilitic involvement of hair follicles

Papular rash on sole of foot

Oral lesions present as mucous patches or split papules

Condylomata lata in moist areas of vulvar or perianal region

JOHN A. CRAIG—AD

FIGURE 10-6 NATURAL PENICILLINS: PENICILLIN G AND PENICILLIN V

Originally obtained from fermentation of the mold *Penicillium chrysogenum*, penicillins are the oldest and still the most widely used of all antibiotics. These agents exert bactericidal activity by interfering with the last step of bacterial cell wall synthesis, which causes rapid cell lysis. Therefore, penicillins are ineffective against organisms that lack a cell wall, such as mycobacteria, protozoa, fungi, and viruses. Natural penicillins target gram-positive and gram-negative cocci, gram-positive bacilli, oral anaerobes, and spirochetes. These drugs have been the cornerstone of therapy for a diverse group of infections including pneumococcal pneumonia, syphilis, meningitis, tetanus, and gonorrhea. Penicillin G and penicillin V have similar spectra of activity, with the latter agent being more acid stable and thus better absorbed by the oral route, whereas penicillin G is administered via injection.

Acute Otitis Media

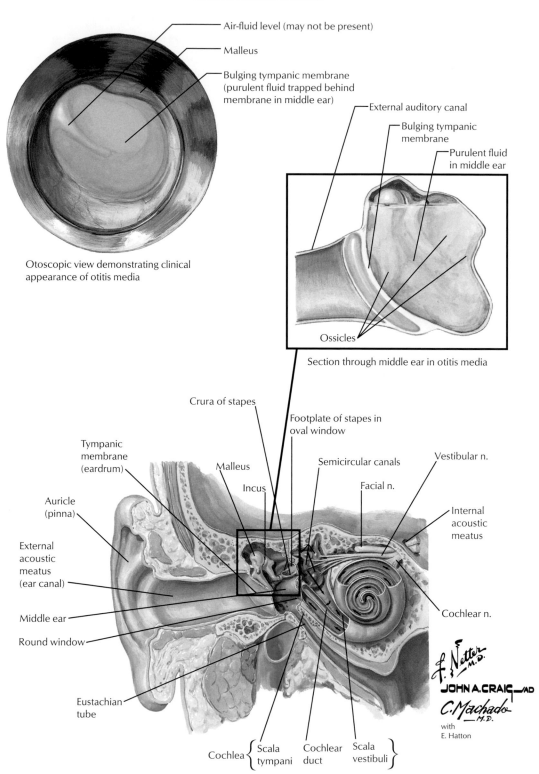

Air-fluid level (may not be present)

Malleus

Bulging tympanic membrane (purulent fluid trapped behind membrane in middle ear)

Otoscopic view demonstrating clinical appearance of otitis media

External auditory canal

Bulging tympanic membrane

Purulent fluid in middle ear

Ossicles

Section through middle ear in otitis media

Crura of stapes

Footplate of stapes in oval window

Tympanic membrane (eardrum)

Malleus

Semicircular canals

Vestibular n.

Auricle (pinna)

Incus

Facial n.

Internal acoustic meatus

External acoustic meatus (ear canal)

Middle ear

Cochlear n.

Round window

Eustachian tube

Cochlea { Scala tympani

Cochlear duct

Scala vestibuli }

with E. Hatton

FIGURE 10-7 AMINOPENICILLINS: AMOXICILLIN AND AMPICILLIN

Aminopenicillins are similar to natural penicillins in spectrum of activity but are also active against many gram-negative organisms (eg, *Helicobacter pylori*) and against *Listeria*. These drugs are used for septicemia; gynecologic, skin, and soft tissue infections; and urinary, respiratory, and GI tract infections. Because these drugs have become inactivated by β lactamase–producing bacteria (eg, *Escherichia coli* and *Haemophilus influenzae*), their use has declined. However, the CDC still indicates amoxicillin as the drug of choice for uncomplicated acute otitis media, despite the presence of drug-resistant *S pneumoniae* (DRSP) and *H influenzae*. The CDC urged use of a high-dose regimen to give amoxicillin a better chance to eliminate DRSP for very young patients with recent exposure to antimicrobials. If amoxicillin fails, antibiotics with activity against DRSP (eg, cefuroxime) or β lactamase–producing strains (ie, amoxicillin-clavulanate) should be tried.

Prevention of Burn Wound Infections, Which Can Be Caused by *P aeruginosa*

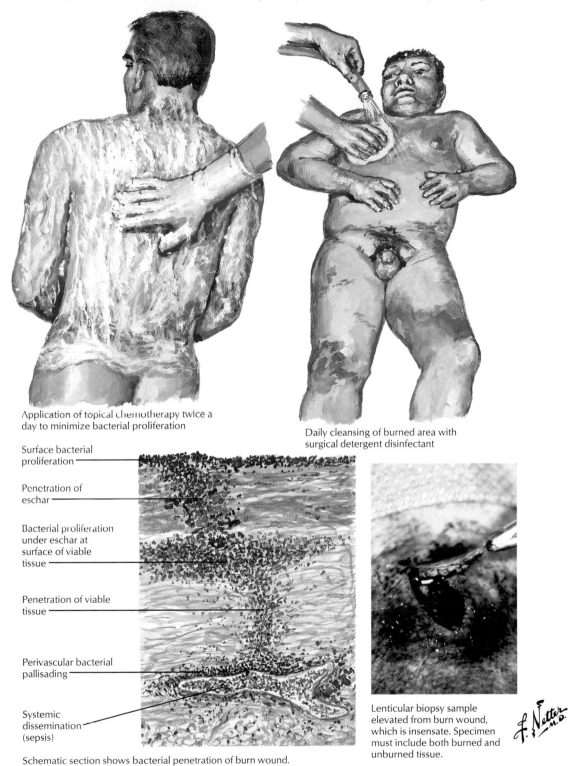

Application of topical chemotherapy twice a day to minimize bacterial proliferation

Daily cleansing of burned area with surgical detergent disinfectant

Surface bacterial proliferation

Penetration of eschar

Bacterial proliferation under eschar at surface of viable tissue

Penetration of viable tissue

Perivascular bacterial pallisading

Systemic dissemination (sepsis)

Schematic section shows bacterial penetration of burn wound.

Lenticular biopsy sample elevated from burn wound, which is insensate. Specimen must include both burned and unburned tissue.

FIGURE 10-8 ANTIPSEUDOMONAL PENICILLINS: CARBENICILLIN, PIPERACILLIN, AND TICARCILLIN

Antipseudomonal penicillins (carbenicillin, piperacillin, and ticarcillin) display improved activity against gram-negative organisms and are usually used in combination with aminoglycosides in patients with febrile neutropenia and in those with hard to treat nosocomial infections caused by strains of *Enterobacter, Klebsiella, Citrobacter, Serratia, Bacteroides fragilis,* and *Pseudomonas aeruginosa.* The antibacterial effects of all β-lactam antibiotics are synergistic with aminoglycosides because the former

inhibit cell wall synthesis, which enhances diffusion of the latter into the bacterium. These drugs should never be placed into the same IV bag because positively charged aminoglycosides can form a precipitate with negatively charged penicillins. Like other penicillins, antipseudomonal agents can be inactivated by β lactamase and are therefore commonly used together with β-lactamase inhibitors (see Figure 10-9).

Drug	Susceptible Organisms	Indications
Amoxicillin-clavulanate 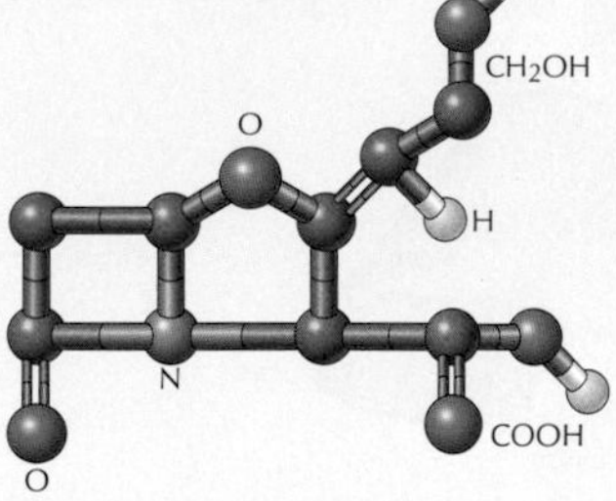	Streptococci, *Escherichia coli*, *Enterococcus faecalis*, *Proteus miribilis*, and β lactamase–producing *Haemophilus influenzae*, *Klebsiella* species, *Moraxella catarrhalis*, and *S aureus* (not MRSA)	Lower respiratory tract infections Otitis media Sinusitis Skin and skin structure infections
Ampicillin-sulbacatam 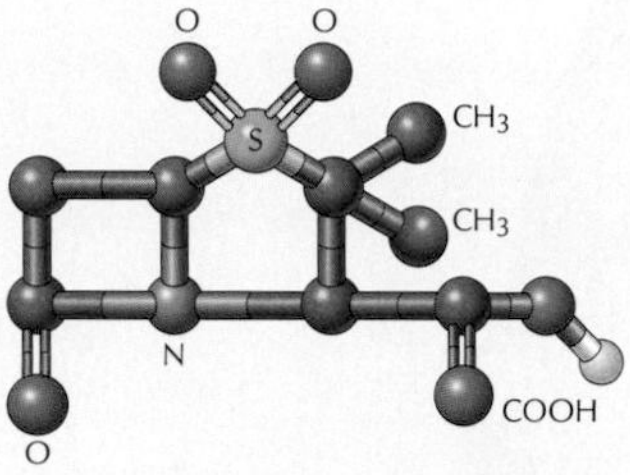	β Lactamase–producing organisms such as *H influenzae*, *E coli*, and *Klebsiella*, *Acinetobacter*, *Enterobacter*, *S aureus*, *Bacteroides* species (anaerobes)	Gynecologic infections Intra-abdominal infections Skin and skin structure infections
Ticarcillan-clavulanate 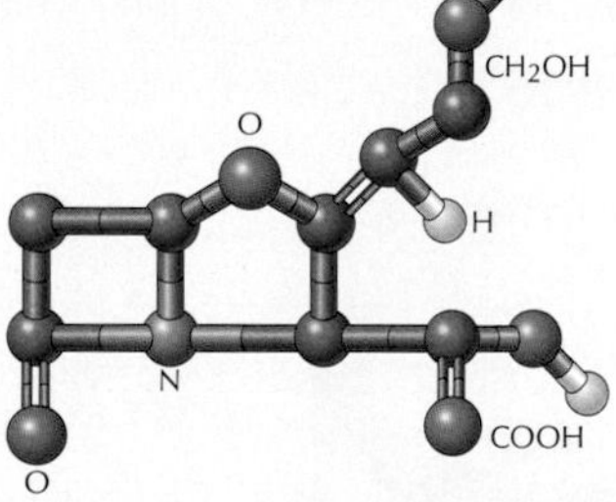	*Pseudomonas*, *E coli*, *Enterobacter* species, *Proteus* species, β lactamase–producing *S aureus*, *M catarrhalis*, *H influenzae*, *Klebsiella* species, *Bacteroides fragilis*	Bone and joint infections Gynecologic infections Intra-abdominal infections Lower respiratory tract infections Septicemia Skin and skin structure infections Urinary tract infections
Piperacillin-tazobactam 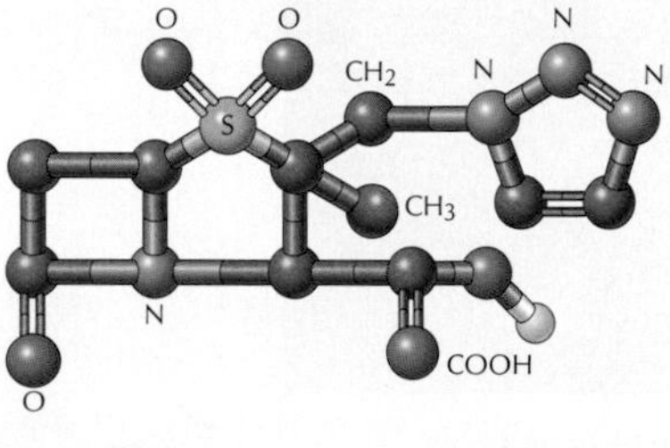	Piperacillin-resistant β lactamase–producing organisms	Appendicitis Pelvic inflammatory disease Peritonitis Pneumonia (community acquired and nosocomial) Postpartum endometritis Skin and skin structure infections including diabetic foot infections

FIGURE 10-9 β-LACTAMASE INHIBITORS

The structures of penicillins and other β-lactam antibiotics have in common a β-lactam ring that is essential to stability and antibacterial activity. After years of exposure to β-lactam antibiotics, a large number of bacterial organisms have developed resistance to the drugs by producing β lactamase, an enzyme that hydrolyzes the β-lactam ring and inactivates the antibiotics.

β-Lactamase inhibitors—clavulanate, sulbactam, and tazobactam—were developed to address this problem. With no antibacterial activity of their own, these inhibitors are used only in combination with β-lactam antibiotics, which creates a product that has extended activity against β lactamase–producing strains.

Etiology and Prevalence of Hematogenous Osteomyelitis

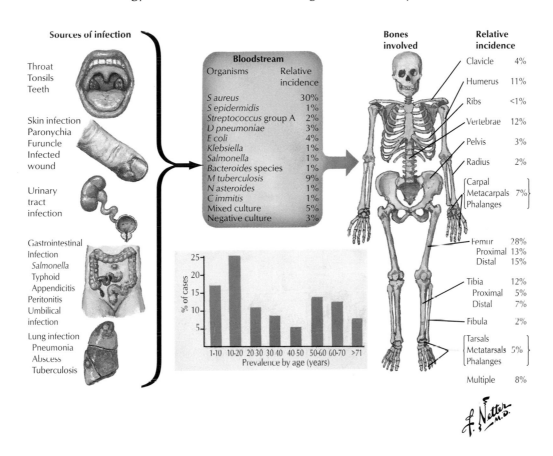

FIGURE 10-10 β LACTAMASE–RESISTANT PENICILLINS: CLOXACILLIN, DICLOXACILLIN, OXACILLIN, AND NAFCILLIN

β Lactamase–resistant penicillins are semisynthetic penicillins that have the same coverage as natural penicillins but are designed to remain stable in the presence of β lactamase–producing staphylococcal organisms. Cloxacillin is used for treatment of septic arthritis; dicloxacillin is used for treatment of skin and soft tissue infections; oxacillin is used for treatment of sepsis, toxic shock syndrome, and infections of wounds and vascular

catheters; and nafcillin is used for treatment of endocarditis, osteomyelitis, skin and soft tissue infections, and encephalitis. Unfortunately, many strains of *S aureus* have developed the ability to inactivate methicillin, leading to the increase of methicillin-resistant *S aureus* (MRSA). This pathogen is considered a serious source of nosocomial infections and produces diseases that are usually treated with vancomycin.

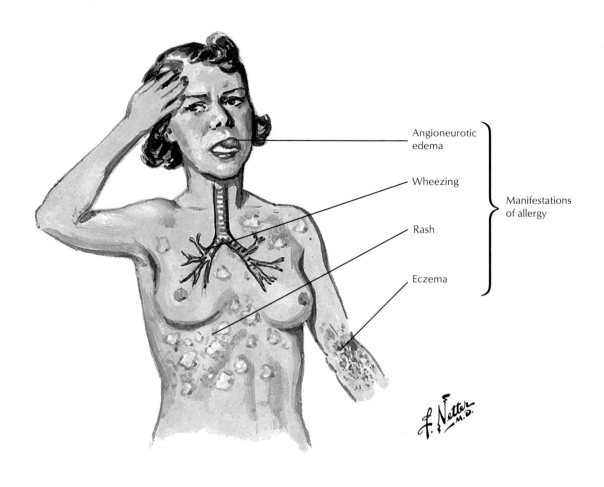

Antibiotic	Adverse Effects
Extended-spectrum penicillins (high doses)	Bleeding, hyperkalemia, hypernatremia
Methicillin	Acute interstitial nephritis
Penicillin G (high doses in renal disease)	CNS effects (confusion, twitching, lethargy, dysphagia, seizures, coma)
Penicillin G (in secondary syphilis)	Jarisch-Herxheimer reaction (fever, chills, myalgia, tachycardia, hypotension)
β Lactamase–resistant penicillins	Hepatotoxicity
Ampicillin	Maculopapular rash (can occur with all penicillins but most common with ampicillin)

FIGURE 10-11 ADVERSE EFFECTS OF PENICILLINS

Although considered the safest of all antibiotics, penicillins can still cause significant adverse effects, with hypersensitivity reactions being most notable. Approximately 5% of patients experience some kind of reaction, which is actually an immune response to the penicillin metabolite penicilloic acid and can range from a maculopapular rash to angioedema and the more significant anaphylaxis. Cross-allergic reactions occur among all β-lactam antibiotics. Other reactions that pertain to specific agents are given in the table.

Strep throat

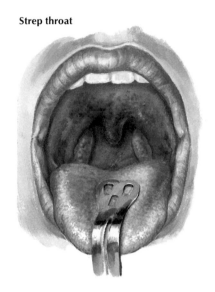

DRAGONFLY MEDIA GROUP

Drug Class and Selected Drugs	Coverage	Organisms
First generation • Cefazolin • Cephalexin • Cefadroxil	+++/− Primarily active against gram-positive organisms, minimally active against gram-negative organisms	Gram positive: β lactamase–producing *S aureus* and *Staphylococcus epidermidis*, *S pneumoniae*, *Streptococcus agalactiae*, *Streptococcus pyogenes*; gram negative: *Klebsiella pneumoniae*, *E coli*, *P mirabilis*, *Shigella*
Second generation • Cefotetan • Cefoxitin • Cefprozil • Cefuroxime • Cefamandole	+/− − Have weaker gram-positive coverage than first-generation agents, but display activity against more gram-negative pathogens than those agents	*M catarrhalis*, *H influenzae*, *Enterobacter*, *Citrobacter*, *Providencia*, *Acinetobacter*, *Serratia*, *Neisseria*
Third generation • Cefixime • Cefotaxime • Ceftazidime • Ceftriaxone • Moxalactam • Cefoperazone • Ceftizoxime	− − −/+ Have minimal gram-positive coverage compared with agents from the first two generations, but excel in activity against gram-negative organisms, especially ones that produce β-lactamase	*Enterobacter*, *Providencia*, *Acinetobacter*, *Serratia*, *Proteus*, *Morganella*, *Neisseria*, possibly *B fragilis*, *Pseudomonas*
Fourth generation • Cefepime	+++ /− − − Is effective against broad spectrum of gram-positive and gram-negative organisms	Generally reserved for severe infections involving gram-negative bacilli and *Pseudomonas* species

FIGURE 10-12 CEPHALOSPORINS

Chemically and pharmacologically similar to penicillins, cephalosporins inhibit cell wall synthesis and cause rapid cell lysis. These antibiotics are classified into first, second, third, and fourth generations on the basis of spectrum of activity and susceptibility to β lactamases. Agents in the first generation tend to have excellent gram-positive coverage but minimal gram-negative coverage, whereas agents in the higher generations tend to possess the reverse spectrum of activity. Also like penicillins, all cephalosporins can produce hypersensitivity reactions, ranging from a mild rash and fever to fatal anaphylaxis. Patients who are allergic to penicillins should avoid these agents because of cross-sensitivity of 5% to 15% between the 2 classes. Other adverse effects include GI disturbances and hematologic reactions including positive Coombs test results, thrombocytopenia, transient neutropenia, and reversible leukopenia.

Lung Abscesses

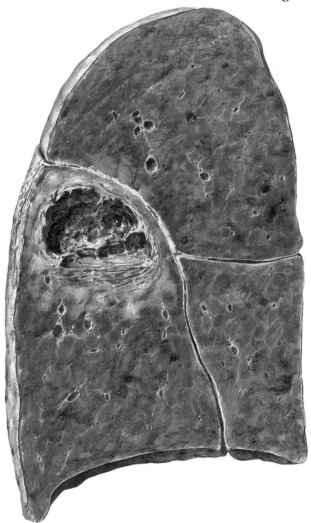

Sagittal section of lung with abscess (cavity in superior segment of lower lobe containing fluid and surrounded by fibrous tissue and pneumonic patches); also pleural thickening over abscess

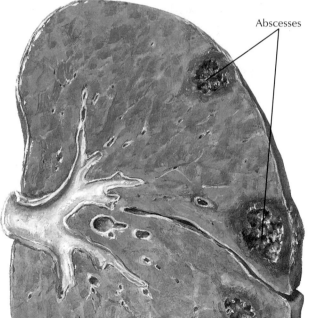

Multiple lung abscesses following septic embolization

Abscesses

FIGURE 10-13 CARBAPENEMS: IMIPENEM-CILASTATIN, ERTAPENEM, AND MEROPENEM

Carbapenems are the broadest spectrum β-lactam antibiotics. They derive potent activity from resistance to bacterial β lactamases, affinity for penicillin-binding protein 2, and lack of permeability barrier. They act against aerobic (gram-positive and -negative) and anaerobic bacteria, including *P aeruginosa*, *B fragilis*, and *Serratia*, *Enterobacter*, *Acinetobacter*, and *Enterococcus* species. Alone or with an aminoglycoside, they are used for severe mixed infections (pulmonary, intraabdominal, soft tissue) caused by multidrug-resistant bacteria. Meropenem is beneficial in febrile neutropenia, urinary tract infections (UTIs), and meningitis. All drugs can have injection site reactions and should be avoided in penicillin-allergic patients. Imipenem-cilastatin (and ertapenem) can cause abnormal liver function test results, thrombophlebitis, and seizures. Imipenem is used with cilastatin to avoid nephrotoxicity. Meropenem can cause agranulocytosis, neutropenia, Stevens-Johnson syndrome, and angioedema.

Factors in Etiology of Cystitis

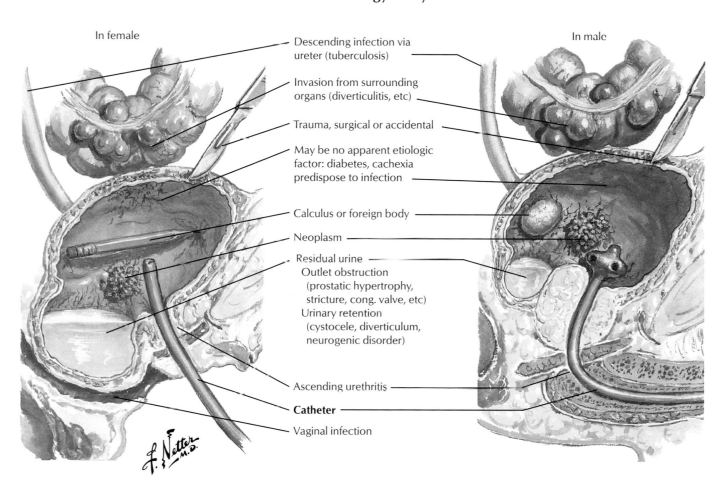

In female

In male

Descending infection via ureter (tuberculosis)

Invasion from surrounding organs (diverticulitis, etc)

Trauma, surgical or accidental

May be no apparent etiologic factor: diabetes, cachexia predispose to infection

Calculus or foreign body

Neoplasm

Residual urine
Outlet obstruction (prostatic hypertrophy, stricture, cong. valve, etc)
Urinary retention (cystocele, diverticulum, neurogenic disorder)

Ascending urethritis

Catheter

Vaginal infection

FIGURE 10-14 MONOBACTAMS: AZTREONAM

Aztreonam is a monobactam antibiotic that inhibits bacterial cell wall synthesis and is resistant to most β lactamases. The agent displays activity only against gram-negative organisms, including *P aeruginosa, E coli, Serratia marcescens, Klebsiella pneumoniae, Proteus mirabilis, H influenzae,* and *Enterobacter* and *Citrobacter* species. Aztreonam is used for treatment of septicemia, lower respiratory tract infections (including pneumonia and bronchitis), and urinary tract, skin and skin structure, intraabdominal, and gynecologic infections. For treatment of mixed infections, aztreonam is combined with other antibiotics to ensure coverage of gram-positive and anaerobic bacteria. Adverse effects include frequent increases in liver function test results, nausea, vomiting, rashes, and phlebitis. The drug may be safe for use in patients who are allergic to cephalosporins and penicillins.

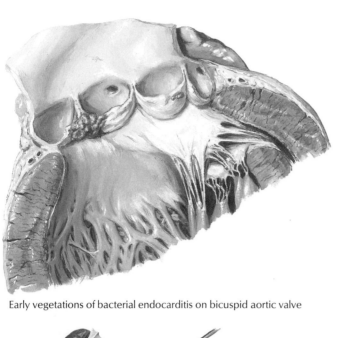

Early vegetations of bacterial endocarditis on bicuspid aortic valve

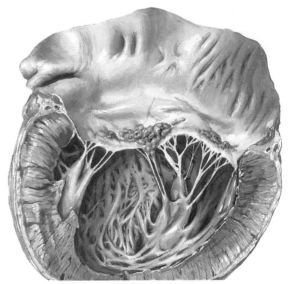

Early vegetations of bacterial endocarditis at contact line of mitral valve

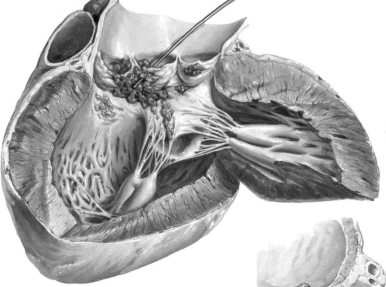

Advanced bacterial endocarditis of aortic valve: perforation of cusp; extension to anterior cusp of mitral valve and chordae tendineae: "jet lesion" on septal wall

Vegetations of bacterial endocarditis on underaspect as well as on atrial surface of mitral valve

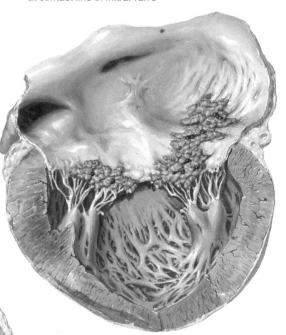

Advanced lesion of mitral valve: vegetations extending onto chordae tendineae with rupture of 2 chordae; also extension to atrial wall and contact lesion on opposite cusp

FIGURE 10-15 VANCOMYCIN

Vancomycin, a glycopeptide, inhibits bacterial cell wall synthesis by binding to cell wall phospholipids and inhibiting polymerase and transpeptidation, which leads to cell wall lysis. Because its site of action is different from that of other β-lactam antibiotics, no cross-resistance occurs. The drug of last resort, vancomycin targets methicillin-resistant staphylococci, *Staphylococcus epidermidis*, *Streptococcus viridans* or *Streptococcus bovis* (alone or with an aminoglycoside), and *Enterococcus faecalis* (with an aminoglycoside). The drug should be used only for serious infections caused by β lactam–resistant gram-positive bacteria, infections caused by gram-positive bacteria in patients with serious allergy to β-lactam antibiotics, antibiotic-associated pseudomembranous colitis that is unresponsive to metronidazole, enterococcal endocarditis, and as prophylaxis for endocarditis after implantation of prosthetic materials or devices at institutions with a high rate of MRSA-related infection.

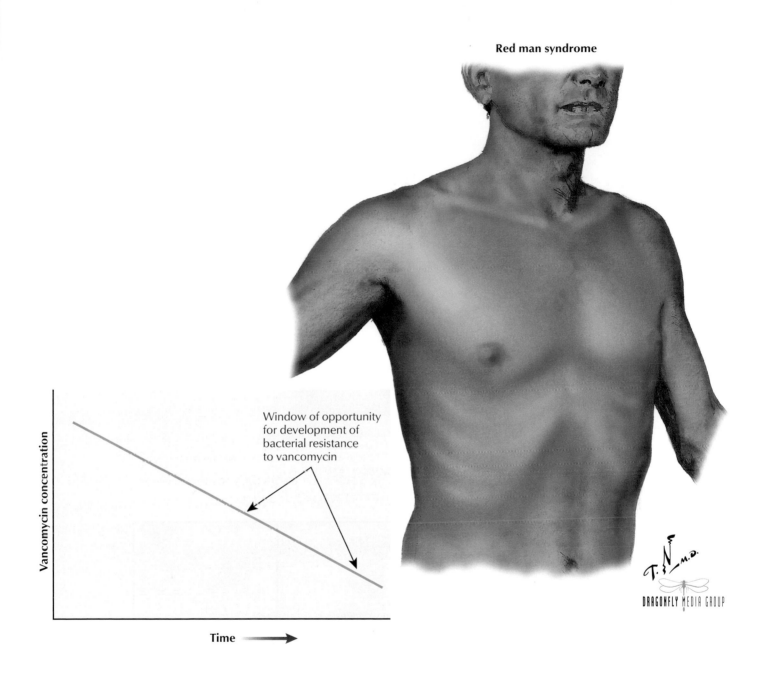

Red man syndrome

Window of opportunity for development of bacterial resistance to vancomycin

Vancomycin concentration

Time

FIGURE 10-16 VANCOMYCIN TREATMENT DIFFICULTIES: RESISTANCE AND ADVERSE EFFECTS

After long-standing efficacy against deadly gram-positive pathogens, resistance of *Enterococcus* and *Staphylococcus* species to vancomycin has begun, such as the case of an *S aureus* isolate from a patient with renal disease that showed intermediate levels of resistance. The patient had undergone long-term peritoneal dialysis and multiple courses of vancomycin for recurring MRSA-associated peritonitis. Patients with renal failure who receive peritoneal dialysis are sometimes given once-weekly vancomycin, which is removed to some extent during each dialysis session. Thus, drug concentrations decrease, and the patient has low drug levels for the latter part of the week. During this time, the organism can mutate and develop resistance. Adverse effects of IV vancomycin include infusion-related events ("red man syndrome": decreased blood pressure, wheezing, urticaria, pruritus, upper body flushing, pain, muscle spasms), thrombophlebitis, hypersensitivity, fever, neutropenia, ototoxicity, and nephrotoxicity.

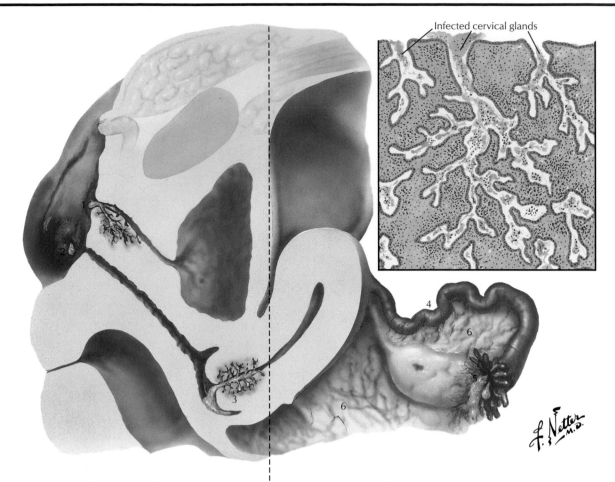

Infected cervical glands

Primary sites of infection
1. Urethra and Skene glands
2. Bartholin glands
3. Cervix and cervical glands

Subsequent sites of infection
4. Fallopian tubes (salpingitis)
5. Emergence from tubal ostium (tubo-ovarian abscess and peritonitis)
6. Lymphatic spread to broad ligaments and surrounding tissues (frozen pelvis)

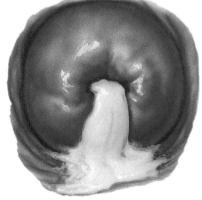

Appearance of cervix
in acute infection

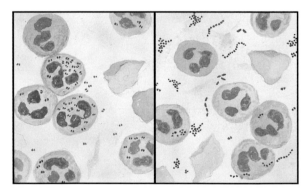

Gonorrheal infection
(Gram stain)

Nonspecific infection
(Gram stain)

FIGURE 10-17 TETRACYCLINES

Tetracyclines bind reversibly to the 30S and 50S subunits of the bacterial ribosome and inhibit protein synthesis, with the broadest spectrum of any antibiotic class: they are bacteriostatic for most gram-positive organisms, many gram-negative organisms, and certain anaerobic bacteria. They are drugs of choice for many animal-borne infections (eg, Lyme disease), sexually transmitted diseases (eg, gonorrhea), and other infections (eg, with *Mycoplasma pneumoniae*). Tetracycline is used for prostatitis,

travelers' diarrhea, acne, *Chlamydia* infections, and *H pylori* infections; doxycycline is used for prophylaxis and treatment of multidrug-resistant malaria. The most common adverse effects target the GI tract; more serious effects include pseudotumor cerebri, superinfections, and hepatotoxicity. These agents should be avoided in children, because of effects on teeth, and in renal disease (except doxycycline); they can render oral contraceptives less effective.

Acute Pyelonephritis: Pathology

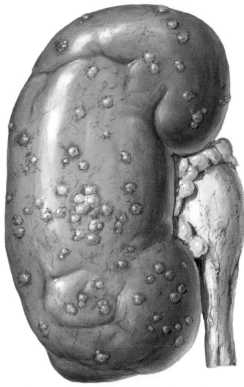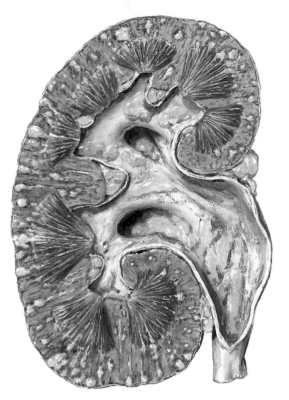

Surface aspect of kidney: multiple minute abscesses (surface may appear relatively normal in some cases)

Cut section: radiating yellowish-gray streaks in pyramids and abscesses in cortex; moderate hydronephrosis with infection; blunting of calyces (ascending infection)

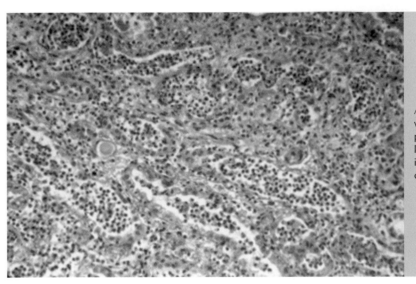

Acute pyelonephritis with exudate chiefly of polymorphonuclear leukocytes in interstitium and collecting tubules

FIGURE 10-18 AMINOGLYCOSIDES

Aminoglycosides are bactericidal agents that bind directly and irreversibly to 30S ribosomal subunits and inhibit bacterial protein synthesis. They target many aerobic gram-negative and some gram-positive organisms but not anaerobes. Monotherapy is limited to infections caused by gram-negative bacilli (eg, septicemia, intraabdominal infections, serious UTIs). The drugs are usually used with other antibiotics for enhanced diffusion. Once-daily higher dosing allows less frequent drug level monitoring. These drugs tend to cause ototoxicity, which is reversible only if noted early and if the drug is stopped. Increased risk for hearing loss can occur when other ototoxic drugs are given. Nephrotoxicity leads to often reversible tubular necrosis. Neuromuscular blockade, causing skeletal weakness and respiratory distress, often occurs after high doses given by an intraperitoneal or an intrapleural route. Safer drugs (eg, third-generation cephalosporins, imipenem-cilastatin) have somewhat replaced aminoglycosides.

Legionnaires Disease
(Pneumonia Due to Legionnaires Bacillus)

A. Small, blunt, pleomorphic intracellular and extracellular bacilli in lung of patient with Legionnaires disease as shown by Dieterle silver impregnation stain, ×1500 (after Chandler et al.)

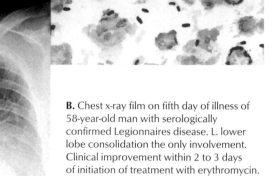

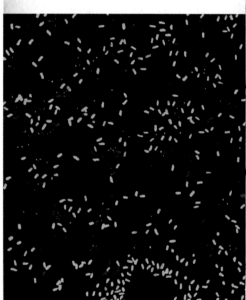

B. Chest x-ray film on fifth day of illness of 58-year-old man with serologically confirmed Legionnaires disease. L. lower lobe consolidation the only involvement. Clinical improvement within 2 to 3 days of initiation of treatment with erythromycin. Radiologic changes did not completely disappear for 2 months.

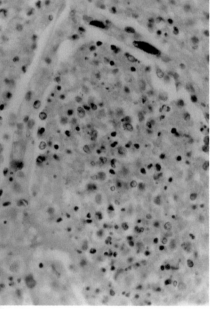

C. Legionnaires bacilli identified by specific fluorescent antibody stain

D. Histologic section of lung (H and E stain) from fatal case of Legionnaires disease; extensive intraalveolar exudate present, containing many large macrophages

FIGURE 10-19 MACROLIDES: ERYTHROMYCIN, AZITHROMYCIN, AND CLARITHROMYCIN

The bacteriostatic macrolides, which bind to the 50S subunit of the bacterial ribosome and inhibit protein synthesis, are effective for sexually transmitted diseases and community-acquired pneumonia. Erythromycin is active against *Chlamydia*, *Treponema pallidum*, *M pneumoniae*, *Ureaplasma*, *Corynebacterium diphtheriae*, and *Legionella*; clarithromycin has greater activity against *Chlamydia*, *Legionella*, and *Ureaplasma* plus coverage for *Haemophilus influenzae*. Erythromycin's spectrum of activity parallels that of penicillin, so it is often used if penicillin allergy exists. Azithromycin is less effective than erythromycin for *Streptococcus* and *Staphylococcus* but better for respiratory infections caused by *H influenza*, *Moraxella catarrhalis*, and *M pneumoniae*. Azithromycin is preferred for *Mycobacterium avium-intracellulare* complex. The most common adverse effect is epigastric pain. Erythromycin can cause cholestatic jaundice and thrombophlebitis; it should be avoided in hepatic dysfunction.

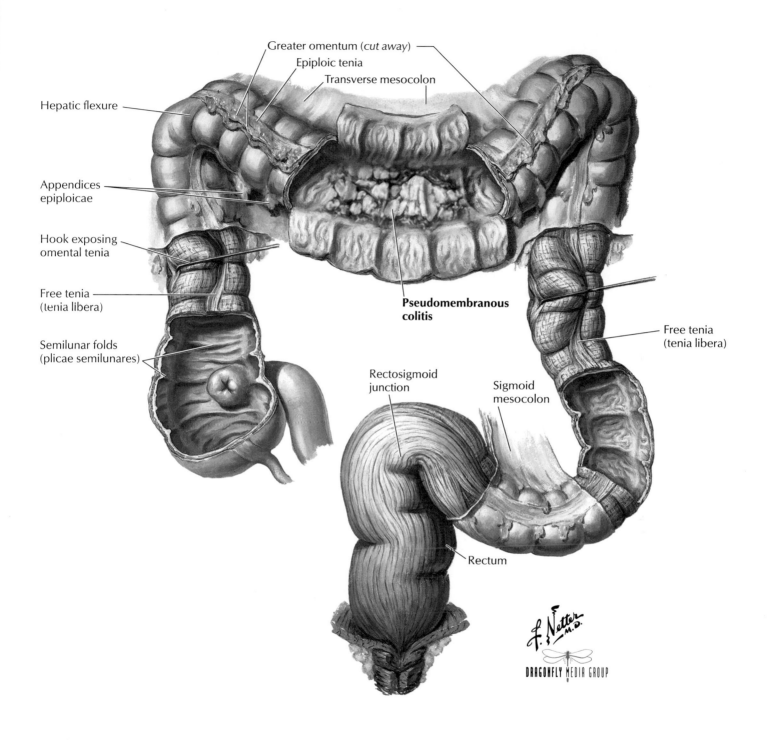

Greater omentum (*cut away*)
Epiploic tenia
Transverse mesocolon

Hepatic flexure

Appendices epiploicae

Hook exposing omental tenia

Free tenia (tenia libera)

Semilunar folds (plicae semilunares)

Pseudomembranous colitis

Free tenia (tenia libera)

Rectosigmoid junction

Sigmoid mesocolon

Rectum

f. Netter
m.s.

DRAGONFLY MEDIA GROUP

FIGURE 10-20 CLINDAMYCIN

Although chemically distinct, clindamycin is similar to erythromycin in mechanism of action and spectrum of activity. It is used mainly for infections caused by anaerobic bacteria such as *B fragilis*, which is responsible for abdominal infections related to trauma. It is also used for aspiration pneumonia and infections caused by streptococci and methicillin-sensitive *S aureus* in patients who are allergic to penicillin. Its most serious adverse effect is pseudomembranous colitis, a possibly fatal superinfec-

tion (*C difficile* overgrowth in the bowel). This complication, which is more likely to occur with clindamycin than with other antibiotics, may present with watery diarrhea, abdominal pain, fever, and leukocytosis. Symptoms begin 3 to 10 days after starting the drug or soon after stopping it. Oral metronidazole and vancomycin effectively eradicate the superinfection, but the latter is usually used only if the former fails. Other adverse effects include nausea, rash, and impaired liver function.

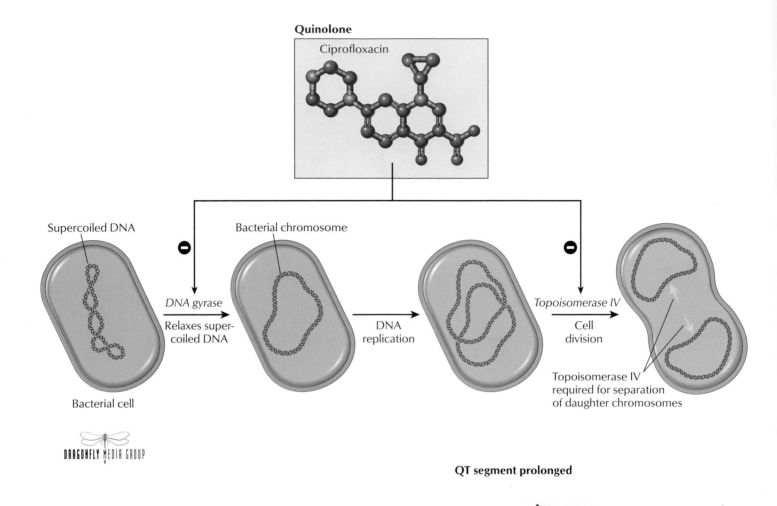

FIGURE 10-21 QUINOLONES

Quinolones (eg, ciprofloxacin), broad-spectrum bactericidal antibiotics that inhibit DNA gyrase or topoisomerase IV (essential for duplication, transcription, and repair of bacterial DNA), target various aerobic gram-positive (eg, methicillin-resistant and β lactamase–producing *Staphylococcus* species, *S pneumoniae*) and gram-negative (eg, *H influenzae, M catarrhalis, P aeruginosa, Legionella, Chlamydia*) organisms. They are used for resistant respiratory infections; chlamydial infections; UTIs; and infections of the GI tract, joints, bones, skin, and skin structures. The most common adverse effects are nausea, headache, phototoxicity, and dizziness; more serious are CNS effects (psychosis, agitation, tremors), hepatotoxicity, interstitial nephritis, tendonitis or joint rupture, and prolonged QTc interval (and thus arrhythmias). Patients with neurologic disorders (eg, seizure), those taking certain antiarrhythmics, and those with a prolonged QTc interval should avoid quinolones.

Empiric Therapy for Patients With Community-Acquired Pneumonia*

Outpatients

- General preferred (not in particular order)
  — Doxycycline
  — A macrolide: erythromycin, azithromycin, clarithromycin
  — A fluoroquinolone: levofloxacin, moxifloxacin, gatifloxacin

- Selection should be influenced by regional antibiotic susceptibility patterns for *S pneumoniae* and the presence of other risk factors for drug-resistant *S pneumoniae*.

- Penicillin-resistant pneumonococci may be resistant to macrolides and/or doxycycline.

- For older patients or those with underlying disease, a fluoroquinolone may be a preferred choice; some authorities prefer to reserve fluoroquinolones for such patients.

- Hospitalized patients (general medical ward)

- Generally preferred are an extended-spectrum cephalosporin combined with a macrolide or a β-lactam/β-lactamase inhibitor combined with a macrolide, or a fluoroquinolone (alone).

- Extended-spectrum cephalosporins: ceftriaxone, cefotaxime, cefepime

- Macrolides: erythromycin, azithromycin

- β-Lactam/β-lactamase inhibitor combination: piperacillin/tazobactam, ampicillin/sulbactam

- Fluoroquinolone: levofloxacin, gatifloxacin, moxifloxacin

Hospitalized patients (intensive care unit)

- Generally preferred are an extended-spectrum cephalosporin or β-lactam/β-lactamase inhibitor plus either fluoroquinolone or macrolide.

- Alternatives or modifying factors

- Structural lung disease: antipseudomonal agents (pipercillin, pipercillin-tazobactam, imiperam or meraperam, or cefepime) plus a fluoroquinolone (including high-dose ciprofloxacin)

- β-Lactam allergy: fluoroquinolone ± clindamycin

- Suspected aspiration: fluoroquinolone with or without clindamycin, metronidazole, or a β-lactam/β-lactamase inhibitor

*Dose may need to be adjusted for weight, or renal or hepatic failure.

Adapted from Bartlett JG, Dowell SF, Mandell LA, File TM Jr, Musher DM, Fine MJ. Practice guidelines for the management of community-acquired pneumonia in adults. Infectious Diseases Society of America. *Clin Infect Dis*. 2000;31:347-382.

Figure 10-22 New-Generation Quinolones

Compared with older quinolones, the newer drugs (eg, levofloxacin, sparfloxacin, grepafloxacin, gaitfloxacin, moxifloxacin) possess enhanced activity against gram-positive organisms, including *S pneumoniae* strains that are resistant to other antibiotics. These agents are thus often used to treat multidrug-resistant community-acquired pneumonia. As with all antibiotics, the new drugs are used excessively and inappropriately in the community setting, which leads to bacterial resistance to the antibiotics.

P aeruginosa Respiratory Infection in Cystic Fibrosis

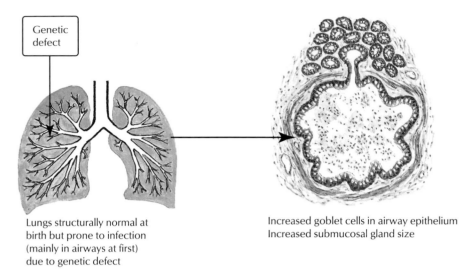

Lungs structurally normal at
birth but prone to infection
(mainly in airways at first)
due to genetic defect

Increased goblet cells in airway epithelium
Increased submucosal gland size

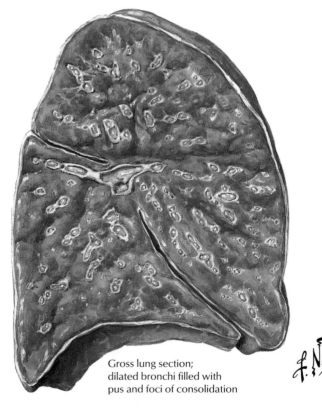

Gross lung section;
dilated bronchi filled with
pus and foci of consolidation

FIGURE 10-22 NEW-GENERATION QUINOLONES (continued)

Ciprofloxacin is a good example of the future for these newer
drugs: although this older quinolone was once 95% effective
against *P aeruginosa*, today it affects only 70% of those isolates.
Older quinolones were also once active against MRSA, but
today, the activity of ciprofloxacin against *S aureus* is variable.
Although new quinolones are quite effective against pneumococci, increased minimal inhibitory concentrations for ofloxacin
against *S pneumoniae* strains have been reported.

Treatment of Septicemia

Clinical Setting	Possible Therapies
Outpatient admission	Third-generation cephalosporin (eg, ceftriaxone, cefotaxime) or piperacillin/tazobactam, or imipenem (or meropenem) each with an aminoglycoside
Intra-abdominal	Piperacillin/tazobactam or imipenem (or meropenem) each with an aminoglycoside
Possible MRSA	Add vancomycin
Hospitalized patient*	Imipenem (or meropenem) or piperacillin/tazobactam (at doses to cover *Pseudomonas aeruginosa*) plus aminoglycoside; ceftazidime, cefepime, and ciprofloxacin are alternatives; use **quinupristin/ dalfopristin** for *Enterococcus faecium* infection
Neutropenic patient	Imipenem (or meropenem), cefepime, ceftazidime alone or with an aminoglycoside; piperacillin/tazobactam (at doses to cover *Pseudomonas aeruginosa*) is an alternative; vancomycin if fevers persist or likelihood of MRSA is high
Possible tick exposure	Add doxycycline

*Local epidemiology of nosocomial infection and antibiotic resistance patterns should be used to guide therapy.

FIGURE 10-23 QUINUPRISTIN/DALFOPRISTIN _____

Perhaps destined to replace vancomycin as the drug of last resort for certain pathogens, quinupristin/dalfopristin is an injectable streptogramin product in which 2 compounds act synergistically to inactivate bacteria via effects on protein synthesis in the bacterial ribosome: dalfopristin inhibits the early phase of synthesis, and quinupristin inhibits the late phase. This drug is used for life-threatening bloodstream infections caused by vancomycin-resistant *Enterococcus faecium* and skin and skin structure infections caused by methicillin-susceptible *S aureus* or *Streptococcus pyogenes*. Identifying *Enterococcus* species (*faecium* and *faecalis*) by blood culture is critical to avoid misuse of this drug (it is active against only the former). The most common adverse effects are pain at the infusion site, arthralgia, and myalgia. Drug interactions may occur, with agents metabolized by the cytochrome P-450 3A4 system (eg, cyclosporine, nifedipine) and with drugs prolonging the QTc interval.

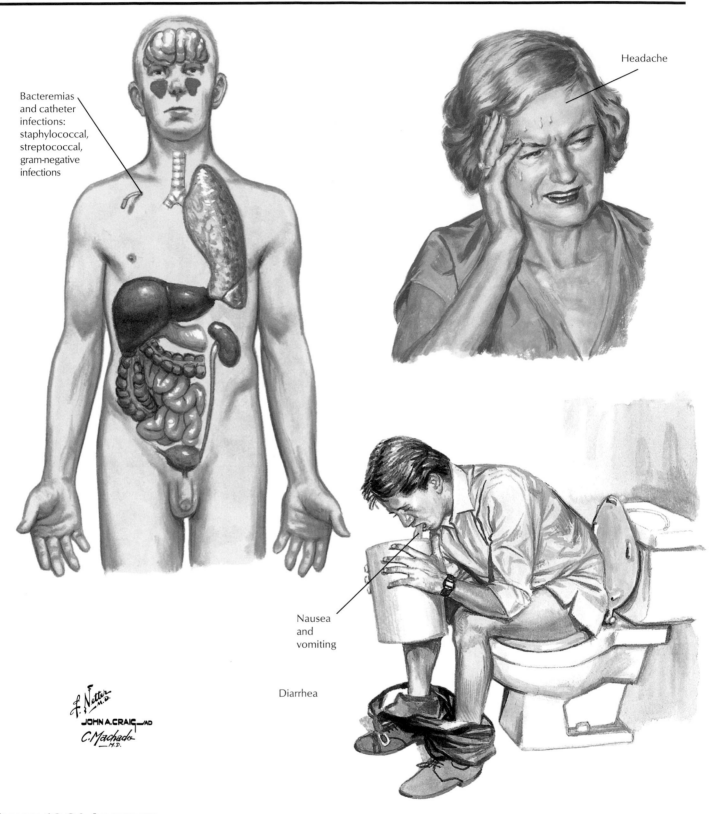

Headache

Bacteremias and catheter infections: staphylococcal, streptococcal, gram-negative infections

Nausea and vomiting

Diarrhea

FIGURE 10-24 LINEZOLID

Another antibiotic for otherwise untreatable infections, linezolid is an oxazolidinone derivative that binds to ribosomal subunits and interferes with bacterial protein synthesis. The drug is intended for treatment of multidrug-resistant gram-positive cocci, particularly as an alternative in infections caused by vancomycin-resistant *Enterococcus*, multidrug-resistant *S pneumoniae* (including vancomycin-ceftriaxone resistant), and MRSA or methicillin-resistant *S epidermidis*. The antibiotic is bacterio-static against *Enterococcus* and staphylococci and bactericidal against most streptococcal strains. The most common adverse effects are nausea, diarrhea, and headache. Linezolid may cause myelosuppression, which could predispose patients to anemia, leukopenia, pancytopenia, and thrombocytopenia. The drug inhibits monoamine oxidase, so consumption of foods with high tyramine content or concomitant use of adrenergic or serotonergic drugs should be avoided.

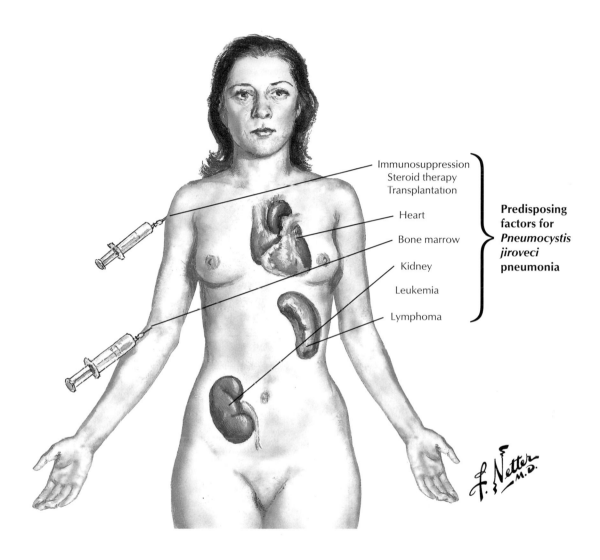

Immunosuppression
Steroid therapy
Transplantation

Heart

Bone marrow

Kidney

Leukemia

Lymphoma

Predisposing factors for *Pneumocystis jiroveci* pneumonia

FIGURE 10-25 SULFONAMIDES

Sulfonamides inhibit synthesis of folic acid and thus synthesis of purines and pyrimidines, so bacteria fail to grow and divide. These bacteriostatic agents are used for trachoma (caused by *Chlamydia*), UTIs caused by *E coli*, and nocardiosis. Trimethoprim, a dihydrofolate reductase inhibitor, is often used with sulfamethoxazole (as co-trimoxazole) for synergy and a broader spectrum of activity. Co-trimoxazole is used for *Pneumocystis jiroveci* pneumonia (a common opportunistic infection in patients with AIDS), chronic UTIs, GI infections (shigellosis and nontyphoid salmonella), and acute gonococcal urethritis. Adverse effects of sulfonamide include crystalluria (minimized by hydration and alkalinization of urine), hypersensitivity reactions (rash, angioedema, and Stevens-Johnson syndrome), and kernicterus in newborns. Adverse effects of trimethoprim (megaloblastic anemia, leukopenia, granulocytopenia) are related to folate deficiency.

Fungal Infections: Antifungal Drugs

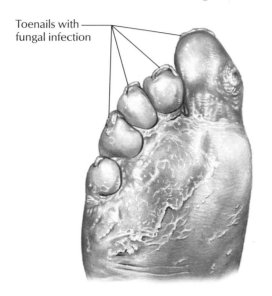

Toenails with fungal infection

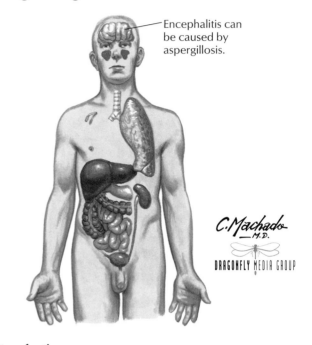

Encephalitis can be caused by aspergillosis.

C. Machado
_M.D.

DRAGONFLY MEDIA GROUP

Mechanisms of action

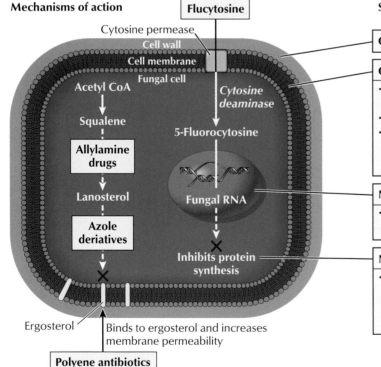

Flucytosine

Cytosine permease
Cell wall
Cell membrane
Fungal cell

Acetyl CoA

Squalene

Allylamine drugs

Lanosterol

Azole deriatives

Ergosterol

Binds to ergosterol and increases membrane permeability

Polyene antibiotics

Cytosine deaminase

5-Fluorocytosine

Fungal RNA

Inhibits protein synthesis

Sites of action

Cell wall

Cell membrane
• Polyenes (amphotericin): bind to membrane ergosterol, altering membrane integrity • Imidazoles (ketoconazole): inhibit cytochrome P-450 • Triazoles (fluconazole): inhibit cytochrome P-450 demethylase–blocks synthesis of ergosterol, necessary for membrane development and maintenance

Nuclear division
• Griseofulvin: inhibits fungal mitosis by binding to intracellular microtubular proteins

Nuclear acid synthesis
• 5-Flucytosine: converted to 5-fluorouracil, which is incorporated into fungal RNA inhibiting protein synthesis; inhibits thymidylate synthase after conversion of flucytosine to 5-fluorodeoxyuridine and fluorodeoxyuridine monophosphate

FIGURE 10-26 NATURE OF FUNGAL INFECTIONS AND THERAPY

Compared with bacteria, fungi have more rigid cell walls and a cell membrane containing ergosterol, they often cause chronic infections, and they are resistant to all antibiotics. Fungal infections, or mycoses, can be superficial, subcutaneous, or systemic. The occurrence of systemic mycoses—the most difficult to treat and usually life threatening—is increasing because there are more immunocompromised patients, such as those with HIV infection, those with cancer, and those who have undergone organ transplantation. In the hospital, complicated surgical procedures, use of implanted devices, and administration of broad-spectrum antibiotics have dramatically increased the incidence of nosocomial fungal infections. The most notable opportunistic fungal pathogens include *Candida albicans* and non-*albicans Candida, Aspergillus, Cryptococcus,* and Zygomycetes species. Agents used to treat systemic fungal infections include amphotericin B, azole derivatives, caspofungin, and voriconazole.

North American Blastomycosis

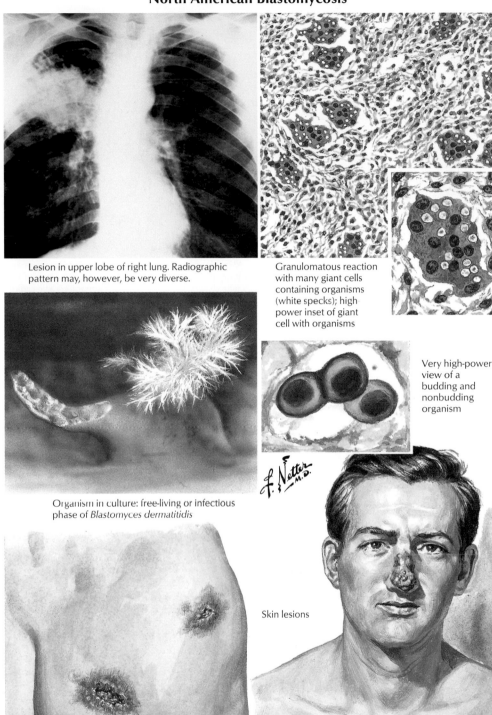

Lesion in upper lobe of right lung. Radiographic pattern may, however, be very diverse.

Granulomatous reaction with many giant cells containing organisms (white specks); high power inset of giant cell with organisms

Very high-power view of a budding and nonbudding organism

Organism in culture: free-living or infectious phase of *Blastomyces dermatitidis*

Skin lesions

FIGURE 10-27 AMPHOTERICIN B

Amphotericin B, a polyene antifungal agent, binds to ergosterol in fungal plasma membranes, interferes with membrane function, and causes cell death. The drug is active against most species including *Cryptococcus neoformans*, *C albicans*, *Sporotrichum*, *Blastomyces dermatitidis*, *Histoplasma capsulatum*, *Coccidioides immitis*, and *Aspergillus fumigatus*. The drug is usually reserved for life-threatening infections (eg, cryptococcal meningitis, histoplasmosis, disseminated candidiasis, coccidioidomycosis, North American blastomycosis, aspergillosis, sporotrichosis). Drug resistance is rare but does occur. Major adverse effects of amphotericin are the reason for its nickname "ampho-terrible." A major adverse effect is renal impairment (reduced by previous sodium loading). Other effects are fever and chills, hypotension, anemia, thrombophlebitis, and neurotoxicity. Lipid-based formulations limit exposure of human cells to the drug and are thus less toxic but are costly and not interchangeable.

Aspergillosis

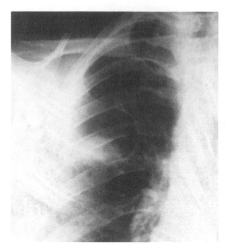

A. Film showing an aspergilloma within a cavity in right lung

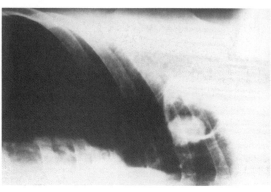

B. Film of same patient as in "A" in l. lateral decubitus position, demonstrating shift of fungus ball to dependent portion of cavity

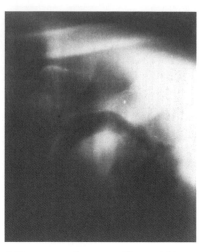

C. Tomogram of an aspergilloma within a cavity in l. upper lobe, demonstrating characteristic radiolucent crescent above fungus ball

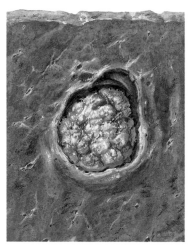

D. Gross appearance of an aspergilloma in a chronic lung cavity

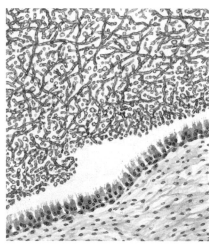

E. Microscopic structure of an aspergilloma composed of a tangled mass of hyphae within a dilated bronchus; no evidence of tissue invasion

FIGURE 10-28 AZOLE ANTIFUNGAL AGENTS AND OTHER ANTIFUNGAL AGENTS

Azole antifungals prevent ergosterol synthesis in fungal cell membranes. Fluconazole is active against *C albicans,* many non-*albicans Candida* species, and *C neoformans* but not *Candida krusei* or *Aspergillus* species. Itraconazole has excellent anti-*Candida* activity; is more effective than fluconazole against *H capsulatum, Sporothrix schenckii,* and *B dermatitidis*; and is fungistatic against *Aspergillus.* Voriconazole has great activity for *Candida* species, is fungicidal for *Aspergillus,* and is active against *Fusarium* species and *Scedosporium apiospermum.* Adverse effects include rash, abnormal liver function (fluconazole); peripheral edema, worsened congestive heart failure (itraconazole); hepatotoxicity (ketoconazole); and transient ocular toxicity (voriconazole). Drug interactions can occur: azoles inhibit metabolism of certain drugs (eg, sulfonylureas, warfarin, digoxin, cyclosporine, tacrolimus); azole serum levels are reduced by other drugs (eg, rifampin, isoniazid, carbamazepine).

Flucytosine is a nucleoside analog that disrupts pyrimidine metabolism in the fungal cell nucleus. The agent is fungicidal for *Candida* species, *C neoformans,* and some strains of *Aspergillus* but not for other commonly encountered fungi. Resistance emerges rapidly during flucytosine monotherapy, so use of this drug is limited to combination therapy (with amphotericin B). Major adverse effects include bone marrow depression, GI toxicity, increased liver function test results, and cutaneous reactions. Caspofungin is a noncompetitive inhibitor of 1,3-β-glucan synthase, an enzyme responsible for formation of an essential cell wall component in many pathogenic fungi and *Pneumocystis carinii* cysts. Caspofungin has good activity against *Aspergillus, Candida,* and *Histoplasma* species. The primary role of this drug is for treatment of refractory invasive aspergillosis and *Candida* esophagitis. The agent is usually well tolerated; rash or GI toxicity occurs rarely.

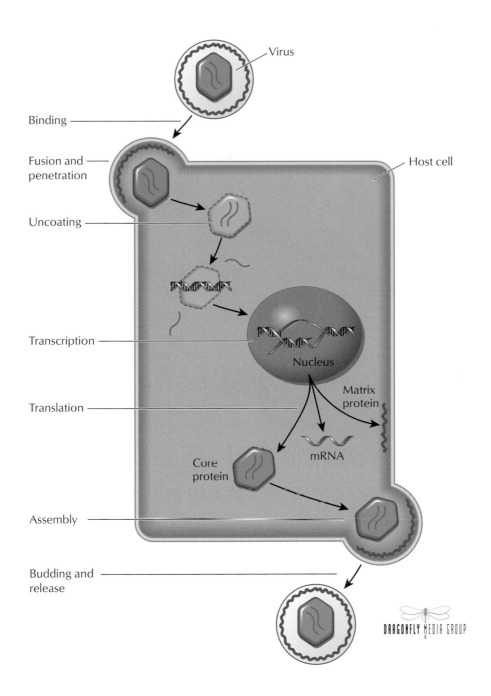

Virus

Binding

Fusion and penetration

Uncoating

Host cell

Transcription

Nucleus

Matrix protein

Translation

mRNA

Core protein

Assembly

Budding and release

DRAGONFLY MEDIA GROUP

FIGURE 10-29 NATURE OF VIRAL INFECTIONS

Unlike fungi and bacteria, viruses lack both cell walls and cell membranes. Viruses consist of either double- or single-stranded DNA or RNA encased in a protein coat (capsid) and can reproduce only by invading a host cell and using its machinery. DNA viruses enter a host cell nucleus and are transcribed into mRNA, which is translated into virus-specific proteins. Infected cells usually die. Most RNA viruses do not depend on host cells for replication but on either enzymes in the virion, which can synthesize its own mRNA, or viral RNA acting as its own mRNA. Influenza virus, however, needs active transcription in a host cell nucleus. Despite a growing arsenal of antiviral drugs, viruses are the most elusive and defiant of all pathogens—as evidenced by the common cold. Immunization against viral infections such as measles, mumps, influenza, and chickenpox is the primary therapeutic approach. Two major infections for which antivirals are often used include influenza and herpesvirus infections.

Clinical Features of HSV Encephalitis

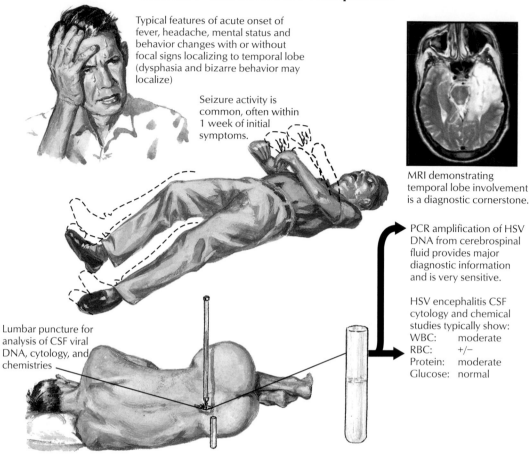

Typical features of acute onset of fever, headache, mental status and behavior changes with or without focal signs localizing to temporal lobe (dysphasia and bizarre behavior may localize)

Seizure activity is common, often within 1 week of initial symptoms.

MRI demonstrating temporal lobe involvement is a diagnostic cornerstone.

PCR amplification of HSV DNA from cerebrospinal fluid provides major diagnostic information and is very sensitive.

HSV encephalitis CSF cytology and chemical studies typically show:
WBC: moderate
RBC: +/−
Protein: moderate
Glucose: normal

Lumbar puncture for analysis of CSF viral DNA, cytology, and chemistries

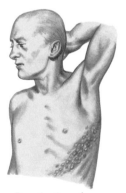

Reactivation of varicella zoster

FIGURE 10-30 HERPESVIRUSES

Human herpesviruses (eg, herpes simplex virus types 1 and 2 [HSV-1 and HSV-2], varicella-zoster virus [VZV], human cytomegalovirus [CMV]) are found worldwide and often infect immunocompetent and immunocompromised patients. HSV-1 causes diseases of the mouth, face, skin, esophagus, or brain; HSV-2 causes diseases of the genitals, rectum, skin, hands, or meninges. HSV infections may be primary or an activation of a latent infection, eg, VZV is a cause of chickenpox first and then herpes zos-ter (shingles). The main physical finding in shingles is a rash that may be preceded by paresthesias or pain along the involved sensory nerve. Herpes encephalitis, a serious infection, is the most common viral infection of the CNS. It presents with general symptoms (fever, headache, decreased consciousness, lethargy) and may be localized to the brain or also involve mucous and cutaneous membranes. Antiviral agents can reduce morbidity, mortality, and duration of symptoms of most HSV infections.

Lesions of Herpes Simplex

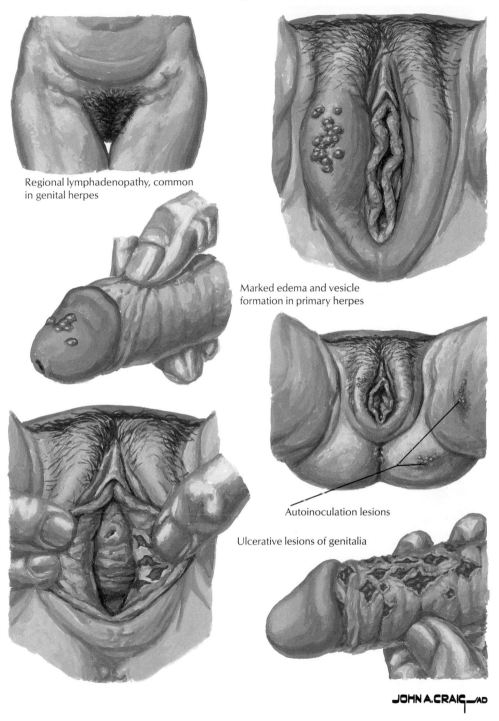

Regional lymphadenopathy, common in genital herpes

Marked edema and vesicle formation in primary herpes

Autoinoculation lesions

Ulcerative lesions of genitalia

JOHN A. CRAIG—AD

FIGURE 10-31 ACYCLOVIR AND FAMCICLOVIR

Acyclovir, an analog of guanosine, is activated by monophosphorylation via viral thymidine kinase and then is phosphorylated via host cell enzymes to a triphosphate form that is a substrate for viral rather than cellular DNA polymerase. It binds to HSV DNA polymerase, is incorporated into viral DNA, and prevents chain elongation. This selective affinity leads to more drug in virus-infected versus healthy cells. Acyclovir is used for initial or recurrent HSV, herpes zoster, and VZV infections. The drug is also used in prophylaxis of HSV and CMV infections in immunocompromised patients but is slightly effective for CMV disease (CMV does not produce thymidine kinase and is thus resistant). Adverse effects depend on route of administration: topical use may cause contact dermatitis, oral use can cause GI effects, and rapid IV infusion may cause renal dysfunction in predisposed patients. Famciclovir is similar to acyclovir but has better bioavailability, which allows for less frequent dosing.

329

Cytomegalovirus Pneumonia

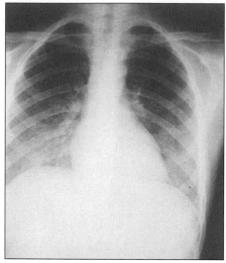

Diffuse densities in both lower lobes

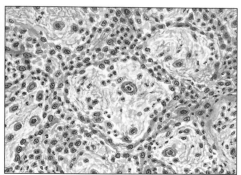

Lung histology in cytomegalovirus pneumonia; cellular and fibrinous exudate in alveoli and in interstitium plus inclusion-bearing cells and epithelial desquamation

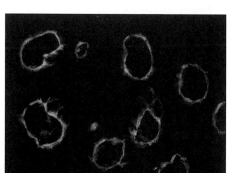

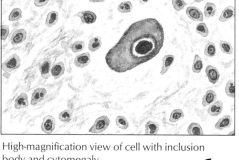

High-magnification view of cell with inclusion body and cytomegaly

Cells infected with cytomegalovirus stained by immunofluorescent technique

Normal tissue culture (HeLa) cells

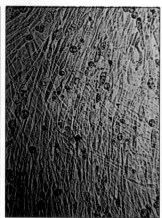

Tissue culture with early rounding of cells due to cytomegalovirus

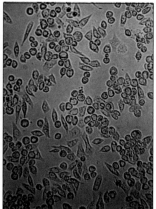

Tissue culture with late cytopathogenic effects due to cytomegalovirus

FIGURE 10-32 GANCICLOVIR

Ganciclovir is similar to acyclovir but somewhat distinct. CMV does not produce thymidine kinase, so ganciclovir is the drug of choice in infections caused by CMV, because enzymes other than thymidine kinase in CMV-infected cells facilitate phosphorylation of the drug. Ganciclovir is used for serious CMV infections, especially retinitis, in immunocompromised patients or patients at risk for CMV disease; it prevents CMV disease in solid organ transplant recipients and HIV-infected patients. The most common adverse effect with IV and oral ganciclovir is bone marrow suppression (anemia, leukopenia, neutropenia, thrombocytopenia). Common adverse effects of intravitreal ganciclovir implants include vitreous hemorrhage and retinal detachments. Valganciclovir is similar to ganciclovir but has better bioavailability, which allows for less frequent dosing.

Influenza Virus and Its Epidemiology

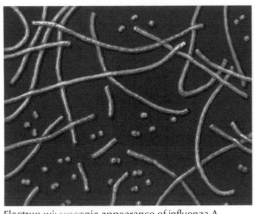

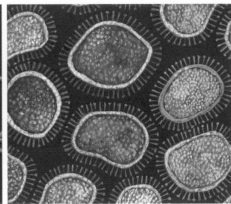

Electron microscopic appearance of influenza A_2 virus; filaments and spherical forms (×10,000)

Virus viewed in section at much higher magnification (×300,000)

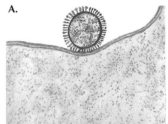

A.

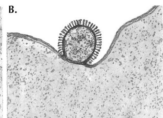

B.

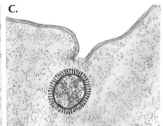

C.

Influenza virus invasion of chorioallantoic membrane cell of chick embryo. **A.** Attachment to cell membrane. **B.** Fusion of viral envelope with cell membrane. **C.** Penetration into cell cytoplasm.

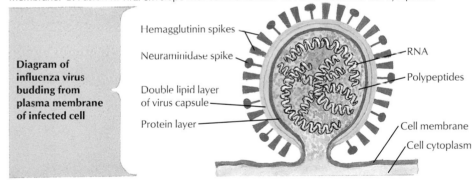

Diagram of influenza virus budding from plasma membrane of infected cell

Hemagglutinin spikes

Neuraminidase spike

Double lipid layer of virus capsule

Protein layer

RNA

Polypeptides

Cell membrane

Cell cytoplasm

FIGURE 10-33 INFLUENZA AND ITS TREATMENT

Influenza, an acute infection, is transmitted by inhalation. Epidemics are usually caused by type A virus; sporadic infections are usually caused by type B. Influenza and the common cold are similar, but the former usually produces more systemic symptoms (eg, high fever, headache, myalgia). Persons at high risk for influenza are the elderly, patients with chronic respiratory and cardiovascular diseases, and health care workers and others who come into contact with high-risk patients. Immunization is preferred to antivirals, which must be given early (within 48 hours). Antiviral drugs do have specific uses, eg, in vaccine-allergic patients and in outbreaks with variants not covered by a vaccine. Amantadine and rimantadine are anti-RNA drugs used for type A virus that block viral penetration of host respiratory epithelial cells; they also block viral uncoating after host cell penetration. Zanamivir (inhaled) and oseltamivir (oral) inhibit viral neuraminidase and are used for type A or B infections.

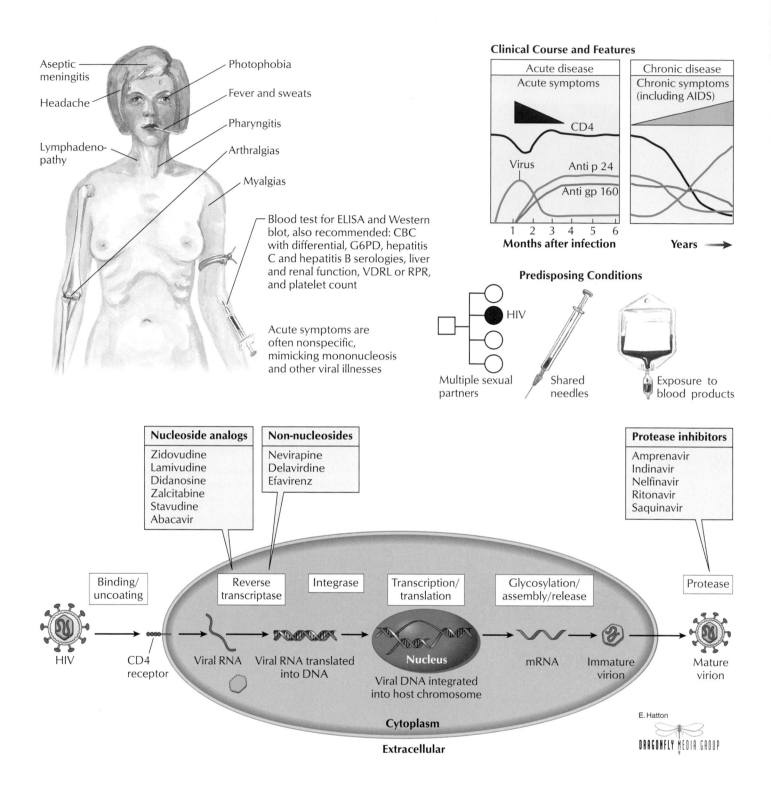

Clinical Course and Features

Acute disease — Acute symptoms

Chronic disease — Chronic symptoms (including AIDS)

CD4

Virus — Anti p 24 — Anti gp 160

Months after infection 1 2 3 4 5 6

Years →

Predisposing Conditions

HIV

Multiple sexual partners — Shared needles — Exposure to blood products

Aseptic meningitis — Photophobia

Headache — Fever and sweats

Pharyngitis

Lymphadeno-pathy — Arthralgias

Myalgias

Blood test for ELISA and Western blot, also recommended: CBC with differential, G6PD, hepatitis C and hepatitis B serologies, liver and renal function, VDRL or RPR, and platelet count

Acute symptoms are often nonspecific, mimicking mononucleosis and other viral illnesses

Nucleoside analogs

Zidovudine
Lamivudine
Didanosine
Zalcitabine
Stavudine
Abacavir

Non-nucleosides

Nevirapine
Delavirdine
Efavirenz

Protease inhibitors

Amprenavir
Indinavir
Nelfinavir
Ritonavir
Saquinavir

Binding/ uncoating — Reverse transcriptase — Integrase — Transcription/ translation — Glycosylation/ assembly/release — Protease

HIV — CD4 receptor — Viral RNA — Viral RNA translated into DNA — **Nucleus** Viral DNA integrated into host chromosome — mRNA — Immature virion — Mature virion

Cytoplasm

Extracellular

E. Hatton
DRAGONFLY MEDIA GROUP

FIGURE 10-34 HIV INFECTION

Acquired through sexual intercourse and exchange of blood, breast milk, and placenta, HIV attacks and binds to the CD4 receptor on CD4+ cells, T helper cells, and T cells. After HIV fuses with the cell, it releases RNA and enzymes needed for replication within the host cell. The single-stranded RNA is transcribed by reverse transcriptase to double-stranded DNA, which is incorporated into the genetic material of host cells via the integrase enzyme. HIV then uses the machinery of the infected cells to produce viral particles that break away from host cells, are cleaved by protease, and can infect other host cells by the same process. Over time, HIV causes host cell lysis and prevents production of new CD4+ cells. AIDS and opportunistic infections arise with decreasing CD4+ cells counts and an increasing viral load. Advances in drug therapy have changed the diagnosis of HIV infection from a death sentence to a life with chronic disease.

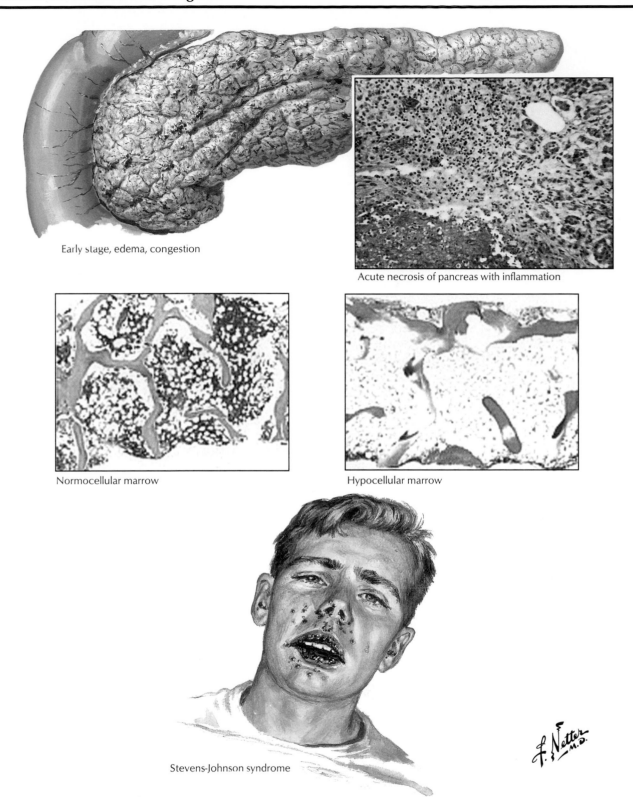

Early stage, edema, congestion

Acute necrosis of pancreas with inflammation

Normocellular marrow

Hypocellular marrow

Stevens-Johnson syndrome

FIGURE 10-35 NUCLEOSIDE REVERSE TRANSCRIPTASE INHIBITORS (NRTIS) AND NON-NRTIS

The first agents developed for HIV, NRTIs suppress viral replication by inhibiting nucleoside reverse transcriptase (converts viral RNA into DNA); non-NRTIs (NNRTIs) also inhibit this enzyme. NRTIs are used with PIs, NNRTIs, or both to treat HIV. NRTIs are also used to prevent maternal-fetal HIV transmission and infection after occupational exposure (eg, needlesticks). Adverse effects are drug specific, eg, zidovudine causes bone marrow suppression and myopathy; didanosine, zalcitabine, and stavudine cause peripheral neuropathy and pancreatitis; lamivudine and abacavir cause fatal hypersensitivity. All NRTIs can cause GI upset and possibly fatal lactic acidosis. NNRTIs can replace a PI in 3-drug regimens that would use 2 NRTIs and a PI. NNRTI adverse effects include rash (eg, Stevens-Johnson syndrome), hepatotoxicity, and CNS effects. All PIs and NNRTIs (not NRTIs) are metabolized by cytochrome P-450 in the liver, and drug interactions may occur with PIs and NNRTIs but are less likely with NRTIs.

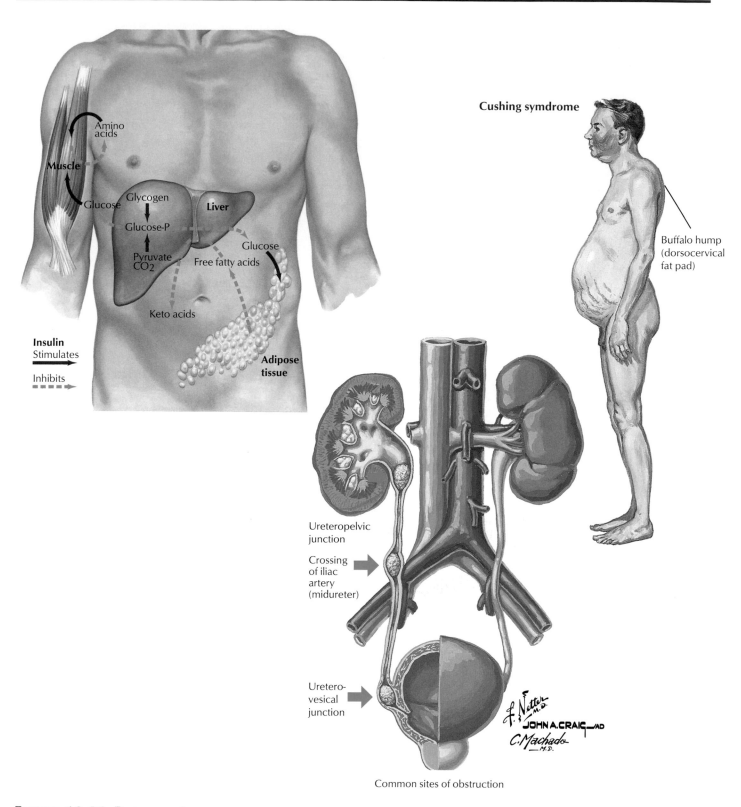

FIGURE 10-36 PROTEASE INHIBITORS

Protease inhibitors inhibit HIV protease, an enzyme needed for proteolysis of viral polyprotein precursors into functional proteins (required for HIV to be infectious). Inhibition leads to formation of noninfectious viral particles. PIs are used with other antiretrovirals to treat HIV; for postexposure prophylaxis, PIs are used with the NRTIs zidovudine and lamivudine. Major adverse effects of PIs include hyperlipidemia; glucose intolerance, insulin resistance, and diabetes; and adipose redistribution syndrome (lipodystrophy,

dorsocervical fat pad [buffalo hump], increased abdominal fat, peripheral lipoatrophy). In addition, ritonavir can cause oral paresthesias and GI upset; indinavir can cause kidney stones and hyperbilirubinemia; nelfinavir can cause diarrhea; and amprenavir can cause rash, GI upset, and oral paresthesias. *Atazanavir* is an azapeptide that can be given once daily and has fewer lipid side effects than other PIs. Its main adverse effect is indirect hyperbilirubinemia with or without jaundice or scleral icterus.

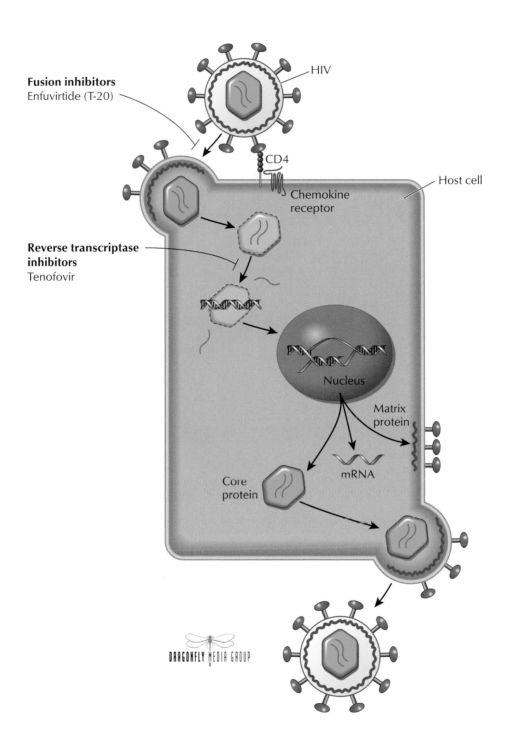

FIGURE 10-37 OTHER ANTIRETROVIRAL AGENTS FOR AIDS: TENOFOVIR AND ENFUVIRTIDE

Tenofovir is a nucleotide analog that, like NRTIs, inhibits nucleoside reverse transcriptase and suppresses DNA viral replication. Unlike NRTIs, it does not require intracellular phosphorylation to an active form; it acts rapidly and is a potent inhibitor of the enzyme. It is active against most NRTI-resistant HIV strains and is reserved for treatment-experienced patients. GI-related adverse effects are common; renal failure and Fanconi syndrome are the more serious effects. *Enfuvirtide*, a peptide that prevents viral fusion with CD4+ cell membranes, is used for HIV infection in treated patients who have HIV replication despite antiviral therapy. The most common adverse effects are injection-site reactions and (in clinical trials) bacterial pneumonia. Because of high cost, complicated dosing, and adverse effects, enfuvirtide is reserved for highly motivated patients who have failed previous regimens and have few options. Both drugs are used in combination with other antivirals.

CHAPTER 11

DRUGS USED IN NEOPLASTIC DISORDERS

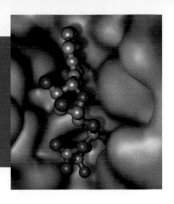

OVERVIEW

The original goal of chemotherapy was not quite as virtuous as that of today, since the first antineoplastic agents (nitrogen mustards) were created to be chemical warfare poisons in World War I. Decades after researchers observed myelosuppressive effects of mustard gas, the goals continue to evolve. At first, the aim was to slow tumor growth, whereas investigators now focus on quality of life, remission, and, sometimes, even cure. Most agents, especially older ones, do not discriminate between normal and abnormal cells and thus affect all proliferating cells, including those found in bone marrow, buccal and GI mucosa, and hair follicles. Most such drugs therefore cause nausea, vomiting, stomatitis, alopecia, and myelosuppression. Newer agents are designed to act more selectively and target components and processes that are unique to cancerous cells, which allows for both safer and more effective treatments.

The pharmacologic principles of chemotherapy are based on the biology of cells, specifically cell division. Antineoplastic agents cause cytotoxicity by targeting events, such as DNA synthesis, that occur during phases of the cell cycle—G_0, G_1, S, G_2, and M. These agents are classified according to these effects on the cell cycle or by other characteristics of their mechanism of action.

Antimetabolites (folate, purine, adenosine, and pyrimidine analogs, and substituted ureas), which are structurally similar to naturally occurring metabolites required for DNA and RNA synthesis, exert their effects either by competing with or by substituting for normal metabolites. Antimetabolites are cell cycle specific; they act during the S phase and are most effective against rapidly growing tumors.

Alkylating agents (eg, nitrogen mustards, nitrosoureas, and platinum compounds) bind to nucleophilic groups on cell constituents, which causes alkylation of DNA, RNA, and proteins. This class is most effective against rapidly dividing cells and is not cell cycle specific.

Popularly known as *spindle poisons*, microtubule inhibitors are plant-derived substances that are cytotoxic because they interfere with the mitotic spindle. The spindle consists of chromatin and microtubules, which are responsible for the metaphase of mitosis. This class includes vinca alkaloids, taxanes, and estramustine.

Steroid hormones affect development of 4 major types of cancer—breast, endometrial, ovarian, and prostate. Breast cancer is classified and treated according to the reactivity of the tumor to estrogen, the main hormone involved in the tumor's growth. Hormone-positive tumors are treated with estrogen antagonists and aromatase inhibitors. A primary treatment method for prostate cancer involves medical androgen ablation via gonadotropin-releasing hormone (GnRH) analogs (with effects on luteinizing hormone [LH] and follicle-stimulating hormone [FSH]) or surgical ablation. Antiandrogens, also used for prostate cancer, block the actions of androgens, whether testicular or adrenal in origin, by interacting with cytosolic androgen receptor sites in all target tissues, including the prostate, hypothalamus, and pituitary.

The aim of antibody-based therapy is to target tumor cells selectively while bypassing healthy cells, thus optimizing efficacy while minimizing toxicity. Monoclonal antibodies are synthetic proteins that can attract immune cells to a tumor or deliver a cytotoxin to a tumor without activating the immune system. Unconjugated antibodies can be used to trigger immune system activation against malignant cells, promote programmed cell death (apoptosis), or interfere with growth factor signals to cancer cells. Conjugated antibodies are attached to radioactive particles or immunotoxins and serve as "guided missiles," delivering their cytotoxic attachments directly to tumors.

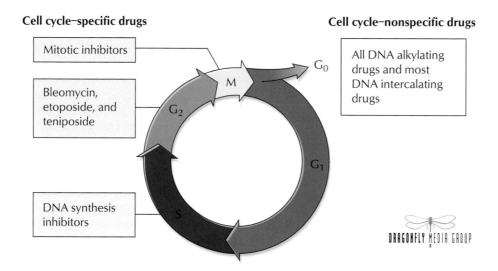

Cell cycle–specific drugs

Mitotic inhibitors

Bleomycin, etoposide, and teniposide

DNA synthesis inhibitors

Cell cycle–nonspecific drugs

All DNA alkylating drugs and most DNA intercalating drugs

G_0

G_1

G_2

M

S

DRAGONFLY MEDIA GROUP

FIGURE 11-1 CELL CYCLE

To replicate, both normal and cancer cells proceed through the cell cycle, which is divided into G_0, G_1, S, G_2, and M (mitosis) phases. In the postmitotic G_1 phase, cells produce many enzymes required for DNA synthesis. In the G_0 phase, cells are resting but are still viable and can enter cell division. During S phase, DNA content doubles in preparation for cell division. In premitotic G_2 phase, additional protein and RNA synthesis occurs. Antineoplastic agents cause cytotoxicity by affecting events occurring during these phases. Drugs that destroy cells only during a certain phase are cell cycle specific; cell cycle–nonspecific agents destroy cells independently of the phases. Chemotherapy is most effective against replicating tumor cells. Cell cycle–nonspecific agents, however, can be useful against tumors with few replicating cells. Chemotherapy is given intravenously, orally, intramuscularly, or subcutaneously or as a bolus injection, a short infusion, or a continuous infusion.

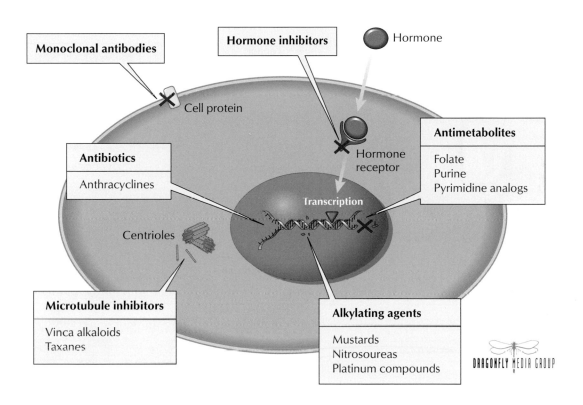

FIGURE 11-2 COMBINATION CHEMOTHERAPY

Aside from a few hematologic malignancies, most tumors show only a partial, fleeting response to monotherapy. Combination chemotherapy provides higher and more durable response rates by displaying efficacy against a broader range of cell lines in heterogeneous tumors, preventing or slowing development of resistance, and providing maximal cell kill (a measure of the number of tumor cells killed by drugs in relation to dose). Combination chemotherapy has thus become the standard for most malignancies. Selection of agents for regimens is based on the following principles: Only agents with demonstrated activity as monotherapy against the specific type of tumor should be selected. All agents within the regimen should have different mechanisms of action (which often has additive or synergistic effects). To minimize unacceptable toxicity, agents should not have overlapping adverse effects. To optimize efficacy and minimize resistance, the optimal dose and schedule of the drugs should be used.

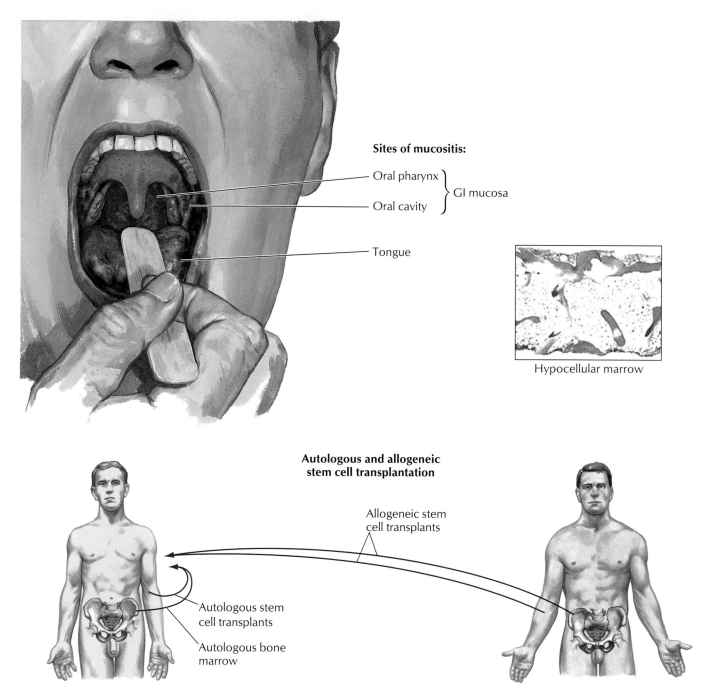

Sites of mucositis:

Oral pharynx
Oral cavity } GI mucosa

Tongue

Hypocellular marrow

Autologous and allogeneic stem cell transplantation

Allogeneic stem cell transplants

Autologous stem cell transplants

Autologous bone marrow

In autologous transplantation the patient is the source of the stem cells (the patient is the donor and the host at the same time). When the stem cells come from another person who is a histocompatible donor, this is called *allogeneic transplantation*.

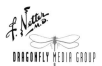

FIGURE 11-3 ADVERSE EFFECTS OF CHEMOTHERAPY

Most agents, especially older ones, do not discriminate between normal and abnormal cells and thus affect all proliferating cells, including those found in bone marrow, buccal and GI mucosa, and hair follicles. This nonselective feature helps to explain toxicities associated with these drugs. To some extent, most such agents cause nausea, vomiting, stomatitis, alopecia, and myelosuppression. Although most adverse effects are transient, certain ones (cardiac, pulmonary, and bladder toxicity) can be

irreversible. Adverse effects can be minimized via supportive care therapy such as antiemetics for nausea and vomiting, erythropoietic agents and hematopoietic colony-stimulating factors for anemia and neutropenia, antihistamines and corticosteroids for hypersensitivity reactions, and chemoprotective agents such as mesna and amifostine for organ toxicity. A more intense measure involves harvesting bone marrow from a patient before myelosuppressive therapy and then reimplanting it after treatment.

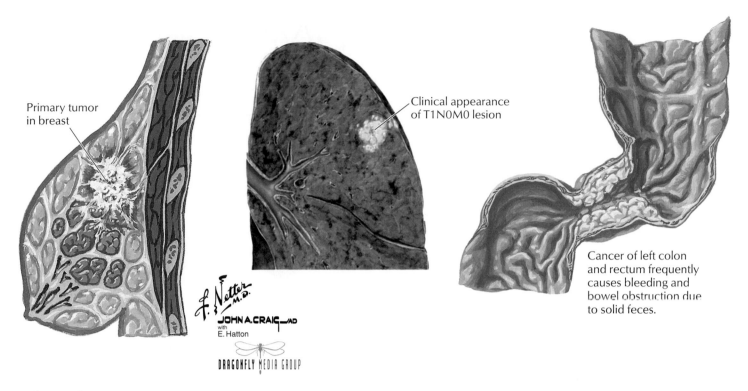

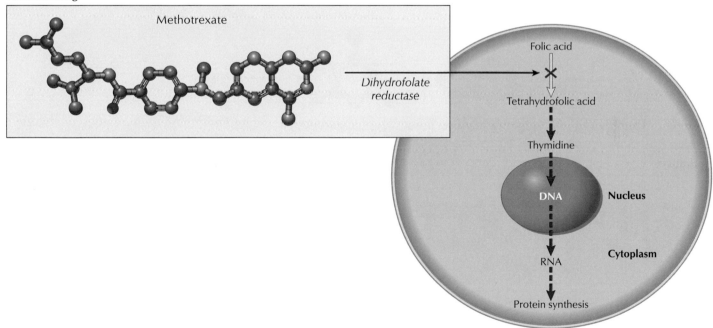

Primary tumor in breast

Clinical appearance of T1N0M0 lesion

Cancer of left colon and rectum frequently causes bleeding and bowel obstruction due to solid feces.

Folate analog

Methotrexate

Dihydrofolate reductase

Folic acid

Tetrahydrofolic acid

Thymidine

DNA   **Nucleus**

RNA   **Cytoplasm**

Protein synthesis

FIGURE 11-4 FOLATE ANALOGS: METHOTREXATE

One of the oldest and most studied antineoplastic drugs, methotrexate (MTX) is structurally related to folic acid and is its antagonist: it inhibits dihydrofolate reductase (converts folic acid to the active tetrahydrofolic acid). Cells' inability to use folate leads to reduced synthesis of thymidine and other building blocks (eg, DNA, RNA, proteins) essential to cell function. Cell death results. MTX is used for different cancers—eg, colorectal carcinoma, hematologic cancers (leukemias, lymphomas), and breast, lung,

head, neck, and ovarian cancers. Common toxicities depend on dose: myelosuppression, erythema, stomatitis, alopecia, nausea, vomiting, diarrhea. More serious effects are hepatotoxicity, renal failure, and neurologic toxicity. Folic acid has no effect on MTX toxicity; leucovorin bypasses MTX-blocked dihydrofolate reductase, replenishes folate stores, and can prevent life-threatening neutropenia and mucositis, but it cannot protect against MTX-induced organ damage.

Acute lymphatic leukemia

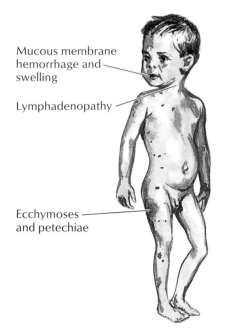

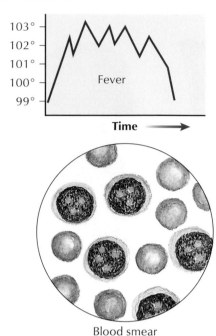

Mucous membrane hemorrhage and swelling

Lymphadenopathy

Ecchymoses and petechiae

Fever

Time

Blood smear

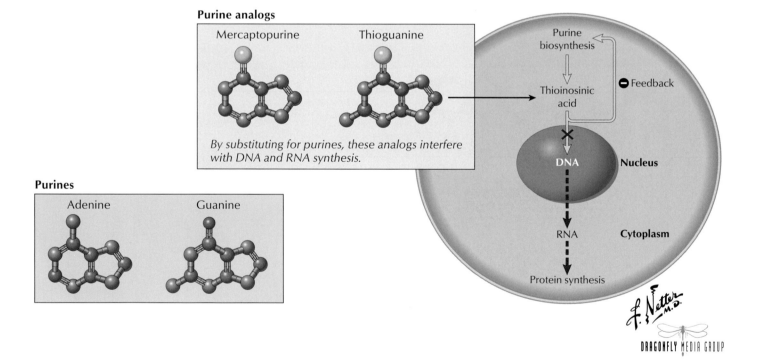

Purine analogs

Mercaptopurine   Thioguanine

By substituting for purines, these analogs interfere with DNA and RNA synthesis.

Purines

Adenine   Guanine

Purine biosynthesis

⊖ Feedback

Thioinosinic acid

DNA   **Nucleus**

RNA   **Cytoplasm**

Protein synthesis

FIGURE 11-5 PURINE ANALOGS: MERCAPTOPURINE AND THIOGUANINE

An analog of hypoxanthine and guanine, *mercaptopurine* (6-MP) is a prodrug that is converted in cells to active nucleotide metabolites. Thioinosinic acid is one such metabolite, which interferes with metabolic reactions needed for RNA and DNA biosynthesis. This metabolite also causes inhibition of the first step in purine biosynthesis or converts to another ribonucleotide that can cause feedback inhibition. 6-MP is primarily used to treat acute lymphatic (lymphocytic, lymphoblastic) leukemia. Adverse effects include dose-related bone marrow suppression, diarrhea, hyperpigmentation, hyperuricemia, and hepatotoxicity (when used with doxorubicin and at certain doses). The toxicity of oral 6-MP is increased when given with allopurinol. *Thioguanine* (6-TG) is also a purine analogue that is structurally and functionally related to 6-MP. Both agents share similar uses and toxicities. Unlike 6-MP, however, 6-TG is not potentiated by allopurinol.

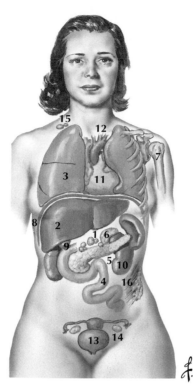

Metastases *from* pancreas
Most common sites:
1. Regional nodes
2. Liver
3. Lung and pleura
4. Intestine
5. Peritoneum

Moderately common sites:
6. Adrenal
7. Bone
8. Diaphragm
9. Gallbladder
10. Kidney

Occasional sites:
11. Heart
12. Mediastinum
13. Bladder
14. Ovary
15. Supraclavicular nodes
16. Muscle or subcutaneous tissue

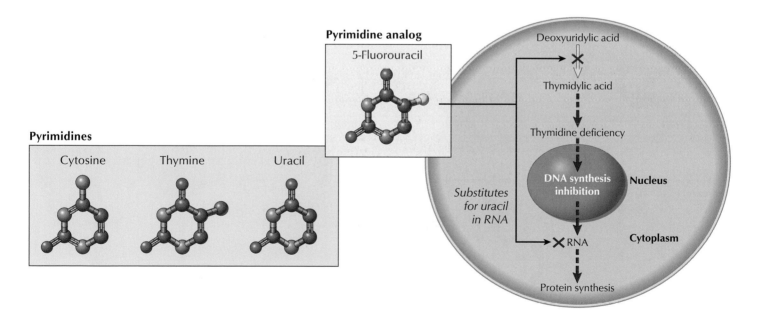

Pyrimidine analog
5-Fluorouracil

Pyrimidines

Cytosine   Thymine   Uracil

Deoxyuridylic acid

Thymidylic acid

Thymidine deficiency

DNA synthesis inhibition   **Nucleus**

Substitutes for uracil in RNA

RNA   **Cytoplasm**

Protein synthesis

FIGURE 11-6 PYRIMIDINE ANALOGS: 5-FLUOROURACIL

5-Fluorouracil (5-FU) is an inactive prodrug that, when converted to its active metabolite, inhibits methylation of deoxyuridylic acid to thymidylic acid, which leads to a lack of thymidine, a nucleoside of DNA. 5-FU also inhibits RNA formation by incorporating itself into the nucleic acid chain. The agent is used to treat solid tumors of the colon, rectum, breast, stomach, and pancreas. 5-FU is poorly absorbed orally and can cause severe GI toxicity, so it is given intravenously, intrahepatically, or topically. Blood dyscrasias, especially leukopenia, are the most common adverse effects; others are stomatitis and diarrhea, which can be severe in certain patients; hand-foot syndrome (painful, erythematous, swollen palms and soles); and cardiac toxicities (chest pain and tightness, dyspnea, cardiogenic shock). Alopecia is uncommon, and nausea and vomiting are usually mild.

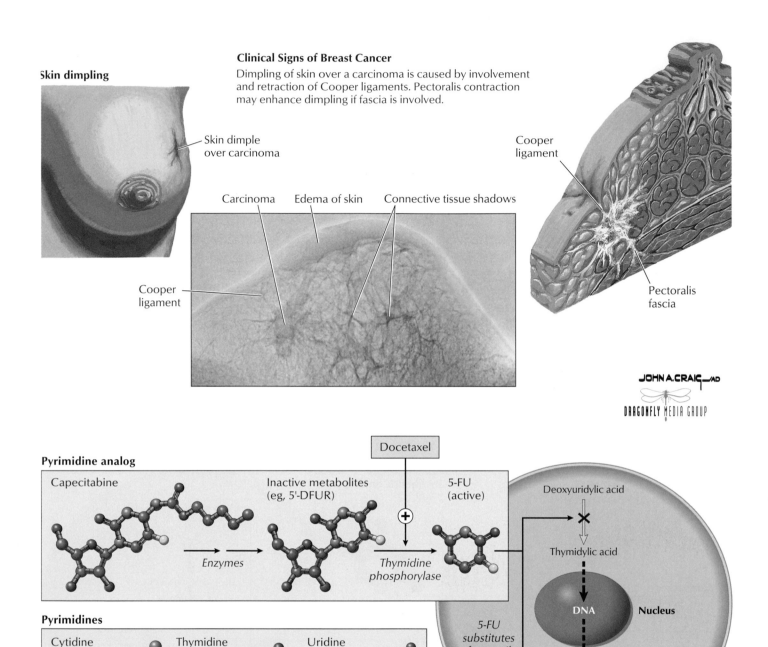

Clinical Signs of Breast Cancer
Dimpling of skin over a carcinoma is caused by involvement and retraction of Cooper ligaments. Pectoralis contraction may enhance dimpling if fascia is involved.

Skin dimpling

Skin dimple over carcinoma

Carcinoma   Edema of skin   Connective tissue shadows

Cooper ligament

Cooper ligament

Pectoralis fascia

JOHN A. CRAIG__AD
DRAGONFLY MEDIA GROUP

Pyrimidine analog

Capecitabine → Enzymes → Inactive metabolites (eg, 5'-DFUR) → Thymidine phosphorylase → 5-FU (active)

Docetaxel

Deoxyuridylic acid ✕ Thymidylic acid

DNA   Nucleus

5-FU substitutes for uracil in RNA

RNA   Cytoplasm

Protein synthesis

Pyrimidines

Cytidine   Thymidine   Uridine

FIGURE 11-7 PYRIMIDINE ANALOGS: CAPECITABINE

An oral, tumor-activated antineoplastic, *capecitabine* is a fluoro-pyrimidine carbamate that undergoes enzymatic conversion to inactive intermediates. When it reaches the tumor, it is converted to active 5-FU by thymidine phosphorylase, an enzyme that is found at high levels in tumors and low levels in normal tissues. This drug, together with docetaxel, is used for patients with metastatic breast cancer and failure to respond to previous anthracycline-containing therapy. It is also indicated as first-line therapy for metastatic colorectal carcinoma. This drug has selective tumor activation, so common drug-related adverse effects (eg, alopecia, bone marrow suppression) are minimized. Its most common side effects include diarrhea, nausea, vomiting, fatigue, stomatitis, and hand-foot syndrome. Potentially serious risks associated with the drug include severe diarrhea, grade 3 or 4 neutropenia, thrombocytopenia, and reduced hemoglobin levels.

Clinical Presentation of Leukemias

Acute myeloid leukemia (AML), acute lymphoblastic leukemia (ALL), chronic myelogenous leukemia (CML), and chronic lymphocytic leukemia (CLL)

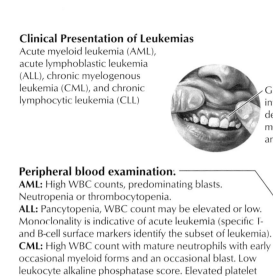

Gum and lung infiltration (AML derived from monocytes M4 and M5)

Peripheral blood examination:

AML: High WBC counts, predominating blasts. Neutropenia or thrombocytopenia.
ALL: Pancytopenia, WBC count may be elevated or low. Monoclonality is indicative of acute leukemia (specific T- and B-cell surface markers identify the subset of leukemia).
CML: High WBC count with mature neutrophils with early occasional myeloid forms and an occasional blast. Low leukocyte alkaline phosphatase score. Elevated platelet count, with dysmorphism and large size. Elevation of basophil count and blasts is seen in accelerated phase of this disorder.
CLL: Elevated WBC count. Mature lymphocytes with "smudge" or broken cells are prevalent.

Hepatomegaly (CML)

Leukemic meningitis, signs of involvement of the central nervous system, cranial nerve abnormalities, headache (ALL)

Fever, weight loss (CML)

Symptoms related to anemia: fatigue, pallor, dyspnea (AML, ALL, CML)

Lymphadenopathy (ALL, CLL)

Abdominal discomfort and early satiety

Splenomegaly (CML, ALL, CLL)

Bone marrow examination:

AML: Hypercellularity with blast count greater than 30%.
ALL: Monoclonality is indicative of acute leukemia (specific T- and B-cell surface markers identify the subset of leukemia). Presence of Philadelphia chromosome (Ph) in a subset of ALL confers a poor prognosis.
CML: Presence of Ph. More than 30% blasts count characterizes blast crisis.
CLL: Diffuse infiltration with mature lymphocytes.

Signs of bleeding, petechiae, purpura (AML, ALL)

C. Machado
—*M.D.*

DRAGONFLY MEDIA GROUP

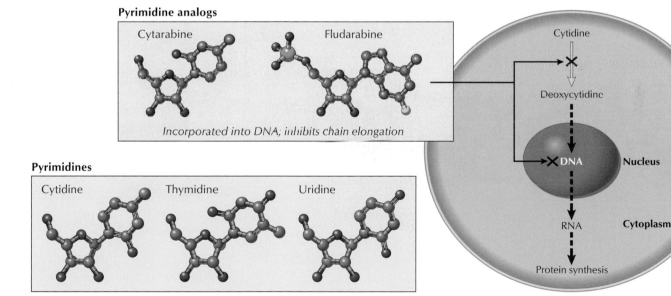

Pyrimidine analogs

Cytarabine   Fludarabine

Incorporated into DNA; inhibits chain elongation

Cytidine

Deoxycytidine

DNA   **Nucleus**

RNA   **Cytoplasm**

Protein synthesis

Pyrimidines

Cytidine   Thymidine   Uridine

FIGURE 11-8 PYRIMIDINE ANALOGS: CYTARABINE AND FLUDARABINE

Cytarabine is a pyrimidine antagonist that inhibits conversion of cytidine to deoxycytidine, which interferes with DNA synthesis. It may also be incorporated into DNA and stop chain elongation. The drug is useful for hematologic malignancies—chronic myelocytic leukemia, lymphoblastic leukemia, acute lympho-cytic and nonlymphocytic leukemias, meningeal leukemia. Cyta-rabine is synergistic with other drugs, including alkylating agents, thiopurines, and anthracycline antibiotics. Although fludarabine is a purine analog, its pharmacologic action is similar to that of cytarabine. It is effective for chronic lymphocytic leukemia, NHL, and acute leukemia. The major toxic effect of both drugs is myelosuppression, which often leads to neutropenia. Other side effects with cytarabine include neuropathies, alopecia, GI dis-tress, hepatic toxicity, hypersensitivity, and corneal toxicity; those of fludarabine include severe neurotoxicity, GI effects, stomatitis, rash, and somnolence.

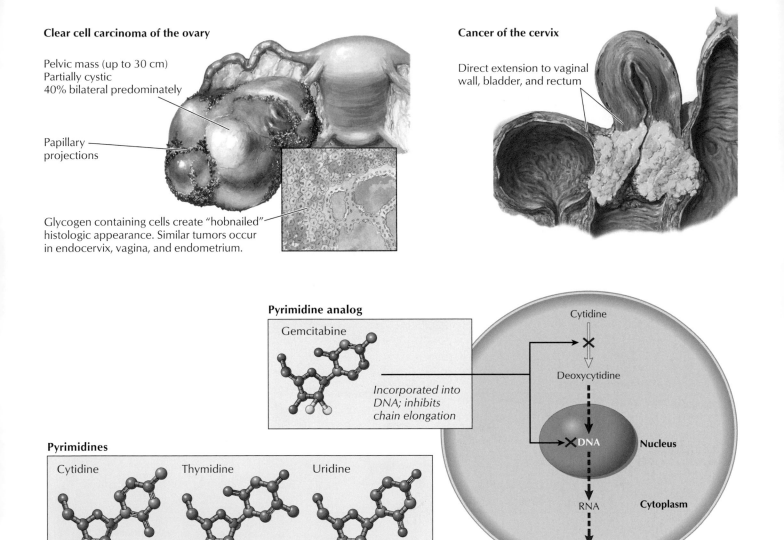

Clear cell carcinoma of the ovary

Pelvic mass (up to 30 cm)
Partially cystic
40% bilateral predominately

Papillary projections

Glycogen containing cells create "hobnailed" histologic appearance. Similar tumors occur in endocervix, vagina, and endometrium.

Cancer of the cervix

Direct extension to vaginal wall, bladder, and rectum

Pyrimidine analog

Gemcitabine

Incorporated into DNA; inhibits chain elongation

Pyrimidines

Cytidine   Thymidine   Uridine

Cytidine

Deoxycytidine

DNA   **Nucleus**

RNA   **Cytoplasm**

Protein synthesis

FIGURE 11-9 PYRIMIDINE ANALOGS: GEMCITABINE

Gemcitabine is structurally and pharmacologically similar to cytarabine. The major distinctions between the two are the longer half-life and higher tissue concentration of gemcitabine. Gemcitabine was specifically developed to extend the activity of cytarabine to nonhematologic malignancies including pancreatic cancer, non–small cell lung cancer, advanced breast cancer, ovarian cancer, and cervical cancer. This drug also has activity as second-line therapy in Kaposi sarcoma. Common adverse effects include myelosuppression (dose limiting), flulike symptoms (occasionally dose limiting), fatigue, fever, peripheral edema, proteinuria, cutaneous reactions (radiosensitizing effects), and GI effects. The drug may also cause adult respiratory distress syndrome and cardiac dysfunction (myocardial infarction, CHF, atrial fibrillation).

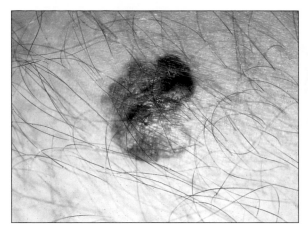

Melanomas

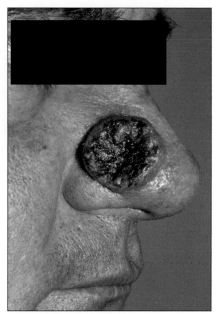

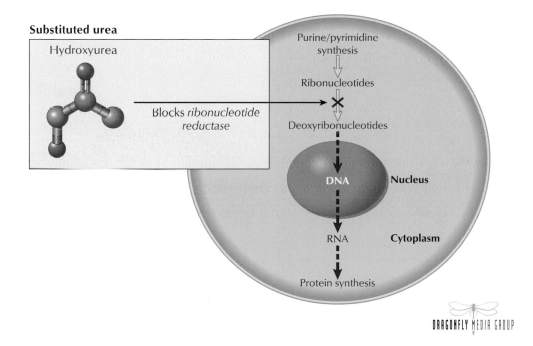

FIGURE 11-10 SUBSTITUTED UREAS: HYDROXYUREA

Hydroxyurea blocks conversion of DNA bases by blocking ribonucleotide reductase; it does not affect RNA or cell proteins. Hydroxyurea causes cells to arrest at the G₁-S interface, which is a period of maximal sensitivity to radiation, so concomitant hydroxyurea and radiation therapy causes synergistic toxicity. Hydroxyurea is used to treat neoplasms including melanoma, chronic myelocytic leukemia, and inoperable ovarian cancer. The agent is given orally to patients with chronic myelogenous leukemia who are in blast crisis (advanced disease in which the number of immature, abnormal leukocytes in bone marrow and blood is quite high). Hydroxyurea is also used as adjunctive therapy to radiation for epidermoid carcinomas of the head and neck. Bone marrow suppression (leukopenia) is the most common adverse effect. Nausea, vomiting, diarrhea, constipation, and mucositis may also occur. Severe and sometimes fatal hepatitis and secondary leukemias have also been associated with this drug.

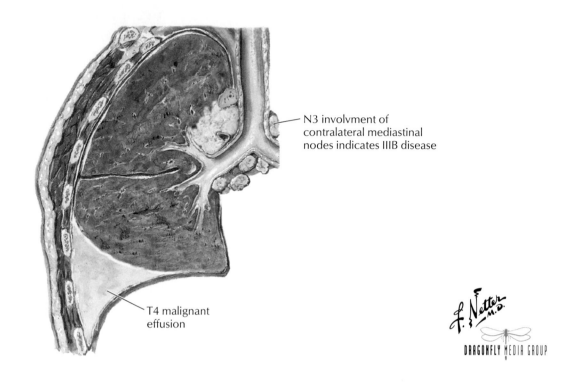

N3 involvment of contralateral mediastinal nodes indicates IIIB disease

T4 malignant effusion

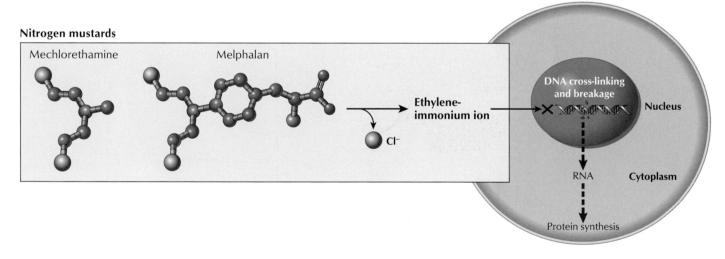

Nitrogen mustards

Mechlorethamine

Melphalan

Cl⁻

Ethylene-immonium ion

DNA cross-linking and breakage

Nucleus

RNA

Cytoplasm

Protein synthesis

FIGURE 11-11 NITROGEN MUSTARDS: MECHLORETHAMINE AND MELPHALAN

Mechlorethamine evolved from its first use as a chemical weapon to medicine, specifically for Hodgkin disease, mycosis fungoides, and malignant pleural effusions. This alkylating agent releases Cl⁻ to form a highly reactive ethylene-immonium ion. In tissues, the ionic form alkylates the nitrogen atom of a guanine residue in DNA, which causes DNA strand cross-linking and then DNA mutation or breakage or both. Proliferating cells, especially cells in G_1 and S phases, are most sensitive to the drug.

Use of this agent is limited by its vesicantlike toxicities, which include nausea, vomiting, skin eruptions, ototoxicity, neurotoxicity, and severe myelosuppression. Melphalan is pharmacologically similar to mechlorethamine but is mainly used for palliation of multiple myeloma and nonresectable epithelial ovarian cancer. Leukopenia and thrombocytopenia are major adverse effects; others include pulmonary infiltrates and fibrosis, nausea and vomiting, amenorrhea, alopecia, sterility, and mucositis.

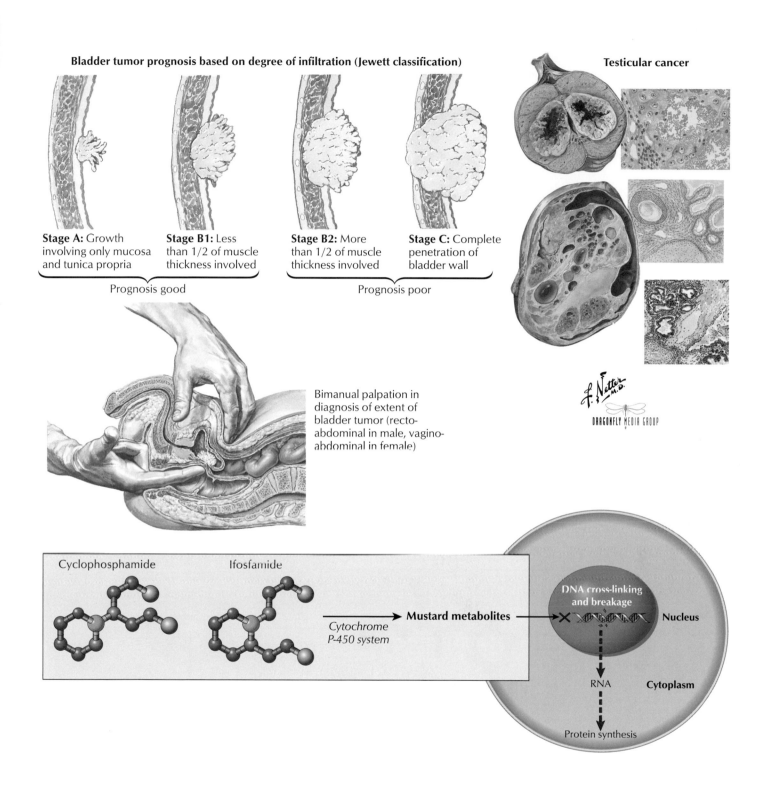

Bladder tumor prognosis based on degree of infiltration (Jewett classification)

Stage A: Growth involving only mucosa and tunica propria

Stage B1: Less than 1/2 of muscle thickness involved

Prognosis good

Stage B2: More than 1/2 of muscle thickness involved

Stage C: Complete penetration of bladder wall

Prognosis poor

Bimanual palpation in diagnosis of extent of bladder tumor (recto-abdominal in male, vagino-abdominal in female)

Testicular cancer

Cyclophosphamide

Ifosfamide

Cytochrome P-450 system → **Mustard metabolites** →

DNA cross-linking and breakage

Nucleus

RNA

Cytoplasm

Protein synthesis

FIGURE 11-12 CYCLOPHOSPHAMIDE AND IFOSFAMIDE

Both cyclophosphamide and ifosfamide are pharmacologically related to nitrogen mustards. These drugs are biotransformed by the cytochrome P-450 system to active mustard metabolites, which act as alkylating agents and form cross-links in the DNA. The first drug is used for a wide variety of cancers—colorectal and cervical cancers, Wilms tumor, pulmonary adenocarcinoma, breast and ovarian carcinoma, leukemias, lymphomas, neuroblastoma, retinoblastoma, bladder carcinoma, and soft tissue sarcomas. Ifosfamide is used in refractory testicular cancer, soft tissue sarcomas, lymphomas, and cancers of the head and neck, breast, lung, cervix, and ovaries. Although ifosfamide has fewer effects, both drugs have similar toxicities, including alopecia, nausea and vomiting, diarrhea, myelosuppression, and hemorrhagic cystitis (can lead to bladder fibrosis). The last can be prevented by hydration and use of mesna, which inactivates toxic metabolites. Ifosfamide can also cause neurotoxicity.

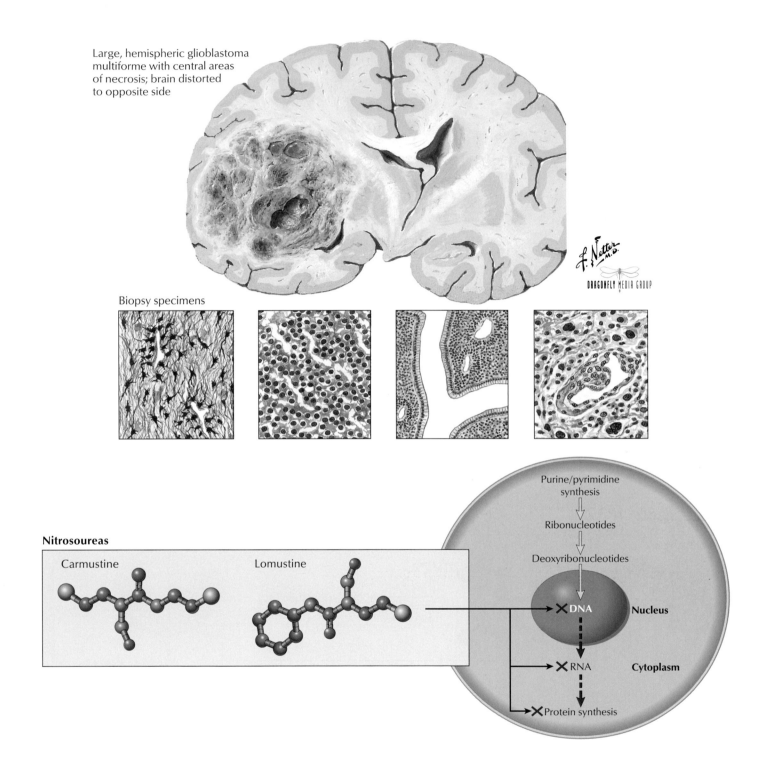

Large, hemispheric glioblastoma multiforme with central areas of necrosis; brain distorted to opposite side

Biopsy specimens

Nitrosoureas

Carmustine

Lomustine

Purine/pyrimidine synthesis

Ribonucleotides

Deoxyribonucleotides

DNA **Nucleus**

RNA **Cytoplasm**

Protein synthesis

FIGURE 11-13 NITROSOUREAS: CARMUSTINE AND LOMUSTINE

Carmustine and lomustine are both nitrosoureas that are cytotoxic via alkylation of DNA and RNA and inhibition of protein synthesis. Both drugs are highly lipid soluble and can therefore enter CSF. As a result, the agents are useful for treatment of brain tumors. Carmustine wafer implants are used as an adjunct to surgery and radiation in patients with newly diagnosed high-grade gliomas and as an adjunct to surgery for patients with recurrent glioblastoma multiforme to prolong survival. Major adverse effects include myelosuppression (delayed with carmustine), pulmonary fibrosis, nausea and vomiting (severe with carmustine), and renal toxicity. Seizures and brain edema are the most common adverse effects associated with carmustine wafer implants. One major difference between the 2 agents is the administration route: carmustine is given intravenously, and lomustine is given orally.

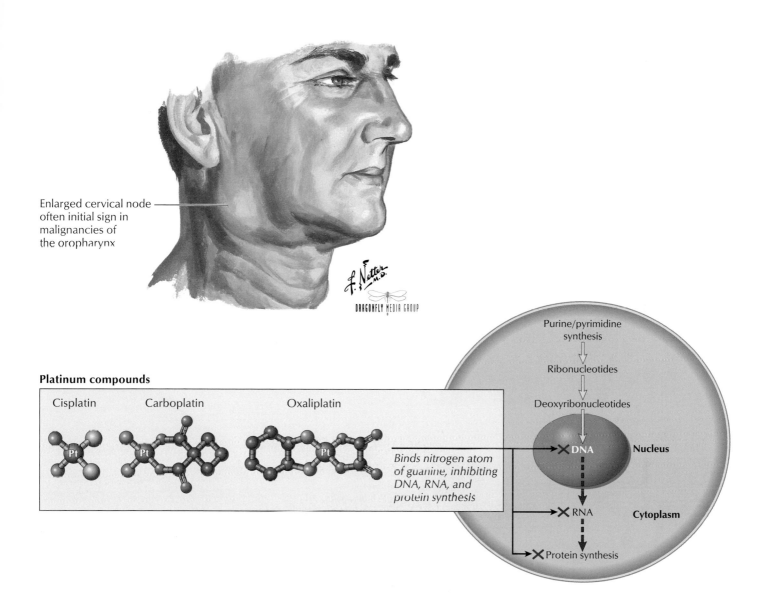

Enlarged cervical node
often initial sign in
malignancies of
the oropharynx

Platinum compounds

Cisplatin   Carboplatin   Oxaliplatin

Binds nitrogen atom
of guanine, inhibiting
DNA, RNA, and
protein synthesis

Purine/pyrimidine
synthesis

Ribonucleotides

Deoxyribonucleotides

DNA   Nucleus

RNA   Cytoplasm

Protein synthesis

FIGURE 11-14 PLATINUM COMPOUNDS: CISPLATIN, CARBOPLATIN, AND OXALIPLATIN

Platinum compounds act as alkylating agents and form covalent bonds with the nitrogen atom of guanine to disrupt DNA, RNA, and protein synthesis. Cisplatin is used for solid tumors—lung, ovarian, head and neck, testicular, and cervical. Adverse effects include neurotoxicity, ototoxicity, GI effects, and nephrotoxicity. Carboplatin, a cisplatin analog with similar activity, is less emetogenic and less nephrotoxic and is used for patients with renal dysfunction. Oxaliplatin, the newest platinum agent, is similar to the other drugs but has a distinct use: combination with 5-FU for metastatic colon or rectal carcinoma after failed therapy with 5-FU and irinotecan. Oxaliplatin causes sensory peripheral neuropathy, neutropenia, GI effects, thromboembolism, and febrile neutropenia. Temozolomide, an imidazotetrazine (a new drug class), forms cytotoxic DNA cross-links. It is used for refractory anaplastic astrocytoma. Myelosuppression, GI distress, fatigue, constipation, and headache are adverse effects of temozolomide.

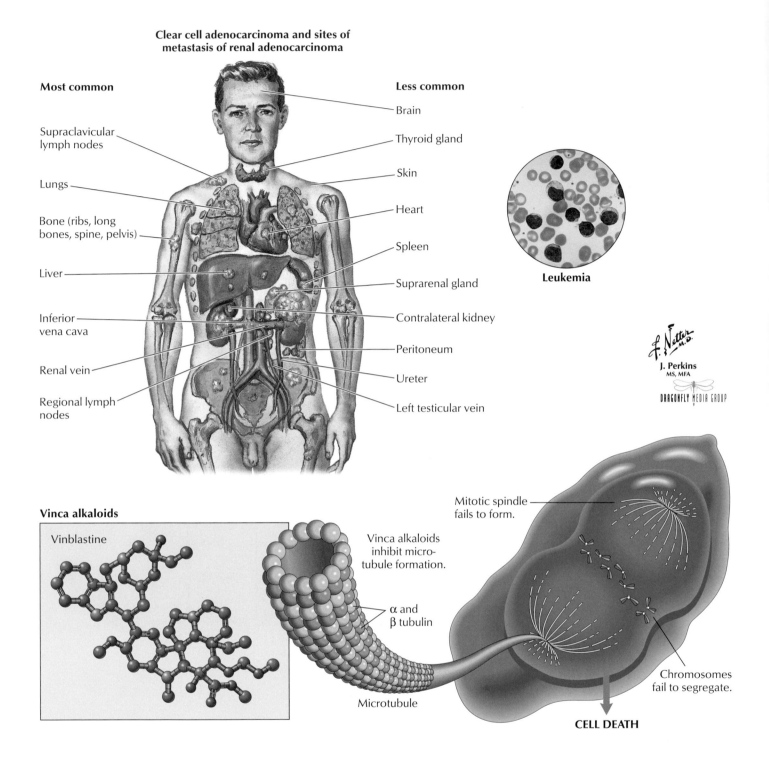

Clear cell adenocarcinoma and sites of metastasis of renal adenocarcinoma

Most common

Supraclavicular lymph nodes

Lungs

Bone (ribs, long bones, spine, pelvis)

Liver

Inferior vena cava

Renal vein

Regional lymph nodes

Less common

Brain

Thyroid gland

Skin

Heart

Spleen

Suprarenal gland

Contralateral kidney

Peritoneum

Ureter

Left testicular vein

Leukemia

J. Perkins
MS, MFA

Vinca alkaloids

Vinblastine

Vinca alkaloids inhibit microtubule formation.

α and β tubulin

Microtubule

Mitotic spindle fails to form.

Chromosomes fail to segregate.

CELL DEATH

FIGURE 11-15 VINCA ALKALOIDS: VINCRISTINE, VINBLASTINE, AND VINORELBINE

These agents, derived from the periwinkle *Vinca rosea*, are cell cycle specific (inhibit mitosis). They bind to tubulin and prevent formation of microtubules (essential part of the mitotic spindle): chromosomes do not segregate correctly, and cell death ensues. CNS functions are also affected, which may account for neurotoxic effects. Vincristine is used for pediatric and adult acute leukemia, Hodgkin disease, lymphomas, multiple myeloma, neuroblastoma, Wilms tumor, and Kaposi sarcoma. Vinblastine,

similar to vincristine, is also used for testicular cancer and renal cell carcinoma. Vinorelbine is mainly used for unresectable, advanced non–small cell lung cancer and breast cancer. All drugs may cause leukopenia, thrombocytopenia, acute uric acid nephropathy, ischemic cardiac toxicity, neurotoxicity, and cellulitis. The dose-limiting toxicities of vincristine include paresthesias, loss of tendon reflexes, neuritic pain, and muscle weakness; the dose-limiting toxicity of vinorelbine is granulocytopenia.

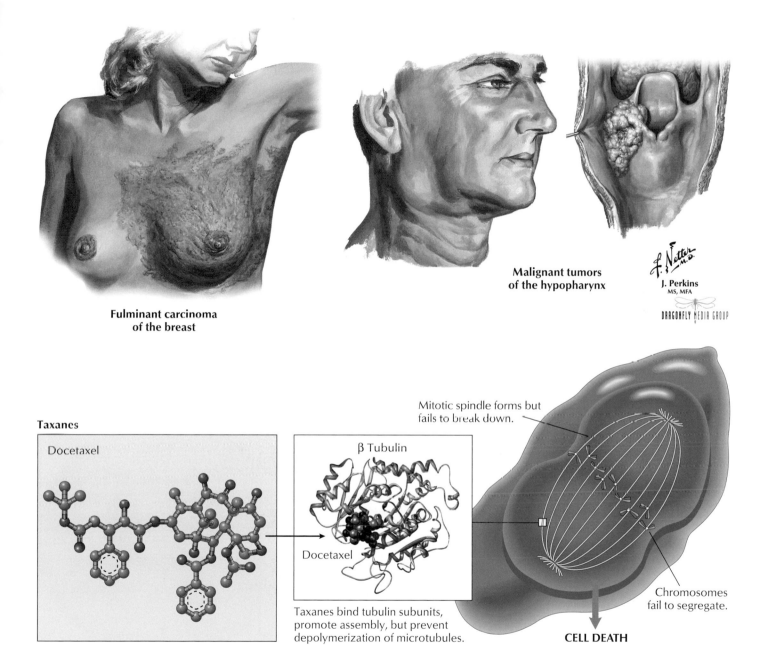

Fulminant carcinoma
of the breast

Malignant tumors
of the hypopharynx

J. Perkins
MS, MFA

DRAGONFLY MEDIA GROUP

Taxanes

Docetaxel

β Tubulin

Docetaxel

Taxanes bind tubulin subunits,
promote assembly, but prevent
depolymerization of microtubules.

Mitotic spindle forms but
fails to break down.

Chromosomes
fail to segregate.

CELL DEATH

FIGURE 11-16 TAXANES

The taxanes docetaxel and paclitaxel both derive their activity from plants. The taxanes bind to tubulin but do not promote microtubule disassembly. Rather, they promote the assembly of microtubules from tubulin dimers and stabilize them by preventing depolymerization. The microtubules formed in the presence of taxanes are dysfunctional because they are too stable; cell death ultimately occurs. Both taxanes are used to treat ovarian cancer, breast cancer, non–small cell lung cancer, head and neck cancer, and AIDS-related Kaposi sarcoma. The drugs cause significant myelosuppression, with neutropenia being the major dose-limiting toxicity. Another important adverse effect is hypersensitivity reaction, which requires premedication with an H_2 blocker, corticosteroid, and diphenhydramine. Other effects include mucositis, alopecia, peripheral neuropathy, relatively mild nausea, and arrhythmias.

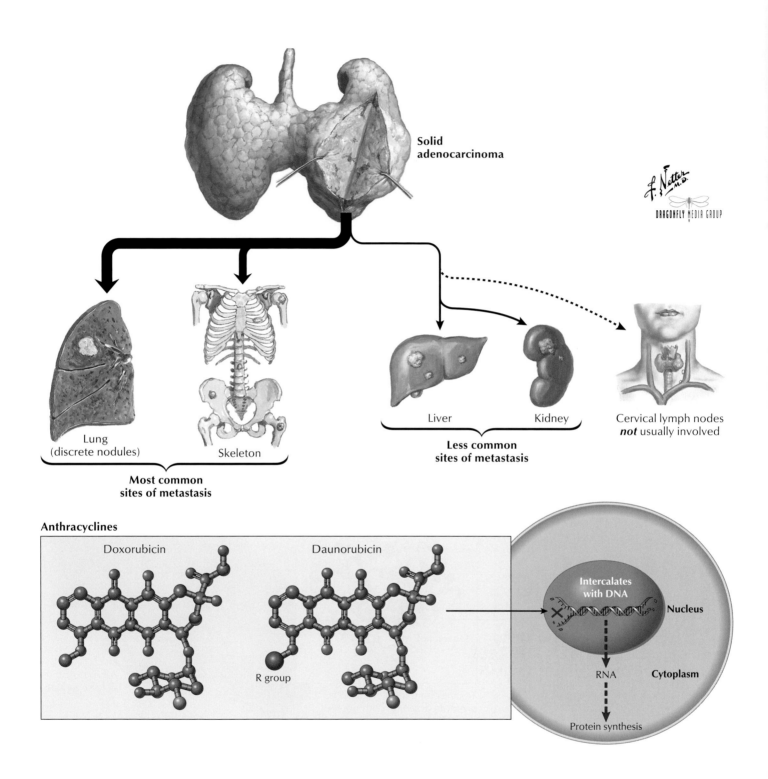

Solid
adenocarcinoma

Lung
(discrete nodules)

Skeleton

**Most common
sites of metastasis**

Liver

Kidney

**Less common
sites of metastasis**

Cervical lymph nodes
not usually involved

Anthracyclines

Doxorubicin

Daunorubicin

R group

**Intercalates
with DNA**

Nucleus

RNA

Cytoplasm

Protein synthesis

FIGURE 11-17 ANTHRACYCLINES: DOXORUBICIN AND DAUNORUBICIN

Isolated from a *Streptomyces* species, anthracyclines are cell cycle–specific antibiotics that bind tightly to DNA by intercalation and cause uncoiling of the double helix, which leads to strand breaks and prevents DNA and RNA synthesis. Another mechanism, which may produce cardiac toxicity, involves conversion of the drugs to toxic oxygen free radicals, to which cardiac tissue and tumors are vulnerable. Doxorubicin, one of the most widely used antineoplastics, has efficacy in various cancers (eg, carcinomas of the breast, prostate, thyroid, and lung; hepatoma; neuroblastoma; Wilms tumor). Daunorubicin is part of many initial remission induction regimens for leukemia (adult and pediatric acute lymphocytic and adult nonlymphocytic). A dose-limiting toxicity of both drugs is irreversible cardiotoxicity, which may be minimized by avoiding use with preexisting cardiac conditions, using dexrazoxane (a cardioprotectant), or using liposomal doxorubicin.

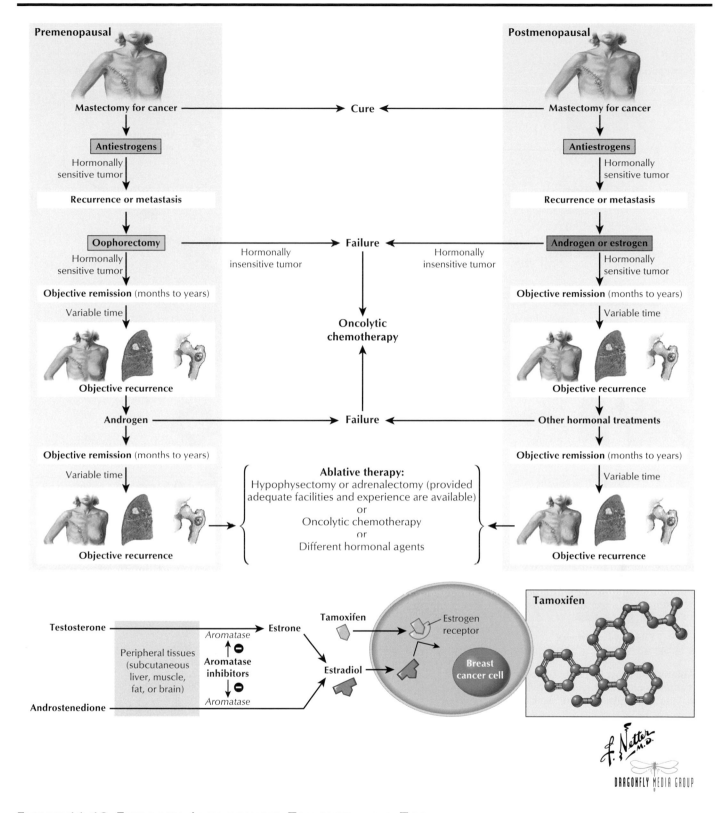

FIGURE 11-18 ESTROGEN ANTAGONISTS: TAMOXIFEN AND TOREMIFENE

The influence of estrogen in breast cancer is so critical that therapy now depends on whether a tumor is hormone dependent or independent. In the former, tumor cells have estrogen (ER) and progesterone receptors (are positive) and need these hormones for growth. In the latter, cells lack these receptors (are negative). Hormone-positive tumors are treated with estrogen antagonists such as tamoxifen, which has dual activity on ERs: antagonistic (inhibits cell proliferation, reduces tumors) and partial agonist

effects (prevents bone demineralization in postmenopausal women). Tamoxifen increases risk of endometrial carcinoma and can cause hot flashes, deep vein thrombosis, pulmonary embolism, and retinal toxicity. Antiestrogens are avoided for ER-negative cancer, which does not respond to these drugs. Low-dose toremifene has similar effects (depletes ERs and is cytostatic for tumor growth), but higher doses produce more antitumor activity; therefore, it is used as second-line therapy after tamoxifen.

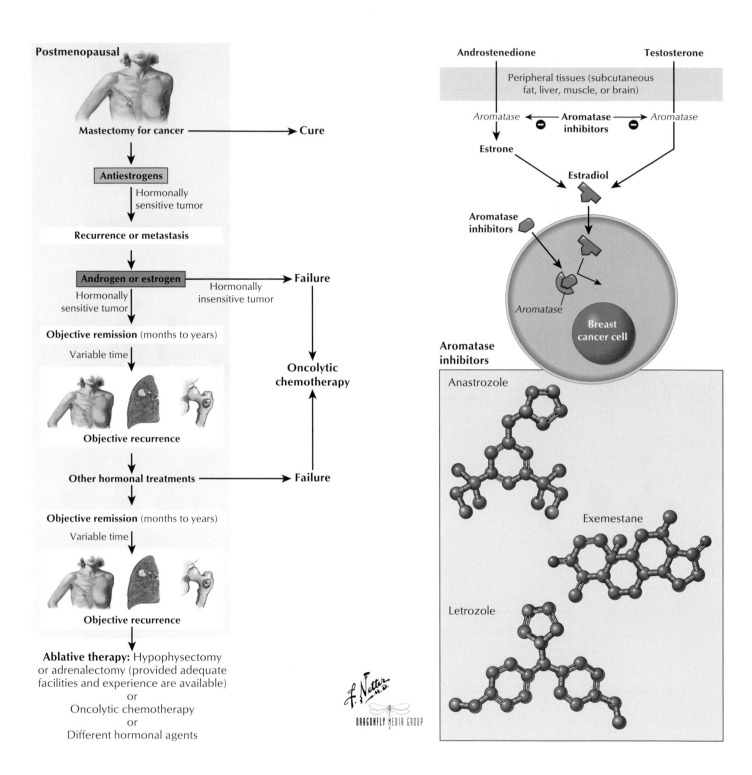

FIGURE 11-19 AROMATASE INHIBITORS: ANASTROZOLE, LETROZOLE, AND EXEMESTANE

Aromatase inhibitors provide a more permanent cutoff of estrogen to cancer cells: they selectively and irreversibly bind to and inactivate aromatase, the main enzyme converting androgens to estrogens. These inhibitors have no partial agonist activity. Adrenal insufficiency caused by aminoglutethimide, the first drug developed, limited its use; the newer anastrozole, letrozole, and exemestane are better tolerated (no effects on corticosteroid or aldosterone biosynthesis). These drugs were first used as second-line therapy, but letrozole and anastrozole are now thought at least as good as, if not superior to, tamoxifen as first-line therapy for advanced breast cancer (and for adjuvant therapy). Adverse effects include hot flashes, musculoskeletal pain, and headache. In contrast to data for tamoxifen, no increased risk of uterine carcinoma or venous thromboembolism exists for the aromatase inhibitors. Premenopausal women with breast cancer and normal ovarian function should avoid aromatase inhibitors.

Androgen Deprivation in Metastatic Disease

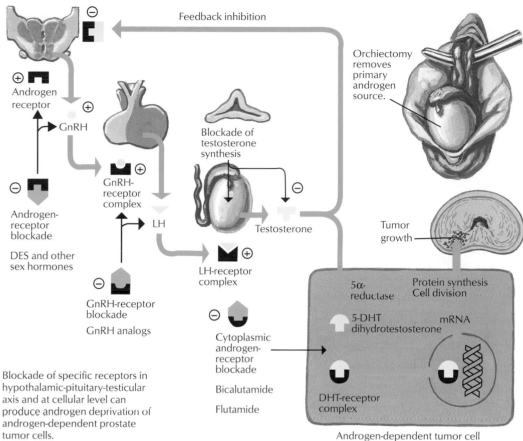

Blockade of specific receptors in hypothalamic-pituitary-testicular axis and at cellular level can produce androgen deprivation of androgen-dependent prostate tumor cells.

"Escape" phenomenon in metastatic disease

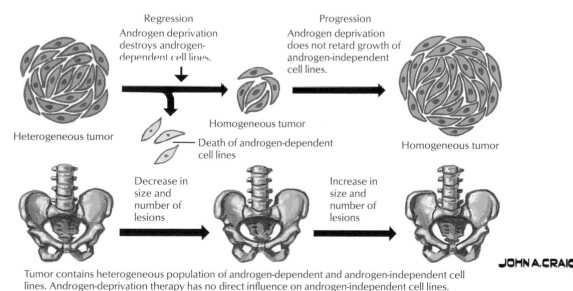

Tumor contains heterogeneous population of androgen-dependent and androgen-independent cell lines. Androgen-deprivation therapy has no direct influence on androgen-independent cell lines.

FIGURE 11-20 GONADOTROPIN-RELEASING HORMONE ANALOGS: LEUPROLIDE AND GOSERELIN

Androgen stimulates prostate cancer cell growth, so main therapies involve medical (GnRH analogs) or surgical (orchiectomy) androgen ablation. Leuprolide and goserelin have paradoxical effects on the pituitary: an initial release of LH and FSH and then down-regulation of GnRH receptors because of repeated dosing (negative feedback). This inhibition leads to reduced testicular steroidogenesis and lower serum testosterone levels. Both drugs are effective for palliation of advanced prostatic carcinoma and may be used in combination with flutamide or instead of diethylstilbestrol and orchiectomy for initial treatment. GnRH may first cause a tumor flare (symptoms and pain) because of initial gonadotropin stimulation. Other adverse effects are hot flashes, blurred vision, injection site pain, and breast swelling. Leuprolide may be given as a depot intramuscular injection or as an implant that releases drug via osmotic-regulated technology. Goserelin is given as a pellet, injected under the skin.

357

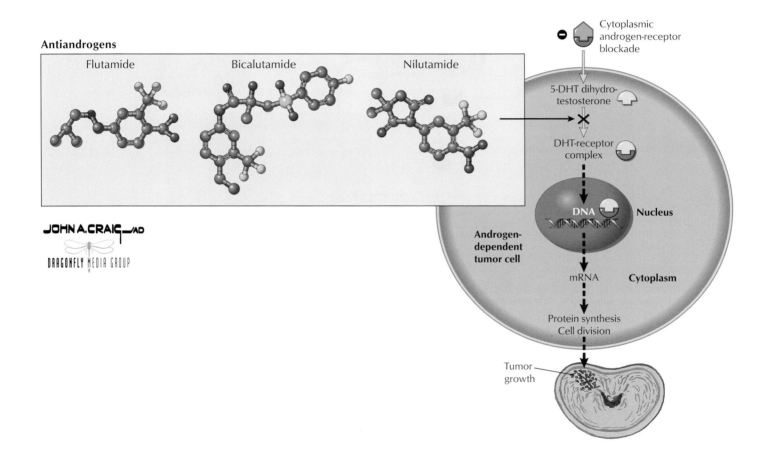

Antiandrogens

Flutamide   Bicalutamide   Nilutamide

JOHN A. CRAIG—AD

DRAGONFLY MEDIA GROUP

Cytoplasmic androgen-receptor blockade

5-DHT dihydro-testosterone

DHT-receptor complex

DNA   Nucleus

Androgen-dependent tumor cell

mRNA   Cytoplasm

Protein synthesis
Cell division

Tumor growth

FIGURE 11-21 ANTIANDROGENS: FLUTAMIDE, BICALUTAMIDE, AND NILUTAMIDE

Antiandrogens achieve total androgen blockade and are useful when GnRH analogs do not produce castration testosterone levels. These drugs block actions of androgens by interacting with cytosolic androgen receptor sites in all target tissues: prostate, hypothalamus, and pituitary. As monotherapy, antiandrogens may cause an increase in plasma testosterone, which may result from increased LH caused by the drugs' interference with negative feedback of androgens at the hypothalamic level. Because this effect could counteract antiandrogen actions in peripheral tissues, these drugs are given mainly to patients receiving GnRH analogs or are used as adjuvant therapy in orchiectomized patients for complete androgen blockade. Adverse effects include diarrhea, breast swelling and tenderness, and hepatotoxicity. Flutamide causes more diarrhea than do bicalutamide and nilutamide. Nilutamide has unique adverse effects: decreased visual accommodation, disulfiram-like reaction, and constipation.

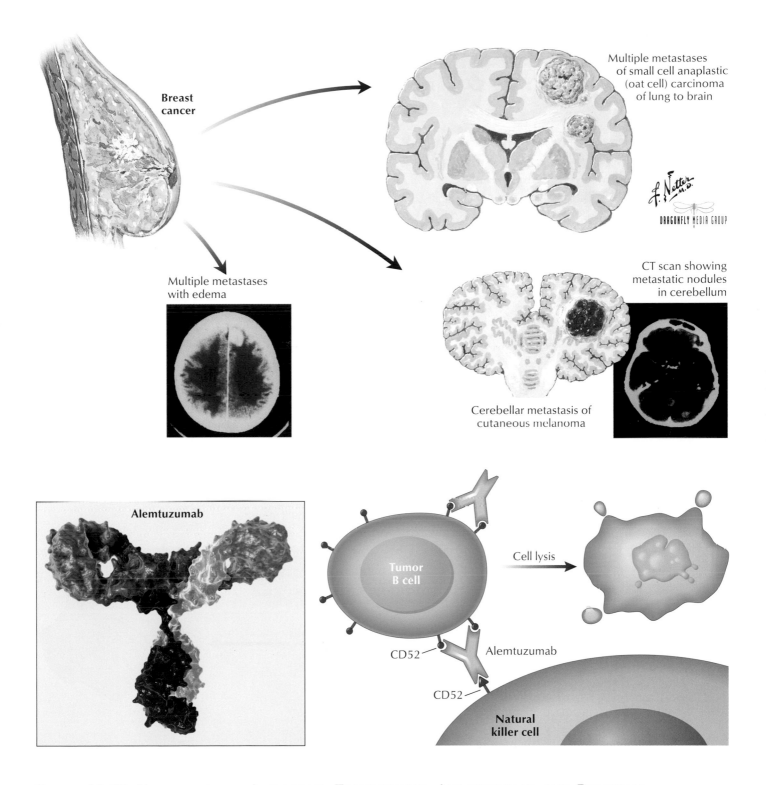

FIGURE 11-22 UNCONJUGATED ANTIBODIES: TRASTUZUMAB, ALEMTUZUMAB, AND RITUXIMAB

Trastuzumab, alemtuzumab, and rituximab are recombinant DNA-derived monoclonal antibodies (MoAbs). The first binds to human epidermal growth factor receptor 2 (HER2), a protooncogene in certain breast tumors. Natural killer (NK) cells identify the drug-MoAb complexes as abnormal, attach to the MoAb, and inhibit tumor growth. Alemtuzumab is directed against CD52 (an antigen on surfaces of normal and malignant B and T lymphocytes, NK cells, monocytes, and macrophages, and male reproductive tissues) and induces cell lysis. It is used for B-cell chronic lymphocytic leukemia in selected patients. Rituximab, a chimeric murine/human MoAb, binds to CD20, a cell cycle–regulating antigen found on more than 90% of B-cell NHL cells but not on stem, pro-B, or normal plasma or other normal tissues. Rituximab induces CD20+ B-cell NHL cell apoptosis and also recruits host immune cells to lyse B cells. These drugs can lead to serious cardiac, hypersensitivity, pulmonary, blood, metabolic, and mucocutaneous effects.

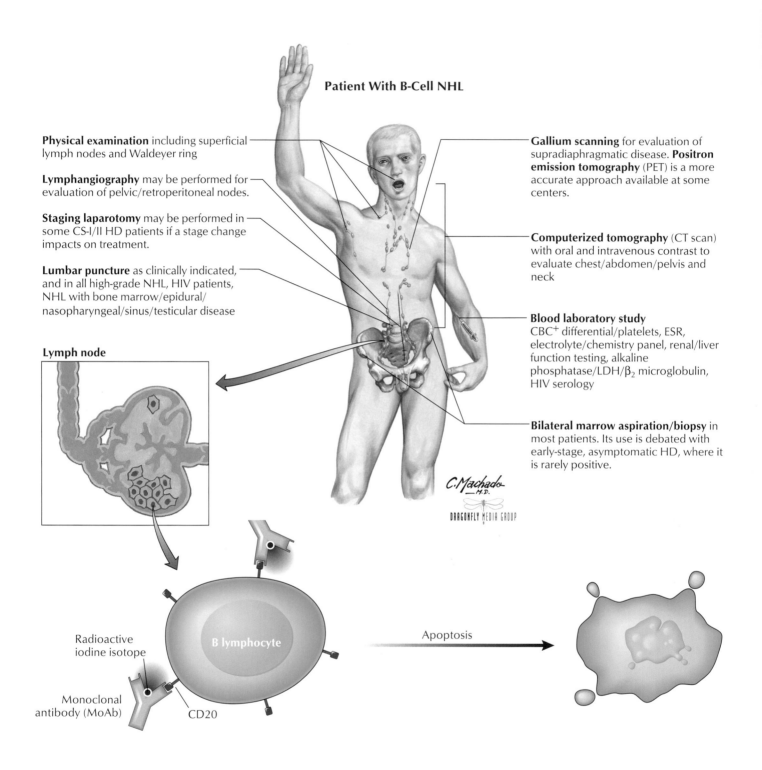

Patient With B-Cell NHL

Physical examination including superficial lymph nodes and Waldeyer ring

Lymphangiography may be performed for evaluation of pelvic/retroperitoneal nodes.

Staging laparotomy may be performed in some CS-I/II HD patients if a stage change impacts on treatment.

Lumbar puncture as clinically indicated, and in all high-grade NHL, HIV patients, NHL with bone marrow/epidural/nasopharyngeal/sinus/testicular disease

Gallium scanning for evaluation of supradiaphragmatic disease. **Positron emission tomography** (PET) is a more accurate approach available at some centers.

Computerized tomography (CT scan) with oral and intravenous contrast to evaluate chest/abdomen/pelvis and neck

Blood laboratory study
CBC^+ differential/platelets, ESR, electrolyte/chemistry panel, renal/liver function testing, alkaline phosphatase/LDH/β_2 microglobulin, HIV serology

Bilateral marrow aspiration/biopsy in most patients. Its use is debated with early-stage, asymptomatic HD, where it is rarely positive.

Lymph node

Radioactive iodine isotope

B lymphocyte

Monoclonal antibody (MoAb)

CD20

Apoptosis

FIGURE 11-23 CONJUGATED ANTIBODIES: IBRITUMOMAB TIUXETAN AND TOSITUMOMAB AND IODINE I 131 TOSITUMOMAB

Ibritumomab tiuxetan and tositumomab and iodine I 131 tositumomab consist of a murine MoAb linked by a chelating agent to a radioisotope. The MoAb delivers the radioisotope to malignant sites, and the drugs, like rituximab, bind to the CD20 antigen. While the antibody induces apoptosis in $CD20^+$ B cells, β emission from the radioisotope induces cell damage through formation of free radicals in target and neighboring cells. Both products are used for relapsed or refractory low-grade, follicular, or transformed B-cell NHL, including follicular NHL that is refractory to rituximab. Both drugs are associated with prolonged and severe cytopenias (thrombocytopenia, neutropenia), which occur in most patients. Therefore, the products should not be given to patients with impaired bone marrow reserve or more than 25% lymphoma marrow involvement. Both drugs may cause serious infusion reactions (fever, rigors or chills, sweating, hypotension, dyspnea, bronchospasm, nausea).

Chronic myeloid leukemia (CML)

Peripheral blood examination:
High WBC count with mature neutrophils with early occasional myeloid forms and an occasional blast. Low leukocyte alkaline phosphatase score. Elevated platelet count, with dysmorphism and large size. Elevation of basophil count and blasts is seen in accelerated phase of this disorder.

Bone marrow examination:
Presence of Philadelphia chromosome. More than 30% blast count characterizes blast crisis.

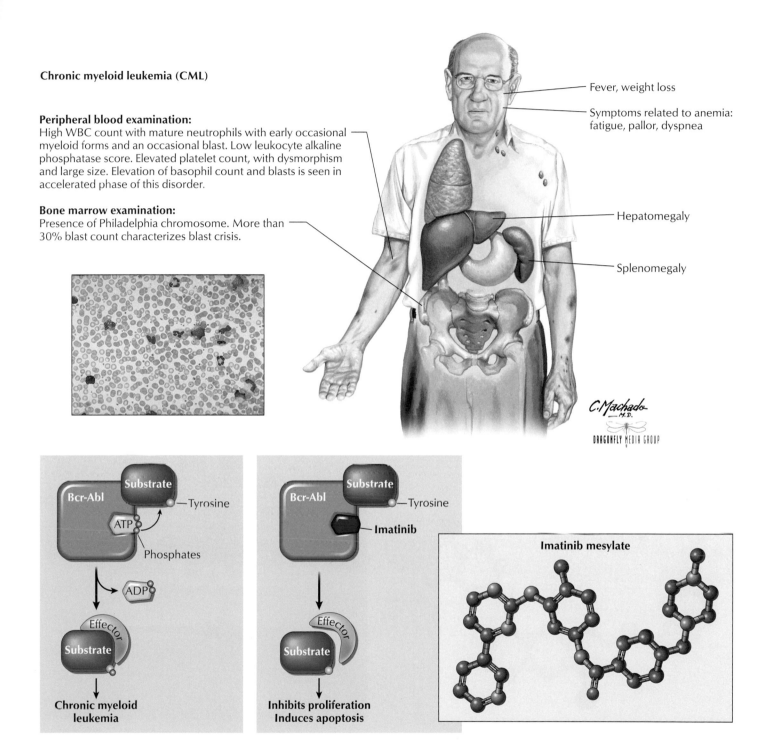

Fever, weight loss

Symptoms related to anemia: fatigue, pallor, dyspnea

Hepatomegaly

Splenomegaly

Bcr-Abl
Substrate
Tyrosine
ATP
Phosphates
ADP
Effector
Substrate
Chronic myeloid leukemia

Bcr-Abl
Substrate
Tyrosine
Imatinib
Effector
Substrate
Inhibits proliferation Induces apoptosis

Imatinib mesylate

FIGURE 11-24 IMATINIB MESYLATE

Imatinib inhibits Bcr-Abl tyrosine kinase, the constitutive abnormal enzyme created by the Philadelphia chromosome (Ph) abnormality in chronic myeloid leukemia (CML). This enzyme is present in almost all patients with CML and some patients with acute lymphoblastic leukemia. Imatinab inhibits proliferation and induces apoptosis in Bcr-Abl+ cell lines as well as fresh leukemic cells from Ph+ CML. The agent, used orally, is indicated as first-line therapy in newly diagnosed patients with Ph+ CML in the chronic phase and after failure of interferon alfa therapy in patients with Ph+ CML in blast crisis, accelerated phase, or chronic phase. Imatinib is also used for patients with Kit+ (CD117+) unresectable and/or metastatic GI stromal tumors. Main adverse effects include thrombocytopenia, neutropenia, liver enzyme increases, edema (responds to diuretics and dose reduction), muscle cramps, nausea (reduced by food and water ingestion), and diarrhea.

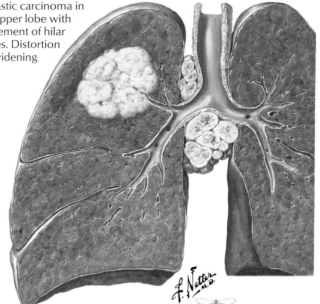

Large cell anaplastic carcinoma in middle of right upper lobe with extensive involvement of hilar and carinal nodes. Distortion of trachea and widening of carina.

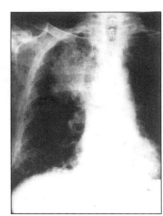

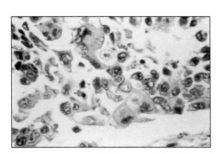

Tumor composed of large multinucleated cells without evidence of differentiation toward gland formation or squamous epithelium. These cells produce mucin (stained red). Some tumors may be composed of large clear cells containing glycogen.

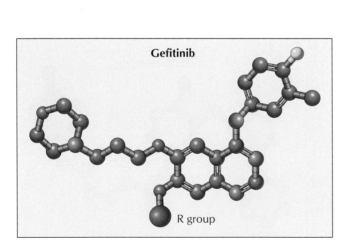

Gefitinib

R group

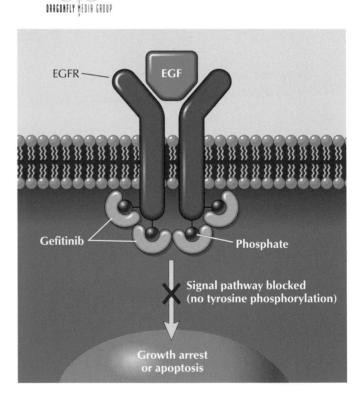

EGFR — EGF

Gefitinib — Phosphate

Signal pathway blocked (no tyrosine phosphorylation)

Growth arrest or apoptosis

FIGURE 11-25 GEFITINIB

Gefitinib is an orally active anilinoquinazoline derivative that inhibits intracellular phosphorylation of several tyrosine kinases, one of which is associated with epidermal growth factor receptor (EGFR). EGFR is expressed on the surface of many normal cells and cancer cells and is thought to play a role in growth, metastasis, angiogenesis, and resistance to apoptosis of non–small cell lung cancer cells. Gefitinib is approved as monotherapy and as third-line therapy (after failure of both platinum-based and

docetaxel regimens) in patients with locally advanced or metastatic non–small cell lung cancer. Main adverse effects are diarrhea, nausea, vomiting, and dermatologic effects. Potentially fatal interstitial lung disease occurs rarely, more often in patients who received previous chemotherapy and, to a lesser extent, previous radiotherapy. Increased mortality has been noted in gefitinib-treated patients with concomitant idiopathic pulmonary fibrosis with worsening lung function.

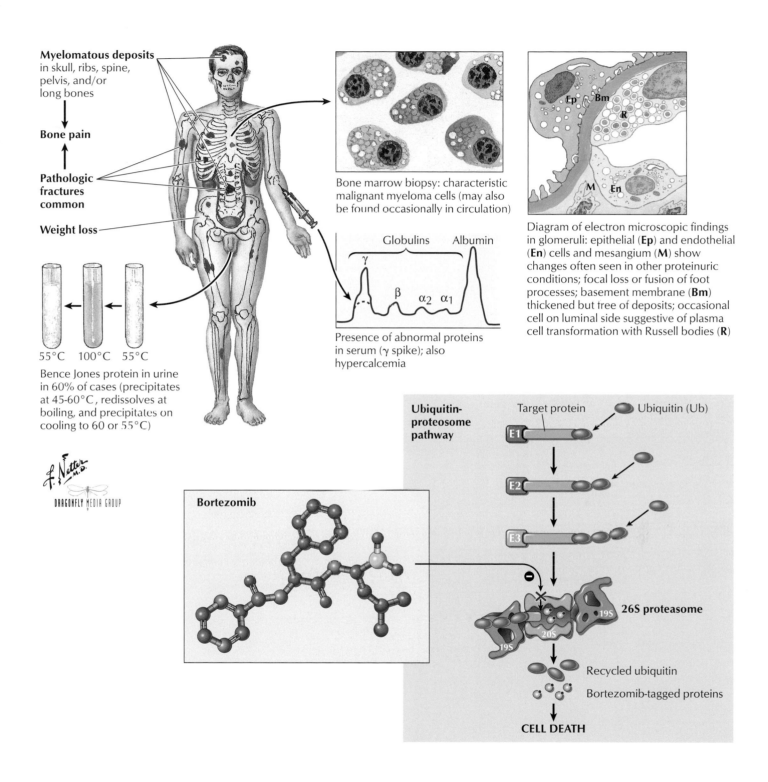

Myelomatous deposits in skull, ribs, spine, pelvis, and/or long bones

Bone pain

Pathologic fractures common

Weight loss

55°C   100°C   55°C

Bence Jones protein in urine in 60% of cases (precipitates at 45-60°C, redissolves at boiling, and precipitates on cooling to 60 or 55°C)

Bone marrow biopsy: characteristic malignant myeloma cells (may also be found occasionally in circulation)

Globulins   Albumin

γ

β   α₂   α₁

Presence of abnormal proteins in serum (γ spike); also hypercalcemia

Diagram of electron microscopic findings in glomeruli: epithelial (**Ep**) and endothelial (**En**) cells and mesangium (**M**) show changes often seen in other proteinuric conditions; focal loss or fusion of foot processes; basement membrane (**Bm**) thickened but free of deposits; occasional cell on luminal side suggestive of plasma cell transformation with Russell bodies (**R**)

Ubiquitin-proteosome pathway   Target protein   Ubiquitin (Ub)

E1

E2

E3

26S proteasome

Recycled ubiquitin

Bortezomib-tagged proteins

CELL DEATH

Bortezomib

FIGURE 11-26 BORTEZOMIB

Bortezomib is a reversible inhibitor of the 26S proteosome, a large protein complex that degrades ubiquitinated proteins. The ubiquitin-proteosome pathway is known to play a major role in intracellular degradation of numerous regulatory proteins involved in cell integrity, such as cell cycle control, cellular apoptosis, transcription factor activation, and tumor growth. Inhibition of the 26S proteosome disrupts cell proliferation and apoptosis, which leads to cell death. Bortezomib is given intravenously and is approved for patients with multiple myeloma who have received at least 2 previous types of therapy but had disease progression after the last therapy. Predominant adverse effects with bortezomib include pyrexia; pneumonia; diarrhea, nausea, and vomiting; dehydration; fatigue, malaise, weakness; thrombocytopenia; peripheral neuropathy; and anemia.

CHAPTER 12

DRUGS USED FOR SKIN DISORDERS

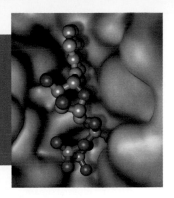

OVERVIEW

Many drugs that are used to treat skin disorders are also administered for systemic disorders, but for skin disorders, the drug formulation is usually designed in a way that limits their absorption and distribution to the skin surface. Systemic distribution in these cases is generally not desirable and can lead to an increased number or severity of adverse effects. In severe skin disease, however, systemic administration is appropriate, and oral preparations are available for such treatment.

Glucocorticoids are a commonly used drug class for treating skin disorders such as dermatoses because of their antiinflammatory, immunosuppressive, and other effects. Glucocorticoids alter gene expression in cells located in the dermis and epidermis by binding to glucocorticoid response elements on DNA. These drugs are transported to the cell nucleus after forming complexes with cytoplasmic receptors. Glucocorticoids include hydrocortisone, beta-methasone, and clobetasol (for psoriasis).

Retinoids, a family of naturally occurring and synthetic vitamin A analogs, affect cell differentiation and proliferation by regulating transcriptional activity mediated by nuclear retinoic acid receptor subtypes. Commonly used retinoids include adapalene, isotretinoin, and tretinoin (for severe acne); acitretin (for severe psoriasis); bexarotene (for early-stage cutaneous T-cell lymphoma); alitretinoin (for cutaneous lesions of Kaposi sarcoma); and naturally occurring β-carotene (for reducing skin photosensitivity).

Other dermatologic agents include antimicrobial, antimalarial, antifungal, and antiviral drugs; drugs (primarily pyrethrins and pyrethroids) used to treat scabies and lice; cytotoxic and immune-modulating drugs; systemic antihistamines (to treat, for example, urticaria, angioedema, and cutaneous mastocytosis); drugs to treat pigmentation disorders; keratolytic agents, such as salicylic acid, urea, lactic acid, and colloidal or precipitated sulfur (to treat excess thickening of the outermost layer of the skin); selenium sulfide (to treat dandruff); and psoralens (eg, 8-methoxypsoralen) and porphyrins (used as photosensitizers to enhance phototherapy).

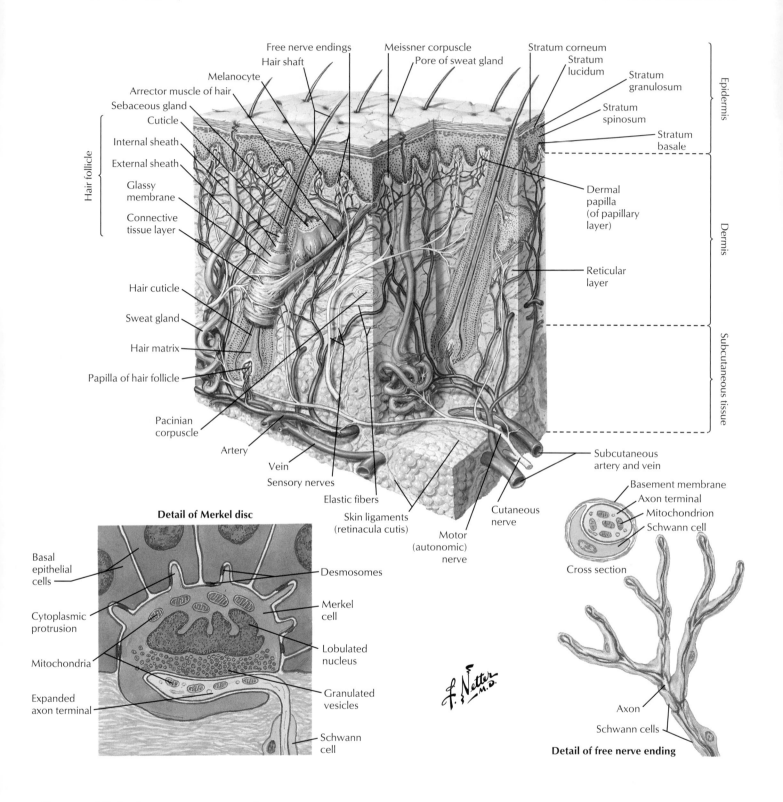

FIGURE 12-1 ANATOMY OF THE SKIN

The skin is a complex, multicomponent organ. It is commonly classified into 3 anatomical regions and multiple subregions: the epidermis, which includes the strata corneum, lucidum, granulosum, spinosum, and basale; the dermis, which includes the papillary and reticular layers; and the subcutaneous tissue, which includes sweat glands. All layers are extensively supplied by blood vessels and innervated by motor and sensory neurons. Disorders of the skin can develop either as primary disease (localized to 1 or more layers of the skin) or as a secondary result of a systemic disease. Drugs for management of these disorders involve topical or systemic administration of medications to treat the dermal or systemic source of the problem. Major classes of drugs used in dermatologic pharmacology include glucocorticoids, antibacterials, antifungals, antivirals, antiparasitics, and retinoids.

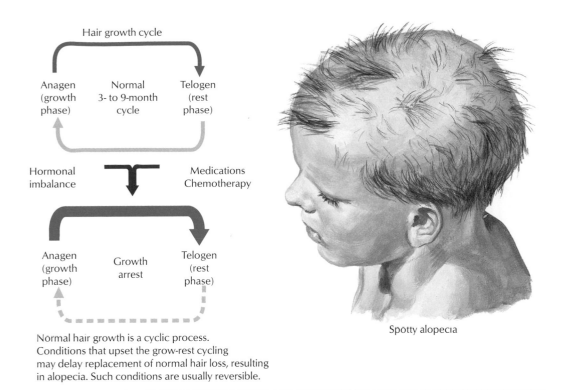

Hair growth cycle

Normal hair growth is a cyclic process.
Conditions that upset the grow-rest cycling
may delay replacement of normal hair loss, resulting
in alopecia. Such conditions are usually reversible.

Spotty alopecia

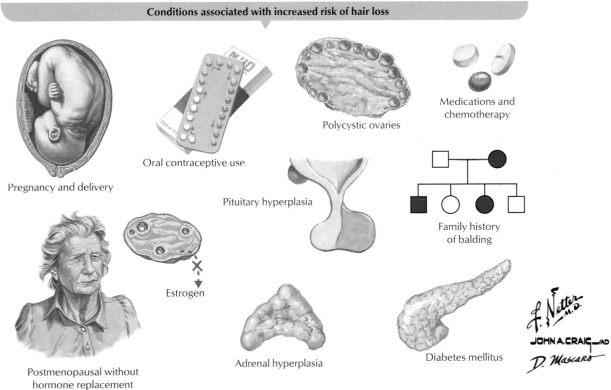

Conditions associated with increased risk of hair loss

Pregnancy and delivery

Oral contraceptive use

Polycystic ovaries

Medications and
chemotherapy

Pituitary hyperplasia

Family history
of balding

Estrogen

Postmenopausal without
hormone replacement

Adrenal hyperplasia

Diabetes mellitus

FIGURE 12-2 ALOPECIA

Alopecia—the loss or absence of hair, especially of the head—can be caused by illness, drugs, endocrine disorders, some types of dermatitis, hereditary factors, radiation, and physiologic processes such as aging. Drug therapy, when appropriate, involves topical steroids (eg, clobetasol) or intradermal injections of triamcinolone for alopecia areata (defined patches, usually on the scalp or beard; occurs most often in children and in autoimmune diseases); minoxidil for androgenic alopecia (affects androgen-sensitive follicles on the scalp of men and women); and griseofulvin, itraconazole, or terbinafine for tinea capitis (fungal infection). Scarring (cicatricial) and permanent alopecias are treated with potent corticosteroids used topically or intralesionally on active inflammatory borders. Systemic drugs (eg, acitretin, chloroquine, doxycycline, low-dose methotrexate, minocycline, prednisone, quinacrine, tetracyclines) may also be used if the disease type and extent warrant them.

Oral Manifestations in Various Skin Conditions

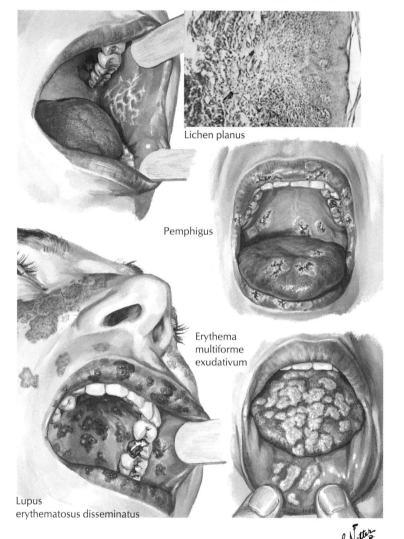

Lichen planus

Pemphigus

Erythema multiforme exudativum

Lupus erythematosus disseminatus

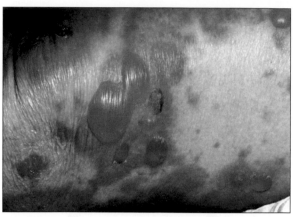

Tense bulla and urticarial plaques in bullous pemphigoid (courtesy of Dr. Walter Barkey)

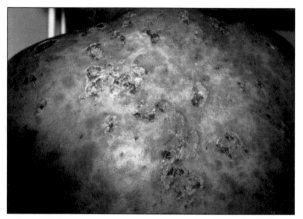

Crusted erosions of the trunk in pemphigus follaceus (courtesy of David S. Rubenstein)

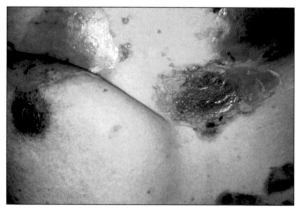

Flaccid vesicles and erosions of pemphigus (courtesy of David S. Rubenstein)

FIGURE 12-3 BULLOUS (BLISTER) SKIN DISEASES

Primary blister diseases are caused by defects in cell adhesion proteins. The defects are either inherited (usually apparent at or soon after birth) or occur in diseases (typically adult onset) in which cell adhesion proteins become target antigens for autoimmune responses. Blisters can also result from infectious, traumatic, or inflammatory processes. Therapeutic drugs include topical, intralesional, or systemic corticosteroids or immunosuppressive agents (eg, azathioprine, cyclophosphamide, cyclosporine, dapsone) for bullous pemphigoid and pemphigoid-like diseases in which IgG autoantibodies attack certain basal keratinocyte proteins; high-dose systemic corticosteroids or mycophenolate mofetil (suppresses lymphocyte proliferation and antibody formation by B cells) for life-threatening pemphigus vulgaris; systemic prednisone for pemphigus foliaceus (affects desmosomes); and dapsone for paraneoplastic pemphigus (associated with lymphoproliferative disorders).

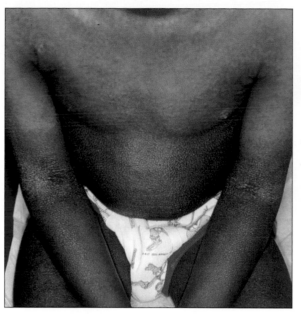

Atopic dermatitis: lichenified plaques of the antecubital fossa are typical (courtesy of David S. Rubenstein)

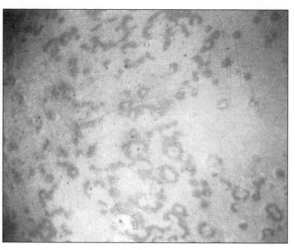

Contact dermatitis: linear distribution of erythematous papules and vesicles characterizes contact dermatitis to poison ivy (courtesy of David S. Rubenstein)

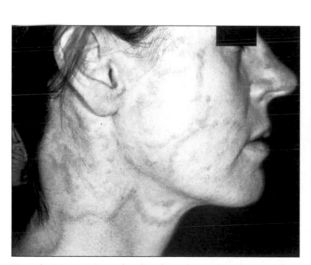

Tinea faciei: serpiginous bordered, erythematous plaque with central clearing (courtesy of David S. Rubenstein)

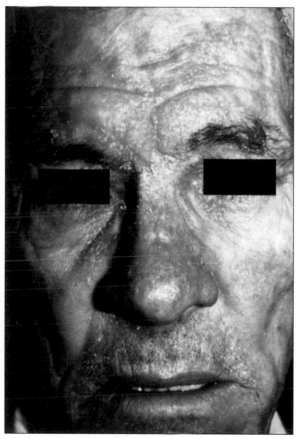

Seborrheic dermatitis: erythema and greasy yellow scale of the forehead, eyebrows, nasal bridge, and nasolabial folds (courtesy of David S. Rubenstein)

FIGURE 12-4 COMMON DERMATOSES INCLUDING ECZEMA

Eczema is an acute or chronic inflammatory skin condition characterized by the presence of 1 or more areas of pruritus (severe itching), erythema (redness), scaling (dry exfoliative shedding), macules (discoloration), papules (pimples), or vesicles (blisterlike sacs). Drugs, when needed, include oral antihistamines or topical corticosteroids for common cases of atopic dermatitis; antibiotics (antistaphylococcal or antistreptococcal) or topical tacrolimus or pimecrolimus for severe or recalcitrant cases of atopic dermatitis; systemic corticosteroids for severe contact dermatitis; topical zinc pyrithione, selenium sulfide, salicylic acid, or ketoconazole for seborrheic dermatitis; topical corticosteroids and emollients for stasis dermatitis (secondary to edema resulting from poor venous return); and antifungal drugs for dermatophytosis (tinea) (ringworm).

369

Typical Distribution

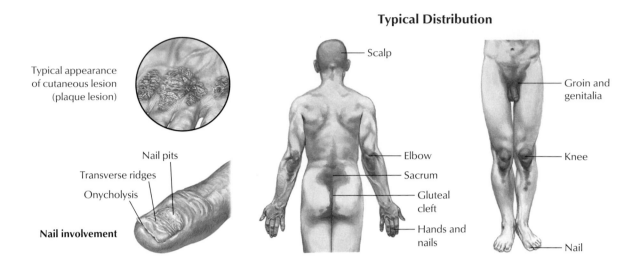

Typical appearance of cutaneous lesion (plaque lesion)

Nail involvement
- Nail pits
- Transverse ridges
- Onycholysis

- Scalp
- Elbow
- Sacrum
- Gluteal cleft
- Hands and nails

- Groin and genitalia
- Knee
- Nail

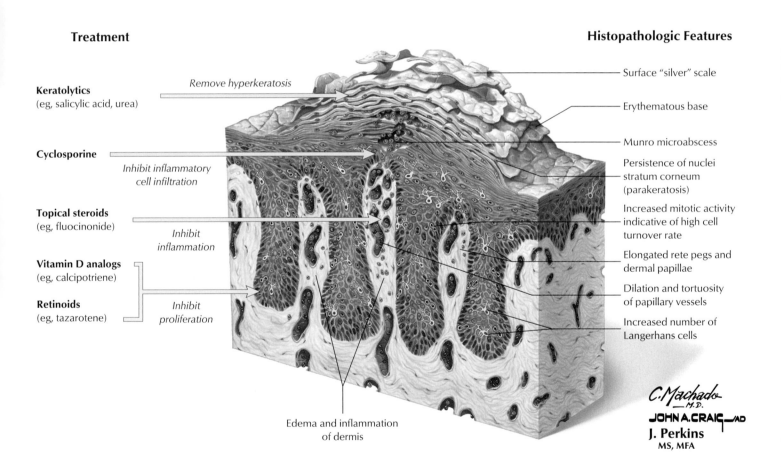

Treatment		Histopathologic Features

Keratolytics (eg, salicylic acid, urea) — *Remove hyperkeratosis*

Cyclosporine — *Inhibit inflammatory cell infiltration*

Topical steroids (eg, fluocinonide) — *Inhibit inflammation*

Vitamin D analogs (eg, calcipotriene)

Retinoids (eg, tazarotene) — *Inhibit proliferation*

- Surface "silver" scale
- Erythematous base
- Munro microabscess
- Persistence of nuclei stratum corneum (parakeratosis)
- Increased mitotic activity indicative of high cell turnover rate
- Elongated rete pegs and dermal papillae
- Dilation and tortuosity of papillary vessels
- Increased number of Langerhans cells

Edema and inflammation of dermis

C. Machado M.D.
JOHN A. CRAIG AD
J. Perkins MS, MFA

FIGURE 12-5 PSORIASIS

Psoriasis is a chronic relapsing skin disorder with distinctive lesions consisting of erythematous papules that coalesce into plaques with sharp borders and silvery, yellow-white scales in patients with advanced disease. It affects approximately 1% to 3% of the population and affects men and women about equally. Management depends on the degree of body surface area affected (topical drugs for <20% body area; systemic drugs for ≥20%), location and sensitivity of affected areas, degree of inflammation, and patient compliance with the therapy regimen. Drugs, when appropriate, include topical steroids (produce a rapid response, but tolerance develops; eg, fluocinonide); vitamin D analogs (eg, calcipotriene), which inhibit proliferation and normalize maturation of keratinocytes; retinoids (eg, tazarotene); and keratolytics (eg, salicylic acid, urea, and lactic acid). Certain drugs—eg, lithium, β blockers, antimalarials, and systemic steroids—can worsen psoriasis and should be avoided.

Dermatoses Secondary to Ectoparasites

Inflammatory excoriated papules (note penile involvement)

Pthirus pubis

Scabies (*Sarcoptes scabiei* in circle)

Pediculosis pubis (exposure of pediculi in hair)

Maculae caeruleae

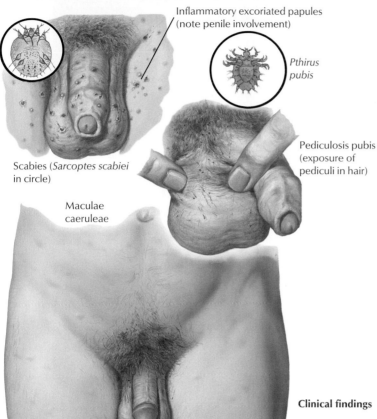

Sexually Transmitted Ectoparasites

Clinical findings

Intense itching in pubic area (often nocturnal) is a hallmark of parasitic infection, and excoriations are common.

Bluish skin discolorations (maculae caerulae) often seen with *Pthirus pubis* infestations

Secondary infection of excoriations or bites may yield eczematoid lesions.

Examination of pubic area and pubic hair may reveal ova and parasites.

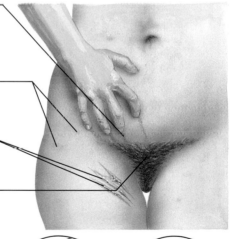

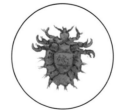
Pthirus pubis

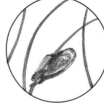
Pthirus pubis egg

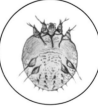
Sarcoptes scabiei

FIGURE 12-6 SCABIES AND PEDICULOSIS

Scabies, a highly communicable skin disease caused by infestation by the mite *Sarcoptes scabiei* var. *hominis* (the itch mite), is characterized by extreme pruritus and widespread inflammatory papules, often scratched (abraded). The mainstay of pharmacologic therapy is the use of topical scabicides, such as permethrin and lindane (although lindane has a higher potential for CNS toxicity), or an oral antiparasitic agent (eg, ivermectin).

Pediculosis is caused by infestation by *Pediculus capitis* (head louse), *Pediculus humanus* (body louse), or *Pthirus pubis* (pubic louse). Head lice and body lice are commonly treated with topical permethrin (but this agent should not be used for infants younger than 2 months or for pregnant or lactating women). Pubic lice (crabs) are treated with topical synergized pyrethrins; eyelashes are treated with petrolatum.

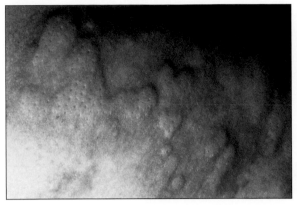

Urticaria

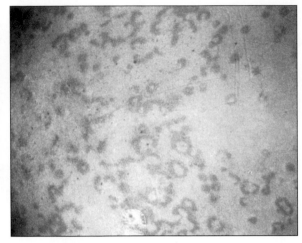

Annular and aerpiginous urticaria

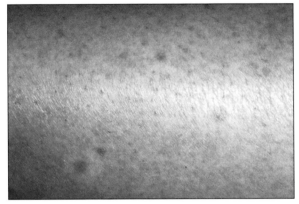

Cholinergic urticaria

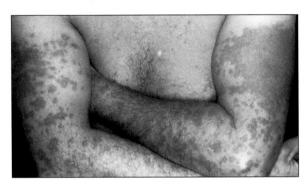

Solar urticaria

Substances Associated With Urticaria or Angioedema

Blood products	Dextran	Shellfish
Contactants	Diuretics	Tomatoes
Animal dander and saliva	Isoniazid	**Food additives**
Arthropods	Nonsteroidal antiinflammatory	Sulfites
Foods	drugs	Tartrazine
Latex	Opioids	**Implants**
Marine forms	Penicillins	Amalgam fillings
Medications (topical)	Polymyxin B	Intrauterine devices
Plants	Quinidine	Orthodontic bands
Textiles	Sulfa drugs	Platinum
Toiletry items	Radiographic contrast media	Tantalum staples
Drugs*	Vancomycin	**Insect/arthropod stings and bites**
Anesthetics	**Foods**	**Inhalants**
Angiotensin-converting enzyme	Berries	Animal dander
inhibitors	Cheese	Cigarette smoke
Antiepileptic agents	Chocolate	Dusts
Aspirin	Eggs	Flour
Bromides	Fish	Mold
Cephalosporins	Milk	Pollen
Chloroquine	Nuts	

*Almost any prescription or over-the-counter medication can cause urticaria.

FIGURE 12-7 URTICARIA

Urticaria, which is characterized by a sudden general eruption of pale evanescent wheals or papules, results from fluid transudation from small cutaneous blood vessels. Histamine and other mediators are released, which leads to severe itching. Acute urticaria is usually treated with antihistamines if it is mild; corticosteroids are used if it is severe. Specific agents include the histamine H1 receptor antagonists cetirizine, cyproheptadine, diphenhydramine, fexofenadine, hydroxyzine, and loratadine. H2-receptor antagonists are sometimes added, or agents having mixed H1/H2-antagonistic action, such as certain tricyclic antidepressants (eg, doxepin), are used. Chronic urticaria is treated with attenuated anabolic steroids, nifedipine, dapsone, sulfasalazine, colchicine, methotrexate, hydroxychloroquine, UV-B light, or PUVA (psoralen plus UV-A light); cyproheptadine is useful for cold urticaria, and β blockers are useful for adrenergic urticaria.

CHAPTER 13

VITAMINS: DEFICIENCIES AND DRUG INTERACTIONS

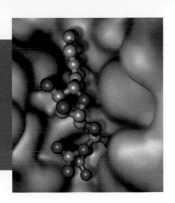

OVERVIEW

Vitamin deficiencies have various causes, including an inadequate supply of the vitamin in the diet, inability of the body to absorb or utilize the vitamin, excessive degradation or excretion of the vitamin, general nutritional deficiency, disease, and vitamin-drug interactions.

Vitamins are commonly classified into those that are water soluble and those that are fat soluble. Water-soluble vitamins include the vitamin B family—thiamine (B_1), riboflavin (B_2), nicotinic acid (niacin) (B_3), pyridoxine (B_6), pantothenic acid, cyanocobalamin (B_{12}), biotin, and folic acid (folacin)—and vitamin C (ascorbic acid). Fat-soluble vitamins include vitamin A (retinol); the vitamin D family—calciferol (D_2) and cholecalciferol (D_3); vitamin E (α tocopherol); and the vitamin K family—phylloquinone (K_1), menaquinones (K_2), and menadione (K_3).

Water-soluble vitamins typically have small body stores, and thus, the concentrations of these vitamins can readily be compromised in the presence of alcoholism, dieting (fads), prolonged anorexia, nausea, dysphagia, diarrhea, weight loss, advanced organ failure, and malabsorption. Fat-soluble vitamins are affected by any chronic deficiency in fat absorption, such as that occurring in short bowel syndrome, pancreatic insufficiency, bacterial overgrowth, celiac sprue, Whipple disease, and primary biliary cirrhosis.

Management of vitamin deficiency disorders can take many forms, including prevention (maintenance of adequate dietary intake), supplementation (usually oral, but the parenteral route is also used), treatment of an underlying disorder, and elimination of interactions with drugs.

Vitamin A Deficiency

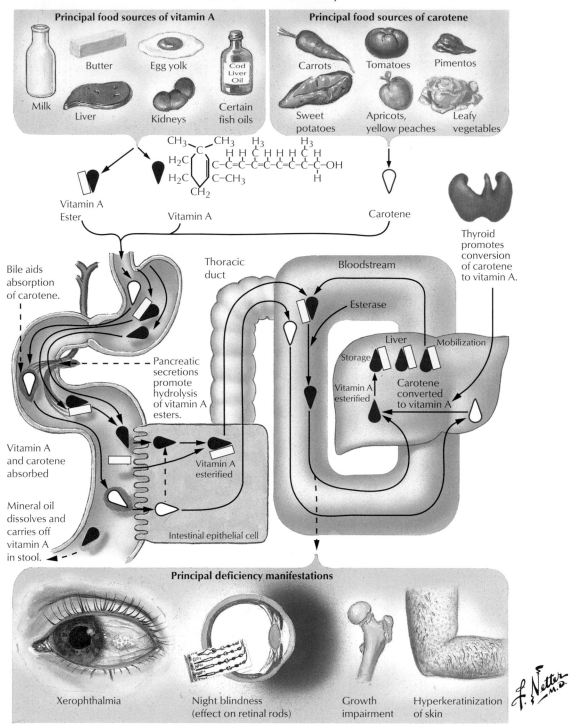

Principal food sources of vitamin A

Milk · Butter · Liver · Egg yolk · Kidneys · Cod Liver Oil · Certain fish oils

Principal food sources of carotene

Carrots · Tomatoes · Pimentos · Sweet potatoes · Apricots, yellow peaches · Leafy vegetables

Vitamin A Ester · Vitamin A · Carotene

Thyroid promotes conversion of carotene to vitamin A.

Bile aids absorption of carotene.

Thoracic duct · Bloodstream · Esterase

Liver · Storage · Mobilization · Vitamin A esterified · Carotene converted to vitamin A

Pancreatic secretions promote hydrolysis of vitamin A esters.

Vitamin A and carotene absorbed

Vitamin A esterified · Intestinal epithelial cell

Mineral oil dissolves and carries off vitamin A in stool.

Principal deficiency manifestations

Xerophthalmia · Night blindness (effect on retinal rods) · Growth impairment · Hyperkeratinization of skin

FIGURE 13-1 DEFICIENCY OF VITAMIN A (RETINOL) AND OTHER FAT-SOLUBLE VITAMINS

Dietary sources of the fat-soluble vitamin A include milk fat, eggs, green leafy or yellow vegetables, and fish oil. Vitamin A is formed from precursors (α, β, and γ carotenes) found in yellow pigments of fruits and vegetables (eg, apples, cabbage, cantaloupes, carrots, oranges, tomatoes). Diseases that result in malabsorption of fat or impaired storage of vitamin A in the liver are characterized by interference with growth, reduced resistance to infections, and disrupted epithelial cell structure and function.

Principal manifestations of this deficiency include xerophthalmia (conjunctival dryness with epithelial keratinization), night blindness, and hyperkeratinization of skin. The main manifestations of other fat-soluble vitamin deficiencies include rickets (vitamin D), excessive steatorrhea (secretion of fat from sebaceous glands of skin; fatty stools) (vitamin E), and increased bleeding time (vitamin K). All these deficiencies are treated via supplementation.

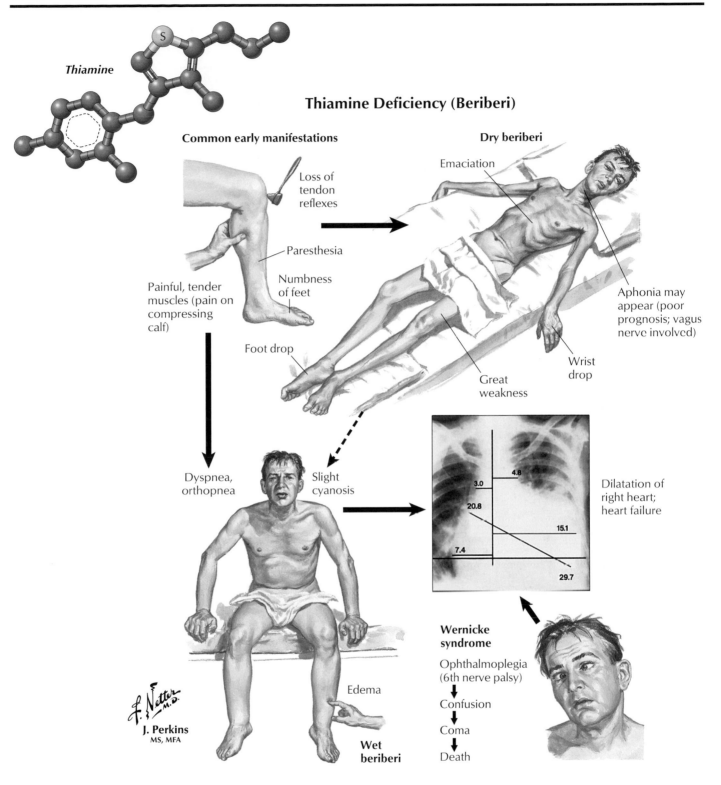

Thiamine

Thiamine Deficiency (Beriberi)

Common early manifestations

Loss of tendon reflexes

Paresthesia

Numbness of feet

Painful, tender muscles (pain on compressing calf)

Foot drop

Dyspnea, orthopnea

Slight cyanosis

Wet beriberi

Edema

Dry beriberi

Emaciation

Aphonia may appear (poor prognosis; vagus nerve involved)

Wrist drop

Great weakness

Dilatation of right heart; heart failure

Wernicke syndrome

Ophthalmoplegia (6th nerve palsy)

↓

Confusion

↓

Coma

↓

Death

J. Netter M.D.

J. Perkins MS, MFA

FIGURE 13-2 DEFICIENCY OF THIAMINE (B₁) AND OTHER B VITAMINS

The B vitamin group includes thiamine (B_1), riboflavin (B_2), nicotinic acid (niacin) (B_3), pyridoxine (B_6), pantothenic acid, cyanocobalamin (B_{12}), biotin, and folic acid (folacin). Major dietary sources are whole grains, whole brown rice, wheat germ, meats, fish, dairy products, and vegetables. Thiamine deficiency (beriberi) is characterized by peripheral neurologic, cerebral, and cardiovascular abnormalities. The disorder is more common in people with alcoholism, whose poor diet can lead to inadequate daily intake of thiamine. The principal manifestations of other vitamin B deficiencies include local seborrheic dermatitis on the face and scrotum (vitamin B_2); alterations in skin, blood, and CNS function (vitamin B_6); pernicious anemia (vitamin B_{12}); anorexia, nausea, vomiting, and dermatitis (biotin); and megaloblastic anemia, diarrhea, and weight loss (folic acid). All of these deficiencies are treated via supplementation.

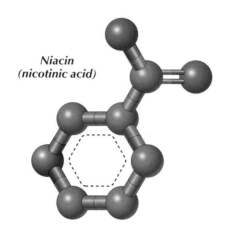

Niacin
(nicotinic acid)

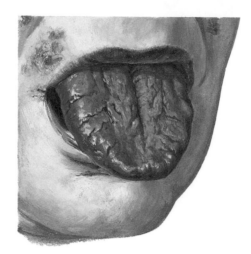

Pellagra tongue

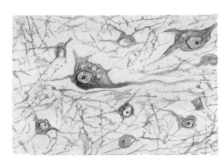

Degeneration of cells of
cerebral cortex

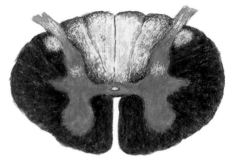

Degeneration in spinal cord

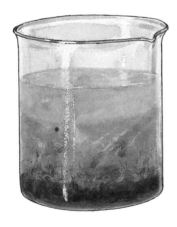

J. Perkins
MS, MFA

Aqueous stool in diarrhea of pellagra

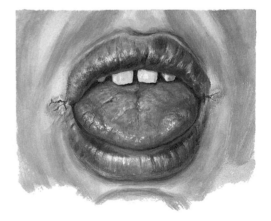

Cheilosis, angular stomatitis, and
magenta tongue in ariboflavinosis

FIGURE 13-3 NIACIN OR NICOTINIC ACID DEFICIENCY (PELLAGRA)

Deficiency of water-soluble niacin (nicotinic acid) or its amide (nicotinamide) results from dietary deficiency or impaired absorption. It is usually associated with diets lacking tryptophan-containing proteins and can occur secondary to gastrointestinal diseases or chronic alcoholism. This deficiency causes pellagra, which is characterized by cutaneous, gastrointestinal, mucosal, neurologic, and cognitive symptoms. The numerous cutaneous symptoms include cheilosis (reddened lips and fissures at the angles of the mouth), angular stomatitis (inflammation and fissures radiating from the corners of the mouth), and magenta-colored tongue (as seen in ariboflavinosis). Involvement of the CNS progresses from general lassitude, disorientation, memory impairment, and confusion to delirium and clouding of consciousness. Treatment is by supplemental intake (parenteral if oral is not possible).

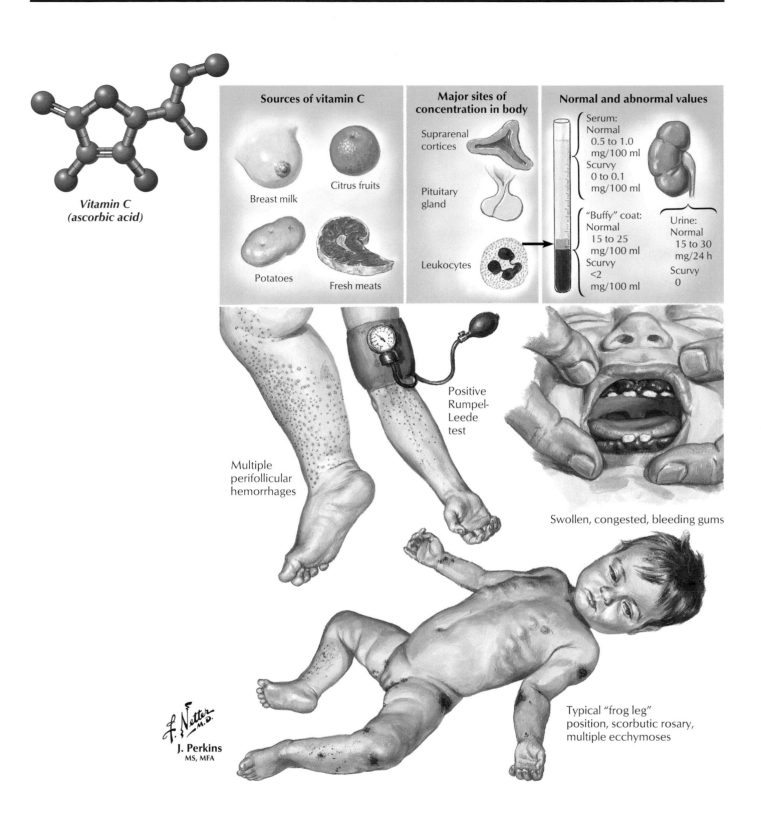

*Vitamin C
(ascorbic acid)*

Sources of vitamin C

Breast milk

Citrus fruits

Potatoes

Fresh meats

**Major sites of
concentration in body**

Suprarenal
cortices

Pituitary
gland

Leukocytes

Normal and abnormal values

Serum:
Normal
0.5 to 1.0
mg/100 ml
Scurvy
0 to 0.1
mg/100 ml

"Buffy" coat:
Normal
15 to 25
mg/100 ml
Scurvy
<2
mg/100 ml

Urine:
Normal
15 to 30
mg/24 h
Scurvy
0

Multiple
perifollicular
hemorrhages

Positive
Rumpel-
Leede
test

Swollen, congested, bleeding gums

Typical "frog leg"
position, scorbutic rosary,
multiple ecchymoses

J. Netter, M.D.

J. Perkins
MS, MFA

FIGURE 13-4 VITAMIN C DEFICIENCY (SCURVY)

Deficiency of water-soluble vitamin C (ascorbic acid) results from impairment of the maintenance of the ground substance that binds cells together and is necessary for the formation and maintenance of collagen in connective tissues. The precise mechanism of this effect is not known but is thought to be due to the ability of vitamin C to participate in oxidation-reduction reactions. Symptoms of vitamin C deficiency (scurvy) include imperfect bone and tooth formation; swollen, congested, bleeding gums; anorexia; multiple ecchymoses (skin discoloration consisting of irregular hemorrhagic areas); and a positive Rumpel-Leede (Hess) capillary fragility test (for thrombocytopenia). Treatment is via supplemental intake.

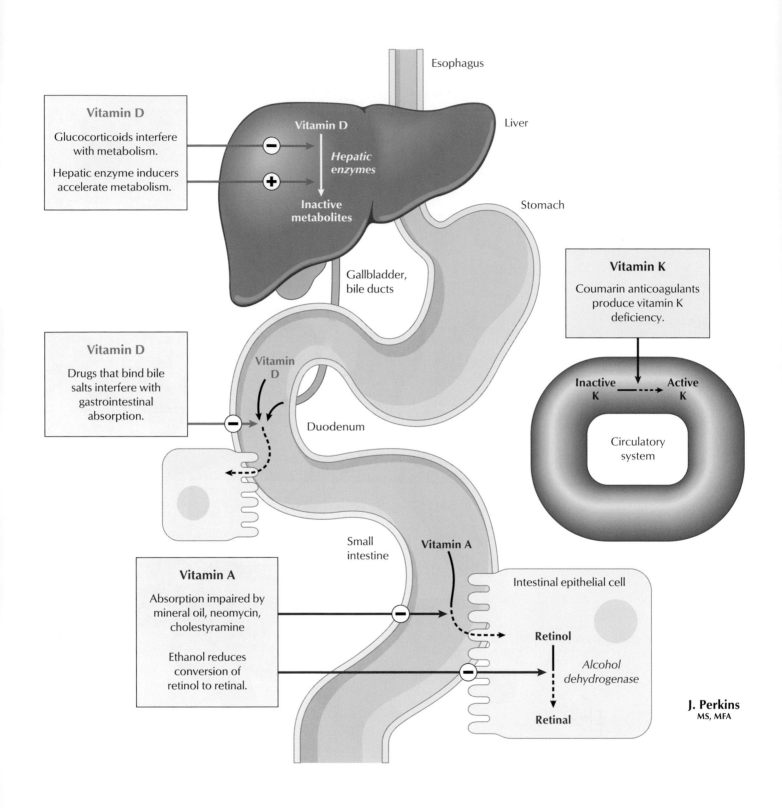

FIGURE 13-5 FAT-SOLUBLE VITAMIN-DRUG INTERACTIONS

Vitamin A: Because dietary fat and pancreatic lipase are necessary for absorption of vitamin A from the small intestine (see Figure 13-1), absorption is impaired by agents that modify this process, such as mineral oil, neomycin, and cholestyramine. Because ethanol competes with vitamin A as a substrate for alcohol dehydrogenase, excess ethanol consumption results in reduced conversion of retinol to retinal (which leads to, for example, night blindness). **Vitamin D:** Drugs that bind bile salts interfere with gastrointestinal absorption of vitamin D; glucocorticoids interfere with hepatic metabolism of this vitamin; and hepatic enzyme inducers can accelerate conversion of vitamin D to its inactive metabolites. **Vitamin K:** Coumarin anticoagulants can produce vitamin D deficiency.

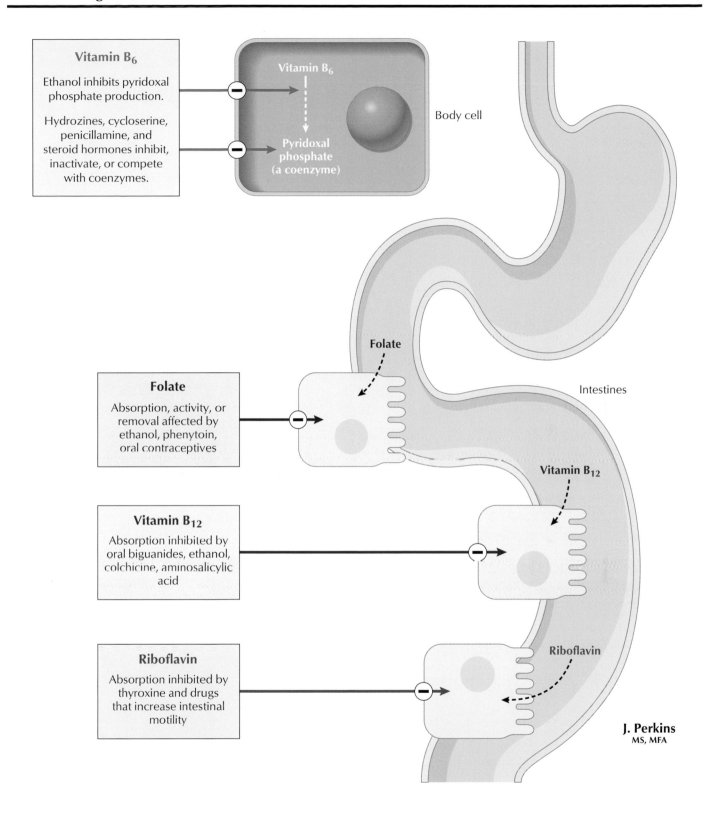

Vitamin B₆

Ethanol inhibits pyridoxal phosphate production.

Hydrozines, cycloserine, penicillamine, and steroid hormones inhibit, inactivate, or compete with coenzymes.

Vitamin B₆

Pyridoxal phosphate (a coenzyme)

Body cell

Folate

Intestines

Folate

Absorption, activity, or removal affected by ethanol, phenytoin, oral contraceptives

Vitamin B₁₂

Absorption inhibited by oral biguanides, ethanol, colchicine, aminosalicylic acid

Vitamin B₁₂

Riboflavin

Absorption inhibited by thyroxine and drugs that increase intestinal motility

Riboflavin

J. Perkins
MS, MFA

FIGURE 13-6 WATER-SOLUBLE VITAMIN-DRUG INTERACTIONS

Vitamin B family: Folate absorption, activity, or removal is affected by ethanol, phenytoin, and oral contraceptives; salicylates (compete with protein-binding sites); and methotrexate (folate antagonist). Vitamin B₆ is affected by ethanol (decreases coenzyme pyridoxal phosphate production); hydrazines (eg, isoniazid) (coenzyme inhibitors); cycloserine and penicillamine (coenzyme inactivators); and steroid hormones (coenzyme competitors). In turn, vitamin B₆ reduces levodopa efficacy or serum phenobarbital and phenytoin levels. Oral hypoglycemic biguanides, colchicine, ethanol, and aminosalicylic acid affect vitamin B₁₂ absorption. Isonicotinic acid hydrazide, 6-MP, and 5-FU cause niacin deficiency; niacin inhibits effects of sulfinpyrazone and probenecid. Riboflavin absorption is inhibited by thyroxine and drugs that increase intestinal motility. **Vitamin C:** Aspirin and oral contraceptives reduce plasma vitamin C levels; this vitamin can alter renal drug excretion.

CHAPTER 14

DRUG ALLERGY, ABUSE, AND POISONING OR OVERDOSE

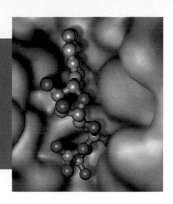

OVERVIEW

Drug allergy, or allergic reaction to drugs, represents a type of adverse drug reaction. The effects are mediated by humoral (involving antibodies) or cell-mediated (eg, T-lymphocyte) immunologic mechanisms and can lead to consequences that are short- or long-term, restricted to a specific organ or involving the whole body, and trivial or life-threatening. The clinical manifestations of allergic reactions to drugs are varied and can include anaphylaxis (anaphylactic shock, ie, life-threatening changes in the vasculature [such as vasodilation and edema] and the bronchioles [such as bronchoconstriction] that are consistent with shock); bronchospasm; dermatitis; fever; granulocytopenia (abnormal reduction of the number of neutrophils, eosinophils, and basophils in the blood); hemolytic anemia (abnormal decrease in red blood cell number); hepatitis; lupus erythematosus–like syndrome; nephritis or pneumonitis (lung inflammation); thrombocytopenia (abnormal decrease in platelet number); and vasculitis (inflammation of blood or lymph vessels). Allergic reactions to drugs are typically characterized by the necessity for previous exposure to the drug or to a drug of similar chemical structure; lack of dose-related effect; similar manifestations independent of the drug (ie, not related to the therapeutic or toxic effects of the drug); and nonresponsiveness to receptor antagonists of the drug.

Drug abuse (addiction) is a multifaceted problem, typically involving a complex combination of psychosocial contributing factors. Hereditary predisposition is also suspected to play a role in some cases. *Drug abuse* is perhaps most succinctly defined as the continued inappropriate nonmedical use of a drug in the face of known negative medical or other consequences. To some extent, every drug that produces a detectable psychic effect is abused by someone, somewhere in the world. In addition, many, perhaps most, drug addicts abuse more than 1 drug. Hence, the list of abused drugs is extensive and includes some substances that are thought of primarily as mood or physique enhancers or as "recreational" drugs (eg, anabolic steroids, mushrooms, designer drugs, hallucinogens, inhalants, marijuana, nicotine). This chapter focuses on some of the major classes of therapeutic drugs that are abused.

Drug poisoning or overdose can be accidental (a result of medical errors or errors in the home) or intentional (suicide attempts). The substances involved include pharmaceuticals (most often analgesics and over-the-counter preparations), cleaning products, cosmetics, and plants or plant extracts. The symptoms and duration of the toxicity depend on the substance involved, the amount, and the site of exposure. The mechanisms can be specific (eg, receptor-mediated reactions) or nonspecific (eg, tissue necrosis). This chapter focuses on toxicity caused by selected pharmacologic agents.

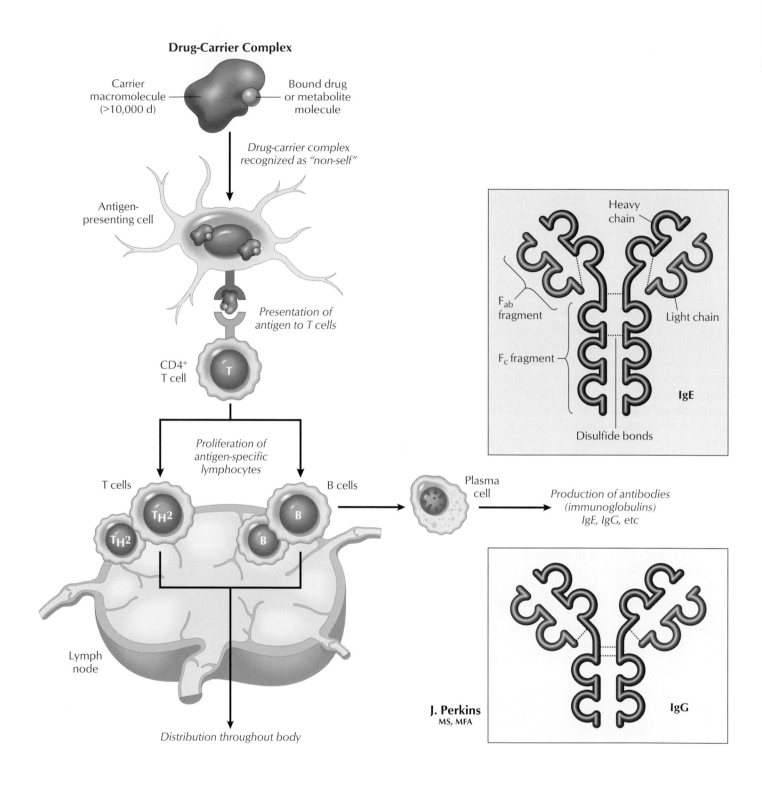

Drug-Carrier Complex

Carrier macromolecule (>10,000 d)

Bound drug or metabolite molecule

Drug-carrier complex recognized as "non-self"

Antigen-presenting cell

Presentation of antigen to T cells

CD4$^+$ T cell

Proliferation of antigen-specific lymphocytes

T cells

T$_H$2

T$_H$2

B cells

B

B

Plasma cell

Production of antibodies (immunoglobulins) IgE, IgG, etc

Lymph node

Distribution throughout body

Heavy chain

F$_{ab}$ fragment

Light chain

F$_c$ fragment

IgE

Disulfide bonds

J. Perkins MS, MFA

IgG

FIGURE 14-1 ALLERGIC REACTIONS TO DRUGS

Only a few drugs have a molecular size (>10,000 d) sufficient to induce an allergic reaction by themselves. Induction of an immune response more often occurs when a small drug molecule, metabolite, or excipient (inert substance in a prescription) covalently binds to some large endogenous macromolecule (carrier), such as a protein, and becomes allergenic. The immune system becomes sensitized during the initial exposure, although the allergic response is not elicited at this time. Antigen-specific antibodies of the T- and B-cell type proliferate in lymphatic tissue, and some remain there (as memory cells) and are clinically silent until reexposure to the antigen (drug-carrier complex). The response to reexposure can be quick and severe, even to a small dose of the drug. Four types of drug allergy are generally distinguished: anaphylactic, cytotoxic, immune complex vasculitis, and cell mediated. Management generally involves treating the symptoms and supporting vital functions.

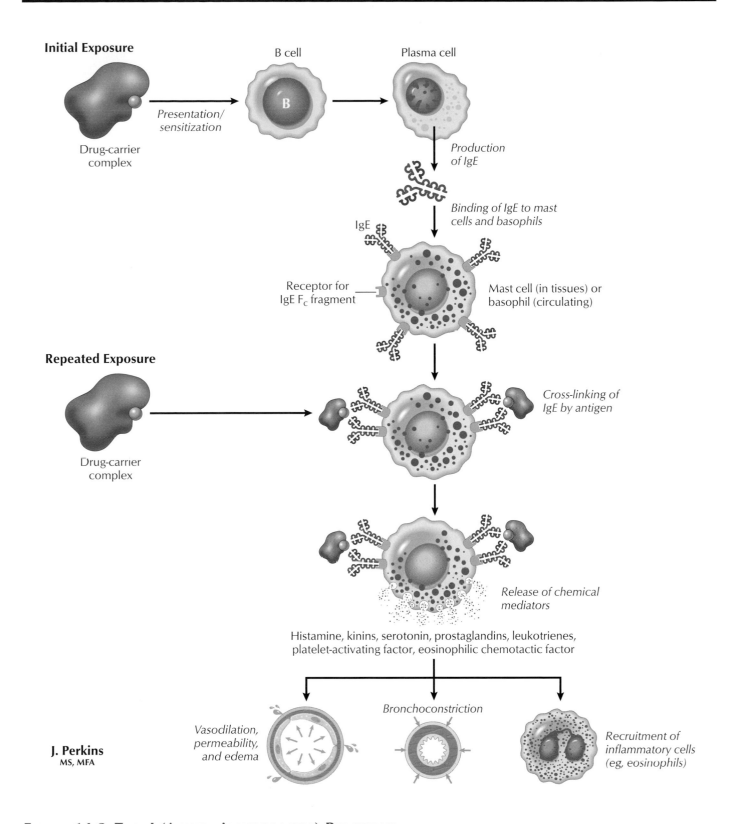

FIGURE 14-2 TYPE I (ACUTE, ANAPHYLACTIC) REACTIONS

After initial exposure to drug antigen (drug-carrier complex), macrophages and interleukins convert B cells into IgE/receptor-expressing cells that circulate in blood (as basophil granulocytes) or reside in tissues (as mast cells). Reexposure to drug antigen results in binding to paired IgE receptors and release of various chemical mediators such as histamine, kinins, serotonin, prostaglandins, leukotrienes, platelet-activating factor, and eosinophilic chemotactic factor. Histamine and other bioactive substances released into the bloodstream cause blood vessels to dilate and tissues to swell. The effect may be life-threatening if airway obstruction, blood pressure decrease, or heart arrhythmias occur. Type I reactions can have a rapid onset (minutes) and are similar to those seen in hypersensitivity reactions to insect stings, extrinsic asthma, and seasonal rhinitis.

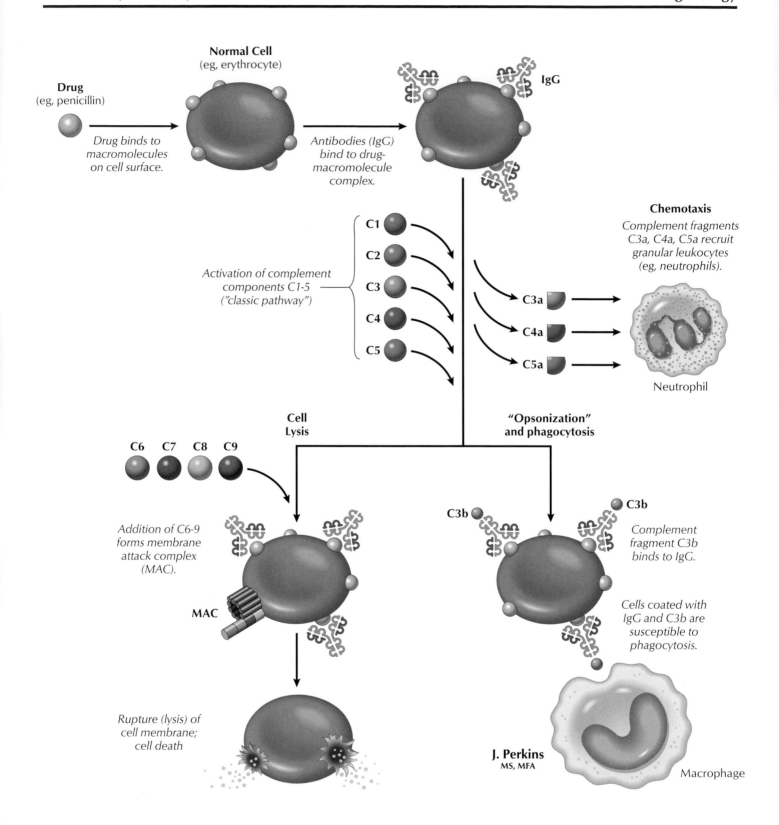

Figure 14-3 Type II (Cytotoxic, Autoimmune) Reactions

If antigen (drug)-antibody (IgG) complexes adhere to a cell surface, the immune response can damage or kill the cell. This effect occurs because the binding of the complex activates complement, which is a family of proteins that circulate in the blood in an inactive form until activated by an appropriate stimulus. Activated complement is normally directed against microorganisms, but when directed against a cell, complement causes lysis and death of the cell, promotes phagocytosis, attracts neutrophil granulocytes (chemotaxis), and stimulates other inflammatory responses. An example is allergy to penicillin. Penicillin binds to red blood cells, antibodies bind to the penicillin, complement is activated, and the cell is damaged or dies, which leads to drug-induced autoimmune hemolytic anemia, agranulocytosis, and thrombocytopenia.

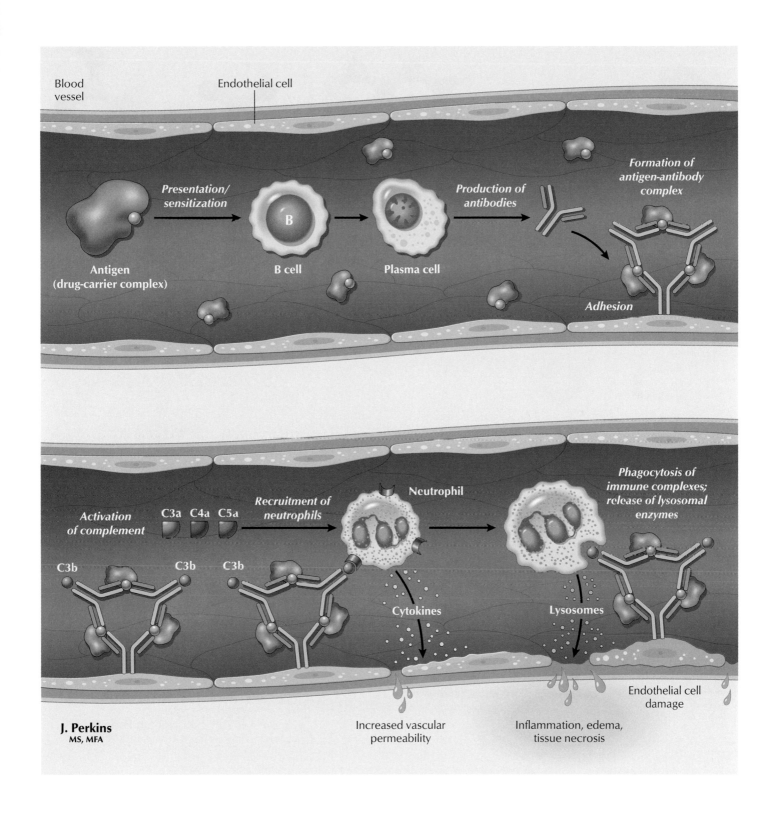

FIGURE 14-4 TYPE III (IMMUNE COMPLEX, SERUM SICKNESS, ARTHUS) REACTIONS

If drug antigen-antibody complexes adhere to cells of vascular tissue, the immune response can attack not only the antigen-antibody complex but also the healthy cells of the vessel to which the complex is attached. This result can cause damage or death of the vessel's cells. Activated complement, inflammation, and vasculitis damage vessel walls and result in the symptoms of serum sickness, which include malaise, fever, rash, arthralgia (pain in a joint), lymphadenopathy, hepatitis, and characteristic rash and eruptions along the sides of the feet and hands.

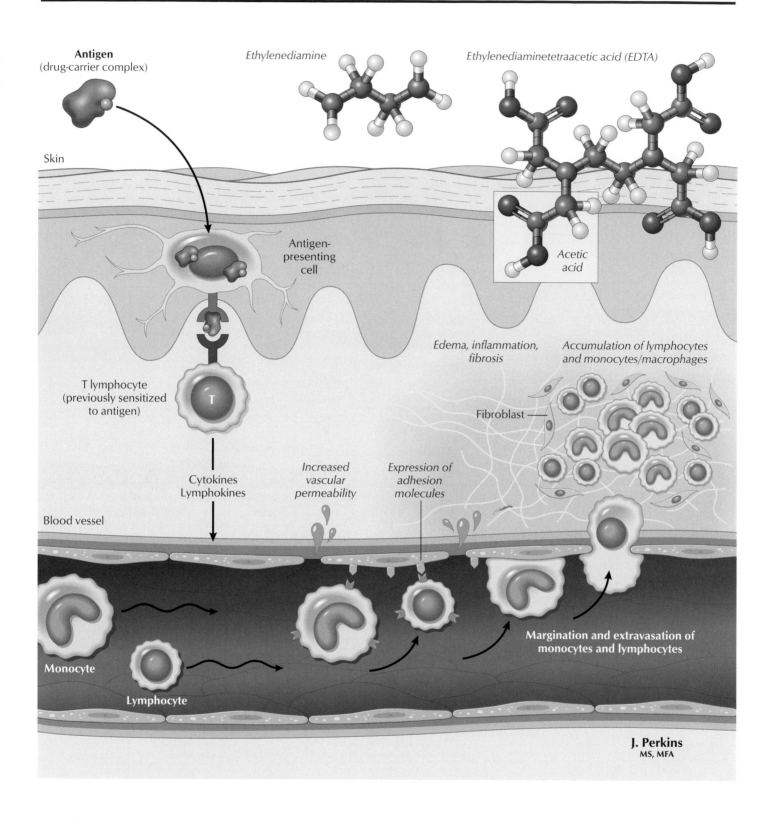

Antigen
(drug-carrier complex)

Ethylenediamine

Ethylenediaminetetraacetic acid (EDTA)

Skin

Antigen-presenting cell

Acetic acid

T lymphocyte
(previously sensitized
to antigen)

Edema, inflammation, fibrosis

Accumulation of lymphocytes and monocytes/macrophages

Fibroblast

Cytokines
Lymphokines

Increased vascular permeability

Expression of adhesion molecules

Blood vessel

Margination and extravasation of monocytes and lymphocytes

Monocyte

Lymphocyte

J. Perkins
MS, MFA

FIGURE 14-5 TYPE IV (CELL-MEDIATED, DELAYED-HYPERSENSITIVITY, CONTACT DERMATITIS) REACTIONS

When drug antigen is administered on or into the skin or mucosa, for example, binding to antigen-specific receptors expressed on T lymphocytes can occur. Binding stimulates lymphocytes to release signal molecules (lymphokines), which activate macrophages and provoke an inflammatory reaction in the surrounding area. This cell-mediated response (involving sensitized T lymphocytes) is slower than humoral immune responses (those involving antibodies). Drug-related substances that can cause type IV reactions include ethylenediamine, which is used as a drug-solubilizing agent, and EDTA, which is used as a preservative in many topical and ophthalmic preparations.

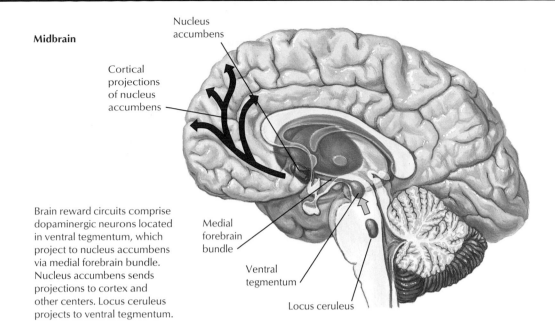

Midbrain

Nucleus accumbens

Cortical projections of nucleus accumbens

Medial forebrain bundle

Ventral tegmentum

Locus ceruleus

Brain reward circuits comprise dopaminergic neurons located in ventral tegmentum, which project to nucleus accumbens via medial forebrain bundle. Nucleus accumbens sends projections to cortex and other centers. Locus ceruleus projects to ventral tegmentum.

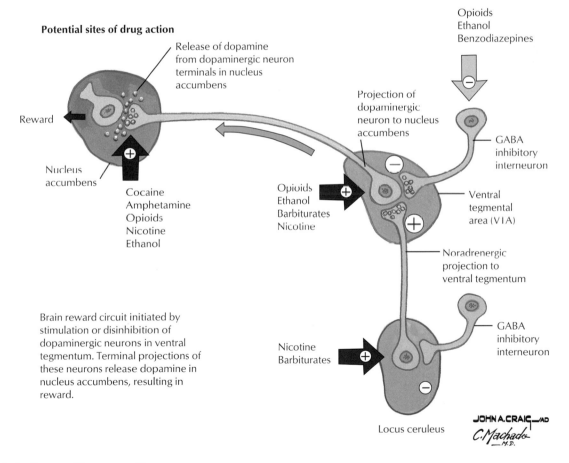

Potential sites of drug action

Release of dopamine from dopaminergic neuron terminals in nucleus accumbens

Opioids
Ethanol
Benzodiazepines

Projection of dopaminergic neuron to nucleus accumbens

GABA inhibitory interneuron

Reward

Nucleus accumbens

Cocaine
Amphetamine
Opioids
Nicotine
Ethanol

Opioids
Ethanol
Barbiturates
Nicotine

Ventral tegmental area (VTA)

Noradrenergic projection to ventral tegmentum

Nicotine
Barbiturates

GABA inhibitory interneuron

Brain reward circuit initiated by stimulation or disinhibition of dopaminergic neurons in ventral tegmentum. Terminal projections of these neurons release dopamine in nucleus accumbens, resulting in reward.

JOHN A. CRAIG—AD
C. Machado—M.D.

Locus ceruleus

FIGURE 14-6 BRAIN REWARD CIRCUIT

Drug abuse involves 2 components: psychosocial (eg, family situation, peer pressure) and endogenous (eg, genetics, enzyme levels). Pharmacologic mechanisms of drug abuse involve CNS neurotransmitter systems that operate for therapeutic drug effects. An endogenous pleasure or reward pathway in the brain is important for motivation and learning (survival) and is thought to be excessively active—because of genetics, overuse, or other factors—in drug abuse. The brain reward circuit consists of

neuronal pathways, cortical sites, and subcortical nuclei, especially within the limbic region. Primary among these are dopaminergic neurons in the ventral tegmentum that project to the nucleus accumbens and then to the cortex and other centers. Also, norepinephrine-containing neurons from the locus ceruleus project to the ventral tegmentum. Stimulation or disinhibition of dopaminergic neurons within the ventral tegmentum may be common to abuse of different substances.

Effects of Alcohol on End Organs

Cellular damage

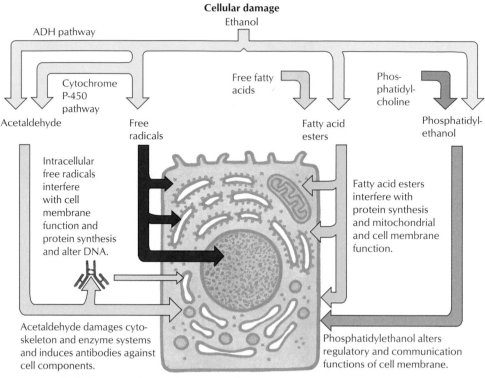

Ethanol

ADH pathway

Cytochrome P-450 pathway

Free fatty acids

Phos-phatidyl-choline

Acetaldehyde

Free radicals

Fatty acid esters

Phosphatidyl-ethanol

Intracellular free radicals interfere with cell membrane function and protein synthesis and alter DNA.

Fatty acid esters interfere with protein synthesis and mitochondrial and cell membrane function.

Acetaldehyde damages cyto-skeleton and enzyme systems and induces antibodies against cell components.

Phosphatidylethanol alters regulatory and communication functions of cell membrane.

Alcohol causes end organ damage via ethanol metabolites and ethanol-generated compounds, which alter structure and function of cell components.

Organ damage

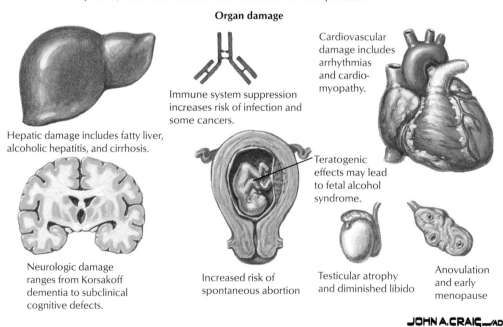

Hepatic damage includes fatty liver, alcoholic hepatitis, and cirrhosis.

Immune system suppression increases risk of infection and some cancers.

Cardiovascular damage includes arrhythmias and cardio-myopathy.

Neurologic damage ranges from Korsakoff dementia to subclinical cognitive defects.

Increased risk of spontaneous abortion

Teratogenic effects may lead to fetal alcohol syndrome.

Testicular atrophy and diminished libido

Anovulation and early menopause

JOHN A. CRAIG—AD

FIGURE 14-7 ETHANOL: DELETERIOUS EFFECTS

Short- and long-term excess ethanol consumption leads to wide-spread problems for the individual and for society. The lifetime prevalence of ethanol dependence is estimated at 10% to 15%, and as many as 30% of male and 10% of female admissions to general hospitals are related to ethanol-associated disorders. Ethanol is rapidly absorbed from the GI tract and distributes to all cells in the body. It readily passes into the fetal circulation.

Low concentrations of ethanol are safely metabolized in a 2-step process: first by alcohol dehydrogenase to acetaldehyde and then by aldehyde dehydrogenase to acetate. High concentrations saturate this pathway and give rise to toxic byproducts of alternative pathways. Because ethanol is so widely distributed throughout the body, the toxic consequences of excess ethanol consumption involve essentially every organ.

Alcohol Withdrawal

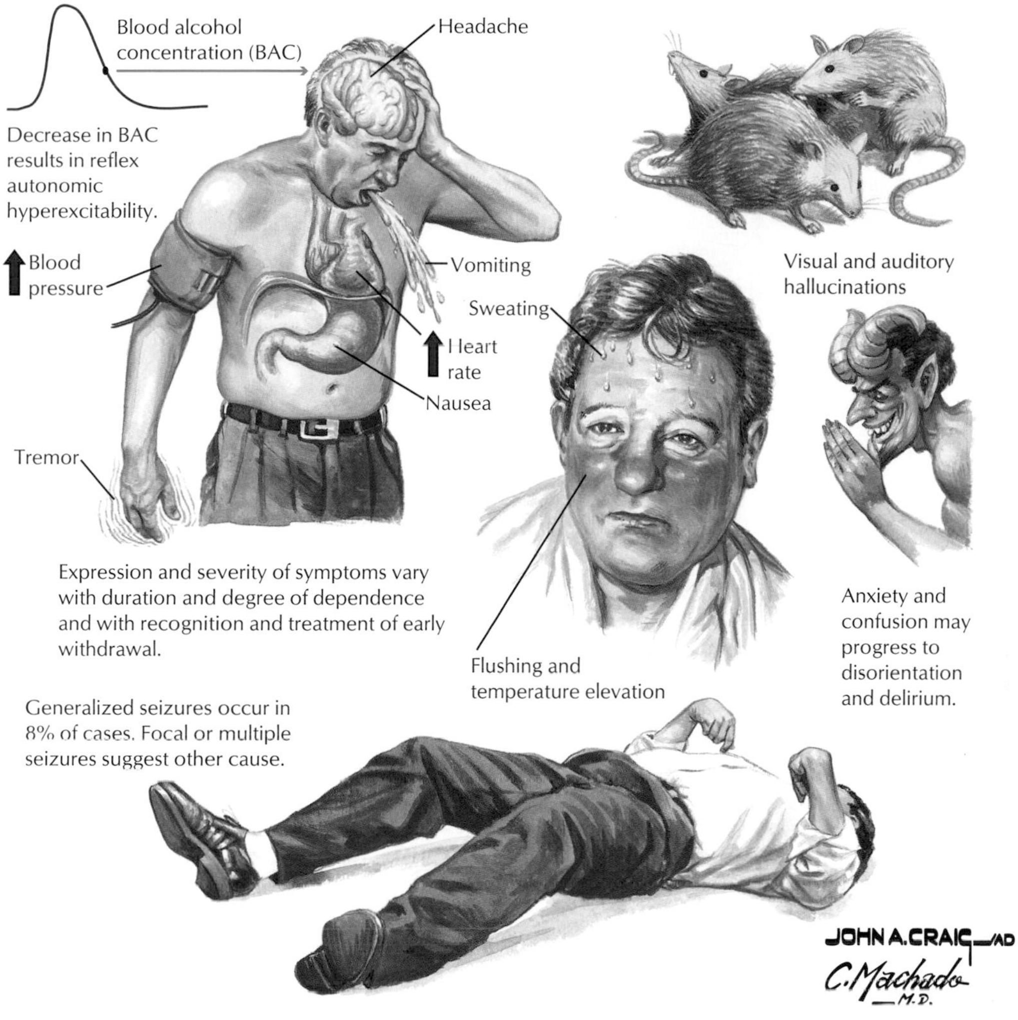

Blood alcohol concentration (BAC)

Headache

Decrease in BAC results in reflex autonomic hyperexcitability.

↑ Blood pressure

Vomiting

Sweating

↑ Heart rate

Nausea

Tremor

Visual and auditory hallucinations

Expression and severity of symptoms vary with duration and degree of dependence and with recognition and treatment of early withdrawal.

Generalized seizures occur in 8% of cases. Focal or multiple seizures suggest other cause.

Flushing and temperature elevation

Anxiety and confusion may progress to disorientation and delirium.

JOHN A. CRAIG—MD
C. Machado—M.D.

Stages of Alcohol Withdrawal

	Stage 1	Stage 2	Stage 3
Hours after alcohol consumption	24 36 (peak) 48	(48-72)	(72-105)
Symptoms	Mild-to-moderate anxiety, tremor, nausea, vomiting, sweating, elevation of heart rate and blood pressure, sleep disturbance, hallucinations, illusions, seizures	Aggravated forms of stage 1 symptoms with severe tremors, agitation, and hallucinations	Acute organic psychosis (delirium), confusion, and disorientation with severe autonomic symptoms

Stage 1 withdrawal usually self-limited. Only small percentage of cases progress to stages 2 and 3. Progression prevented by prompt and adequate treatment.

FIGURE 14-8 ETHANOL ABUSE: TREATMENT

Abrupt withdrawal from ethanol is accompanied by excitatory CNS signs such as delirium tremens and potentially lethal seizures. Medication management in the past was limited to disulfiram, which inhibits aldehyde dehydrogenase. The buildup of acetaldehyde produces an unpleasant reaction when ethanol is consumed and thereby provides a deterrent to excess ethanol use. Naltrexone and acamprosate (in Europe) are newer alternative choices. Naltrexone is an opioid receptor antagonist that seems to have the additional (perhaps independent) property of reducing the chance of relapse when used in conjunction with psychosocial treatment. Acamprosate seems to enhance abstinence by a modulatory effect on the NMDA subtype of the glutamate receptor.

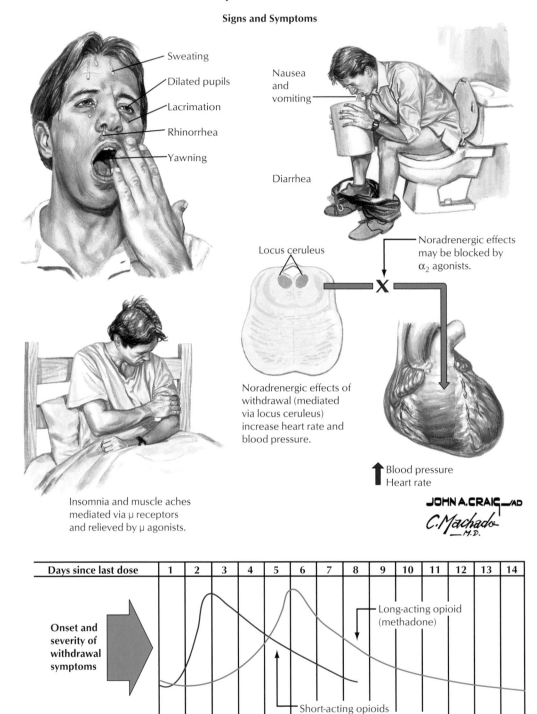

Opioid Withdrawal

Signs and Symptoms

Sweating

Dilated pupils

Lacrimation

Rhinorrhea

Yawning

Nausea and vomiting

Diarrhea

Locus ceruleus

Noradrenergic effects may be blocked by α_2 agonists.

Noradrenergic effects of withdrawal (mediated via locus ceruleus) increase heart rate and blood pressure.

Blood pressure
Heart rate

Insomnia and muscle aches mediated via μ receptors and relieved by μ agonists.

JOHN A. CRAIG—MD
C. Machado—M.D.

Days since last dose	1	2	3	4	5	6	7	8	9	10	11	12	13	14

Onset and severity of withdrawal symptoms

Long-acting opioid (methadone)

Short-acting opioids (morphine, hydromorphone)

Severity of opioid withdrawal varies with dose and duration of opioid use. Onset and duration of symptoms after last drug dose depend on half-life of particular drug.

FIGURE 14-9 WITHDRAWAL: OPIOIDS, BENZODIAZEPINES, AND BARBITURATES

Abrupt discontinuation of drugs used for long-term abuse results in withdrawal signs. In general, these signs are the opposite of those induced by the drug: withdrawal from CNS excitatory drugs is inhibitory, and withdrawal from CNS depressants is excitatory. The rate and severity of withdrawal are lessened by tapered cessation of drug use rather than abrupt cessation. Withdrawal that is too rapid, particularly from CNS depressant drugs such as ethanol and barbiturates, can be life-threatening.

Benzodiazepine Withdrawal

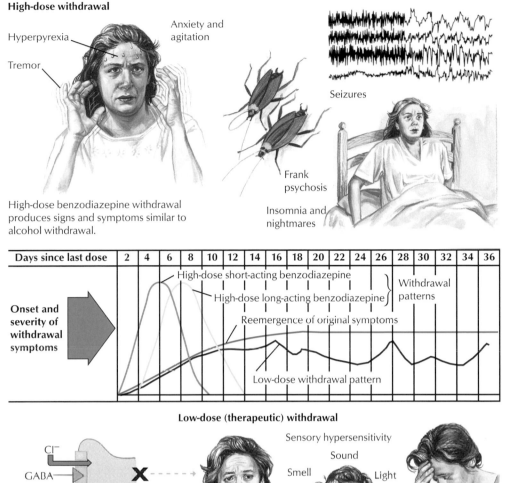

High-dose withdrawal

Hyperpyrexia

Tremor

Anxiety and agitation

Seizures

Frank psychosis

Insomnia and nightmares

High-dose benzodiazepine withdrawal produces signs and symptoms similar to alcohol withdrawal.

Days since last dose	2	4	6	8	10	12	14	16	18	20	22	24	26	28	30	32	34	36

Onset and severity of withdrawal symptoms

High-dose short-acting benzodiazepine
High-dose long-acting benzodiazepine } Withdrawal patterns
Reemergence of original symptoms
Low-dose withdrawal pattern

Low-dose (therapeutic) withdrawal

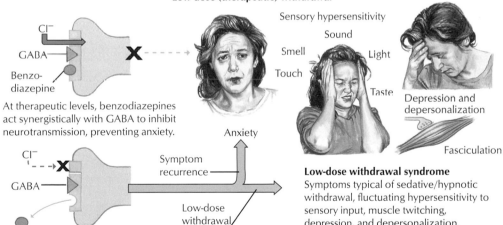

Cl^-

GABA

Benzodiazepine

At therapeutic levels, benzodiazepines act synergistically with GABA to inhibit neurotransmission, preventing anxiety.

Cl^-

GABA

Benzodiazepine

Symptom recurrence

Anxiety

Low-dose withdrawal syndrome

Sensory hypersensitivity
Sound
Smell
Touch
Light
Taste
Depression and depersonalization
Fasciculation

Low-dose withdrawal syndrome
Symptoms typical of sedative/hypnotic withdrawal, fluctuating hypersensitivity to sensory input, muscle twitching, depression, and depersonalization.

Withdrawing long-term benzodiazepine causes loss of synergism with GABA inhibition, resulting in recurrence of original symptoms and low-dose withdrawal syndrome.

JOHN A. CRAIG—MD
C. Machado
—M.D.

FIGURE 14-9 WITHDRAWAL: OPIOIDS, BENZODIAZEPINES, AND BARBITURATES (continued)

Withdrawal from opioids involves influenzalike symptoms, diarrhea (rather than the opioid-induced constipation), and effects mediated through adrenoceptors. Opioid withdrawal can be ameliorated by opioid substitution (eg, with methadone) or with α_2-adrenoceptor agonists. Withdrawal from benzodiazepines is generally mild after therapeutic (low) doses but can be severe (eg, tachycardia) after long-term abuse of high doses.

Physiology of the Specialized Conduction System

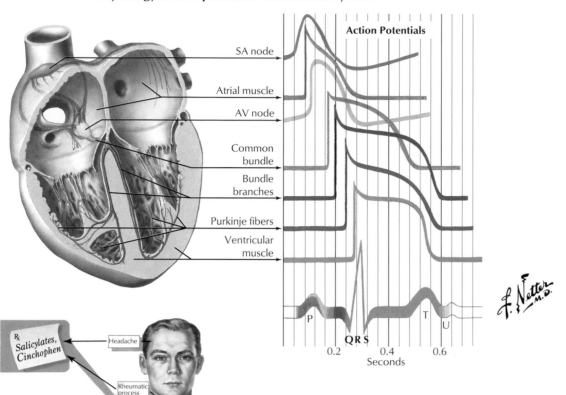

Toxic Syndromes

Syndrome	Clinical Manifestations	Associated Toxins
Sympathomimetic	CNS excitation, seizures, tachycardia, hypertension, mydriasis, diaphoresis	Cocaine, caffeine, theophylline, amphetamines
Anticholinergic	Delirium, hallucinations, dry mucosa, mydriasis, decreased bowel sounds, dry skin, tachycardia, seizures	Atropine, tricyclic antidepressants, antihistamines, phenothiazines
Cholinergic	CNS excitation or depression, bradycardia or tachycardia, miosis or mydriasis, diarrhea, salivation, diaphoresis, lacrimation, paralysis	Organophosphates, pilocarpine, acetylcholine
Opiate	CNS depression, miosis, hypoventilation hypotension, response to naloxone	Heroin, codeine, propoxyphene, pentazocine, oxycodone
Serotonin	Altered mental status, increased muscle tone, hyperreflexia, hyperthermia, tremors	MAOI + SSRI, MAOI + meperidine, SSRI + tricyclic, SSRI overdose

FIGURE 14-10 SYMPATHOMIMETIC DRUGS

Accidental or intentional overdose of sympathomimetics produces symptoms that mimic, in an exaggerated fashion, activation of the sympathetic subdivision of the ANS. Therefore, common effects of moderate overdose of these drugs include mydriasis, diaphoresis (profuse sweating), tachycardia, and hypertension; CNS excitation and seizures are common consequences of severe overdose. The sympathetic nervous system can be overstimulated either by drugs that act directly by binding to adrenergic receptors (eg, α- or β-adrenoceptor agonists) or by drugs that act indirectly by enhancing release of norepinephrine (eg, amphetamines), inhibiting the reuptake of norepinephrine (eg, cocaine), or inhibiting the breakdown of adrenergic receptor–associated second messengers (eg, inhibition of phosphodiesterase by high doses of xanthines such as caffeine and theophylline). Management of effects produced by overdose of these drugs typically involves supportive care.

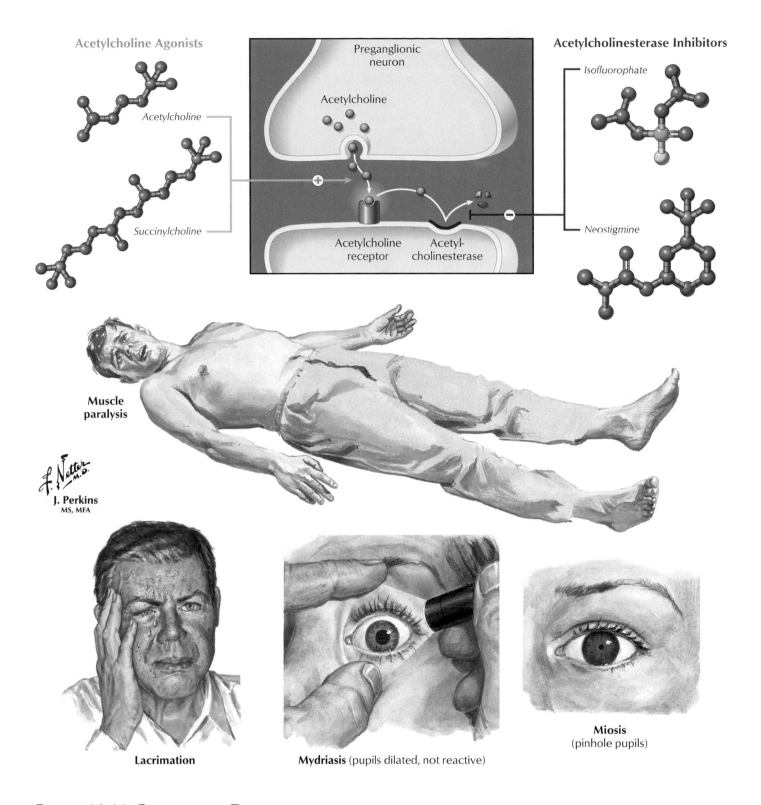

Acetylcholine Agonists

Acetylcholine

Succinylcholine

Preganglionic neuron

Acetylcholine

Acetylcholine receptor   Acetyl-cholinesterase

Acetylcholinesterase Inhibitors

Isofluorophate

Neostigmine

Muscle paralysis

J. Perkins
MS, MFA

Lacrimation

Mydriasis (pupils dilated, not reactive)

Miosis
(pinhole pupils)

FIGURE 14-11 CHOLINERGIC DRUGS

Accidental or intentional overdose of cholinergic drugs produces symptoms that mimic, in an exaggerated way, activation of the SNS and the ANS. Because of excess stimulation at the site of preganglionic cholinergic receptors in both the sympathetic and parasympathetic subdivisions, the action on the ANS is mixed. Thus, overdose can cause muscle paralysis, miosis or mydriasis, bradycardia or tachycardia, CNS stimulation or depression, salivation, lacrimation, diaphoresis, and diarrhea.

Cholinergic receptors can be overstimulated by direct-acting agonists (eg, acetylcholine, succinylcholine) or indirect-acting drugs that enhance the action of acetylcholine, such as organophosphates that inhibit acetylcholinesterase (eg, physostigmine, neostigmine, edrophonium, certain insecticides, nerve gases). Management of the effects produced by overdose of these drugs involves supportive care, especially of the respiratory system, and other measures.

393

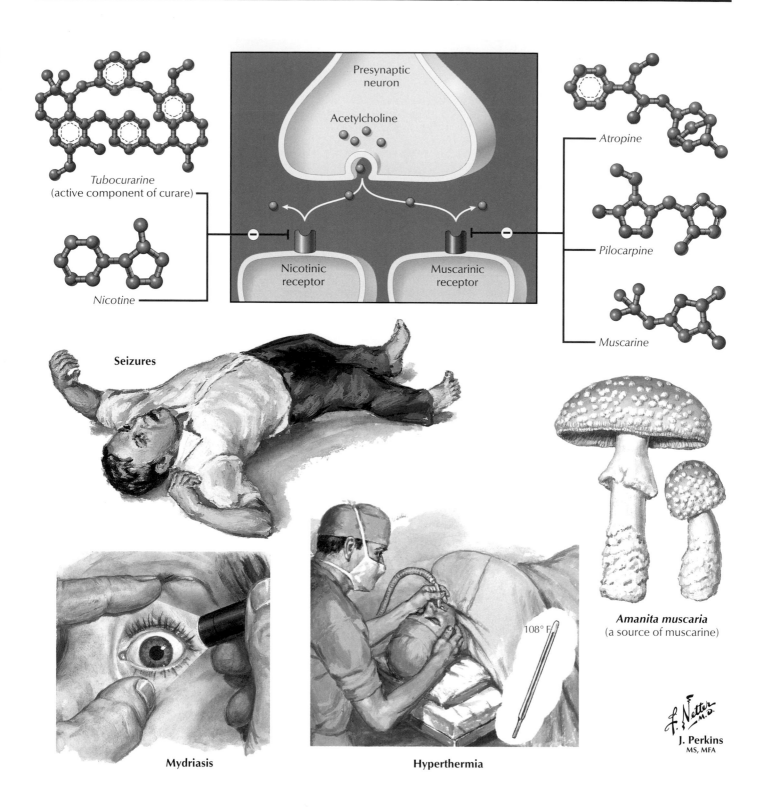

Presynaptic neuron

Acetylcholine

Tubocurarine
(active component of curare)

Nicotine

Nicotinic receptor

Muscarinic receptor

Atropine

Pilocarpine

Muscarine

Seizures

Mydriasis

Hyperthermia

108° F

J. Perkins
MS, MFA

Amanita muscaria
(a source of muscarine)

FIGURE 14-12 ANTICHOLINERGIC DRUGS

Accidental or intentional overdose of anticholinergic drugs produces effects that result from blockade of nicotinic cholinergic receptors located on skeletal muscles in the SNS (eg, effects of curare) and synapses of preganglionic neurons in the ANS (eg, effects of nicotine), and/or from blockade of muscarinic cholinergic receptors located on smooth muscles, cardiac muscles, or glands in the ANS (eg, effects of atropine and pilocarpine).

Overdose signs include skeletal muscle paralysis, mydriasis, tachycardia, decreased gastrointestinal activity, dry mucosa, dry skin, delirium, hallucinations, and seizures. Management of the effects produced by overdose of these drugs usually involves supportive care, particularly of the respiratory system, and other measures (for the autonomic signs).

Hepatic Coma

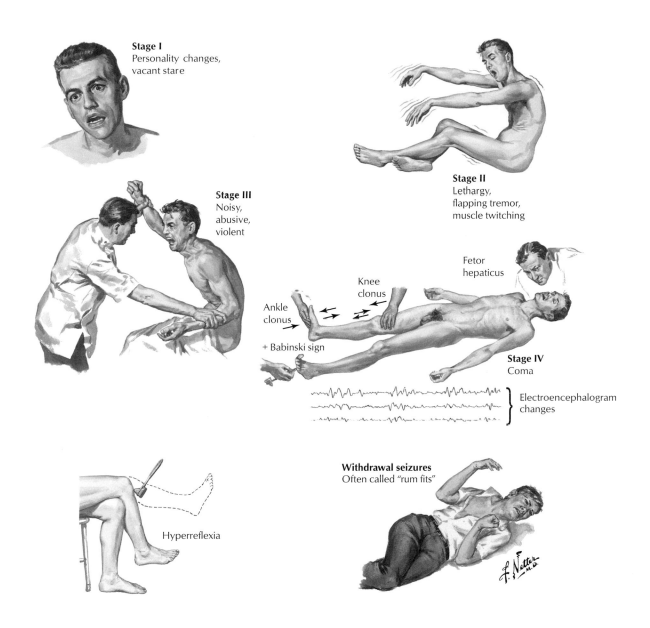

Stage I
Personality changes,
vacant stare

Stage II
Lethargy,
flapping tremor,
muscle twitching

Stage III
Noisy,
abusive,
violent

Fetor
hepaticus

Knee
clonus

Ankle
clonus

+ Babinski sign

Stage IV
Coma

Electroencephalogram
changes

Hyperreflexia

Withdrawal seizures
Often called "rum fits"

FIGURE 14-13 SEROTONERGICS

Excess serotonin can result from the accidental or intentional overdose of drugs that directly activate serotonin receptors or, more commonly, from drugs that indirectly enhance serotonin levels by inhibiting presynaptic neuronal reuptake of serotonin or by inhibiting serotonin breakdown by monoamine oxidase. The latter category includes selective serotonin reuptake inhibitors, nonselective serotonin reuptake inhibitors, and MAOIs. Excessive serotonin activity produces a serotonin syndrome, which may include akathisialike restlessness, muscle twitches and myoclonus, hyperreflexia, sweating, shivering and tremor, and possibly life-threatening seizures or coma.

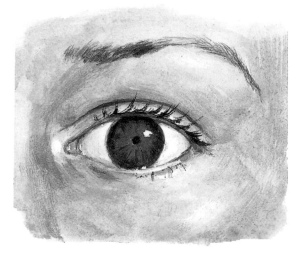

Miosis (pinhole pupils)
Seen in poisoning by morphine and morphine derivatives, some types of mushrooms, cholinesterase inhibitors, parasympathomimetics, nicotine, chloral hydrate, sympatholytics, and some other compounds

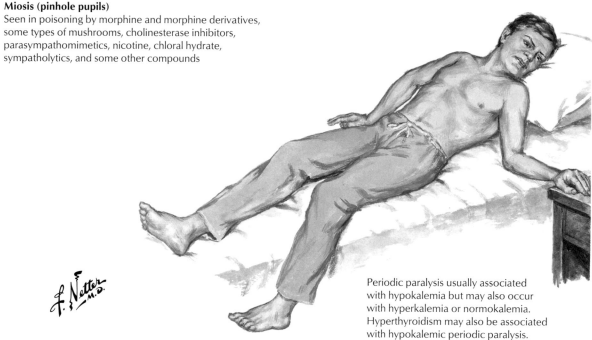

Periodic paralysis usually associated with hypokalemia but may also occur with hyperkalemia or normokalemia. Hyperthyroidism may also be associated with hypokalemic periodic paralysis.

FIGURE 14-14 OPIOIDS

Accidental or intentional overdose of opioid agonists, such as morphine, codeine, or oxycodone, results in overstimulation of opioid receptors that are located throughout the CNS and in the periphery. Overdose of these drugs is characterized by miosis, constipation, hypothermia, hypotension, pulmonary edema, and possibly life-threatening respiratory depression, among other signs. Seizures can also occur. Metabolites of the drugs can produce additional toxicity (eg, neuromuscular excitability by normeperidine and myocardial depression by norpropoxyphene). All effects that are produced by excess opioid receptor activation are reversed by administration of an opioid receptor antagonist such as naloxone. Multiple treatments with an antagonist may be required if the half-life of the antagonist is shorter than that of the agonist. High doses of antagonist may be needed against propoxyphene (and reversal of the toxic effect may still be incomplete).

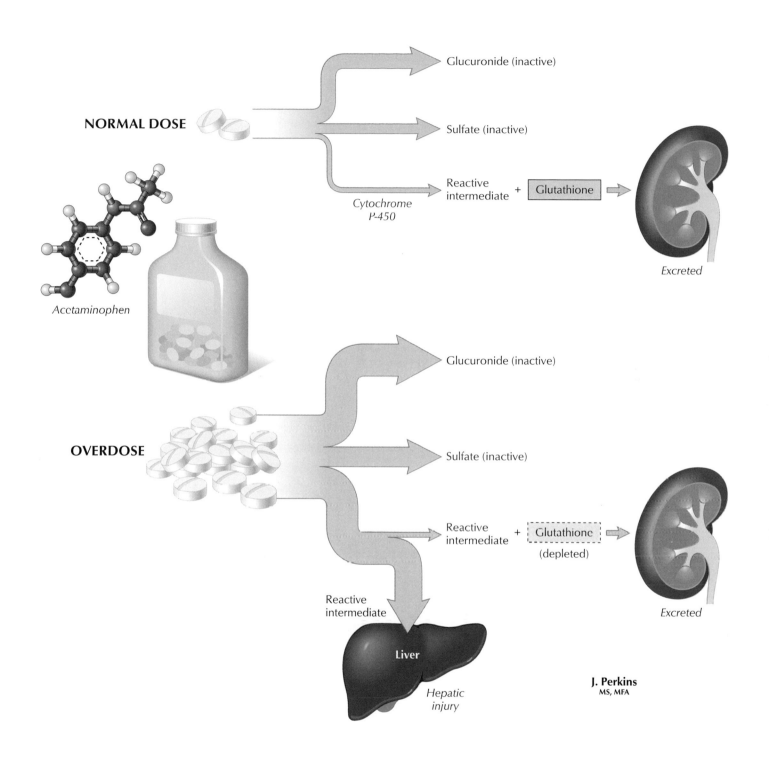

Acetaminophen

FIGURE 14-15 OVER-THE-COUNTER PRODUCTS

Many products on the market have pharmacologic activity and can be obtained without a prescription. Some of these products contain single or multiple ingredients, such as antihistamines, decongestants, analgesics (eg, nonsteroidal antiinflammatory drugs or acetaminophen). These drugs, as well as vitamins, health aids, and herbals, can produce toxicity in overdose or when taken together (too numerous to list here). An overdose scenario that highlights an important pharmacologic principle is that associated with acetaminophen (paracetamol). It is one of the safest drugs at therapeutic doses because it and its potentially toxic intermediate metabolites are rapidly metabolized in a glutathione-dependent pathway and then excreted. However, in overdose, depletion of glutathione allows accumulation of reactive metabolites that cause hepatic injury. If treatment with a glutathione substitute is initiated early enough, it provides a successful antidote.

Emesis

Vomiting induced by the emetic syrup of ipecac is occasionally recommended for pediatric ingestions, being managed at home, in consultation with the poison center. It no longer has a role in the hospital management of poisonings.

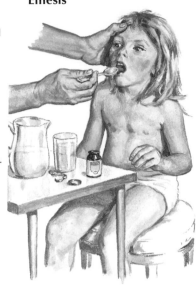

Gastric Lavage: Specialized Equipment

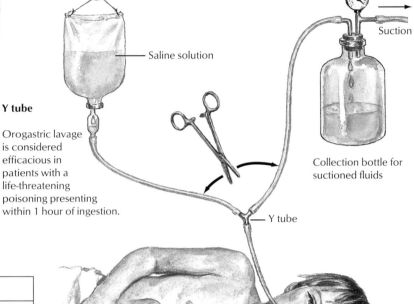

— Saline solution

Suction

Y tube

Orogastric lavage is considered efficacious in patients with a life-threatening poisoning presenting within 1 hour of ingestion.

Collection bottle for suctioned fluids

— Y tube

Toxins With a Specific Antidotal Therapy

Toxin	Antidote
Acetaminophen	N-acetylcysteine
β Blockers	IV glucagons
Calcium channel blockers	IV calcium, glucagons
Cholinesterase inhibitors	Atropine, pralidoxime
Cyanide	Cyanide kit
Cyclic antidepressants	Sodium bicarbonate
Carbon monoxide	Oxygen
Digitalis	Digibind
Ethylene glycol	Ethanol, 4-methylpyrazole
Fluoride	IV calcium, magnesium
Hypoglycemics	IV glucose
Isoniazid	IV pyridoxine
Iron	Deferoxamine
Methanol	Ethanol, 4-methylpyrazole
Methemoglobin producers	IV methylene blue
Narcotics	Naloxone, naltrexone
Salicylates	Sodium bicarbonate

FIGURE 14-16 MANAGEMENT OF POISONING AND OVERDOSE

Specific antidotes are available for only a limited number of drugs. However, most drug overdoses or poisonings can be successfully managed by using a combination of drugs (eg, a receptor antagonist for opioids) and/or supportive care, with particular attention to vital organ functions, breathing, circulation, cardiac arrhythmias, seizures, and altered mental status.

Benefit may also be derived from surface decontamination and, under certain restricted conditions, use of emetic agents or gastric lavage. Forced diuresis has unproven efficacy, but alkalinization of the urine may delay gastric absorption of weak acidic drugs and enhance their urinary excretion (eg, salicylates and barbiturates).

INDEX

Page numbers followed by "f" indicate figures, "t" indicate tables, and "b" indicate boxes.